Systemic Pathology

Authors

C. W. M. Adams

B. S. Cardell

J. B. Cavanagh

*K. G. A. Clark

C. A. G. Cook

T. Crawford

A. R. Currie

P. M. Daniel

*W. M. Davidson

I. M. P. Dawson

I. Doniach

B. Fox

I. Friedmann

H. Haber

D. G. F. Harriman

B. E. Heard

*Kristin Henry

R. E. B. Hudson

P. E. Hughesdon

*M. L. Lewis

R. B. Lucas

W. H. McMenemey

J. A. Milne

G. Morgan

B. C. Morson

D. A. Osborn

K. A. Porter

H. A. Sissons

J. C. Sloper

W. Thomas Smith

Sabina J. Strich

*W. St C. Symmers

A. C. Thackray

K. Weinbren

C. P. Wendell-Smith

E. D. Williams

G. Payling Wright

A. H. Wyllie

* Contributors to Volume 2

Editor

W. St C. Symmers

Systemic Pathology

SECOND EDITION

by THIRTY-EIGHT AUTHORS

VOLUME 2

Blood and Bone Marrow
Lymphoreticular System
Thymus Gland

CHURCHILL LIVINGSTONE
Edinburgh London and New York 1978

CHURCHILL LIVINGSTONE

Medical Division of Longman Group Limited

Distributed in the United States of America by Longman Inc., 19 West 44th Street, New York, N.Y. 10036, and by associated companies, branches and representatives throughout the world.

First Edition (edited by G. Payling Wright and W. St Clair Symmers) 1966

Second Edition 1978

ISBN 0 443 01331 4

British Library Cataloguing in Publication Data

Main entry under title:

Systemic pathology.

First ed. edited by G. P. Wright and W. St C. Symmers.
Includes bibliographical references.
CONTENTS: v. 1. Cardiovascular system, respiratory system.
1. Pathology. I. Wright, George Payling,
1898-1964, ed. Systemic pathology. [DNLM:
1. Pathology. QZ4 S995]
RB111.W76 1976   616.07   75-35746

Printed in Great Britain
by T. & A. Constable, Edinburgh

Contents

CONTENTS

Volume 4

Volume 5

Authors of Volume 2

K. G. A. CLARK, MD (London), MRCPath

Consultant Haematologist, Guy's Hospital Health District, London.

W. M. DAVIDSON, MD (Aberdeen), FRCPath, FRS (Edinburgh)

Emeritus Professor of Haematology in the University of London; Consulting Haematologist, King's College Hospital, London.

KRISTIN HENRY, MB, BS (London), MRCP (London), FRCPath

Reader in Pathology in the University of London at Westminster Medical School; Honorary Consultant Pathologist, Westminster Hospital, London.

M. L. LEWIS, MB, BS (London), MRCPath

Consultant Haematologist to the Bromsgrove General Hospital, Bromsgrove and Redditch Health District, Bromsgrove, Worcestershire.

W. St C. SYMMERS, MD (Belfast), PhD (Birmingham), FRCP (London), MRCP (Ireland and Edinburgh), FRCPA

Professor of Histopathology in the University of London at Charing Cross Hospital Medical School; Honorary Consultant Pathologist, Charing Cross Hospital, London.

*Acknowledgements**

The publishers and the editor thank Dr T. R. Mitchell, Dr S. Shaw and Professor J. Henry Wilkinson, CBE, Charing Cross Hospital Medical School, University of London, for advice on the use of SI units (*Système international d'unités*) and other units of measurement that have been introduced since Volume 1 went to press.

They thank also Mrs S. Godbolt, Librarian to Charing Cross Hospital Medical School, and other members of the staff of the Library, particularly Mr H. Hague and Mr P. Morrell, for their interest in the book and for help in tracing and checking certain references.

Note: The editor is responsible for all mistakes in the calculation and presentation of SI and other units and in the content of the lists of references.

* Please see also the Preface to Volume 1 of this edition.

8: *The Blood and Bone Marrow*

by W. M. DAVIDSON, K. G. A. CLARK *and* M. L. LEWIS

CONTENTS

8: *The Blood and Bone Marrow*

by W. M. Davidson, K. G. A. Clark *and* M. L. Lewis

Note

Abbreviations.—The following abbreviations are used in this chapter:

DNA, deoxyribonucleic acid
G6PD, glucose-6-phosphate dehydrogenase
IgG, IgM, etc., immunoglobulin of class G, class M, etc.
MCH, mean red cell haemoglobin content
MCHC, mean red cell haemoglobin concentration
MCV, mean red cell volume.

Units of Measurement.—SI units (*Système international d'unités*) are used in this chapter. In accordance with the practice current at the time of writing (December 1975), the mass concentration of haemoglobin is still expressed in grams per decilitre (g/dl). All other concentrations are expressed in molecular units—moles (molecular weight in grams) or a submultiple (for example, millimoles)—per litre or (in the case of proteins) in grams or submultiples of grams per litre.

THE NORMAL BLOOD AND BONE MARROW

BLOOD VOLUME

The volume of the blood, and of its cell and fluid components, can be measured with much accuracy during life. The methods chiefly used depend on the degree of dilution of known amounts of some vital dye (such as Evans blue) or of isotope-labelled plasma proteins or erythrocytes after their injection into the circulation. In the average normal adult, the blood volume is about four litres in women and almost five litres in men (some 70 ml per kilogram of body weight); some variation is associated with differences of weight and height and in the amount of fatty tissue.

Much detailed work has been done on devising methods for determining total blood volume, in view of its importance in disease and in the circulatory failure that may follow severe trauma.[1]

Minor variations in blood volume result from changes in posture or in bodily activity, or through heavy sweating. A striking increase—even as much as 40 per cent—occurs during pregnancy, due mainly to a rise in plasma volume.[2] Considerable changes can also occur in disease.[3] Acute severe haemorrhage, extensive burns and prolonged dehydration through vomiting or diarrhoea may result in such a marked reduction in the volume of the blood that the systemic blood pressure falls dangerously. In cases of cardiac failure[4] and of polycythaemia[5] the blood volume may be substantially raised. These changes frequently affect the red cells and the plasma differentially. In cases of severe anaemia there is a relative loss of cells. In disorders accompanied by marked splenomegaly the plasma volume may be greatly increased:[5a] the resulting 'haemodilution anaemia' augments the severity of any anaemia that is associated with the condition responsible for the splenomegaly. The blood volume may rise by 1 to 2 per cent for each centimetre of enlargement of the spleen below the costal margin. The explanation of the increase in the volume of the plasma in association with splenomegaly is unknown; it does not appear to be accompanied by any significant abnormality of the plasma proteins.

THE CELLS OF NORMAL BLOOD

The composition of the blood depends largely on a dynamic equilibrium between its constituents (cells and plasma) and the tissues and tissue fluids. The blood can be regarded as a solution of colloids and crystalloids in which the cellular elements are

References to Other Chapters.: A list of the chapters in each of the five volumes is on page v at the front of this volume.

430

suspended in osmotic equilibrium. Many of its constituents—red cells, white cells, platelets and plasma proteins—are too large to escape freely through capillary walls, and can be regarded as belonging to the blood. In fact this statement is not strictly true—for example, the majority of the leucocytes in the body are in the tissues, although for our present purpose they may be considered as part of the blood. Other substances in the blood are merely in transit between tissue cells and sites of absorption or excretion. Some of these substances (such as iron and copper, trace metals, small amounts of haemoglobin, lipids and bile pigments) are temporarily bound to particular plasma proteins (see page 445);[6] others (including some of the hormones, sugars, fatty acids, amino acids and electrolytes) are more or less uniformly partitioned between the plasma and the tissue fluid.

All the constituents of the blood, including the water in which they are suspended or dissolved, are constantly undergoing replacement. There are wide differences in the rate at which their turnover occurs: information on this aspect of the various types of cells and plasma proteins that are specifically part of the blood is essential for an understanding of the pathology of the blood diseases. As all these elements are formed outside the circulation proper, most blood diseases are the reflection of some disturbance in the tissues of their origin—the bone marrow, the lymphoreticular tissues, the spleen and the liver.

The Red Cells

The red cells (see Table 8.1) are non-nucleate, discoid structures, composed of a lipoprotein envelope and a fluid interior that normally is saturated with haemoglobin. Their typical biconcave shape facilitates the rapid gaseous exchanges that occur in the capillaries of the lungs and of the tissues; at the same time, their ready distortability allows free movement through small vessels.

Enumeration of Cells and Measurement of Haemoglobin Content.—Since quantitative determinations figure prominently in haematological diagnosis, it is necessary to define the normal limits of the numbers of the various types of blood cells. Formerly, a visual count of red cells and an estimation of the amount of haemoglobin in a sample of blood were regarded as the only practical, simple, quantitative investigations needed for the diagnosis of anaemia or polycythaemia. It has become realized, however, that the errors inseparable from

the visual methods of red cell counting make these unreliable. Greater accuracy is obtained by the use of electronic counting instruments.

Separation of the red cells by centrifugation provides a valuable measure of the relative proportions of cells and plasma—the packed-cell volume (PCV) or haematocrit value.

Modern automated instruments measure the haemoglobin level, count the red cells and measure the mean red cell volume (MCV) automatically. They may measure or compute the packed cell volume (PCV) and calculate the mean cell haemoglobin (MCH) and the mean cell haemoglobin concentration (MCHC).[7] While the total red cell mass is the ultimate measure of whether an individual is normal or polycythaemic or anaemic, in practice it is the haemoglobin level and the related indices that are used in making the initial diagnosis of disorders affecting the red cells. The normal range of these parameters in men and in women is shown in Table 8.1.

Table 8.1. *The Normal Parameters of the Red Blood Cells in Adults (SI Units)**

	Men	Women
Number ($\times 10^{12}$/l)	$5\cdot4\pm0\cdot8$	$4\cdot8\pm0\cdot6$
Haemoglobin (g/dl)	16 ± 2	14 ± 2
Packed cell volume (%)	47 ± 5	42 ± 5
Mean cell volume (fl)	87 ± 5	
Mean cell haemoglobin (pg)	29 ± 2	
Mean cell haemoglobin concentration (g/dl)	34 ± 2	
Mean cell diameter (μm)	$7\cdot5\pm0\cdot3$	

* Based on: Wintrobe, M. M., *Clinical Hematology*, 6th edn, page 86. London, 1967.

Blood Films.—In addition to the investigations noted above, study of the red cells requires examination of thin films of blood stained by one of the Romanowsky methods, such as those of Leishman, Wright, May and Grünwald, Jenner, and Giemsa. This study should include observation of the size, shape and staining of the cells and the presence of any inclusions (Fig. 8.9).

Red Cell Diameter.—It may be helpful to determine the distribution of variation in the diameter of the red cells, especially in certain macrocytic anaemias (see page 458). This was formerly done by the laborious method of Price Jones;[8] similar information can now be obtained by use of an automatic instrument that determines the distribution of the red cells according to their volume.[9]

Reticulocytes

When the red cells first enter the circulation they are not fully mature, and they appear a slaty blue in Romanowsky-stained films. By staining blood films, while the blood is still moist, with vital dyes, such as brilliant cresyl blue or Nile blue sulphate, the remains of a basiphile material (ribonucleic acid) within these immature cells can be precipitated as a conspicuous reticulum (see Fig. 8.9N, page 450). It is from this reticulum, which disappears in a day or two in the circulation, that the reticulocyte derives its name. A large number of reticulocytes in the blood indicates that erythropoiesis is currently proceeding at an unusually active level or that there is a gross marrow disturbance. A constant reticulocytosis indicates a shortening of the life span of the red cells (see page 472).

Red Cell Life Span

In mammals, the red blood 'cell' is not a cell in the usual sense of a nucleate unit, but rather an envelope filled almost entirely with a nearly saturated solution of haemoglobin. Under ordinary circumstances, the red cells remain in the circulation for about four months, at the end of which their remnants are ingested and destroyed by the reticulo-endothelial cells of the marrow, spleen, liver and other organs.[10] In some diseases of the blood, however, they may disappear from the circulation much more rapidly (see page 472).

The White Cells

The white cells have a lower specific gravity than the red cells, and consequently they sediment less rapidly on centrifugation. In a haematocrit tube, therefore, they come to form, together with the platelets, a layer normally about a millimetre deep —the 'buffy coat'—between the plasma above and the packed red cells below. Although the depth of this layer varies with the number of white cells in the blood, the relationship is not very close. For the determination of the white cells in a specimen of blood, total and differential counts are required.

Accepted values for the numbers of the various types of white cells are given in Table 8.2. The criteria used for their differentiation in Romanowsky-stained films are indicated in Table 8.3.

Table 8.2. *The Normal Total and Differential White Cell Count per Litre (SI Units)*

	Average count ($\times 10^9/l$)	Normal range ($\times 10^9/l$)
Total cell count	7·0	4·0 to 11·0
Neutrophils	4·5 (65%)	2·5 to 7·5
Lymphocytes	1·8 (25%)	1·5 to 4·0
Monocytes	0·55 (8%)	0·2 to 1·0
Eosinophils	0·15 (2%)	0·05 to 0·5
Basiphils	'occasional'	0 to 0·1

Young neutrophile granulocytes can be identified by the incomplete segmentation of their nucleus. In the earliest stage the nucleus is reniform, but segmentation into two, three, four or more lobes soon follows. Attempts have been made to ascertain the rate of formation of granulocytes by determining the relative numbers of cells showing the various degrees of lobation. In the case of the neutrophils, the presence of many bilobate cells—the so-called

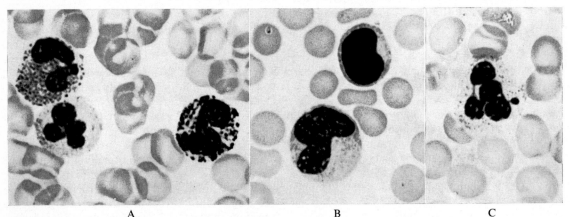

A   B   C

Fig. 8.1. Normal leucocytes in blood films. *Jenner–Giemsa stain.* × 1250.

A. Left to right: an eosinophil, a neutrophil and a basiphil.
B. Above, a lymphocyte; below, a monocyte.
C. A neutrophil from a female, showing a sex 'drumstick', which is believed to be formed from the inactive X chromoso me.

Table 8.3. *Appearance of White Blood Cells in Romanowsky-stained Films* (Fig. 8.1)

	Size (μm)	Nucleus	Chromatin	Cytoplasm	Granules
Neutrophils	12–14	2–5 lobes	Heavy clumps	Abundant; yellow	Fine; purple
Eosinophils	12–17	2–3 lobes	Heavy clumps	Overlaid with granules	Coarse; orange-red
Basiphils	10–12	Indented	Heavy clumps	Overlaid with granules	Coarse; purple-blue
Small lymphocytes	8–11	Unlobed	Heavy clumps	Clear; blue	Clumps of 5–6 red granules
Large lymphocytes	11–18	Unlobed	Heavy clumps	Clear; blue	Clumps of 5–6 red granules
Monocytes	14–25	Overlapping	Fine lacework	Abundant; cloudy; blue	Fine red stippling

'shift to the left'—implies active leucopoiesis, while an unusually large proportion of cells with four or five lobes—the 'shift to the right'—indicates the persistence of senescent cells in the circulation. Determinations of the frequency of these differing lobate forms are known as Arneth counts; they may have some value in estimating the responsiveness of the marrow in some forms of infection. No criteria have yet been recognized by which to estimate the age of the other types of white cells in man; in animals, this can be done by isotopic labelling methods.

Measurement of the life span of the leucocytes in the blood[11] is complicated by the fact that the great majority of these cells are in the tissues, where they cannot be examined readily. By labelling the mature granulocytes with diisopropylfluorophosphonate containing radioactive phosphorus (^{32}P) it has been found that their life span in the blood is about one day. However, about four days may be spent in the bone marrow and rather longer in the tissue compartment, the total life span being therefore, perhaps, 10 days. In contrast, the lymphocytes, which recirculate through the lymph nodes and thoracic duct, appear to consist of two populations, one of which survives for many years (see page 519).

Neutrophils from donors with the Pelger–Huët neutrophil nuclear anomaly (Fig. 8.25C, page 476) are easily recognized in the circulating blood of recipients: they survive at most only six hours in the circulation of normal recipients.[12]

The Platelets

In the stained films that are used for differential leucocyte counts, platelets are seen lying either singly or in small clumps, and a rough estimate of their number can thus be made. Accurate platelet counts are obtained by using electronic counting equipment. The normal number is from 200×10^9/l to 400×10^9/l.

The platelets, which are merely fragments of the cytoplasm of the marrow megakaryocytes, exhibit some reduction in their size and a gradual diminution of their stickiness as they age in the circulation. Their life span, measured by labelling with radioactive isotopes, is about nine days.

THE BONE MARROW

Since most of the so-called blood diseases are in reality diseases of the bone marrow, a general knowledge of haemopoiesis is essential for an understanding of their pathogenesis. Moreover, while these diseases were formerly diagnosed merely by an examination of the peripheral blood, nowadays much use is made of cytological studies of samples of marrow obtained by needle puncture of the sternum or of the crest of the iliac bone.

In the healthy newborn infant, haemopoietic marrow is present in the cavities of all the bones of the body. With time, the extent of haemopoietic marrow recedes; in the adult it is confined mainly to the bones of the skull and the vertebrae, ribs and pelvic bones, with small remnants in the head of the humerus and of the femur. In health, even the haemopoietic portions of the marrow are composed mainly of adipose cells, bands of haemopoietic cells lying between them (Fig. 8.20A, page 461). It is estimated that the medullary cavity of the bones of an adult contains in all about 2 kg of marrow, the greater part of which consists of adipose tissue. When haemopoiesis is stimulated, as may happen in widely differing types of disease, the haemopoietic tissue becomes progressively more abundant. In the severer forms of haemolytic anaemia the adipose tissue is almost wholly replaced by erythropoietic cells, and the rate of production of red cells is increased five-fold or more. At the other extreme, in depression of marrow activity, as in aplastic anaemia, the haemopoietic elements may be so diminished that the medullary cavities are wholly filled by adipose cells (Fig. 8.20B); sometimes, in such cases, the marrow may be replaced by fibrous tissue (Fig. 8.22).

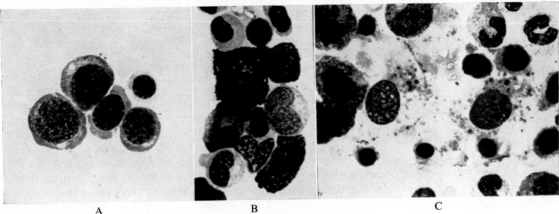

| A | B | C |

Fig. 8.2. Normal marrow. *Film preparations: Jenner–Giemsa stain.* ×1000.

A. Erythropoiesis. A group of normoblasts—in order of decreasing nuclear size and increasing nuclear density the cells are early, intermediate and late normoblasts.

B. A mast cell, above the centre, on the left. The nucleus appears pale in comparison with the heavily stained cytoplasmic granules.

C. Two macrophages, one on each side of the centre of the field. The abundant, ill-defined, pale cytoplasm contains ingested granules; the nucleus is oval and its chromatin has a net-like pattern.

The haemopoietic cells comprise two main series, the red cell precursors (Fig. 8.2A) and the precursors of the granular leucocytes (Fig. 8.3A). In normal marrow, the precursors of the granulocytes predominate over the precursors of the red cells in a ratio of about four to one. The marrow also contains megakaryocytes (Fig. 8.3B), fat cells and other supporting tissue cells, macrophages (Fig. 8.2C), plasma cells and mast cells (Fig. 8.2B). The haemopoietic cells are conventionally regarded as arising from a common ancestor, sometimes called the haemohistioblast, which supposedly is also the ancestral cell of lymphocytes and monocytes (see below). After birth, these primitive cells ('colony-forming units') are very scanty, both in the haemopoietic tissues of the marrow and in the lymphoreticular tissues elsewhere.

Division of a haemohistioblast gives rise to two daughter cells: one of these may retain the attributes of the parent cell while the other is able to differentiate toward any of the definitive cell series. The first of the specific cells in each series is the 'blast' cell, characterized by the relatively large size and uniform chromatin content of the nucleus, which

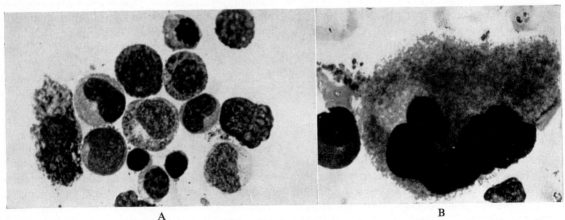

| A | B |

Fig. 8.3. Normal marrow. *Film preparations: Jenner–Giemsa stain.* ×1000.

A. Leucopoiesis. Clockwise from the left, clustered round an early myelocyte in the centre of the field, a myeloblast, a late myelocyte, a promyelocyte, a myelocyte and a metamyelocyte.

B. A megakaryocyte, with a group of platelets to the left.

contains one or more nucleoli, and by the absence
of granules in the cytoplasm (Fig. 8.3A). The blast
cell that is the precursor of the red cell series, the
proerythroblast, is recognizable from the blast cells
of the other series by the granular appearance of its
chromatin, the poor definition of its nucleoli and
the greater opaqueness of its cytoplasm. The earliest
blast cell of the granulocyte series, the myeloblast,
can be distinguished morphologically from the
megakaryoblast, and by cytochemical methods
(especially the periodic-acid/Schiff reaction) from
the earliest precursors of the non-granular leucocytes—lymphoblasts (Fig. 8.4C) and monoblasts.[13]
Lymphoblasts and monoblasts are commoner in
the lymphoreticular tissues elsewhere in the body
than in the bone marrow. In practice, the main
guide to the identification of the nature of any
particular blast cell is the character of the mature
cells that are associated with it and that presumably
are its derivatives.

Recently, doubt has been raised about the occurrence of the elusive haemohistioblasts. When
leucocytes are cultured in the presence of phytohaemagglutinin (a substance extracted from beans),
lymphocytes, although apparently adult cells, revert
to a more primitive type and undergo mitosis.[14]
This may not happen in the case of other cell types,
but the fact that it occurs at all suggests that the
principle of differentiation is not absolute and that
it is, perhaps, not necessary to postulate the
presence of ancestral cells to account for expansion
of the lymphoreticular and haemopoietic tissues
(see page 522).[15]

Erythropoiesis

The *proerythroblast* divides by mitosis, and this
initiates a series of developmental steps, leading by
further mitotic divisions and progressive maturation to the orthochromatic red cells found in the
peripheral blood. These stages are defined according
to the state of the nucleus and the degree to which
haemoglobin synthesis has taken place in the cytoplasm (Fig. 8.2A). The proerythroblast gives rise to
the *early normoblast*, which differs from the former
in being rather smaller and in having no nucleoli.
The next stage, the *intermediate normoblast*, has a
smaller and more compact nucleus; a more important distinguishing feature is the commencing
haemoglobinization of the cytoplasm. The final
nucleate stage is the almost completely haemoglobinized *late normoblast*. This cell eventually
extrudes its pyknotic nucleus, and passes into the
blood stream as a *polychromatic red cell* (*reticulocyte*
—see page 432). It matures into the *orthochromatic
red cell* and loses its mitochondria after being in
the circulation for a day or two. Occasionally, particularly after splenectomy, some of the red cells
in the circulation still contain coarse basiphile
nuclear fragments: these are known as Howell–
Jolly bodies (Fig. 8.9K, page 450).

During the nucleate stages of development a series
of enzyme-controlled reactions is needed both to
build up deoxyribonucleic acid (DNA) in the
chromatin, preparatory to cell division, and to effect
the synthesis of haemoglobin. In addition to its
constituent pyrimidines (thymine and cytosine),
purines (adenine and guanine) and phosphates, the

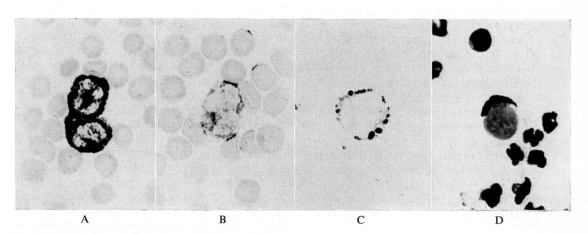

Fig. 8.4. Leucocytes—special staining and other techniques.
A and B. Demonstration of alkaline phosphatase in neutrophils (grades 4 and 1 respectively). × 1000.
C. Periodic-acid/Schiff reaction in a leukaemic lymphoblast. × 1000.
D. Lupus erythematosus: the neutrophil at the centre of the field has engulfed a large spheroidal mass of pale,
    degenerate nuclear material ('LE cell'). *Incubated leucocyte preparation; Jenner–Giemsa stain.* × 700.

formation of DNA requires vitamin B_{12},* ascorbic acid (vitamin C) and folinic acid (the active derivative of folic acid). Lack of these essential substances hinders the enzymatic synthesis of the nucleoproteins of chromatin and consequently interferes with the further multiplication of the cells. As a result, while maturation and haemoglobinization can advance in the cytoplasm, nuclear development is delayed or prevented. Under these conditions, the cells grow abnormally large, and have a delicate expanded nucleus: they are then known as *megaloblasts* (Fig. 8.5C). A defect in the action of one of the enzymes would impair development of the nucleus: this may account for some of the cases of megaloblastic anaemia that are refractory to treatment.

Formation of Haemoglobin

The formation of haemoglobin takes place within the cytoplasm of the developing cells. The haemoglobin molecule is built in two parts: a large protein mass, the globin, and the porphyrin ring structures of the four haem molecules. The globin acts as a vehicle for the four haems, which each contain an atom of iron in a union suited to rapid uptake and liberation of oxygen. The many amino acids that form the four long polypeptide chains of the globin are linked in a specific order in accordance with the hereditary pattern of the DNA (see page 468). Enzymes control each step in the synthesis of the haem, from the union of relatively simple materials, glycine and succinate, through the intermediary stages of delta-aminolaevulic acid and porphobilinogen, to the final chelation of the iron atoms into the porphyrin ring by chelatase.[16]

The synthesis of haemoglobin may be impeded at any stage, either through some congenital or acquired enzymatic defect, or through a lack of an essential substance, particularly iron. Deficiency of iron generally follows prolonged loss of blood but may be due to malabsorption. Non-utilization of iron can be due to an enzyme defect in the red cell precursors or to interference with the transport of iron from the reticuloendothelial cells to the erythropoietic tissues.[17] Whatever the cause of diminished haemoglobin synthesis, it results in poor development of the cytoplasm. The abnormal red cell precursors that are found in these circumstances

* For some years vitamin B_{12} was believed to be cyanocobalamin; cyanide was later found to have become incorporated accidentally in the cobalamin molecule during the course of the purification of the vitamin (E. Lester-Smith, *Vitamin B_{12}*, 3rd edn, page 26; London, 1965).

are known as *micronormoblasts*, and are characterized by having only a narrow and ragged rim of cytoplasm and a rather over-developed, pyknotic nucleus (Fig. 8.5B). The red cells that develop from these micronormoblasts are small (MCV below 80 fl) and deficient in haemoglobin (MCH below 27 pg) (see page 452 and Figs 8.9C and 8.11A).

When the stroma of the red cells is also defective the cells may vary in size (anisocytosis) or shape (poikilocytosis) (Fig. 8.9C, page 450).

Metabolism of the Mature Red Blood Cell

In comparison with its nucleate precursors, the fully formed red blood cell shows little metabolic activity and its aerobic respiration is negligible.[18] Nevertheless, it has to expend energy to preserve its integrity, to keep its water-repellent lipoprotein surface intact, to retain its biconcave shape, to hold the haemoglobin in the active ferrous state, and to maintain a higher concentration of potassium and a lower concentration of sodium within its envelope than is present in the plasma. Most of the energy that is needed for these purposes is derived from anaerobic glycolysis. During the serial enzymatic degradation of diphosphoglycerate to pyruvate in that part of the main Embden–Meyerhof pathway that includes the activity of the enzyme pyruvate kinase, adenosine diphosphate (ADP) is phosphorylated to adenosine triphosphate (ATP) to provide a considerable amount of potential energy (see Fig. 8.6). A smaller amount is produced in the pentose phosphate shunt and at the same time nicotinamide adenine dinucleotide phosphate (NADP) is reduced ($NADPH_2$) by the activity of the enzymes glucose-6-phosphate dehydrogenase and 6-phosphogluconate dehydrogenase. This maintains glutathione in the reduced state and in turn prevents the degradation of the haemoglobin in the living red cells. In the region between the glyceraldehyde-3-phosphate and the diphosphoglycerate not only is some energy produced to help maintain haemoglobin in its reduced form, but there is also a small side shunt involving the synthesis of the important substance 2,3-diphosphoglycerate. This substance controls the release of oxygen from haemoglobin: its increased production helps to compensate for relative hypoxia at high altitudes and for anaemia. When stored blood is transfused its capacity for oxygen release is defective during the first 24 hours because its content of 2,3-diphosphoglycerate diminishes progressively during storage and time is needed for it to form again.

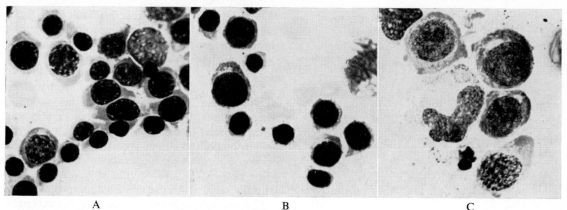

Fig. 8.5. Abnormal erythropoiesis. *Film preparations of marrow: Jenner–Giemsa stain.* × 1000.
A. Over-active normoblastic erythropoiesis in haemolytic anaemia.
B. Micronormoblastic erythropoiesis in iron-deficiency anaemia.
C. Megaloblastic erythropoiesis in pernicious anaemia (Addisonian anaemia). A giant metamyelocyte is also seen, at the centre of the field, surrounded by the megaloblasts.

Once the developing red cell has lost its nucleus, production of further enzyme molecules probably ceases. Recent investigations of these enzyme systems have provided much information regarding disorders of red cell metabolism (see page 468).

The constant replacement of senile red cells through erythropoiesis involves the continuous synthesis of haemoglobin. Studies on the metabolism of iron have been of particular importance in throwing light on the problems of haemoglobin formation: in recent years, use of the radioactive isotope, ^{59}Fe, has much advanced knowledge of the absorption, transportation, utilization and excretion of iron, both in health and in disease.

The amount of iron normally present in the body is from 4 to 5 g. Of this, about 2·5 g are combined organically in haemoglobin (1 g of haemoglobin contains 3·39 mg of iron). From 1 to 1·5 g of iron is stored in the reticuloendothelial cells; a small quantity (about 200 mg) is present in the myoglobin of muscle, and in respiratory enzymes such as the peroxidases, and a trace (about 3 mg) is bound to a plasma globulin, transferrin (siderophilin). Despite its small quantity, the iron present in the transferrin fraction of the plasma proteins represents a vital link in the chain of iron metabolism.[19]

Although the quantity of iron in the plasma is so small, its turnover is rapid. Every day, a number of red cells equivalent to the normal red cell content of over 40 ml of blood is replaced, and this means that about 20 mg of iron have to be made available for the synthesis of the appropriate amount of haemoglobin. Some 18 mg of this comes from the recycling of haemoglobin iron released during the degradation of effete red cells in the reticuloendothelial system. Only 1 to 2 mg of iron are lost from the body daily, mainly in enzymes of cells desquamated from the skin and from the mucosa of the gastrointestinal and urinary tracts: to maintain a balance, this amount of iron must be absorbed daily from the alimentary canal. Menstruation accounts for the equivalent of a regular loss of 1 mg of iron daily throughout reproductive life. While this additional loss is ordinarily made good by a corresponding increase in iron absorption, a comparatively slight excess of blood loss during menstruation or a slight deficiency in the amount of iron absorbed may suffice to upset the balance. Even in the poorer diets in a country such as Britain there are probably about 15 mg of iron in the food consumed daily. In iron-deficiency anaemia iron administered therapeutically may raise the amount absorbed to over 20 mg a day.

Before it can be absorbed, much of the iron in food must be liberated from its combination with organic substances; this is effected by digestion in the stomach. Conversion of the iron into the ferrous form precedes its absorption through the mucosa of the duodenum and the upper part of the jejunum. Some foods contain large amounts of phosphates and phytic acid, which impair iron absorption. Achlorhydria does not itself block the absorption of therapeutically-administered iron, or even of iron in the food,[20] but indirectly it probably hinders the increased degree of absorption from the food that would be needed to prevent develop-

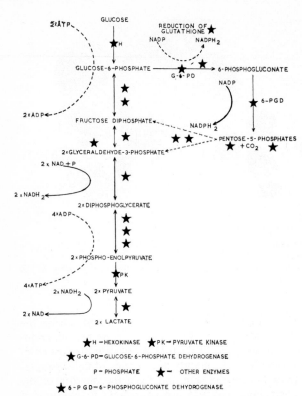

Fig. 8.6. The Embden–Meyerhof pathway, with pentose phosphate shunt. In addition to the reactions indicated in the diagram there is a lesser, but important, shunt at the first of the three steps in the conversion of diphosphoglycerate to phosphoenolpyruvate. In the direct pathway, 3-phosphoglycerate is formed by means of phosphoglyceric acid kinase while adenosine diphosphate (ADP) is converted to high energy adenosine triphosphate (ATP). In contrast, in the side pathway 2,3-diphosphoglycerate is formed as an intermediate product and energy is lost. These pathways are believed to alternate, when needed, to maintain the appropriate level of ADP–ATP conversion.

ment of hypochromic anaemia when there is excessive loss of iron from the body.

When iron is absorbed by the epithelial cells of the intestinal mucosa, it is converted into the ferric form and bound to an intracellular protein, apoferritin, to form ferritin. The subsequent passage of the iron across the cell membrane to the iron-binding plasma globulin, transferrin, requires conversion from the ferric through the ferrous and back to the ferric form. Although the turnover of transferrin-bound iron is rapid, this transportation mechanism, operating from the intestine and from sites of haemoglobin degradation, may not suffice to supply all the 20 mg of the element required for the daily production of haemoglobin. It is possible that the macrophages in the marrow may transfer

iron liberated from ingested effete red cells directly to nearby maturing erythropoietic cells (Fig. 8.15A, page 455).[21] But the iron from haemoglobin broken down in macrophages in the liver, spleen and other organs must be returned to the marrow by way of the plasma.

Although it is the metabolism of iron that has naturally received most attention in studies of erythropoiesis, there is evidence that certain trace metals, among them copper, cobalt and manganese, are also needed. Erythropoietic disorders may appear in farm animals grazing on soils deficient in these elements; there is little evidence that man, with his very mixed diets, is ever similarly affected.

Certain vitamins are intimately concerned in erythropoiesis; of great importance is the cobalamin, vitamin B_{12}. This has a complex tetrapyrrole molecule with a linking cobalt atom. The principal form used in therapy is hydroxocobalamin. In health nearly 0·5 μg of vitamin B_{12} is bound to protein (transcobalamins I and II) in the plasma for transport to the tissues, where it enters the cells, including the red cell precursors, and participates in nucleic acid synthesis. Ample quantities of this vitamin are present in the average diet, but a mucoprotein secreted by the mucosa of the fundus of the stomach—the intrinsic factor of Castle—is needed for its absorption from the small intestine. This factor may be missing as a result of atrophy of the mucosa (Fig. 8.17, page 457) or after extensive resection of the stomach. Alternatively, absorption of vitamin B_{12} may be impaired by disease of the lower part of the ileum, or by a change in the bacterial flora of the small intestine, such as may be brought about by the presence of a blind loop, diverticulum or stricture. The normal daily requirement of the vitamin is about 1 to 2 μg, and as about 3 mg are ordinarily stored in the body, even complete lack of intake of the vitamin would have little effect on haemopoiesis for several years. Usually, evidence of abnormal haemopoiesis is the first manifestation of a deficiency of vitamin B_{12}, although, as with iron deficiency, other types of cell may suffer before those of the marrow. Soreness and ulceration of the tongue, and even subacute combined degeneration of the spinal cord, may precede the development of anaemia.

Folic acid, which is a pteroylglutamic acid, is now known to be of fundamental importance in many metabolic processes, among them those concerned in erythropoiesis.[22] The daily requirement of this substance is much greater than that of vitamin B_{12}, and is measured in milligrams. In the body, folic acid is converted into folinic acid, which is required for deoxyribonucleic acid metabolism. The sites at which vitamin B_{12} and folinic acid participate in the metabolic activities must be very close, for, up to a point, the one can be replaced by the other. The two substances are not interchangeable, however: in cases of vitamin B_{12} deficiency, a period of 'false recovery' may be induced by folic acid, and this may result in exhaustion of the last traces of stored vitamin B_{12} and lead suddenly to a disastrous relapse. Not only does the anaemia then return quickly, but subacute combined degeneration of the spinal cord may develop in a fulminating manner.

Vitamin B_{12} appears to act as a co-enzyme, either alone or in conjunction with folic acid derivatives. In the formation of ribonucleic acid in the central nervous system it appears to act alone. In general, vitamin B_{12} is concerned in the transfer of single carbon units in the synthesis of ribonucleic acid and deoxyribonucleic acid. When there is a deficiency of vitamin B_{12} one effect is that succinate cannot be formed from methylmalonic acid, which therefore accumulates and may pass into the urine. The rare condition of methylmalonicaciduria in children with neurological abnormalities, but no deficiency of vitamin B_{12} and no anaemia, has been attributed to an enzyme defect in the same pathway.[23]

Other vitamins required for erythropoiesis are normally present in adequate amounts in the diet and are readily absorbed. Ascorbic acid (vitamin C) plays a part in the formation of folinic acid, but even in cases of scurvy the development of anaemia is only of secondary importance.[24] Pyridoxine (vitamin B_6) is necessary for the union of glycine and succinate during the formation of haem. Ascorbic acid, folinic acid and pyridoxine are also concerned in the enzymatic reactions in amino acid metabolism. Anaemia due to a block in haemoglobin synthesis caused by pyridoxine deficiency, although well recognized, is rare.[25, 26]

Leucopoiesis

The white cell precursors in the marrow (Fig. 8.3A) undergo a series of developmental changes comparable with those of the cells of the erythroblastic series. The *myeloblasts* divide to form *promyelocytes*, which have a smaller nucleus; with further divisions, the nucleus becomes smaller still, the nucleoli disappear, and a layer of faintly acidophile 'endoplasm' grows out from it and eventually, by the time the *myelocyte* stage is reached, fills the cytoplasm. In the maturer myelocytes the definitive

granules appear (see Table 8.3, page 433); in Romanowsky-stained preparations the cytoplasm of the neutrophile myelocytes is peppered with small purple-staining granules, that of the eosinophile myelocytes is filled with coarse, refractile granules that stain orange-red, and the basiphile myelocytes contain granules that stain an intense purple-blue.

Once the late myelocyte stage is reached, no further cell division takes place. The cell continues to mature: the nucleus becomes sausage-shaped in the *metamyelocyte* stage, and then develops progressively into its final multilobate form at about the time of its entry into the circulation. Mature *neutrophils* have three or possibly four lobes; old ones may have more (Fig. 8.9D, page 450). The *eosinophils* have two, sometimes three, clearly separated lobes, while the *basiphils*, in contrast, have an indented nucleus that only rarely shows definite lobation. The cytoplasmic granules, which are so conspicuous a feature of the mature leucocytes, appear to be concerned with functions of the cell—the production of histamine antagonists by the eosinophils and of heparin by the basiphils.[27–29] Other organized structures in the cytoplasm of the leucocytes, especially the mitochondria, are centres of enzyme activity; the enzymes that have been recognized include peroxidases and alkaline phosphatases.

Eosinophils are conspicuous in many types of infestation by metazoan parasites and in many allergic reactions. *Basiphils* possibly play a part in the prevention of intravascular clotting of plasma. The *neutrophile leucocytes* (the microphages of Metchnikoff) ingest and may destroy bacteria and other small foreign particles. The *monocytes* are the blood macrophages, capable of engulfing larger particles, and active in the later stages of acute infections and throughout the course of chronic inflammatory reactions. The *lymphocytes* are of two types: the T cells, modified by the thymus, are concerned with tissue immunity, including delayed hypersensitivity; the B cells form antibody globulins and may themselves undergo transformation into plasma cells (see page 522).

In the circulating blood, there are, on average, 7000 white cells to every 5 000 000 red cells, a ratio of one to about 700: in contrast, the ratio of the white cell precursors to the red cell precursors in the marrow is four to one. This 3000-fold difference in the two ratios is partly attributable to the difference in the life span of the two types of cell once they have entered the circulation, and partly to the huge reserves of leucocytes that are maintained in the marrow and in various other tissues.[30]

Platelet Formation

The *platelets*, or thrombocytes, are formed in the marrow by the shedding of small portions of the cytoplasm of the *megakaryocytes*. The latter develop from a precursor cell, the *megakaryoblast*, which is rather larger than the other blast cells. The growth of the megakaryoblasts is peculiar in that nuclear division is not accompanied by cytoplasmic division: as a result, the nucleus of the megakaryocyte has multiple lobes—their number is represented by powers of two.[31] As the megakaryocyte matures it develops a richly granular cytoplasm, parts of which eventually break away to form platelets, which pass into the circulation (Fig. 8.3B); this sequence eventually leaves the nuclei of the mega-karyoblast bare and degenerating. The platelets play an important part in maintaining the integrity of the capillary walls: a reduction in their number below about $50 \times 10^9/l$ (the so-called 'critical number') usually results in purpura. The platelets are also closely concerned with the formation of intravascular thrombi (see page 491). Their sudden disruption, which may occur in some forms of allergic reaction, leads to the release of 5-hydroxy-tryptamine and possibly of other vasoactive substances.

The Marrow Macrophages and Red Cell Destruction

In addition to adipose and haemopoietic tissues, the marrow contains 'fixed' macrophages (Fig. 8.2C, page 434), plasma cells and mast cells (Fig. 8.2B), and small numbers of endothelial cells and fibro-blasts in the supporting stroma.

The marrow macrophages actively remove senile or abnormal red cells from the blood. They are also concerned with the removal and destruction of moribund white cells and of the nuclear remnants extruded by maturing normoblasts (Fig. 8.15C, page 455). The haemoglobin liberated from the ingested red cells is split into globin and haem: the amino acids of the former are returned to the general metabolic pool while the latter is further broken down. The first stage in the catabolism of haem is the opening of the porphyrin ring to form a straight linkage of four pyrrole rings. The second stage is the removal of the iron: in this way the bile pigment, bilirubin, is formed. The iron continues in the closed circuit of the iron metabolism, while the bilirubin is bound to plasma albumin and carried to the liver for conjugation and conversion to the water-soluble form, preparatory to its excretion in the bile. In the macrophages of normal marrow, iron can be demonstrated by Perls's Prussian blue reaction to be present partly in a diffuse form, ferritin, and partly in a granular form, haemosiderin (Fig. 8.15).[32–34] Ferritin and haemosiderin are iron–protein complexes; they form respectively the labile and the more permanent stores of iron. This stored iron is of great importance, not only in the daily turnover of the element, amounting to some 20 mg, but also for meeting any sudden demand for haemoglobin, such as may follow a large haemorrhage. The reticuloendothelial system of the body normally stores a reserve of about 1 to 1·5 g of iron. With persistent small haemorrhages, this reserve gradu-ally becomes depleted, but it is only after it has become exhausted that an iron-deficiency anaemia develops. At the other extreme, there is excessive storage of iron in conditions in which grossly abnormal amounts have been absorbed from the in-testine—as in haemochromatosis (see page 1270)—or when large quantities of iron or iron-containing materials, including blood, have been administered parenterally.

Control of Haemopoiesis

The mechanisms that control the production of the various types of blood cell are still incom-pletely understood. There is little doubt that hypoxia stimulates erythropoiesis, but its effect seems to be indirect and is probably mediated by the erythropoiesis-stimulating factor (ESF, ery-thropoietin) which is believed to be formed in the kidneys, and which operates directly on the red cell precursors in the bone marrow.[35] The adrenal cortex and, possibly, the thyroid gland are also concerned: for this reason, certain endocrine dis-orders are accompanied by anaemia that is refrac-tory to the usual methods of treatment.

Certain hormones can affect the white cell and platelet counts, a notable example of such activity being the fall in the eosinophil count that follows the administration of cortisone. White cell mobiliza-tion and production appear to be sensitive to certain tissue breakdown products (leucocytosis-stimulating factors), and the leucocytosis that often accompanies infection or myocardial infarction may be brought about by some substance released at the site of inflammation or from the necrotic tissue.[36]

A humoral factor controlling platelet production ('thrombopoietin') has been postulated.[37]

The Spleen and Haemopoiesis.—It has been suggested, but remains unproved, that the spleen may produce a hormone-like substance that has an inhibitory effect on haemopoiesis, particularly on the release of cells—red cells, leucocytes and platelets—from the marrow into the circulation.

The concept of *hypersplenism*[38] is related to this hypothesis. Hypersplenism is the supposedly causative association between splenomegaly and anaemia, leucopenia and thrombocytopenia, in any combination and of any degree, usually in the presence of very active haemopoiesis. The evidence that the enlarged spleen is responsible for the deficiencies in the blood picture is the beneficial effect of splenectomy in some cases. It is conceivable that such changes result from overproduction of the hypothetical inhibitory agent or agents by the enlarged spleen, as a factor of the increase in splenic cellularity, irrespective of the cause of the splenomegaly. Alternatively, the large spleen may be capable of sequestering a larger number of blood cells than a normal spleen, and the anaemia, leucopenia or thrombocytopenia may result simply from such excessive sequestration. Haemodilution may accentuate these effects (see page 448). Finally, there is the possibility that the changes in the blood are due to increased destruction of blood cells by increased phagocytic activity in the enlarged spleen.

THE BLOOD GROUPS[39]

In addition to providing the envelope and supporting stroma, the fraction of the protein of the red cell that is not a constituent of the haemoglobin carries the principal antigens of the cell. The most important of these antigenic components is the species-specific human antigen, but there are, in addition, a number of genetically-determined blood group isoantigens that separate the human race into many overlapping subdivisions. These isoantigens differ from one another biochemically and immunologically because the protein is associated with different mucopolysaccharides.[40] With the nine major blood groups and a number of minor groups there are many possible combinations. As additional groups come to light it is conceivable that the pattern of the blood group antigens may prove to be as individually distinctive as the finger print.

The ABO Blood Group System

The first blood group antigens to be discovered, and the most important, are the antigens of the ABO system of Landsteiner:[41] they are A, B and H.

H is present in all human red cells and is apparently a precursor from which A and B are formed. In group O, strictly speaking, the H antigen alone is present while in groups A and B, H is associated with the specific antigen of the group. The ABO system differs from many of the other blood group systems in that the plasma of the individual always contains a natural antibody to those antigens that are missing from the red cells. Thus, a group A plasma contains an anti-B antibody, which agglutinates group B red cells, while group B plasma contains anti-A; group O plasma contains both anti-A and anti-B. The results of mixing the cells and plasma of the different groups are shown in Table 8.4 (it may be noted that in practice it is better to use serum to avoid interference with the agglutination reactions by clotting factors). For transfusions, it is always best to give blood of the same ABO group, and under no circumstances should the donor's red cells be incompatible with the recipient's plasma. The reverse situation, when there is an antibody in the donor's plasma that can react with the recipient's cells, is generally less important, for any antibodies that are present in the relatively small volume of plasma transfused are so much diluted and neutralized by soluble antigens in the plasma of the recipient that they would ordinarily cause no serious reaction; only if the donor's plasma contains the agglutinin at an exceptionally high titre, or if the recipient is unusually anaemic, or if a very large transfusion, especially an intra-arterial transfusion, is required, are untoward results at all likely. In general, therefore, group O blood can be given to any recipient in an emergency, in spite of the presence in its plasma of both anti-A and anti-B agglutinins; however, it should not be obtained from a donor with a very high titre of agglutinins. In this connexion it should be noted that anti-A agglutinins may rise to dangerous levels after active immunization with various vaccines and after passive protection with tetanus antitoxin.[42]

The frequency of the ABO groups varies throughout the world. In Britain, group O and group A are almost equally frequent, and account for nearly 90 per cent of the population (Table 8.4). Group B accounts for 8 per cent, and its frequency is increasing with the immigration of people of African and Asian origin. AB is rare, being found in no more than 3 per cent of the population.

In theory, all who belong to group AB can receive blood from any donor. In practice, however, difficulties may arise because of subgroups of A (A_1 and A_2). Individuals belonging to group AB may,

Table 8.4. *The ABO Blood Group System*

ABO GROUP ———→	Natural Antibodies in Serum			O	A		B	AB		
					A₁	A₂		A₁B	A₂B	
				Antigens in Red Cells						
				OO	A₁O,A₁A₁ or A₁A₂	A₂O or A₂A₂	BO or BB	A₁B	A₂B	Antigens (genotype)
				47	34	8	8	2·5	0·5	Incidence per cent
	Anti-A	Anti-A₁	Anti-B	Reaction between red cells and serum antibodies†						
O	+	+	+	—	Agg	Agg	Agg	Agg	Agg	
A　A₁	—	—	+	—	—	—	Agg	Agg	Agg	
A　A₂	—	—/+*	+	—	—/Agg	—	Agg	Agg	Agg	
B	+	+	—	—	Agg	Agg	—	Agg	Agg	
AB　A₁B	—	—	—	—	—	—	—	—	—	
AB　A₂B	—	—/+**	—	—	—/Agg	—	—	—/Agg	—	

Key: † = At room temperature.　 * = in 5 per cent of sera.　 ** = in 25 per cent of sera.　 Agg = Agglutination.

therefore, be either A₁B or A₂B. An A₂B individual may have a natural or an acquired anti-A₁ antibody. The natural anti-A₁ antibodies are of little significance in relation to transfusion as they are usually cold antibodies and therefore not active at body temperature.

The genes that determine the main blood groups (ABO system) are located as allelomorphs (that is, in the same position on the homologous chromosomes), but it seems that the genes for the other systems are situated in different pairs of chromosomes. In the ABO system, the genes for A and B dominate over that for O, so that an individual whose phenotype is group A may have the genetic structure (genotype) AA or AO. Similarly, a group B person may be BB or BO. People of group AB and group O can be only of the genotypes AB and OO respectively.*

The H antigen is important in relation to the secretor state and to the Lewis blood groups system (page 444). Anti-H antibody is found as a cold agglutinin in all sera and as a warm agglutinin in

the serum of a small proportion of people of groups A₁, A₁B and B: it reacts preferentially with group O and group A₂ cells. A rare suppressor gene inhibiting the formation of the inherited ABO antigen has been described as the Bombay gene.

The Rhesus or CDE/cde Blood Group System

In addition to the ABO system, the rhesus or CDE/cde system is important in transfusion practice (Table 8.5). There are no natural antibodies in this system: instead, immune antibodies may be present that have formed in response to exposure to the particular antigen. Antibodies to five of the major antigens of the system and to a number of the minor antigens are known; no anti-d antibody has been observed yet. The term 'rhesus positive' is applied to those people who possess the antigen D and have the genetic structure DD (homozygous) or Dd (heterozygous). In Britain, about 85 per cent of the population are rhesus positive; the remaining 15 per cent have the genetic structure dd and are described as 'rhesus negative'.

In transfusion practice and in obstetrics the CcEe antigens and their corresponding antibodies must be taken into account. It is very important that blood for transfusion should be matched for com-

* When the subgroups A₁ and A₂ are involved, the combinations A₁A₁, A₁A₂, A₁O, A₂A₂, A₂O, A₁B and A₂B are all possible. In Britain, the gene for the group A₁ is about three times as common as that for A₂ (see Table 8.4). Several other subgroups of A are also known.

Table 8.5. *Three Further Blood Group Systems of Clinical Importance—The Rhesus (CDE/cde), Kell and Duffy Groups*

RHESUS GROUP	POSITIVE						NEGATIVE	
Red Cell Antigens (genotype)	CDE/cde	CDe/CDe	CDe/cDE	cDE/cde	cDE/cDE	Including C^{w}De, CDE and cDe	cde/cde	Including Cde, cdE and CdE
Incidence per cent	35	18	13	11	3	3	15	2
Serum Antibodies	Reaction between red cells and serum antibodies†							
Anti-D	Agg	Agg	Agg	Agg	Agg	Agg	–	–
Anti-E	–	–	Agg	Agg	Agg	–/Agg	–	–/Agg
Anti-c	Agg	–	Agg	Agg	Agg	–/Agg	Agg	–/Agg
Anti-C	Agg	Agg	Agg	–	–	–/Agg	–	–/Agg
Anti-e*	Agg	Agg	Agg	Agg	–	–/Agg	Agg	–/Agg

KELL GROUP	POSITIVE		NEGATIVE
Red Cell Antigens (genotype)	KK	Kk	kk
Incidence per cent	0·2	9	91
Serum Antibodies	Reaction between red cells and serum antibodies†		
Anti-K	Agg	Agg	–
Anti-k*	–	Agg	Agg

DUFFY GROUP	POSITIVE		NEGATIVE	
Red Cell Antigens (genotype)	Fy^{a}Fy^a	Fy^{a}Fy^b	Fy^{b}Fy^b	Fy$^-$Fy$^-$
Incidence per cent	17	49	34	**
Serum Antibodies	Reaction between red cells and serum antibodies†			
Anti-Fy^a	Agg	Agg	–	–
Anti-Fy^b*	–	Agg	Agg	–

Key: † = Incubated at 37°C under appropriate conditions using saline suspensions or albumin suspensions of red cells, enzyme-treated red cells, or the indirect antiglobulin test where necessary.
  * = Rare antibody.
  ** = Genotype found only in Africans.
  Agg = Agglutination.

patibility within this grouping system as well as within the ABO system; this is necessary in order to avoid the formation in the recipient of specific agglutinins that might be a danger during a subsequent transfusion with blood containing the same antigens. The rhesus system is of particular importance in pregnancy, for if the mother is rhesus negative, and the father rhesus positive, the fetus may be heterozygous positive. Red cell antigen passing to the mother through the placenta, especially during labour, can induce specific antibody formation. In the later stages of a subsequent pregnancy, these antibodies may in turn cross the placenta, enter the fetal circulation, and cause serious, even fatal, injury (hydrops fetalis; erythroblastosis fetalis) (see page 464).

Other Blood Group Systems

Of the other known blood group systems the Kell (K), Duffy (Fy), and Kidd (Jk) are the most important in relation to transfusion complications and haemolytic disease of the newborn (Table 8.5). Red cell destruction *in vivo* may be caused by antibodies in the Lewis, MNS, P, Lutheran, Auberger, Diego and Sutter systems: screening and cross-matching techniques must be designed to detect such antibodies, especially when the prospective recipient has received previous transfusions or is multiparous. As 90 per cent of the population of Britain are Kell negative, acquired anti-K antibodies are not very rare. With the Duffy group the position is more complex. Most Europeans are positive: half are Fy(a+b+), with the genotype Fy^aFy^b, one-third Fy(a−b+) and the remainder Fy(a+b−); in contrast, two-thirds of Africans are Duffy negative, Fy(a−b−). The commonest antibody is anti-Fy^a (Table 8.5). Positivity in the Kidd group is widely distributed. In Britain, half the population is Jk(a+b+), a quarter is Jk(a+b−) and a quarter is Jk(a−b+). Jk(a−b−) appears to have been recognized only once. Anti-Jk^a, the commonest antibody, has caused a number of cases of severe haemolytic disease, with kernicterus.

The Lewis system, which is closely related to the ABO system and to the secretor state, is also of practical importance as the antibodies in the system have caused transfusion reactions. The antigens Le^a and Le^b are really serum and saliva antigens that attach themselves to red cells, including transfused red cells. Lewis antibodies are usually of the naturally occurring complete type, more active at room temperature than at 37°C, and complement-binding, but they may be incomplete and detectable only by the indirect anti-globulin test. The system is controlled directly by the genes Le and le and less directly by the genes Se and se, which determine whether the ABH blood group substances are secreted in the saliva or not. Seventy-five per cent of the population who inherit the Se gene (the secretors) and who have the appropriate ABH blood group antigens in their saliva are Lewis(a−) (see Table 8.6). The ABH and Lewis antigens arise from a common mucopolysaccharide precursor: in the serum this is transformed under the influence of the Le gene to Le^a substance. If the gene Se is also present the Le^a substance, together with some of the common precursor, is then converted to Le^b substance.

In addition to these 12 main blood group systems there are some rarer antigens, such as Levay and Wright, which are virtually confined to particular families and are sometimes called the 'private' antigens. Others have a very high incidence and individuals lacking the antigen, and therefore liable to make the antibody, are rare. Such 'public' antigens are Vel, Yt^a, I and Ge. The I system is important in that a powerful cold antibody found in the serum of certain patients with acquired haemolytic anaemia has been demonstrated to have anti-I specificity.

Table 8.6. *Relationship Between the Lewis System and the Secretor State*

	Antigens present								
	Serum		Saliva			Cells			
Genotype*	Le^a	Le^b	ABH	Le^a	Le^b	Le^a	Le^b	Phenotype
(1) Le/Se	(±)	+	+	+	+	(±)	+	Le(a−b+) 70%
(2) Le/se	+	−	−	+	−	+	−	Le(a+b−) 25%
(3) le/Se	−	−	+	−	(±)	−	(±)	Le(a−b−) 5%
(4) le/se	−	−	−	−	−	−	−	Le(a−b−) 5%

* These may be homozygous or heterozygous for the factor—that is Le/Le or Le/le, Se/Se or Se/se. (±): possible reaction.

The ABO, MN and P antigens are also present in leucocytes and platelets; curiously, those of the rhesus system do not occur in either of these types of cell. The other leucocyte antigens are less well understood but they and the serum antigens of the Ag system appear to be responsible for certain reactions after repeated blood transfusions.

Detection of Blood Group Antibodies

Detection of the natural ABO antibodies is easy, for they are active at room temperature and are complete agglutinins—that is, they agglutinate the corresponding red cells in a saline suspension. Rhesus antibodies, in contrast, are active only at body temperature, and they may be 'incomplete', so that they require special techniques, such as the addition of albumin to the test mixture, pretreatment of the red cells with enzymes, or the use of an anti-human-globulin serum (the Coombs test)[43] to demonstrate them.* Antibodies to the Kell, Duffy

* In this test, the donor's red cells are incubated with the recipient's serum at body temperature. If an incomplete antibody is present, it will not agglutinate them: however, each red cell becomes coated with immune globulin. If such 'sensitized' red cells, well washed, are now exposed to the serum of a rabbit that has been immunized with human globulin, the antibody to human globulin in the rabbit serum brings about the agglutination of the cells.

and similar systems are detected if the appropriate antiglobulin test is included in the cross-matching procedures. These investigations are especially important when the recipient has been transfused previously. When caring for patients, such as haemophiliacs, who are likely to need repeated transfusion, it is wise to carry out a full genotyping of their cells, and as far as possible to choose donors with cells of the same antigenic structure.

Genetical and Ethnological Importance of Blood Groups

In the past, blood groups have been studied mainly from the point of view of ensuring the safety of transfusions. As the determining genes and their alleles for each group are carried on separate pairs of chromosomes, it is now recognized that they provide markers of considerable genetical and ethnological significance.[44] The discovery of the Xg group, carried on the X chromosome and therefore sex-linked, is of particular genetical importance.[45] In addition excellent markers are provided by the inherited leucocyte anomalies,[46] the Gm serum antigen system, and inherited differences in the haptoglobins and transferrins.[47]

Immunoglobulins[48]

Although antibodies, including those of the blood group systems, are not limited to the gamma globulin band but may be found with the alpha and beta globulins on electrophoresis, the use of immunoelectrophoresis* has shown that this is an artificial subdivision and that they belong to a more homogeneous system—the immunoglobulins (see Table 8.7). Ultracentrifugation, with the sedimentation constant recorded in Svedberg units (S), chemical analysis and the physicochemical dissection of the constituent polypeptides have shown that the antibodies can be grouped into five main classes and a number of subclasses. The commonest class, immunoglobulin G (IgG), includes most of the incomplete blood group antibodies of the ABO system. These, because of their smaller molecular size, can pass the placental barrier with ease. The

---

* Immunoelectrophoresis entails first submitting the mixed protein to electrophoresis in a transparent gel. Then, when the proteins have migrated and separated into albumin and globulin fractions, antiserum is poured into an elongated trough parallel to the axis of the migration. The antigens and antibodies diffuse into the gel: arcs of specific precipitation are formed where they meet. Analysis of these showed the immunological relationships among the antibodies and led to the concept of immunoglobulins.

other complete antibodies, including most of the natural ABO antibodies, belong to the large molecule IgM class. Antibodies of the third class, IgA, account for a small proportion of the naturally occurring anti-A and anti-B antibodies. Neither of the remaining classes of immunoglobulin, IgD and IgE, is involved in blood group serology.

Each immunoglobulin consists of two 'heavy' and two 'light' polypeptide chains. The heavy chains are specific—gamma, mu or alpha—for each of the three classes; two varieties of light chain—kappa and lambda—are shared and subdivide each class.

Table 8.7. *Characteristics of Immunoglobulins*

	IgG	IgM	IgA
Molecular weight	150 000	1 000 000	150 000
Sedimentation coefficient	7S	19S	7S
Carbohydrate content	2·5%	10%	10%
Polypeptide chains:			
Heavy	γ	μ	α
Light	κ or λ	κ or λ	κ or λ

Crude anti-human-globulin sera contain anti-IgG and anti-complement factors. When used in antiglobulin tests, red cells coated with almost any incomplete antibody are agglutinated, although sometimes only if coated in the presence of complement. More specific antiglobulins separate most of the antibodies into their respective immunoglobulin classes; those requiring complement react with anticomplement globulin by virtue of the complement bound by the antibody to the cells.

THE BLOOD PLASMA

A variety of methods—among them salt precipitation, electrophoresis (Fig. 8.7; Fig. 8.37, page 490) and gravitational sedimentation—have helped to distinguish the various plasma proteins and to disclose the variations that may be found in them in diseases of the blood. Since they pass through the capillary wall with difficulty, these proteins, and especially albumin, are responsible for the colloidal osmotic pressure of the plasma and the distribution of water between the blood and the tissue fluids. Some of the plasma proteins have a distinctive role in the transport of other substances in the circulation—transferrin (a β_1 globulin) for iron, caeruloplasmin for copper, globulins for vitamin B_{12} and for cholesterol and other lipids, and albumin for bile pigments. Others, the haptoglobins, are capable of binding and transporting small quantities of free haemoglobin in the plasma. In addition there are the immunoglobulins, which include the specific antibodies, the various antigenic fractions and the haemostatic factors. Normally there are from 1·5 to 4 g of fibrinogen, the precursor of fibrin, in each litre of plasma. When the amount of fibrinogen present is increased, the large, asymmetrical molecules induce the formation of red cell rouleaux, which is the basis of the increase in the erythrocyte sedimentation rate in such cases.

Under some circumstances, distinctive proteins, among them macroglobulins and cryoglobulins, may appear in the blood (see page 498).

HAEMOSTASIS AND BLOOD COAGULATION

The haemostatic mechanisms of the blood are complex. From time to time, capillaries and other small vessels are injured by minor trauma, and any breaks in continuity of their endothelium require to be sealed to prevent the development of a small haemorrhage. Haemostasis, under these circumstances, is achieved mainly by prompt contraction of the capillary endothelium, followed by the formation of a plug of platelets and fibrin. It is suggested that the injury to the capillary endothelium causes increased local permeability and adherence of the platelets to the exposed collagen fibrils in the vessel wall. The attached platelets then release adenosine diphosphate which causes the aggregation of further platelets to form a definite mass. After a time the platelets, first at the periphery and later throughout the aggregation, lose their structure and swell. This change, known as viscous metamorphosis, leads to permeation of the mass by fibrin and the formation of a more permanent thrombus.[49] When the damage is greater, and involves bleeding from arteries or veins, the haemorrhage is arrested partly by contraction of the muscle in the vessel wall and partly by activation of the clotting factors on the exposed injured surface, leading to local coagulation of the blood.

Avoidance of the no less serious condition of spontaneous thrombosis is accomplished by a balanced system of plasma factors that either promote or inhibit intravascular coagulation.[50, 51] These factors include the platelets, calcium (factor IV) and a series of protein substances. The protein factors are: fibrinogen (factor I); prothrombin (factor II); the labile factor (factor V); the stable factor (factor VII); antihaemophiliac globulin (factor VIII); Christmas factor (factor IX); Stuart–Prower factor (factor X); plasma thromboplastin antecedent (factor XI); Hageman factor (factor XII) and the fibrin-stabilizing factor (factor XIII). Factors III (thromboplastin) and VI have disappeared from the accepted hypothesis,[52] but the former is still used as a convenient concept.

In the process of clotting, the soluble fibrinogen is simplified to a monomer that subsequently polymerizes to relatively insoluble fibrin (Fig. 8.8). This forms a spongework of long, interlacing threads that enmesh red cells and later retract toward incorporated platelets, so drawing the surrounding structures together. The conversion of fibrinogen to fibrin takes only a few seconds, and is effected by the enzyme thrombin, but the entire process of clotting extends over nearly 10 minutes at body temperature: most of this time is taken up by the successive protein conversions that lead eventually to the formation of thrombin. These conversions have been described aptly as a cascade of proenzyme-enzyme transformations (Fig. 8.8).[52] The process starts when blood comes into contact with a surface other than normal endothelium, possibly with the slow transformation of a trivial amount of factor XII, although even in the absence of demonstrable amounts of this factor there may be no disorder of coagulation. The activated material then converts a rather larger amount of factor XI to its active state. Factor XII has a wide range of other biological activities, including activation of the fibrinolytic, complement and kinin systems. Activated factor XI converts factor IX to its active form by an enzymatic process involving calcium ions. Factor IX, with a molecular weight of about

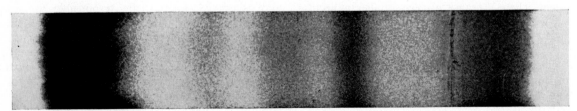

Fig. 8.7. Paper-strip electrophoresis of normal serum. The bands from left to right are: albumin; alpha$_1$-globulin; alpha$_2$-globulin; beta globulin; gamma globulin. The line of origin, where the serum was applied, lies between the beta and gamma globulin bands.

110 000, is relatively stable; it is synthetized in the liver, together with the other vitamin-K-dependent factors (factors II, VII and X). Factor VIII is a glycoprotein with a very high molecular weight (about 2 000 000). It appears to join with activated factor IX, calcium ions and platelet phospholipid to activate factor X. In an alternative pathway—the extrinsic or tissue pathway—activation of factor

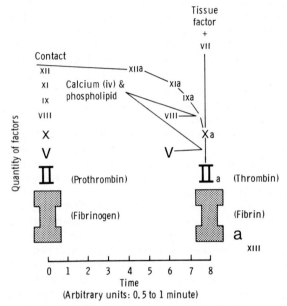

Fig. 8.8. The clotting mechanism. The units of time and quantity are arbitrary, and depend on variable physical conditions: their purpose is to indicate that during the clotting process the serial alteration of the plasma factors (left of diagram) to produce their active forms (indicated by the letter 'a') increases in speed (time curve) and quantity (progressively larger numerals) to culminate in the sudden conversion of a relatively large amount of fibrinogen to fibrin. The subsequent stabilization of the fibrin requires factor XIII. The activated form of factor V is doubtful. At the right of the diagram an alternative pathway is indicated: this pathway is initiated by a tissue factor, requires plasma factor VII, and obviates the initial stages of the main pathway (factors XII to VIII). It is this alternative pathway that is tested in measuring the 'prothrombin time'. Factors V and VIII do not appear to be directly in the pathway.

X occurs when extravasated blood comes into contact with tissue factor (a lipoprotein derived from the microsomal fraction of tissue cells). Factor VII probably acts as a catalyst in this reaction. The existence of such an alternative pathway explains why haemophiliac blood clots in the tissues in spite of the lack of factor VIII.

Activated factor X has the properties of a hydrolytic enzyme. On the platelet phospholipid micelles

it forms a complex with factor V, calcium and prothrombin and it cleaves the prothrombin molecule to form thrombin. Factors V and VIII are heat labile; they are entirely consumed during clotting. Their activity is enhanced by thrombin. The fibrinogen molecule, with a molecular weight of 330 000, has an elongated structure, composed of three pairs of polypeptide chains linked by disulphide bonds. Thrombin, which is a protease, removes the A and B terminal portions of the alpha and beta chains of fibrinogen by disrupting arginyl–glycine bonds. The resulting loss of negative charges allows polymerization, with the formation of insoluble fibrin threads that show ultramicroscopical cross striation. Through the action of factor XIII, a transamidating enzyme, the fibrin is stabilized to form the tough framework of the clot.

The formation of fibrin is not the end of the process, for after about 20 minutes the clot begins to retract and continues to do so during the next 24 hours, with the extrusion of clear, yellow fluid—the serum.[53] Platelets are an essential factor in the retraction of the clot and during this stage the prothrombin is used up. During clot formation the platelets that are dispersed throughout the fibrin network become linked together by pseudopodia; activation of their contractile protein, thrombasthenin, causes retraction of the clot.

Lack of any of these essential clotting factors may result in excessive bleeding after minor injuries (see pages 495–498). However, some factors cannot be reduced in vivo to a level sufficiently low to impede clotting: in the case of calcium, for instance, the effects of hypocalcaemia on the nervous system and on the heart would prove fatal before the concentration of calcium ions fell to a level at which the clotting mechanism would fail.

A series of naturally occurring inhibitors, complementary to the coagulation cascade, helps to localize fibrin formation to the site of injury. Some of these have been identified as inhibitors of the activated forms of factors II, X, XI and XII. There are at least six inhibitors of thrombin, including antithrombin III and α_2-macroglobulin. Antithrombin III is probably the co-factor that combines with heparin to block the action of thrombin on fibrinogen. Heparin can be extracted from the liver and is present in other organs and particularly in the granules of the basiphile leucocytes and of the tissue mast cells.[54] The lessened coagulability of the blood in anaphylaxis may be attributable to the release of heparin from these cells. Despite the inhibitors, small amounts of fibrin are formed from time to time. This fibrin, however, adsorbs plasminogen and its activator from the plasma. Protected from the antiplasmins of the plasma by adsorption, the plasminogen is converted to the proteolytic enzyme plasmin. This splits the fibrin into soluble fragments that are washed away in the circulation.[55]

DISORDERS OF THE BLOOD AND BONE MARROW

The blood and marrow are subject to a wide variety of disorders, both primary and secondary, and their classification necessarily presents numerous problems. For convenience they are considered here under the headings of disturbances in blood volume, disorders that affect the red cells, disorders that affect the white cells, disorders that affect the platelets, disorders of the coagulation mechanism, and disorders of the plasma proteins. It must be recognized that this classification involves considerable simplification, and that in practice more than one of these constituents of the blood may be affected at the same time.

DISTURBANCES OF BLOOD VOLUME

The commonest cause of a sudden change in blood volume is the fall that follows a sudden, severe haemorrhage, such as may accompany serious trauma or complicate chronic peptic ulceration, oesophageal varices or parturition. This is always a serious emergency and demands prompt treatment.

Haemorrhage

A small, sudden loss of blood is immediately followed by widespread, compensatory vasoconstriction, with the result that there is little or no fall in blood pressure. When the amount of blood lost is not great (up to half a litre), the volume is quickly restored, mainly through the withdrawal of tissue fluid from the extravascular space. The reserves of red cells in the marrow and spleen are mobilized and, with only slightly increased marrow activity, the volume and the composition of the blood are regained within a short time. When three quarters of a litre are lost suddenly, pallor and faintness develop;[56] with the rapid loss of larger volumes, the clinical signs are correspondingly severer. The loss of a litre and a half to two litres may cause death within a few hours; this outcome can often be averted by prompt and adequate transfusion of blood or even of physiological fluids.

The main sequels of sudden, severe haemorrhage are deficient cardiac filling, reduced cardiac output and a fall in systemic arterial blood pressure. This gives rise to giddiness and loss of consciousness through inadequacy of the cerebral circulation. The pulse is rapid and thready, respiration rapid and shallow, and the temperature soon becomes subnormal. The decrease in the circulation through the eyes causes blurring of vision and may even lead to permanent retinal damage. Later, the effects of renal ischaemia may supervene, with anuria leading to acute uraemia.

In cases of acute and severe haemorrhage, the danger lies in the sudden fall in the blood volume and not in the decrease in the oxygen-carrying capacity of the blood itself. Should death follow, it results from acute cerebral ischaemia due to the circulatory failure. After a single, non-fatal haemorrhage, the composition of the peripheral blood alters over a period of several hours as its volume is gradually restored by dilution with tissue fluid.[57] When this restoration is completed, the blood shows the simplest of all forms of anaemia—a normochromic, normocytic anaemia in which the haemoglobin concentration and the packed cell volume are equally lowered. The degree of anaemia does not provide an exact measure of the amount of blood lost, for certain changes other than dilution with tissue fluid may have taken place, including the mobilization of sequestered red cells; this possibly accounts for the leucocytosis that is often seen early in the post-haemorrhagic state. The effects of the hypoxia on the marrow soon begin to stimulate the multiplication of the cells of the erythropoietic series. As these cells proliferate and mature, the number of reticulocytes in the peripheral blood rises (Fig. 8.9N), to reach a peak after 7 to 10 days that is proportional to the amount of blood lost. This reticulocytosis is followed by a return of the count to the normal value of under one per cent when recovery is well established.

In young, healthy adults, the haemoglobin concentration of the blood will quickly recover, and even after severe haemorrhage will be normal in three to four weeks. In older people, or in patients who have lost their iron stores through earlier, small, intermittent haemorrhages or from long maintenance on a restricted diet, the recovery period may be more prolonged. Final restoration of all the blood constituents takes much longer; only when the immature red cells that were released prematurely into the circulation during the early stages of recovery are replaced at the end of their life span of several months does the peripheral blood again become normal as regards the size and haemoglobin content of its red cells. Restoration of the iron stores, depleted to form new haemoglobin, may take longer, perhaps even a year.

Dehydration and Acute Haemolysis

In some diseases in which vomiting and diarrhoea are severe, large amounts of water and electrolytes may be lost from the body very quickly, and even the large extravascular reserves of fluid in the cellular and tissue fluid compartments of the body may fail to maintain the normal blood volume. Acute enteritis in infants and cholera[58] in adults are two diseases in which grave dehydration is particularly likely to supervene. In cholera, the terminal collapse may be associated with the loss of a litre or more of fluid from the normal three litres of the plasma, and there is a corresponding increase in the number of the red cells per litre and in the viscosity of the blood.[58]

A sudden fall in the blood volume can also result when rapid haemolysis causes the destruction of a significant proportion of the red cells, which ordinarily occupy about two litres. There is only a slight diminution in blood volume in other forms of anaemia.

An increase in blood volume occurs physiologically in pregnancy and pathologically in polycythaemia.

DISORDERS THAT AFFECT THE RED CELLS

The disorders of red cells can be divided into two major groups—anaemia and polycythaemia. Of these, anaemia is much the commoner, and can arise from many causes.

Anaemia.—In some forms of anaemia the red cells are reduced in number but normal in their character —the immediate post-haemorrhagic state is the classic example (see above). In other forms, the cells may be both reduced in number and in some respect abnormal in structure (Fig. 8.9). There may be evidence that the anaemia arose from a disorder affecting the marrow: the cells then show such

abnormalities of appearance as *anisocytosis* (variation in size), *poikilocytosis* (variation in shape), *hypochromasia* (reduced haemoglobin content, with in extreme instances only a peripheral ring of staining), '*target cell*' *change* (hypochromic cells with a central as well as a marginal area of staining), *punctate basiphilia*, and the presence of inclusions, such as chromatin (*Howell–Jolly bodies*) and iron granules (in the so-called *siderocytes*).

In other instances the cells are formed normally and changes develop only after they enter the circulation. As the result of a latent defect in the structure of the envelope, or through damage to it by toxins or antibodies, the cells shrink and become rounded (*spherocytosis*); or, because of a change in the plasma the cells become enlarged and thinned ('target cell' change accompanying cholaemia), or develop irregular spiking of their surface ('*burr cells*' in uraemia), or undergo fragmentation in cases of intravascular coagulation (for instance, in the haemolytic-uraemic syndrome— see page 493). Finally, toxic denaturing of haemoglobin—particularly in cells already deficient in glucose-6-phosphate dehydrogenase, or having an unstable haemoglobin—can result in the formation of inclusion bodies (*Heinz bodies*) that stain supravitally with methyl violet.

In the marrow erythropoiesis may be interfered with in various ways. There may be a deficiency of some substance that is essential for the formation of haemoglobin or of deoxyribonucleic acid or for control of their synthesis (iron, vitamin B_{12}, folic acid, ascorbic acid, pyridoxine, erythropoietin and various hormones). An inherited fault may inhibit the development of a red cell enzyme system or lead to the production of a haemoglobin of abnormal structure and physical properties. Toxic substances or ionizing radiation may inhibit cell growth and multiplication. The haemopoietic tissue may be replaced in the course of extensive invasion of the marrow by metastatic tumour or through the proliferation of leukaemic or myelomatous cells; the same effect may be produced by overgrowth of the fibrous tissue of the marrow (*myelosclerosis*).

After entering the circulation normal red cells may be lost randomly through chronic bleeding or because of the destructive action of a toxic agent or of an antibody, or by overactivity of the cells of the reticuloendothelial system. Defective red cells may be destroyed prematurely in the course of normal wear and tear or because of abnormal sensitivity to certain chemicals.

This formidable array of potential causes has to be considered and evaluated in the investigation of

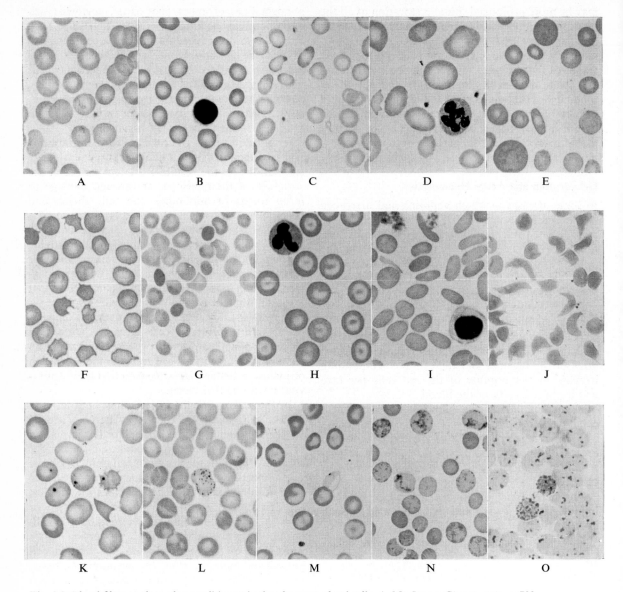

Fig. 8.9. Blood films to show abnormalities and other features of red cells. A–M: *Jenner–Giemsa stain*. × 700.

A. Normal red blood cells.
B. Normochromic microcytic red cells, and a lymphocyte.
C. Hypochromic microcytic red cells, with slight poikilocytosis.
D. Macrocytic red cells, and a 'senile' neutrophil.
E. Gross anisocytosis of red cells.
F. Burr cells.
G. Spherocytes—the small, darkly stained cells.
H. Target cells, and a neutrophil.
I. Elliptocytes (ovalocytes), and a lymphocyte.
J. Sickle cells.
K. Howell–Jolly bodies (nuclear chromatin) in red cells.
L. Punctate basiphilia.
M. A very thin red cell (leptocyte) with a Howell–Jolly body (target cell change in transfused cells).
N. Reticulocytes. *Nile blue sulphate*. × 700.
O. Heinz bodies in red cells. *Crystal violet*. × 700.

every case of anaemia (Fig. 8.10). The various forms of anaemia are considered below.

Polycythaemia.—In polycythaemia the number of circulating red cells is greatly increased. This may be the manifestation of a primary disorder of the marrow; oftener, it arises as an adaptation of the erythropoietic tissue to physiological or pathological hypoxia (see page 474).

The Deficiency Anaemias

Anaemia Due to Iron Deficiency

The commonest cause of an iron-deficiency anaemia is chronic haemorrhage, which may take the form of small, frequently recurring losses of blood—for instance, from excessive menstruation, peptic ulcers or haemorrhoids. In the tropics, chronic, debilitating blood loss is often due to infestation by blood-sucking intestinal parasites, of which the hookworms *Ancylostoma duodenale* and *Necator americanus* are the most widely distributed.

When small haemorrhages are repeated over a long time the stress falls on the iron stores of the body. For a time, cell production can proceed normally, or even at an increased rate; eventually, when the iron reserves are exhausted, the precursor cells cannot procure enough iron to saturate their cytoplasm with haemoglobin. In consequence, the red cells are small and thin, and stain palely; in the severest degrees of iron-deficiency anaemia they appear as mere rings, which are often distorted, forming poikilocytes (Figs 8.9C, 8.11A and B). To diagnose such an iron-deficiency anaemia it is helpful to calculate the mean cell haemoglobin (see page 431), for this indicates whether the cells are saturated with haemoglobin or not.

During the early stages of an anaemia due to chronic blood loss the marrow becomes hyperplastic. If the condition is balanced by an adequate iron intake, the haemopoietic tissues may extend along the medullary cavity of the long bones and replace a large part of the adipose tissue that normally is present there in adults. Since the precursors of the red cells are stimulated more than those of the white cells, the leucopoietic-erythropoietic ratio falls from its normal value of about four to one to nearly one to one. Nevertheless, the overproduction of red cells is accompanied by increased formation of white cells and platelets, which is reflected in leucocytosis and thrombocytosis in the peripheral blood. Should the iron stores become depleted, the production of red cells begins to fail. Yet, under these circumstances, the body is not wholly dependent upon its iron reserves (which in health suffice for the replacement of the haemoglobin contained in about two litres of blood), for as the reserves fall a larger fraction of the iron in

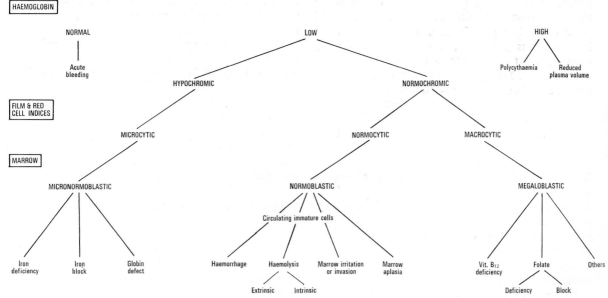

Fig. 8.10. Scheme for the diagnosis of disorders that affect the red cells. The steps that are indicated in the diagram illustrate the sequence that leads to diagnosis. They are not an absolute guide—for example, if there is a marked production of large, immature red cells following a haemorrhage, a macrocytic blood picture may be associated with a normoblastic marrow.

salt, usually accelerates recovery. The onset of improvement is heralded by a rise in the number of reticulocytes in the blood; later, the reappearance in the blood films of many normal cells, contrasting with the hypochromic cells, indicates that regeneration is proceeding vigorously (Fig. 8.11B).

Iron-Refractory Hypochromic Anaemia.—Rarely, hypochromic, microcytic anaemia proves to be refractory to iron administered by mouth.[60] An iron absorption test* and an examination of the bone marrow for iron (Fig. 8.15) will indicate whether the anaemia is due to failure of absorption or to failure of utilization of the iron administered. Many patients with the former defect also have difficulty in absorbing fats owing to changes in the mucosa of the jejunum. Extensive resection of the stomach can interfere with the absorption of iron. When the uptake of iron is found to be defective, or when severe gastrointestinal irritation makes administration of iron by mouth impossible, it may be necessary to give it parenterally.

Should the utilization of iron be defective, the cause of the deficient haemoglobin formation may be lack of an enzyme essential to the synthesis of haem: this is the case, for example, in *congenital sideroblastic anaemia*. Alternatively, there may be a fault in the synthesis of globin (see page 436). Such a defect underlies the red cell changes in the inherited condition of *thalassaemia*, found originally in people of Mediterranean origin (see page 469). The spectrum of the manifestations of thalassaemia extends from a trivial red cell defect to a grave form in which there are skeletal changes (resulting from marrow hyperplasia), splenomegaly, haemosiderosis and a rapidly fatal course, in spite of blood transfusions.

In other conditions, haem formation may be blocked by some metabolic disorder.[61] Such disorders are present in acquired sideroblastic anaemia, pyridoxine-responsive anaemia, lead poisoning, and various chronic disorders and 'toxic states', including uraemia and Hodgkin's disease. Sections or films of marrow, stained for iron, show that there is an excess of iron, stored in the macrophages, instead of a deficiency. The failure may lie in the transfer of iron from the macrophages to the developing red cells, but in some instances the blockage is within the normoblasts, and an accumu-

lation of iron-containing granules in the cytoplasm of these cells has earned them the name of *sideroblasts*.[62] In the ring variety of sideroblast the iron, located in the mitochondria, is grouped round the nucleus (Fig. 8.16). In these disorders the concentration of iron in the serum may be low, despite the large stores. More frequently, it is at the upper limit of normal. In contrast to the findings in cases of iron deficiency, the plasma transferrin is reduced in amount and nearly saturated,* and usually the amount of ferritin is raised.

Anaemias Due to Vitamin Deficiency

The introduction by Minot and Murphy,[63] in 1926, of a successful treatment for pernicious anaemia at once led to a much closer study of the biochemical aspects of erythropoiesis. It is now known that vitamin B_{12} and folic acid and, to a smaller extent, ascorbic acid are dietary constituents essential for normal haemopoiesis. All these substances are needed for the synthesis of deoxyribonucleic acid, any deficiency of which interferes with the development of the nucleus of the precursor cells in the marrow, and leads to a disparity between the evolution of the nucleus and that of the cytoplasm (see page 435). Consequently, the abnormal precursor cells—*megaloblasts*—differ from the normal proerythroblasts and early, intermediate and late normoblasts in that they are larger, have a looser nuclear chromatin and are prematurely haemoglobinized (see page 436 and Fig. 8.5C, page 437). Although the marrow proliferates actively in an apparent attempt to increase erythropoiesis, there is evidence that the maturation of the red cell series becomes arrested in its more primitive stages. The failure of the marrow to deliver red cells into the circulation gradually becomes more and more evident, until, in untreated cases, the haemoglobin falls to very low values (even below 2·5 g/dl) and signs of severe tissue hypoxia appear.

Anaemia Due to Deficiency of Vitamin B_{12}

This form of anaemia was first described by Combe,[64] in 1824, and then independently by Addison,[65] in 1849, and by Biermer,[66] in 1872. Addison's account brought the disease to the

---

* In this test, the serum iron is estimated before and two hours after the administration of a dose of about 100 mg of iron in the form of ferrous gluconate or ferrous fumarate by mouth. A rise to a level of over 18 μmol/l (100 μg/dl) should follow if the iron is absorbed.

* Transferrin is also nearly saturated, and the serum iron raised, during the development of haemochromatosis (see page 1270), a disorder in which the absorption of iron exceeds the losses. A similar condition ('siderosis') can be produced artificially by numerous transfusions, or by the parenteral administration of very large quantities of iron in the absence of blood loss.

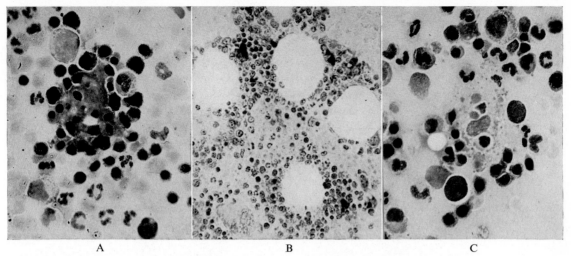

Fig. 8.15. Iron stores in the macrophages of the bone marrow. *Perls's reaction.*
A. A macrophage with ill-defined, iron-laden cytoplasm; round it a cluster of normoblasts. *Film preparation.* × 500.
B. A section of marrow with fat cells among the haemopoietic cells. The dark cellular masses, which were stained blue in the original preparation, are collections of iron-laden macrophages. × 100.
C. In the centre, a large macrophage with pale, irregular cytoplasm containing granules and cellular debris. It is partly surrounded by micronormoblasts. No iron was demonstrated in this cell. *Film preparation.* × 500.

general attention of doctors in Britain and elsewhere and it goes appropriately by his name. Because of its then invariably progressive course and fatal outcome, it became widely known as *pernicious anaemia.* The fact that the condition can now be treated successfully has taken the meaning from this ominous term.

Aetiology and Pathogenesis.—Although the essential nature of the pathogenesis of this type of anaemia is now known, the cause of the gastric atrophy that leads to the deficiency of vitamin B_{12} remains largely speculative. As it is not uncommon for more than one case to occur in a family, in the same and successive generations, it is possible that there may be an underlying genetical abnormality,[67, 68] possibly manifested through an autoimmune mechanism.[69] This view is supported by the fact that antibodies to gastric parietal cells are to be found in over 80 per cent of the cases;[70] antibodies to intrinsic factor (see below) are found in about 50 per cent.[71]

Vitamin B_{12} is a common constituent of human food, especially animal products. Only rarely does its concentration in the diet prove to be so low that anaemia results: this has been observed in a proportion of Vegans—vegetarians so strict that their diet contains no constituents whatever that are of animal origin. Usually, deficiency of vitamin B_{12} is attributable to a failure of absorption. Before absorption can take place, the vitamin has to be conjugated with a mucoprotein of small molecular size that normally is secreted by the stomach:[72] this mucoprotein has become known as the intrinsic factor of Castle,[73] in recognition of his discovery that pernicious anaemia results from its lack.

In adults with true pernicious anaemia the failure of secretion of the intrinsic factor is accompanied by complete achlorhydria. The defects of gastric secretion are associated with structural changes in the mucosa of the fundus of the stomach (see page 1023). It is not yet certain whether the extreme atrophy of this part of the gastric lining that is found in most fully developed cases (Fig. 8.17) precedes or follows the vitamin deficiency;[74] the fact that there is a pure defect in secretion of intrinsic factor in the very rare condition of pernicious anaemia of childhood suggests that the atrophy is secondary. The secretion of intrinsic factor may be diminished or abolished by extensive gastric resection, and more rarely by damage to the fundus by chemical substances or irradiation. As the daily requirement of vitamin B_{12} is only 1 to 2 μg, the fact that the amount of the vitamin stored in the body is ordinarily 3 mg or more means that two to three years pass in such cases before the store falls to the point at which anaemia develops.

Sometimes deficiency of vitamin B_{12} results from its destruction within the intestine. This can occur through some permanent alteration in the bacterial

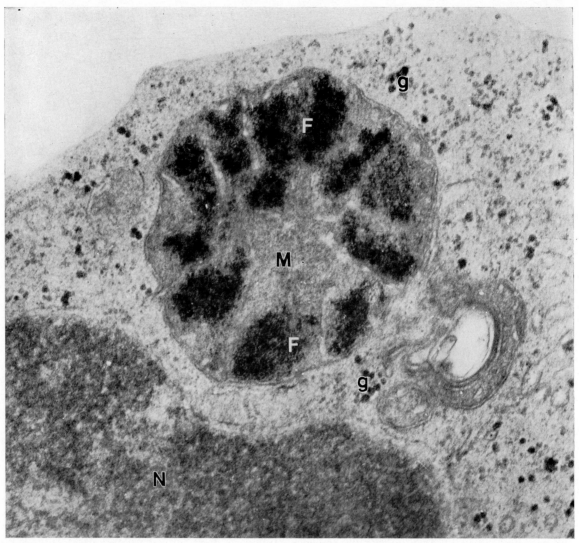

Fig. 8.16. Electron micrograph of a normoblast in a case of refractory sideroblastic anaemia. A mitochondrion (M) containing conspicuous intercristal deposits of iron (F) is seen adjacent to the nucleus of the cell (N). There are glycogen particles (g) in the cytoplasm. × 75 000.

flora of the small intestine, such as may accompany stenosis, diverticulosis or the presence of a blind loop of bowel following a surgical procedure. As vitamin B_{12} is absorbed from the ileum, extensive resection of this part of the bowel and Crohn's disease may lead to deficiency. In parts of the world where the fish tapeworm, *Diphyllobothrium latum*, is a frequent parasite of man—notably the Baltic states (particularly Finland), parts of Siberia and Japan—anaemia due to vitamin B_{12} deficiency may be a considerable clinical problem: the deficiency is due to the extent to which the worm

absorbs the vitamin from its host's intestinal contents.[75]

The Schilling test, in which a physiological dose of vitamin B_{12} in the form of a preparation labelled with radioactive cobalt ([58]Co or [57]Co) is given by mouth, has provided much information on the metabolism of this vitamin (see also page 459). After absorption, it is transported to the tissues where, in its active forms, it participates as a co-enzyme in the transfer of carbon in the synthesis of ribonucleic and deoxyribonucleic acids (see page 435).

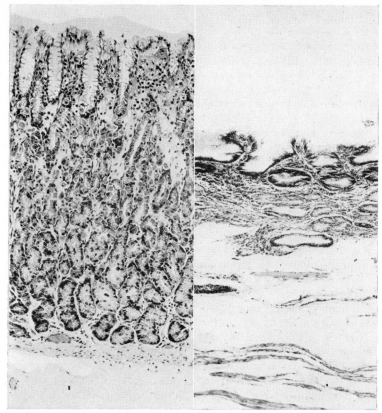

Fig. 8.17.§ The stomach wall in pernicious anaemia. Left, normal gastric mucosa for comparison with the pathological specimen. Right, atrophic gastric wall in pernicious anaemia, showing atrophy of both the mucosa and the muscularis. *Haematoxylin–eosin.* × 30.

Unlike folic acid, vitamin B$_{12}$ is essential for the maintenance of the motor and sensory pathways in the spinal cord (see Chapter 34).

Clinical Manifestations.—Pernicious anaemia is rare before the fifth decade, presumably in part because of the large stores of vitamin B$_{12}$. The patients tend to have blue eyes and prematurely grey hair, their skin may be mottled with patchy pigmentation and depigmentation (vitiligo), purpura may occur, morning diarrhoea may be troublesome, and some personality change is common. The symptoms of pallor, palpitation and lassitude are common to all forms of anaemia, but with vitamin B$_{12}$ deficiency three distinctive features, when present, direct attention to the correct diagnosis: lemon-yellow tinting of the skin; a red, smooth, painful tongue; and paraesthesiae in the legs. The paraesthesiae are due to subacute combined degeneration of the spinal cord (see Chapter 34); on occasion their appearance provides the earliest evidence of vitamin B$_{12}$ deficiency. In established cases of subacute combined degeneration of the cord, vibration sense is lost and, at first, there is some exaggeration of the tendon reflexes. Later, with progressive loss of muscle tone from interruption of the proprioceptive impulses, the reflexes disappear. The changes begin symmetrically in the lower parts of the legs and gradually ascend until the trunk is paralysed and numbed. If the condition has not advanced too far, the parenteral administration of vitamin B$_{12}$ leads to marked improvement, but the neurological signs and symptoms regress much more slowly than does the anaemia: neurological recovery takes up to two years, compared with two months for haematological recovery, and may never become complete.

Blood Picture.—Many of the haematological descriptions of pernicious anaemia date from the days before its effective treatment was known: they tend to present a picture of a degree of abnormality that is greatly exaggerated in comparison with that usually found nowadays, when the disease is generally arrested earlier. However, they do include details of the extraordinarily complete, if temporary, natural remissions that sometimes occurred.[76] In the disease as it is now seen the haemoglobin may be under 7·0 g/dl (48 per cent); the number of red cells is proportionately more reduced—sometimes to two million or less per microlitre. The cells are, on average, large (macrocytic—Fig. 8.9D), with a mean cell volume above 100 fl and mean cell haemoglobin above the normal range of 27 to 31 pg. In advanced, untreated cases, the red cells vary widely in size (anisocytosis—Fig. 8.9E) and shape (poikilocytosis)—oval forms are common (Fig. 8.11C). Occasionally megaloblasts (see page 436) appear in the peripheral blood. The abnormal red cells have a short life span; some never reach the circulation, being destroyed prematurely in the marrow ('ineffective erythropoiesis').[77] The excessive rate of destruction is responsible for the slight hyperbilirubinaemia and the distinctive lemon-yellow colour of the skin. When vitamin B_{12} is injected, large numbers of reticulocytes appear in the peripheral blood; the peak count is reached after about a week.

The leucocytes and the platelets are often reduced in number, and the presence of many-lobed neutrophils—a shift to the right in the Arneth count—indicates impairment of leucopoiesis. Sometimes the thrombocytopenia is sufficiently severe for purpura and retinal haemorrhages to result.

The diagnosis of pernicious anaemia may be suspected from the changes in the blood. Its confirmation largely rests on the marrow picture and on the occurrence of a reticulocyte crisis in response to specific treatment. The most typical feature on examination of films or biopsy sections of the bone marrow is the presence of megaloblasts, which may outnumber all the other haemopoietic cells together (Figs 8.5C and 8.18A). Leucopoiesis and platelet formation are also disturbed: giant metamyelocytes and multinucleate megakaryocytes are found.

The megaloblasts are strikingly affected by vitamin B_{12}: their number falls rapidly, and within hours of starting treatment they are changing to normal forms. Erythropoiesis is normal within two to three days of starting treatment. Provided that treatment is maintained for the rest of the patient's life, the macroscopical and microscopical appearances of the marrow remain normal.

The amount of vitamin B_{12} in biological fluids and in the tissues is normally very small. It can be measured by means of biological tests that depend on the fact that some micro-organisms, such as the green pond alga, *Euglena gracilis*, have an essential requirement of vitamin B_{12}. The normal range in serum is from 160 to 925 ng/l.

The demonstration of histamine-fast achlorhydria may be useful in the recognition of true pernicious anaemia. The critical test in distinguishing the classic disease from other causes of vitamin B_{12}

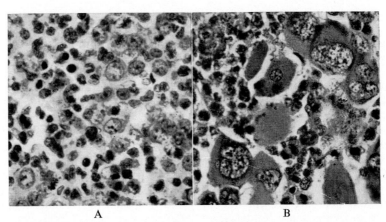

A   B

Fig. 8.18. Histological sections of grossly abnormal bone marrow. *Haematoxylin–eosin.* × 400.

A. The marrow in pernicious anaemia. The large, pale megaloblasts are conspicuous.
B. Increased numbers of immature megakaryocytes in idiopathic thrombocytopenic purpura.

deficiency is the Schilling test, with or without factorintrinsic .*

Post-Mortem Findings.—At necropsy, there may be widespread visceral changes. Many of the features that were usual in the advanced, untreated cases of former days are now rarely seen. Death is now almost always due to intercurrent causes. In untreated cases the most frequent changes, in addition to the characteristic atrophy of the gastric mucous membrane, were replacement of the fatty marrow by hyperplastic red marrow, and fatty change causing 'tigering' or 'tabby-cat striation' of the myocardium. The presence of large amounts of iron pigment in the liver, spleen and kidneys, and often in other organs, was well shown by the intense positive reaction that it gives with Perls's Prussian blue test.

In correctly treated cases, in which death has occurred from other causes, there are no specific changes except in the stomach. In cases of subacute combined degeneration of the spinal cord there is little macroscopical change in the cord, but histological examination shows degeneration of the posterior and pyramidal tracts (Fig. 8.19).

Anaemia Due to Deficiency of Folic Acid

A dietary deficiency in folic acid (pteroylglutamic acid) may cause a megaloblastic anaemia comparable to that brought about by a lack of vitamin B_{12}, except that subacute combined degeneration of the spinal cord does not occur. In countries with a good standard of living, dietary deficiency of folic acid affects mainly the elderly. However, it may occur as an important complication of pregnancy, in which a combination of insufficient diet, lack of appetite, and possibly some previously inapparent malabsorption, reduces the folic acid intake to below that needed to meet the combined demands of mother and fetus. The mother develops anaemia that for a time may be difficult to diagnose. Often the peripheral blood shows only a moderate degree of anisocytosis of the red cells and a tendency for

* In the Schilling test a physiological dose of vitamin B_{12}, labelled with radioactive cobalt, is given by mouth. Deficient absorption is revealed when less than 10 per cent of the dose is excreted in the urine in 24 hours. In a modification of the test, two doses of vitamin B_{12} are given simultaneously, one bound to intrinsic factor and the other free. The two doses are labelled with different isotopes (^{57}Co and ^{58}Co). If there is a failure of absorption due to lack of intrinsic factor, only the vitamin B_{12} that is administered bound to intrinsic factor will be absorbed and therefore appear in the urine. In cases of intestinal malabsorption neither dose of the vitamin is absorbed.

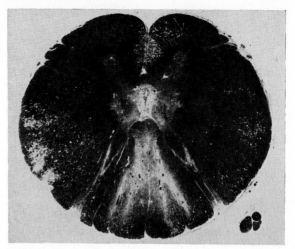

Fig. 8.19.§ The spinal cord in advanced subacute combined degeneration. Demyelination of the posterior and lateral columns is shown by the pale areas. *Weigert–Pal method for myelin.* × 4.

the neutrophils to have excessively lobed nuclei; it is only when the marrow is examined that the megaloblastic reaction is disclosed. The condition is soon reversed by the administration of folic acid; it can be prevented by the daily administration of some 300 μg of folic acid, which is usually given in combination with iron. Occasionally, there is a deficient intake of folic acid in infancy and in alcoholics.

Folic acid is absorbed from the jejunum along with iron, sugars and fats. Lack of folic acid may result from a failure in absorption; this is usually associated either with malabsorption of fat or with an abnormal intestinal flora in blind loops of bowel or above strictures of the small intestine. Rarely the deficiency is caused by the administration of drugs that chemically resemble folic acid sufficiently closely to be incorporated during synthesis of nucleic acid, with consequent blockage in its further development. These so-called folic acid antagonists include methotrexate, which is used in the treatment of acute leukaemia and of some other forms of cancer, particularly choriocarcinoma. The anticonvulsant drugs phenytoin and primidone, certain barbiturates, and such antimalarials as pyrimethamine, can also interfere with folic acid metabolism and cause a megaloblastic anaemia.

Folic acid deficiency differs from vitamin B_{12} deficiency in that the quantity of the former substance required for normal haemopoiesis is measured in milligrams rather than in micrograms, with the consequence that the amount normally stored in the body—about 5 mg—is exhausted quickly. After absorption, folic acid is converted to its active derivative, folinic acid, through a reaction stabilized by ascorbic acid. Folic acid derivatives are necessary, along with vitamin B_{12}, for the synthesis of the nucleic acids (see page 436). They are not involved in the metabolism of the nervous system; however, administration of folic acid to patients with pernicious anaemia, instead of vitamin B_{12}, may precipitate the development of subacute combined degeneration of the spinal cord.

The folic acid in the serum can be assayed, as folate, using the organism *Lactobacillus casei*. The normal range varies according to the methods of estimation used: it is usually accepted that a concentration of less than 3 μg/l is low, that from 3 to 5 μg/l is equivocal, and that the normal level is above 5 μg/l. The upper limit of the normal range differs considerably from laboratory to laboratory but usually is at some point between 7 and about 30 μg/l. Folic acid derivatives are necessary for histidine metabolism: a deficiency blocks this process at the intermediate stage of formation of forminoglutamic acid ('FIGLU'), which is then excreted in the urine. This forms the basis of a test for folic acid deficiency; its results are not specific.

Anaemia Due to Deficiency of Ascorbic Acid

Lack of ascorbic acid (vitamin C), although a cause of macrocytic anaemia in monkeys, rarely, if ever, produces megaloblastic anaemia in man. The mechanism seems to be closely concerned with folic acid metabolism.

Anaemias Due to Other Deficiencies

Although some trace metals, notably cobalt, copper, manganese and zinc, are needed for certain enzyme systems, and their absence from the diet in animals may result in anaemia, all human diets contain them in amounts sufficient to supply the needs of the body. There is no evidence that disorders of haemopoiesis can be ascribed to lack of any of them.

Even when man has to subsist on a diet that is poorly balanced, the protein intake usually suffices for haemopoiesis: any accompanying anaemia is likely to have a complex origin in which infections and infestations may play a part. However, alterations in the pattern of the plasma proteins, such as that present in chronic rheumatoid arthritis, may contribute to the development of a severe refractory type of anaemia in which iron is not re-utilized.

Certain diseases of the liver, notably obstructive

jaundice, tend to be accompanied by the formation of red cells with a central thickening, known as 'target cells' (Fig. 8.9H, page 450). This alteration in the appearance of the cells occurs after they have entered the circulation: cells transfused from normal people may become similarly affected. It may be noted that similar appearances are seen in the red cells in cases of thalassaemia and of some of the other haemoglobinopathies (see page 469).

Anaemia accompanies some diseases of the endocrine glands, notably myxoedema,[78] Addison's disease, and Simmonds's disease.[77]

Anaemia Due to Primary and Secondary Hypoplasia of the Bone Marrow

Primary Hypoplasia

In certain conditions, the marrow fails to produce sufficient red cells to replace those lost through normal ageing, and a normocytic normochromic anaemia develops that may be so severe that repeated transfusions are needed to keep the patient alive. In many cases, the granular leucocytes and the platelets are also involved (*pancytopenia*) and the diagnosis of *aplastic anaemia* can be made.

The condition may be irreversible and can result from an inherited defect or from damage by a toxic agent or by ionizing radiation (Fig. 8.20B).

The inherited form of hypoplasia, which is conveyed by a recessive gene, is sometimes accompanied by defects in other organs; most of these are associated with abnormalities in the excretion of amino acids and electrolytes by the kidneys (the Fanconi syndrome—see Chapter 24).[79]

The acquired forms of hypoplasia are commoner. They may follow exposure to industrial and domestic poisons, among which are benzene and some of its derivatives, some heavy metals, the antibiotics chloramphenicol and streptomycin, certain insecticides, and the hair-dye, paraphenylenediamine. Ionizing radiation, either X-rays or from bone-seeking radioactive isotopes (phosphorus, ^{32}P; calcium, [45]Ca; strontium, ^{89}Sr), is particularly damaging to the marrow (radioactive phosphorus has been used deliberately to destroy abnormal cells in polycythaemia and in leukaemia). Inhibition of marrow activity, even amounting to hypoplasia, can be caused by uraemia. Although usually due to chronic renal disease and, therefore, irreversible, the uraemic state may follow urinary obstruction and it may then be cured by relief of the cause, for example by prostatectomy. Long-

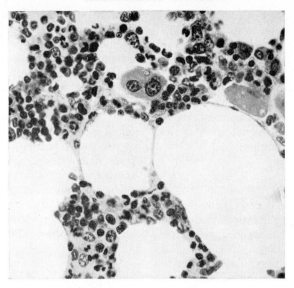

A. Normal marrow, to show the relative proportions of haemopoietic cells and fat cells. Leucopoietic and erythropoietic cells can be distinguished; there is a conspicuous megakaryocyte.

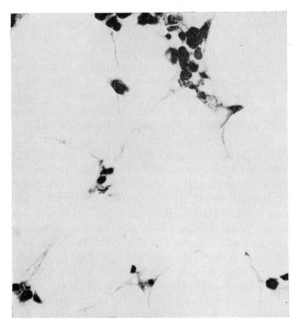

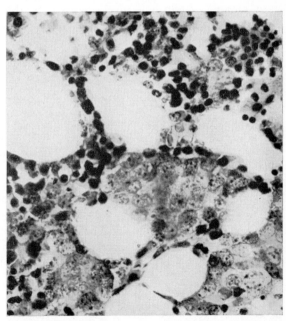

B. Severe hypoplasia of the marrow.

C. Invasion of the marrow by a carcinoma. The tumour cells in this case are larger and paler than the marrow elements.

Fig. 8.20. Destruction of bone marrow (histological sections). *Haematoxylin–eosin.* × 250.

standing iron deficiency also causes hypoplasia of the marrow, which, when the cause is treated, is reversible. Often, however, there is no demonstrable cause for the hypoplasia: recovery in these 'idiopathic' cases is rare. Occasionally, hypoplasia of the marrow precedes the development of paroxysmal nocturnal haemoglobinuria or of leukaemia. The demonstration of a chromosomal abnormality (see page 479) may be helpful in the detection of cases in which leukaemia might develop.

Secondary Hypoplasia

Secondary hypoplasia of the haemopoietic elements is a complication of the proliferation of abnormal cells in the marrow, as in leukaemia, myelomatosis and metastatic carcinoma (Figs 8.20C and 8.21). Under these circumstances many immature cells— myelocytes and normoblasts—appear in the peripheral blood: the picture is therefore described as *leucoerythroblastic anaemia*.

Myelosclerosis (Myelofibrosis)

A similar leucoerythroblastic blood picture is found in a number of other disorders of the marrow, the most notable of which is myelosclerosis. In this condition, the marrow is ultimately replaced

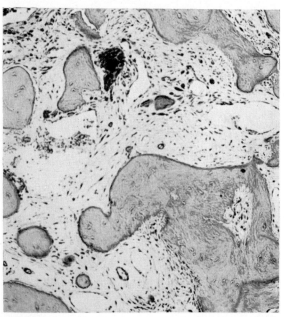

Fig. 8.21. Destruction of bone marrow by carcinoma. There is extensive invasion of the marrow by scirrhous carcinoma; the primary growth was in a breast. *Haematoxylin–eosin.* × 100.

entirely by fibrous tissue containing distorted megakaryocytes (Fig. 8.22). Normal medullary haemopoiesis is suppressed, but blood formation continues in the massively enlarged spleen. The reticuloendothelial cells of the spleen proliferate, and phagocytosis of the red cells that stagnate in the distended sinusoids is a prominent feature. In some cases, anaemia dominates the clinical picture; a diminution in the number of platelets (thrombocytopenia) and extensive bruising may herald death from haemorrhage. The presence of many pear-shaped red cells in the peripheral blood may suggest the possibility of myelosclerosis. A number of variants of this condition are known but all ultimately lead to fibrosis. The cause is unknown and the condition is fatal.

Other Causes of Leucoerythroblastic Changes

Leucoerythroblastic changes may be seen also in hypoxic states, severe anaemia (especially in childhood), acute pneumonia, polycythaemia and cyanotic congenital heart disease.

Anaemia Due to Excessive Haemolysis[80]

It is characteristic of the many different forms of haemolytic anaemia that the red cells are either lysed while still in the circulation or destroyed prematurely by the cells of the reticuloendothelial system. Iron deficiency is not usually a feature of the haemolytic anaemias, because the iron liberated from the lysed cells is not lost to the body unless the concentration of haemoglobin in the plasma rises so high that haemoglobinuria develops.

There are many causes of haemolysis (see Table 8.8). For the most part they may be classified into three main categories: haemolysis due to the action on normal red cells of some haemolytic chemical or biological agent; haemolysis due to specific antibody action; and haemolysis due to an intrinsic defect of the red cells that leads to their premature destruction. Many of the abnormalities in the third of these groups are inherited: in some of these— for example, certain defects of the enzyme glucose-6-phosphate dehydrogenase—the cells are abnormally susceptible to damage by exogenous agents.

Much information about the haemolytic processes has been obtained by labelling red cells with radioactive isotopes,[81] particularly ^{51}Cr, ^{59}Fe and ^{14}C. By determining the radioactivity of a series of daily or weekly samples, the life span of the red cells can be ascertained. Further, by the application of surface counters to various parts of

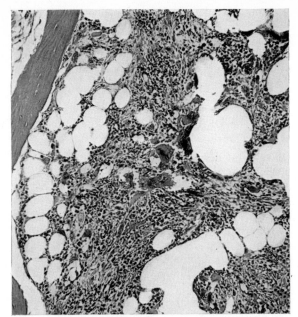

Fig. 8.22. Destruction of the bone marrow in myelosclerosis. Part of the marrow has been replaced by cellular fibrous tissue, leaving only a few haemopoietic cells, among them megakaryocytes. *Haematoxylin–eosin.* × 100.

Table 8.8. *Classification of the Causes of Haemolytic Disorders*

A. Chemical, Physical and Biological Agents
  1. Toxic chemicals and drugs—for example, lipid solvents, phenylhydrazine, phenacetin, sulpha-salazine, dapsone
  2. Physical agents:
    burns
    synthetic grafts replacing arteries
    march haemoglobinuria
    microangiopathic haemolytic anaemia (thrombotic thrombocytopenic purpura and haemolytic-uraemic syndrome)
  3. Bacterial toxins
  4. Protozoal, bacterial and other parasitic infections of the red cells
  5. Haemolysis secondary to malignant tumours, chronic infections, renal disease, rheumatic disorders, and splenomegaly
  6. Lipoprotein deficiencies

B. Antibodies
  1. Isoantibodies:
    haemolytic disease of the newborn (erythroblastosis fetalis)
    reaction to transfused antibodies
  2. Autoantibodies:
    Warm antibodies—
     idiopathic
     drug-induced—for example, caused by methyldopa, penicillin
     secondary to other diseases—for example, leuk-aemia, systemic lupus erythematosus, ulcerative colitis
    Cold antibodies—
     idiopathic
     secondary to infection—for example, glandular fever (anti-i antibody), mycoplasma pneumonia (anti-I antibody)
     secondary to lymphosarcoma or lymphocytic leukaemia
     paroxysmal cold haemoglobinuria (anti-P antibody)

C. Defective Red Cells
  1. Paroxysmal nocturnal haemoglobinuria
  2. Hereditary spherocytosis
  3. Hereditary elliptocytosis
  4. Inherited enzyme abnormalities:
    defects in the pentose-phosphate pathway
    defects in the Embden–Meyerhof pathway
  5. Haemoglobinopathies:
    molecular abnormalities of globin polypeptides
    thalassaemias
  6. Erythropoietic porphyria

the body, the distribution of isotopes producing gamma rays can be traced. These techniques have made it possible to determine the time needed for the formation of red cells in the marrow and to locate the sites of their destruction.

Haemoglobinuria.—When intravascular haemolysis occurs, haemoglobin will appear in the urine if more than about 3 g of haemoglobin (roughly the amount in 20 ml of normal blood) are released rapidly: this amount saturates the haemoglobin-binding capacity of the haptoglobins and any excess of haemoglobin appears in the urine.

A. Haemolysis Due to Chemical, Physical and Biological Agents

Chemical Causes

Many of the agents in this group are frankly haemolytic *in vitro* as well as *in vivo*. They include volatile lipid solvents, such as benzene, and some toxic substances, such as phenylhydrazine, that cause haemolysis when absorbed in sufficient quantity. In cases of anaemia due to the direct action of drugs and other chemicals, the red cells often appear irregularly contracted or fragmented; when the cells are stained supravitally with basic dyes

they may show the presence of Heinz bodies (Fig. 8.9, part O, page 450), which are inclusions of denatured globin.*

---

* Heinz bodies should not be confused with Howell–Jolly bodies (Fig. 8.9K, page 450), which are nuclear fragments, or with the iron-containing Pappenheimer bodies that are found in 'siderocytes' (see page 449).

Physical Causes

It has been suggested that the fragmentation of the red cells that is a feature of microangiopathic haemolytic anaemias results from their passage through small blood vessels that are partially obstructed by fibrin strands or microthrombi (see page 493).[82] Red cells circulating through the dilated vessels of the soles of the feet may be damaged by prolonged tramping or running on hard surfaces, causing *march haemoglobinuria*.[83] Damage to the red cells as they circulate past artificial cardiac valves or through grafts of synthetic materials replacing arteries sometimes results in haemolytic anaemia. Damage to the red cells in vessels in the immediate vicinity of severe burns is another physical cause of haemolysis; toxic products of the burnt tissues may be a factor in these cases.[84]

Biological Agents

Among the biological agents that may cause haemolysis, malarial parasites and the toxins of some clostridia and of *Streptococcus pyogenes* are especially important. The list of such lysins is long, and includes such diverse agents as snake venoms and toxic products released by neoplasms or accumulating in renal disease. The degree of the haemolysis depends mainly on the quantity of the lytic agent that reaches the blood. The haemolytic reaction may be acute or chronic, and sometimes the same agent may be responsible at different times for both acute and chronic haemolysis.

Lipoprotein Deficiency.—Acanthocytosis, which is a peculiar spiky distortion of the red cells, and mild haemolysis are features of *familial abetalipoproteinaemia*, a rare disorder that is inherited as an autosomal recessive defect.[85] Familial *alphalipoprotein deficiency* (Tangier disease) is characterized by the formation of target cells (see page 449), mild haemolysis and a moderate anaemia.[86]

B. Haemolysis Due to Antibodies

Many of the antibodies that are capable of lysing red cells are group-specific. Some, such as those of the ABO blood group system, can effect haemolysis *in vitro*, the sensitized cells being haemolysed through the action of complement. Others, among them the rhesus antibodies, merely cause agglutination of the cells *in vitro*, or do no more than sensitize them ('incomplete antibodies'), although they are haemolytic *in vivo*. When a transfusion reaction takes place, it is usually the wrongly matched donor cells that are destroyed; only rarely is an antibody in the transfused blood of sufficient strength, after dilution and partial neutralization by circulating antigen, to haemolyse the recipient's cells (see page 441).[87]

Haemolytic Disease of the Newborn (Erythroblastosis Fetalis)

Haemolytic disease of the newborn is a special instance of haemolysis due to the operation of an antibody.[88] The condition may occur when a mother's blood contains an antibody that can cross the placental barrier, react with a blood group antigen on her child's red cells, and thereby initiate their destruction. Haemolysis continues after the birth of the child while the maternal antibody persists in its circulation. The incompatible antigen is inherited from the father, and affected infants are therefore heterozygous. Haemolytic disease of the newborn has been recognized in association with a number of blood group systems, but it is the variety caused by rhesus incompatibility that is of the most practical importance (see Table 8.5, page 443). Antibodies may appear in the blood of a rhesus-D-negative woman as a result of immunization by rhesus-D-positive fetal cells, which enter her circulation during pregnancy and labour. Because the main stimulus to the formation of anti-D antibody occurs at or soon after delivery, the first rhesus-D-positive child is usually unaffected. Thereafter, antibodies form more readily in subsequent pregnancies and are liable to cause fetal haemolytic disease. Occasionally, the initial stimulus for antibody formation is blood transfusion. During pregnancy, the presence of antibodies in the serum of a woman who is likely to give birth to an affected baby may be demonstrated by appropriate serological techniques. The acid elution method for the cytochemical demonstration of cells that contain fetal haemoglobin has been extensively employed to show the presence of fetal erythrocytes in the maternal circulation[89] and to assess their number.

Complete agglutinating antibodies of the IgM class appear not to pass across the placenta. The antibodies that cause haemolytic disease of the newborn are for the most part of the IgG class and react *in vitro* as typical incomplete antibodies. They are of comparatively small molecular size, and, if a sufficient titre is reached, enough pass back across the placenta to cause a severe haemolytic reaction in the fetus. Before birth, the breakdown products of the affected red cells return to the maternal circulation; a compensatory increase in erythropoiesis in the fetus helps maintain the haemoglobin level. At birth, the anaemia is characterized by the presence of many nucleate red cells in the peripheral blood ('erythroblastosis') and by the fact that the cells are sensitized by the antibody and—apart from some instances associated with ABO system antibodies—give a positive direct antiglobulin reaction (see page 444). In severe cases, a marked degree of anaemia develops; this may be accompanied by widespread oedema (hydrops fetalis), and the fetus may die in utero. If born alive, the infant, whose hepatic function is not fully developed, has difficulty in disposing of the breakdown products of haemoglobin. The ability to form water-soluble conjugates with aldobiuronic acid or related compounds[90] is insufficient: consequently, unconjugated bilirubin accumulates in the plasma and in the tissues instead of being excreted in the bile. The depth of jaundice indicates the severity of the haemolysis. Death may occur within a day or two of birth; in less severe cases the disorder is self-limiting and recovery follows, because the cessation of the placental circulation at birth removes the maternal source of the antibody. Nevertheless, if the jaundice is severe (serum bilirubin above 340 μmol/l) the prolonged presence of excess bile pigment in the blood leads to the development of Kernikterus (see Chapter 34).[91] Hypoxia due to anaemia increases the risk of cerebral damage. Treatment by exchange transfusion, using donor blood that will not react with the maternal antibody, greatly reduces the amount of haemolysis. This procedure, which removes the circulating antibody, sensitized red cells and bilirubin, decreases the likelihood of permanent injury to the brain.

The occurrence of haemolytic disease of the newborn due to anti-D antibody can be prevented by passive immunization of the rhesus-D-negative woman who has given birth to a rhesus-D-positive baby. Immediately after the delivery, the mother is given an intramuscular injection of anti-D immunoglobulin to prevent her from forming her own antibodies to any fetal cells that have entered her circulation.[92] This procedure is of value only if the mother has not already been immunized as the outcome of a previous pregnancy or by transfusion.

Acquired Autoimmune Haemolysis

Autoantibodies may form in the body and attack the individual's own red cells. This may arise as a primary condition, or it may complicate other diseases, including systemic lupus erythematosus (Fig. 8.4D) and, especially, chronic lymphocytic leukaemia (see page 487). The sensitization of the red cells can be demonstrated by appropriate methods, particularly by a direct anti-human-globulin test (the Coombs test—see footnote on page 444). In many instances, the autoimmune antibodies that coat the cells and give rise to a positive direct antiglobulin reaction are of a 'warm' type (that is, they are most active at 37°C) and are immunoglobulins of the IgG class (see page 445). Often such antibodies are group specific, especially against the antigens of the rhesus system. The haemolytic anaemia caused by 'warm' antibodies usually runs a chronic course, but there may be acute haemolytic episodes with accompanying haemoglobinuria.

In vitro, some autoantibodies are active mainly at or below room temperature; others cause agglutination over a wide thermal range. Such complete antibodies may be present in high titre; they are usually of the IgM class. They are sometimes associated with cryoglobulin fractions in the serum, and occasionally with the occurrence of Raynaud's syndrome. Those that are haemolytic in vivo bind complement to the red cells; they frequently show blood group specificity within the Ii system. The presence of such antibodies may indicate the underlying presence of a lymphosarcoma or of leukaemia.

Mycoplasma pneumonia is sometimes associated with the formation of an auto-anti-I cold agglutinin. Infection with the Epstein–Barr virus may stimulate the production of an anti-i antibody (anti-i is always an autoantibody). In rare instances these antibodies cause haemolytic anaemia. Occasionally, other viruses provoke the formation of similar autoantibodies.

Paroxysmal Cold Haemoglobinuria.—Paroxysmal cold haemoglobinuria is another disorder due to the formation of an autoantibody. It is often associated with a positive Wassermann reaction, but this is usually non-specific and not due to syphilis. In this condition, the antibody becomes attached to the red cells when they are at a relatively low temperature, as while they circulate through the distal parts of the limbs when these are chilled. Complement is also bound to the red cells: when, in the course of circulation, they are again warmed to normal body temperature, lysis takes place and liberated haemoglobin is passed in the urine (see page 463). Episodic haemoglobinuria after exposure to cold (the Donath–Landsteiner reaction) is characteristic of the disease. The autoantibodies react with the P antigen of normal red cells (see page 444).

C. Haemolysis Due to Defective Red Cells

Haemolysis may result from abnormalities of the structure and composition of the red cells. The mechanisms involved are not fully understood in all instances.

Paroxysmal Nocturnal Haemoglobinuria
(Marchiafava–Micheli Syndrome)[92a, 92b]

The red cells in cases of paroxysmal nocturnal haemoglobinuria are abnormally sensitive to the lytic action of activated complement. Ham's test, which is specific for the condition, depends on the fact that the abnormal cells are lysed by complement that has been activated by acidification.[92c] The level of acetylcholinesterase activity in the red cells is less than normal.[93] The cells may also be unduly susceptible to lysis by hydrogen peroxide. These findings may be the results of an underlying defect in the composition of the cell membrane.

The haemoglobinuria is not necessarily nocturnal. Why some of the patients are peculiarly liable to haemolysis at night is not known. The intravascular lysis of the red cells is probably mediated by complement in conjunction with properdin and ions of magnesium. More haemoglobin is liberated than can be bound by plasma haptoglobins: the excess escapes into the urine (see page 463). Methaemalbumin is also formed.

In some cases the disorder follows, or is associated with, hypoplasia of the marrow (see page 462): a relation to the myeloproliferative diseases has been suggested.[94]

Thrombosis of small blood vessels and the development of infarcts in the viscera are features of paroxysmal nocturnal haemoglobinuria. They probably account for many of the episodes of severe abdominal pain that are common in this disease.

Hereditary Spherocytosis

The most important of the anaemias that are due to defective structure of the red cells is the condition now called hereditary spherocytosis. Formerly it was known as acholuric jaundice, because the unconjugated bilirubin derived from lysis of red cells is bound to albumin and therefore not excreted by the kidneys. Only the colourless derivative, urobilinogen, escapes into the urine.

The red cells in this disease are excessively permeable to sodium ions and have to maintain a very high rate of glycolysis in order to provide enough energy to keep the 'sodium pump' fully active in expelling sodium from the cell. The condition is inherited as an autosomal dominant characteristic. The nature of the primary abnormality that causes the biochemical and morphological changes is unknown. Many of the red cells in the peripheral blood are small, darkly staining spherocytes (Fig. 8.9G, page 450). Compared to the normal biconcave red cell these spheroidal cells have a reduced ratio of surface area to volume. The osmotic fragility of the cells is abnormal:* this is a characteristic of spherocytes irrespective of the cause of the spherocytosis. The fragility test may be useful in the recognition of mild cases of hereditary spherocytosis when the appearances in blood films are indecisive: however, in such cases the changes in fragility tend to be minor and the test must be particularly precisely carried out.

Large numbers of prematurely senescent red cells are removed from the circulation by the reticuloendothelial cells, particularly in the spleen: this leads to splenomegaly. To compensate for the excessive destruction of the abnormal cells, the marrow proliferates and extends far along the shaft of the long bones of the limbs (Fig. 8.23A). Histological examination of the marrow shows that the fat cells are almost wholly replaced by erythropoietic elements; most of these are normoblasts (Fig. 8.36A, page 489). The reticulocyte count ranges from 5 per cent in the mildest cases to over 30 per cent in severe cases.

Because of the excessive haemolysis, increased amounts of iron are present throughout the reticuloendothelial system and in the parenchymatous cells of the liver and kidneys. This excess is readily demonstrated by Perls's Prussian blue test, which may be applied grossly to the organs during necropsy and to histological sections.

The correspondingly excessive production of bile pigments by the liver often results in the formation of pigment stones in the gall bladder (see page 1311). In a few cases gall stone colic is the first clinical manifestation of hereditary spherocytosis. The

---

* The osmotic fragility test is performed by exposing the red cells to a series of saline solutions ranging in concentration from 0·72 to 0·28 per cent. Normally, haemolysis begins in about 0·48 per cent saline and is complete at 0·28 per cent. In cases of hereditary spherocytosis it may begin in 0·68 per cent or even higher concentrations of saline; it tends to be incomplete in 0·28 per cent saline because there is a high proportion of young, and therefore more resistant, cells in the blood.

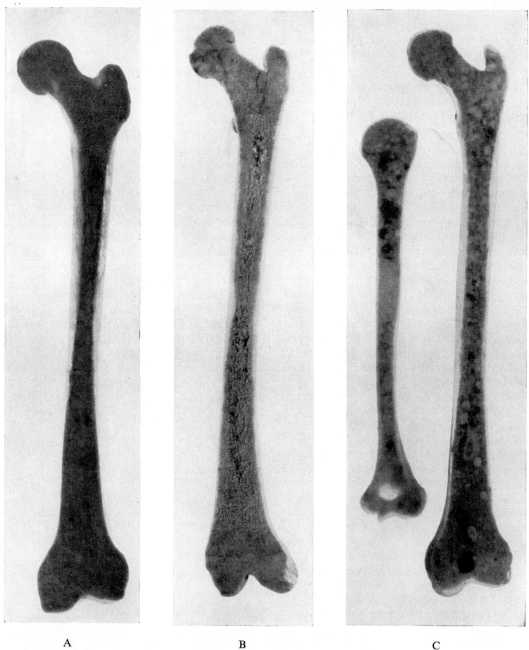

A   B   C

Fig. 8.23. Changes in the long bones in haematological disorders.
A. Extension of erythropoietic tissue throughout the shaft of a femur in a case of hereditary spherocytosis.
B. Diffuse infiltration of the marrow cavity by neoplastic neutrophil precursors in chronic myeloid leukaemia.
C. Multiple myelomatous foci in the shaft of a humerus and femur.

stones may be present from a comparatively early age; their long persistence appears to predispose to carcinomatous change in the mucosa of the gall bladder in some cases (see page 1314).

Elliptocytosis (Ovalocytosis)
The name of this uncommon inherited anomaly of the red cells indicates the distinctive shape of the affected cells (Fig. 8.9I, page 450). In a small

proportion of cases the cells may be fragile: excessive haemolysis may then result, but only rarely is it sufficient to cause anaemia.

Elliptocytosis is genetically linked to the rhesus blood group.[95]

Inherited Enzyme Abnormalities (Familial Non-Spherocytic Haemolytic Anaemias)

Glucose-6-Phosphate Dehydrogenase Deficiency.— Glucose-6-phosphate dehydrogenase (G6PD) is a key enzyme of the hexose-monophosphate shunt. Metabolism of glucose by this pathway is important for the formation of reduced nicotinamide adenine dinucleotide phosphate, which in turn maintains the glutathione in the red cells in the reduced state. Reduced glutathione appears to protect the sulphydryl groups of haemoglobin and of membrane components from oxidation.

The commonest metabolic defect of red cells is an abnormality of G6PD that is inherited as a sex-linked characteristic. Over 75 molecular variants are known: not all of them cause clinical disease. The chief manifestation of abnormality is sensitivity to haemolysis by drugs and other substances.[96] In Caucasoids, particularly Italians, the variant known as G6PD Mediterranean is responsible for the syndrome of *favism*, in which the red cells are lysed following the ingestion of an unidentified substance present in the broad bean, *Vicia fava*.

Episodes of haemolysis in cases of G6PD deficiency may occur spontaneously or as a complication of intercurrent infections, or be provoked by drugs, such as sulphonamides. For instance, the 'A-type' of G6PD deficiency, which is commonly found in people of African origin, predisposes to haemolysis induced by drugs, particularly antimalarials and especially primaquine. Neonatal jaundice is sometimes attributed to G6PD deficiency; this has been observed most frequently in the Chinese and the enzyme variant usually involved is known as G6PD Canton.[97]

Pyruvate Kinase Deficiency.[98]—Pyruvate kinase catalyses a step in the Embden–Meyerhof pathway (see page 436)—the conversion of phosphoenolpyruvate to pyruvate, with the formation of adenosine triphosphate from adenosine diphosphate. Compared with G6PD deficiency, pyruvate kinase deficiency is rare. It may present with neonatal jaundice, anaemia or splenomegaly. It is inherited as an autosomal recessive trait.

Other Deficiencies.[99]—Haemolytic anaemia may be associated with some very rare abnormalities of other enzymes involved in the glycolytic pathways.

Haemoglobinopathies (Hereditary Abnormalities of Haemoglobin Constitution)

In adult haemoglobin (haemoglobin A, Hb A) the globin is composed of two pairs of polypeptide chains that differ in their amino acid sequences. These are described as alpha and beta chains: the formula of adult haemoglobin can therefore be designated $\alpha_2\beta_2$. Instead of a pair of beta chains, fetal haemoglobin (haemoglobin F, Hb F) and haemoglobin A_2 (Hb A_2) have, respectively, a pair of gamma polypeptide chains and a pair of delta polypeptide chains in their molecule. The gamma and delta polypeptides also have their own characteristic amino acid sequences. The formation of the polypeptides is determined by corresponding alpha, beta, gamma and delta genes. The loci of the beta and gamma chains are closely linked; they are separate from the alpha chain locus. In man there appear to be at least two, and probably more, gamma chain loci on each member of a pair of chromosomes.[100] It is possible that the alpha chain locus is also duplicated;[101] the beta chains probably have a single locus (see Table 8.9).

Table 8.9. *Structural Features of Some Varieties of Haemoglobin*

Haemoglobin	General formula; position and type of amino acid abnormality
Normal varieties:	
A	$\alpha_2\beta_2$
F	$\alpha_2\gamma_2$
A_2	$\alpha_2\delta_2$
Lacking alpha chains:	
H	β_4
Barts	γ_4
Abnormal alpha chains:	
I	$\alpha_2^{16\ \text{lysine}\rightarrow\text{glutamine}}\beta_2$
Constant Spring	$\alpha_2^{\text{additional amino acids}}\beta_2$
Abnormal beta chains:	
S	$\alpha_2\beta_2^{6\ \text{glutamic acid}\rightarrow\text{valine}}$
C	$\alpha_2\beta_2^{6\ \text{glutamic acid}\rightarrow\text{lysine}}$
D Punjab	$\alpha_2\beta_2^{121\ \text{glutamic acid}\rightarrow\text{glutamine}}$
E	$\alpha_2\beta_2^{26\ \text{glutamic acid}\rightarrow\text{lysine}}$
Abnormal gamma chains	
Hb F Hull	$\alpha_2\gamma_2^{121\ \text{glutamic acid}\rightarrow\text{lysine}}$
Abnormal delta chains	
A'_2	$\alpha_2\delta_2^{61\ \text{glycine}\rightarrow\text{arginine}_1}$
Composite non-alpha chain	
Lepore haemoglobins	$\alpha_2$non-$\alpha_2$sequence—part δ, part β

The Thalassaemias.[102]—Inherited abnormalities of the molecular structure of globin, or of the production of globin, may be associated with haemolytic anaemia. Genetic defects that cause deficiencies of one or other type of globin chain lead to the various syndromes that are known as the thalassaemias. These are classified according to the nature of the polypeptide deficiency.

The red cells of patients with *heterozygous beta-thalassaemia* are usually hypochromic and microcytic; target forms and punctate basiphilia are often seen in blood films; there may be a mild degree of anaemia. An increased proportion of Hb A_2 is demonstrated by electrophoresis; a small amount of Hb F is often detectable also.

In *homozygous beta-thalassaemia* the anaemia is much severer than in the heterozygous form of beta-thalassaemia and the changes in the red cells are more marked. A substantial amount of Hb F is present and the proportion of Hb A_2 is increased. There is hyperplasia of the erythropoietic tissue and the spleen and liver are enlarged. Many of the patients die in infancy or childhood.

Homozygous alpha-thalassaemia is characterized by the formation of large amounts of haemoglobin Barts (Hb Barts), which contains only gamma chains and is unable to deliver oxygen to the tissues efficiently. This severe disability is incompatible with extrauterine life. It is a cause of fetal hydrops and stillbirth.

Haemoglobin H disease is another form of alpha-thalassaemia. Electrophoresis shows a considerable amount of haemoglobin H (Hb H). The condition varies in clinical severity. It is probably the manifestation of heterozygosity for two types of alpha-thalassaemia—or similar—genes. The red cells are hypochromic. There is splenomegaly accompanying the anaemia. Less severe forms of *heterozygous alpha-thalassaemia* may be difficult to detect in adults, although suspected from family studies. The presence of Hb Barts in samples of cord blood suggests that an infant has inherited one or more genes for alpha-thalassaemia.

Thalassaemias are far more widely distributed than was thought at first, when they were recognized mainly in people of Mediterranean origin. They are commonest among the population of a broad stretch of land that extends from the Mediterranean through the Levant and northern India to the Far East.

Over a hundred structural variants of haemoglobin are now known. Many of these have no clinically important effects and only a few are common. Some examples are given in Table 8.9.

They are identified in practice by their electrophoretic mobility and by their solubility, resistance to alkaline denaturation, heat stability, and reaction to various special tests, such as the ability of the cells to sickle under appropriate conditions. The precise characterization of rare haemoglobins may require peptide mapping and amino acid analysis. The most frequent of the abnormal haemoglobins are all beta-chain variants. Haemoglobin S (sickle cell haemoglobin, Hb S) is commonest in tropical Africa but has become quite widespread elsewhere. Haemoglobin C is commonest in West Africa. Haemoglobin E is found predominantly in south eastern Asia. Haemoglobin D Punjab appears to have originated in the north west of India.

Sickle Cell Anaemia.[103]—Sickle cell anaemia (haemoglobin SS disease) is due to the homozygous inheritance of the genes determining the abnormal beta chains of Hb S (see Table 8.9). The reduced form of Hb S has only about 2 per cent of the solubility of the oxygenated form, and tends to crystallize inside the cells, which then undergo the characteristic distortion that produces the sickle-shaped form (Fig. 8.9J, page 450). When sickling occurs the viscosity of the blood rises sharply. The abnormal cells do not pass through the small vessels readily. Obstruction of the blood supply to viscera, bones and other tissues may lead to infarction, causing fever and pain, which may be severe. Such ischaemic lesions may be fatal. Hemiplegia, renal papillary necrosis, infarction of the head of the femur simulating Perthes's disease (see Chapter 37), and pulmonary hypertension following vascular obstruction are among the serious pathological consequences of the disease. Interestingly, there are distinct differences in the pathology of sickle cell anaemia as seen in North America[104] and in Africa. For instance, chronic ulcers of the legs are commoner in American patients, and the great shrinkage of the spleen through fibrosis following multiple episodes of infarction that is so often described as a classic morbid anatomical stigma of the condition is less frequently observed in Africa, perhaps because the coexistence of stable malaria tends to maintain a measure of splenomegaly in these patients.[105] Splenomegaly is almost invariably present during the earlier years of the disease, but is demonstrable with diminishing frequency in older children and adults.

Patients with sickle cell anaemia are commonly of asthenic build and stunted in growth. The skull is often large, sometimes showing frontal and parietal bosses; the diploë is widened in consequence of the greater volume of erythropoietic marrow, and the formation of fine, vertically oriented spicules of periosteal new bone may give a characteristic radiological appearance. Similar changes may be seen in some cases of thalassaemia. Painful swelling of the extremities in small children causes the condition that is referred to as the 'hand-foot' syndrome.

There is often severe anaemia as a result of premature destruction of cells that are irreversibly damaged by sickling. Sickle cells, target cells and polychromasia may be seen in the blood films.

Haemoglobin A is absent from the blood of patients with sickle cell anaemia. Electrophoretic analysis of red cell lysates from adult patients shows the presence of haemoglobin S, a normal proportion of haemoglobin A_2 and a variable, but usually small, amount of haemoglobin F. At birth, most of the haemoglobin is Hb F and therefore symptoms of sickle cell disease do not occur in the neonate. As the infant matures the proportion of Hb F falls, though somewhat more slowly than is normally the case; it is replaced by Hb S. The persistence of even a small proportion of Hb F appears to be advantageous. Serious crises often occur in the second or third year of life; they are the cause of a number of deaths at that age. Comparatively few of the patients reach puberty. Anaemia, ischaemic visceral lesions and intercurrent infection are causes of death.

Sickle Cell Trait.—Individuals who are heterozygous for haemoglobin A and haemoglobin S (haemoglobin AS trait) are not anaemic and rarely suffer from overt ischaemic complications. Some of them are subject to episodic haematuria; there may be impairment of the concentrating power of the kidneys (see Chapter 24). Rarely, renal papillary necrosis develops. The blood film shows no diagnostic changes. *In vitro* exposure of the red cells to low oxygen tension induces sickling.

'Haemoglobin SC Disease'.—Those who are heterozygous for haemoglobin S and haemoglobin C often have an enlarged spleen and may be mildly anaemic. Contrary to expectation, a high haematocrit reading in a case of this condition may not be relied on as an index of the unlikelihood of thrombotic crises, for this combination of haemoglobins proves capable of making the blood especially viscous when deoxygenated. Progressive retinopathy is an occasional complication, the sequel of local sickling.

Women with haemoglobin SC disease are at increased risk from thrombotic crises during pregnancy. An attack of pain may herald infarction of bone marrow, and this may be followed by rapidly fatal marrow embolism. At necropsy, fatty marrow and, sometimes, haemopoietic marrow are found in the capillaries of the lungs, brain, kidneys and other organs.

Haemoglobin C Disease and Haemoglobin AC Trait.—People who are homozygous for haemoglobin C (haemoglobin C disease) have a mild haemolytic anaemia with splenomegaly. Those who are heterozygous for haemoglobin A and haemoglobin C (haemoglobin AC trait) have no clinical manifestations.

Miscellaneous Haemoglobinopathies.—No symptoms are observed in those who are heterozygous for haemoglobins A and E or for haemoglobins A and D.

Double heterozygosity for abnormal haemoglobins and thalassaemias leads to a variety of conditions that may vary widely in their features. Family studies are sometimes necessary to distinguish patients with—for example—*sickle cell thalassaemia* from those who have true homozygous sickle cell anaemia.

A few rare haemoglobins, such as haemoglobin C Harlem, show the characteristic amino acid substitution of sickle cell haemoglobin and, in addition, an alteration elsewhere in the beta chain. These variants also possess the property of sickling, but their electrophoretic mobility differs from that of haemoglobin S.

Uptake and release of oxygen are influenced by the composition of those parts of the haemoglobin molecule that embrace the haem groups, and by the ability of the protein structure to undergo the changes in shape that are associated with these processes. The introduction of amino acids that alter the nett charge in the neighbourhood of the haem groups increases the likelihood of methaemoglobin formation followed by denaturation of the globin. A number of congenital types of methaemoglobin may result from such substitutions. Others cause the formation of unstable haemoglobins that are associated with haemolysis and the production of Heinz bodies (see page 449). Some unstable variants are sensitive to the action of certain drugs —for instance, sulphonamides provoke haemolysis in carriers of haemoglobin Zürich.

Some mutant haemoglobins have an abnormally high oxygen affinity and are therefore associated with polycythaemia (for instance, haemoglobin Chesapeake).

Porphyria[106]

The porphyrias are diseases associated with primary abnormalities of porphyrin synthesis and metabolism. They may be considered in two main groups: in one the erythropoietic tissue is the seat of the disturbance in porphyrin metabolism or is conspicuously involved in it (the *erythropoietic porphyrias*) and in the other the liver is primarily at fault (the *hepatic cutaneous porphyrias*, so called because of the involvement of the skin in the clinical symptomatology of many of the varieties of porphyria that are assigned to this group). *Acute intermittent porphyria* (Swedish porphyria) is sometimes separated from other forms of hepatic porphyria because of its striking clinical picture and particularly the absence of skin involvement. Significant haematological abnormalities occur only in the group of erythropoietic porphyrias; only these are considered here. Other aspects of porphyria are considered on page 1272 and in Chapters 34 and 35.

Congenital Erythropoietic Porphyria (Günther's Disease[107]).—This rare disorder of porphyrin metabolism is inherited as an autosomal recessive trait. The synthesis of haem in the erythropoietic tissue is markedly disturbed, porphyrins, haem and bile pigment being produced in excessive quantities. Much of the surplus uroporphyrin and coproporphyrin formed by these patients consists of series I isomers, which are by-products of porphyrin synthesis that cannot be utilized in the metabolic pathway that leads to the formation of haem: they are for the most part excreted, both in the urine and in the faeces. The urine is characteristically the colour of burgundy. Porphyrins are deposited in the bones and teeth, which acquire a reddish brown tint. The skin becomes sensitive to light. This photosensitivity may result in the appearance of blisters and bullae (porphyria is one of the causes of the conditions formerly grouped by dermatologists under the name hydroa aestivale); scarring, deformation and, ultimately, total destruction of exposed parts, such as fingers, nose and ears, are the outcome (see Chapter 39).

Haemolysis is sometimes a feature, although the osmotic fragility of the red cells is normal (see page 466), even when their life span is shortened. Ineffective erythropoiesis contributes to the anaemia that accompanies the disease; hypersplenism may

be important in some cases (see page 441). Their porphyrin content renders some of the red cells fluorescent.

The erythroblasts show nuclear vacuolation; the vacuoles are bounded by deeply staining chromatin (heterochromatin) and contain haem and ribonucleic acid, and often an excess of porphyrins. The proportion of the cells that show these anomalies is not constant, being dependent on the rate of erythropoiesis. Cells that contain large amounts of porphyrin are strongly fluorescent, the nucleus often particularly so. After extrusion, the nuclei disintegrate and the liberated porphyrins probably account for a major proportion of these substances and of the bile pigment in the urine and faeces.

Erythropoietic Protoporphyria.[108]—In this condition, which is inherited as a dominant defect, the red cells contain abnormally large amounts of protoporphyrin and are fluorescent (Fig. 8.24). The marrow is not fluorescent, or at most shows slight porphyrin

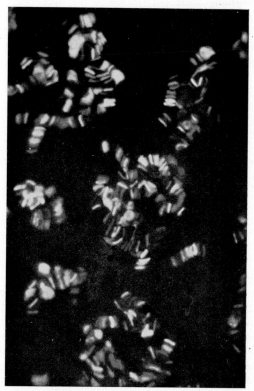

Fig. 8.24. Erythropoietic protoporphyria. There is porphyrin fluorescence of almost all of the red cells (fluorocytes); the most brilliant cells are young cells. It may be noted that the majority of the red cells in cases of lead poisoning also become fluorescent: the appearances are usually less striking than in erythropoietic protoporphyria.

fluorescence, confined to the cytoplasm of normo-blasts. The patients are not usually anaemic. The commonest presenting symptom is photosensitivity, manifested by an urticarial eruption following exposure and the gradual development of chronic eczematous changes. Bulla formation, scarring and loss of tissues do not occur, in contrast to the severe mutilation that eventually accompanies congenital erythropoietic porphyria (see above). The photosensitivity in erythropoietic protoporphyria is to light of the wavelengths that excite fluorescence of porphyrins. These wavelengths, notably the Soret band (410 nm), pass through ordinary window glass, unlike the light that tans the skin of normal people.

Erythropoietic protoporphyria is probably due to an abnormality of ferrochelatase, the enzyme that catalyses the formation of haem from iron and protoporphyrin.[109] Much protoporphyrin is excreted in the bile, but there is usually little or no excess of porphyrins or their precursors in the urine in uncomplicated cases. Some of the patients eventually develop cirrhosis of the liver. There is also an increased incidence of cholelithiasis. During periods of impairment of hepatic function there is an increase in the amount of protoporphyrin in the plasma and of porphyrinuria.

Erythropoietic Coproporphyria.[110]—Erythropoietic coproporphyria presents clinical and pathological findings similar to those of erythropoietic protoporphyria, except that the porphyrin that is present in excess in the red cells and in the faeces is a coproporphyrin. The inherited anomaly is presumed to be an enzyme defect at the stage in the pathway of haem synthesis at which coproporphyrinogen should undergo decarboxylation to form protoporphyrin.

The General Responses to Acute and Chronic Haemolytic Anaemia

In acute haemolytic crises in man, as in experimental animals, the outcome depends on the amount and nature of the haemolytic agent, the susceptibility of the individual,[111, 112] particularly his red cells, and whether the destruction is intravascular or takes place outside the circulation, in the spleen, liver or other tissues. When small amounts of haemoglobin (about 100 mg/dl) are liberated into the circulation, they combine with an α_2 fraction of the plasma globulins (haptoglobin). If more haemoglobin is released from lysed red cells than can be bound by haptoglobin and the

plasma albumin, it circulates in the free form until excreted by the kidneys. After a time, the circulating bound haemoglobin is altered to the ferric complex, methaemalbumin, which has a single spectroscopic absorption band at 624 nm. This complex can be converted to a haemochromogen with an absorption band at 558 nm by the addition of ammonium sulphide (Schumm's test).* Should the haemolysis be severe, death follows from the circulatory crisis caused by the sudden loss of blood volume, the rise in colloidal osmotic pressure of the plasma and the effects of the sudden liberation of large amounts of potassium from the disrupted red cells. In animals with experimentally induced haemolytic anaemia it has been shown that a haemolytic crisis is followed by a considerable fall in blood volume, due to the loss of cells, and that replacement of the lost volume—even by plasma or plasma substitutes—protects such animals from an otherwise fatal dose of the haemolytic agent.

In less acute haemolytic reactions, the remains of the lysed red cells and their liberated contents are removed from the circulation over a period of several days. The fall in blood volume is substantially made good by an increase in plasma volume. With slower haemolysis there is time for hyperplasia of the marrow to occur, and in this response both the erythropoietic and the leucopoietic tissues share, so that the increased production of red cells, which reaches a peak after about eight days, is accompanied by leucocytosis. In time, the increased production compensates for the loss of red cells, the lost haemoglobin is replaced, and recovery takes place.

In chronic haemolytic anaemia, recovery is less complete: instead, a balance between destruction and replacement is reached, there is a constant reticulocytosis, and the haemoglobin level tends to become stabilized in a fairly closely maintained range. If this is above 8·5 g/dl the patient can lead a fairly normal life; if it is below 7·5 g/dl treatment may be required, but it is remarkable how well these patients can adjust to low haemoglobin levels.

Variation in individual sensitivity, and particularly in the adequacy of regeneration, is commonly seen when investigating a family for some inherited form of haemolytic anaemia. Some of its members will be severely anaemic, some may have died in a haemolytic crisis, and there will also be some who,

* In Schumm's test the plasma is covered with ether, and one-tenth of its volume of a concentrated solution of ammonium sulphide is added. If methaemalbumin is present it will be converted to haemochromogen, which can be recognized by spectroscopy.

though affected and with red cells of abnormally short life span, can maintain nearly normal haemoglobin levels. Those who belong to the last of these three categories owe their relatively normal haemoglobin concentration to the effectiveness of their hyperplastic bone marrow in compensating for the losses due to haemolysis. However, in any case of chronic haemolytic anaemia, a crisis of either a haemolytic or a hypoplastic nature may occur—the former due to exacerbation of the haemolytic process and the latter to a recession in red cell production. In both types of crisis, the haemoglobin level falls: they can be distinguished by the fact that if the crisis is due to bone marrow hypoplasia, the reticulocyte count also decreases.

With the great hyperplasia characteristic of all forms of chronic haemolytic disease, the haemopoietic marrow extends far into the shaft of the limb bones. Foci of haemopoiesis may even reappear in the sites where blood formation occurs during fetal life—the liver and spleen and the hilum of the kidneys. Examination of the marrow shows replacement of much of the adipose tissue of the fatty marrow by erythropoietic cells, often in foci of 20 or more normoblasts grouped round an iron-laden macrophage (Figs 8.15A and 8.36A). The increase in the red cell precursors is usually so great that the leucoerythroblastic ratio falls to unity or is even reversed. Occasionally, an increase in the proportion of the earlier red cell precursors—the proerythroblasts and early normoblasts—suggests that there is some concomitant arrest in maturation. The macronormoblastic change that is sometimes found in cases of haemolytic anaemia indicates some interference at a later stage of erythropoiesis—possibly as a result of a relative deficiency of folic acid, or of some other essential factor, induced by the prolonged duration of the excessive red cell production.

In the congenital forms of haemolytic anaemia, well-marked marrow hyperplasia is present while the bones are developing. Changes may therefore be visible in radiographs of the skeleton, and particularly of the skull: the 'hair-on-end' appearance of the external surface of the calvarium is characteristic of some cases of the thalassaemias and of sickle cell anaemia (see page 470).[113]

Enlargement of the spleen is found in many cases of chronic haemolytic anaemia and results from sequestration of the abnormal red cells in its pulp, hyperplasia of its reticuloendothelial elements, and, often, the presence of foci of erythropoiesis.[114] Focal splenic infarction, with subsequent scarring, is common. Large amounts of iron are present in the reticuloendothelial cells and free in the interstitial tissue. The liver and kidneys also contain large amounts of iron, and, like the spleen, give a strongly positive Perls's reaction. Necrosis of bone may follow infarction of the marrow, which is particularly liable to occur in sickle cell anaemia (see page 469).

Haemolytic Episodes in Other Diseases

Haemolytic episodes are also a feature of some disorders that primarily affect the lymphoreticular system. The most striking examples are Letterer-Siwe disease and conditions related to it (see page 858), in which there is a remarkably widespread proliferation of reticulum cells. If these abnormal cells are able to function as macrophages, as is not seldom the case, excessive destruction of red cells takes place, especially in the spleen and lymph nodes. Other conditions in which haemolysis may develop include Hodgkin's disease, chronic lymphocytic leukaemia and some forms of carcinomatosis and of chronic inflammation. Abnormal antibodies—perhaps autoantibodies—are a possible cause of the haemolysis in these conditions, with proliferation of the reticuloendothelial cells and consequent augmentation of phagocytosis as a contributory factor.

Effects of Therapeutic Measures on Haemolytic Anaemias

The successful treatment of many forms of haemolytic anaemia by corticosteroids possibly depends on the capacity of these substances to depress antibody formation and on their general inhibitory action on the reticuloendothelial system.

The almost specific effect of removal of the spleen in cases of congenital spherocytic anaemia is probably to be explained by the functional effects of the removal of the main site of destruction of the abnormal red cells in this disease. Splenectomy has no effect on the defective erythropoiesis, for abnormal red cells persist in the circulation after the operation. In many other haemolytic conditions, however, splenectomy is less effective, probably because the affected red cells are not removed so predominantly in the spleen, and may be destroyed mainly in the liver and bone marrow, or even perhaps in the lungs.

Repeated transfusions may be necessary and there is then the ultimate danger of siderosis (see footnote, page 454). Iron therapy is useless and increases this risk.

Polycythaemia

The term polycythaemia is applied to the condition in which the number of red cells in the peripheral blood substantially exceeds the normal upper limit of about $6 \times 10^{12}/l$. In polycythaemia, the number may rise to $9 \times 10^{12}/l$ or even more, and the packed cell volume may reach 80 per cent. The number of red cells in the circulation is even larger than these figures suggest, for the volume of the blood is materially raised—sometimes to twice its normal value. It is the combination of raised red cell count, increased blood volume, engorgement of skin capillaries and slight cyanosis that produces the plethoric habitus typical of the condition. The viscosity of the blood is increased: this can often be demonstrated clinically by the peculiarly sluggish flow of the blood as it refills superficial veins that have been emptied by digital stroking in the Harveian manoeuvre. It is also responsible for the difficulty that may be experienced in drawing off a sample of venous blood.

Polycythaemia occurs in both primary and secondary forms. Primary polycythaemia is known as *polycythaemia vera*, erythraemia or Vaquez–Osler disease:[115, 116] its cause is unknown. Secondary polycythaemia is known as *erythrocytosis*; the rise in the red cell count is due to some pre-existent disturbance, generally some cardiac or pulmonary disease, in which the oxygenation of the tissues is impaired. Erythrocytosis may be regarded as the pathological counterpart of the physiological polycythaemia that develops in people who live at high altitudes, for instance, in the Andes (see page 287).

Polycythaemia must be distinguished from haemoconcentration resulting from diminution of the plasma volume accompanying dehydration, a condition now commonly seen in patients under treatment with diuretics.

Polycythaemia Vera

Little is known of the aetiology of polycythaemia vera except that the disease has sometimes been found in several members of a family, and in more than one generation. It is uncommon, and usually becomes clinically manifest in middle life, with symptoms of a protean nature that usually include fatigue, headache and dizziness. Generally, the engorgement of the vessels of the face and the presence of a much enlarged and sometimes painful spleen are strong diagnostic leads, indicating the need for an examination of the blood.

The red cells, apart from being greatly increased in number, often show much polychromasia, even though the haemoglobin level is above normal; nucleate forms are not uncommon in the circulating blood. Although fully haemoglobinized, the cells are often small and hypochromic, with the result that both the haemoglobin level of the blood and the packed cell volume are lower than the count would suggest. The white cell count is generally much raised, with many early forms of granulocytes. The number of platelets may be three or more times the normal figure.

At necropsy, dark red, haemopoietic marrow is found to have extended far into the medullary cavity of the limb bones. Extramedullary foci of blood formation may be present. All varieties of blood-forming cells are seen, and there is a particularly striking increase in the number of megakaryocytes. The spleen is greatly enlarged and often contains infarcts.

Thrombosis is a frequent complication of polycythaemia vera. Its occurrence may be accounted for by the combination of a high platelet count and the tendency to slowing of the circulation that results from the raised viscosity of the blood. Curiously, haemorrhage, especially from the gastrointestinal tract, is also common. These features greatly increase the risk of postoperative complications in untreated patients.

It is noteworthy that myelofibrosis and leukaemia sometimes develop in cases of polycythaemia vera. Aberrant forms of chromosome may appear in advance of such a transformation.

Erythrocytosis (Secondary Polycythaemia)

An increase in the red cell count is a common feature of a wide variety of congenital and acquired diseases of the heart and lungs. The changes in the blood are essentially a physiological adaptation to hypoxia of the tissues. Hypoxia has various causes: inadequate oxygenation of the blood as it passes through the lungs; a considerable reduction in the circulation rate; shunting of venous blood from the right side of the heart to the left; the presence of much abnormal haemoglobin, such as methaemoglobin and sulphaemoglobin, and the rare haemoglobin Chesapeake, which are incapable of releasing oxygen to the tissues; and tumours that produce erythropoiesis-stimulating substances (erythropoietin—see page 440), such as some primary adenocarcinomas of kidney (see Chapter 24). The number of red cells in the blood is seldom as large in erythrocytosis as in polycythaemia vera, and erythrocytosis is rarely associated with an increase in the number of white cells or platelets. An important difference between the two conditions is that the oxygen saturation of arterial blood is decreased in most instances of erythrocytosis (the exceptions are those cases in which the increase in the number of circulating red cells is associated with an erythropoietin-secreting tumour).

Erythraemic Myelosis (Di Guglielmo's Syndrome[117])

Erythraemic myelosis is a rare form of malignant neoplasm of the primitive cells of the erythropoietic series. The syndrome comprises anaemia, with many nucleate red cells in the blood, and splenomegaly. The marrow abounds in early precursors of the red cells, but the appearance differs from that seen in haemolytic anaemia in the marked irregularity in the size and character of these cells. In the usual, acute, form of the disease, the illness runs a rapid, fatal course, comparable with that of acute leukaemia. Sometimes erythraemic myelosis and acute leukaemia are associated. A more chronic form of erythraemic myelosis has also been described.

The Effects of Anaemia and Polycythaemia on the Circulation

The maintenance of the blood volume, and with it of the arterial blood pressure, is of first importance in ensuring the adequacy of the circulation: even a marked reduction in the haemoglobin concentration in the blood, especially if the rate of fall has been gradual, can occur without serious danger to life, provided the blood volume is maintained. When there is chronic anaemia, the effects of the lowered oxygen-carrying power of the blood, notably the lack of reserve energy for sustained physical effort, begin to appear when the haemoglobin concentration falls to about 9 g/dl; they do not become serious until the haemoglobin concentration reaches about 4 g/dl. At this level, the patient may develop rapidly progressive cardiac failure.

In severe, chronic anaemia, two compensatory mechanisms operate to minimize tissue hypoxia. First, the circulation rate increases considerably— with a haemoglobin concentration of about 5 g/dl the cardiac index may be increased threefold.[118] This accelerated circulation rate does not entail quite the expected addition to the work of the heart, because the fall in the red cell count is accompanied by a decrease in the viscosity of the blood, and consequently in the peripheral resistance to the circulation. The second means of compensa-

tion is a proportionate increase in the difference in the oxygen content between the arterial and venous blood in the systemic circulation, an increase that reflects the greater fraction of its oxygen that is abstracted from the blood as it passes through the tissue capillaries. It is possible that the ability to increase production of 2,3-diphosphoglycerate and bind it to haemoglobin is a factor in the individual patient's capacity to compensate (see page 436).

In polycythaemia, the viscosity of the blood is increased, and the rise is disproportionately large in comparison to the increase in the packed cell volume.[119] It is worthy of note that the work required of the heart in supplying the oxygen needed by the tissues is minimal when the packed cell volume is normal (about 45 per cent). Above that value, increased viscosity, and below it, an increased circulation rate, result in less economical working by the heart and hence in an added strain upon it.

DISORDERS THAT AFFECT THE WHITE CELLS

The upper and lower limits of the normal white cell count may be regarded as, roughly, $11 \times 10^9/l$ and $4 \times 10^9/l$ respectively. A rise in the white cell count occurs in a wide variety of circumstances: two main forms must be clearly distinguished— *leucocytosis* and *leukaemia*. A fall in the number of leucocytes in the blood is known as *leucopenia*.

Leucocytosis and Leucopenia

Leucocytosis

Leucocytosis is a common feature of pyogenic infections. It also occurs in other conditions that stimulate leucopoiesis, such as haemorrhage and burns, or other severe forms of tissue damage, as well as in such physiological states as digestion, muscular exercise and pregnancy. White cell counts of up to $20 \times 10^9/l$ are common, but much higher figures may sometimes be met with, and leucocytosis can then be mistaken for leukaemia, particularly if many immature white cells are present (*leukaemoid reaction*).

An increase in the number of neutrophils is the commonest form of leucocytosis, and particularly suggests the existence of an overt or occult pyogenic infection (Fig. 8.25A). The presence of young or frankly immature forms of neutrophils (a 'shift to the left'—Fig. 8.25B), toxic enhancement of the granulation (Fig. 8.26A), and the development of

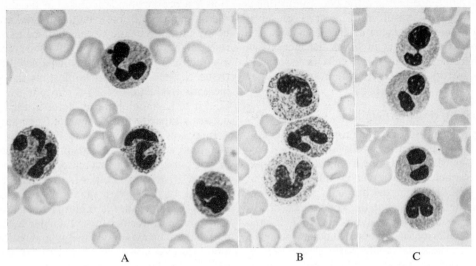

A   B   C

Fig. 8.25. Abnormalities of the leucocytes, as seen in the peripheral blood (see also Fig. 8.26). *Jenner–Giemsa stain.* × 1000.

A. Leucocytosis, with toxic granulation of the neutrophils.

B. 'Left shift', with toxic granulation.

C. The Pelger-Huët anomaly.

Döhle bodies (blue staining areas in the cytoplasm) are all evidence of acute infection, even when there is no leucocytosis.

It may be noted that the Pelger–Huët inherited anomaly (Fig. 8.25C) must not be mistaken for a 'left shift', that toxic granulation and the Alder anomaly* should not be confused, and that Döhle bodies also occur in the May–Hegglin disorder.[120]†

A mixed leucocytosis, with an increase in the number of monocytes and lymphocytes as well as of neutrophils, is more typical of subacute and chronic pyogenic infections.

Lymphocytosis is most characteristic of viral infections, including the viral exanthemas. Eosinophilia (Fig. 8.26B) suggests an underlying allergic condition and is found in bronchial asthma and in some cases of infestation by metazoan parasites.

Infectious Mononucleosis

Infectious mononucleosis (glandular fever) is considered to be a viral infection almost certainly caused by the Epstein–Barr virus. It is characterized by a distinctive form of leucocytosis in which peculiar mononuclear cells, variously regarded as abnormal lymphocytes or abnormal monocytes, are associated with neutrophile leucocytes that show a 'shift to the left' (see page 433) (Fig. 8.26C). The illness is usually accompanied by headache and ulceration of the throat, and there may be a transient skin rash. Rather less often there is enlargement of the lymph nodes (page 650) and of the spleen; rarely, jaundice may appear. The disease varies in severity from a mild malaise, which does not oblige the patient to stop working, to a severe and prostrating febrile illness that may last for several weeks before recovery takes place. The diagnosis may be suspected clinically, and is strongly supported by the finding of the abnormal white cells in a blood film. It is established beyond doubt by the demonstration of a positive Paul–Bunnell reaction (heterophile antibody test) in the serum.‡

* The Alder anomaly is characterized by the presence of abundant abnormal granules in the cytoplasm of all varieties of leucocytes.

† The May–Hegglin disorder is characterized by the presence of Döhle bodies (see above) in the cytoplasm of mature granulocytes, and by thrombocytopenia with the formation of abnormally large platelets.

‡ In the Paul–Bunnell test, the patient's serum, after destruction of its complement by heating to 56°C for 20 minutes, is examined for the presence of an antibody that agglutinates fresh sheep red cells. The specificity of the test is made certain by demonstrating that any heterophile antibody present is absorbable by bovine red blood cells and not by suspensions of guinea-pig kidney. This antibody absorption test distinguishes between the heterophile (anti-sheep-red-cell) antibody of infectious mononucleosis and heterophile antibodies that may, occasionally, occur naturally or follow serum sickness.

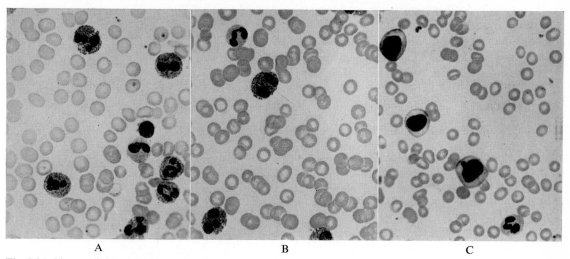

Fig. 8.26. Abnormalities of the leucocytes, as seen in the peripheral blood (see also Fig. 8.25). *Jenner–Giemsa stain.* × 500.
A. Neutrophil leucocytosis, with toxic granulation and 'left shift', including the presence of a metamyelocyte.
B. Eosinophilia; a neutrophil at the top, for comparison.
C. Infectious mononucleosis (glandular fever): abnormal lymphocytes, and a neutrophil.

Leucopenia

A reduction in the number of leucocytes below $4.0 \times 10^9/l$—the condition of leucopenia—is associated with so many clinical conditions that it has little diagnostic value. It may, however, have considerable prognostic significance, especially if it develops in the course of an infection. Leucopenia is a characteristic feature of starvation and of overwhelming infections, and also of such diseases as measles, typhoid fever, disseminated histoplasmosis, malaria and dengue fever. It is sometimes met with after the use of certain drugs, especially amidopyrine and the 'anti'-drugs (anti-thyroid, anti-convulsant, anti-histamine, anti-bacterial and anti-metabolic agents), or as a reaction to foreign protein, and after exposure to some toxic chemicals or to ionizing radiations. The reaction to drugs often appears to depend on idiosyncrasy and is probably of an immunological nature. Diseases in which the haemopoietic tissues are seriously involved, such as aplastic anaemia, Addisonian anaemia, Hodgkin's disease, and leukaemia in its aleukaemic stage, may also be associated with a secondary leucopenia. Leucopenia—possibly as a manifestation of 'hypersplenism' (see page 441)—may accompany splenomegaly resulting from various causes, including the Still–Felty syndrome (see page 724). It also occurs as a primary, often cyclical, condition. The role of leucocyte agglutinins as a cause is still not clear.

An extreme form of leucopenia, in which the granulocytes virtually disappear from the blood, is known as *agranulocytosis*. This is a very grave condition, for without the normal defence mechanism of phagocytosis by neutrophils the body becomes peculiarly liable to bacterial invasion. Infection of mucous membranes are characteristic and they result in the development of areas of necrosis without any accompanying suppuration. The mouth (especially the tonsils), the intestines and the genital tract are particularly liable to such spreading ulcerative infections. The subsequent haematogenous dissemination of the invading organisms is often the cause of death.

Those patients in whom leucopoiesis has been arrested in a late stage of maturation have more chance of recovery than those in whom the marrow is hypoplastic, for with antibiotic treatment it may be possible to prevent infection from spreading during the period in which the marrow is recovering. Leucopenia can be treated by the transfusion of leucocytes, but this procedure is of limited value because the cells survive in the recipient for so short a time that frequent repetition of the treatment is needed (see page 433). The most important step in treatment is—if possible—to prevent exposure to the causative agent, if such exists.

Agranulocytosis may be a feature of the acute forms of leukaemia. Differentiation between agranulocytosis and aleukaemic leukaemia may be difficult or impossible without examination of the marrow.

The Leukaemias[121, 122]

The leucopoietic cells of the marrow are particularly liable to undergo neoplastic transformation, and their subsequent unrestrained multiplication generally leads to the flooding of the circulating blood with white cells in varying stages of maturity. It was the pallor of the blood seen at necropsy in such patients,[123] due to a combination of a low red cell count and a high white cell count, that led Virchow, in 1845, to introduce the name leukaemia.[123a] The neoplastic transformation can take place in any of the three varieties of leucocyte —granulocytes, lymphocytes and monocytes—and at an early or later stage in their development. The blood picture of each form of leukaemia is characteristic.

Incidence

Reliable statistics of the occurrence of leukaemia in England and Wales before 1931 are not available. Since that year, a steady and general rise in incidence has been recorded. In 1959, 2534 deaths from the various forms of leukaemia were reported in England and Wales; the two sexes were affected about equally. The number of deaths has remained nearly constant at about 2600 since then. Since 1931, the recorded mortality has almost trebled, a rate of increase comparable only with that of bronchial cancer and coronary thrombosis. As with these diseases, the rise in the leukaemia mortality may be partly attributable to improvements in diagnostic facilities in recent years[124] and to the prevention of death from intercurrent infection before the diagnosis is established. An increase, however, seems to have been world-wide, for similar rises in mortality from leukaemia have been reported from North America, Europe and Australia. In England and Wales, where the types of leukaemia have only recently been distinguished in the Registrar General's returns, acute leukaemia is found to be the commonest, chronic lymphocytic leukaemia and chronic myeloid leukaemia are more or less equal in incidence, and monocytic leukaemia is much less frequent. In considering the figures relating to the incidence of the different types of leukaemia, it must be appreciated that their accurate differentiation may be difficult, especially in the acute cases.

In Britain, deaths from leukaemia tend to have a bimodal age distribution, with a relatively high incidence of the acute lymphoblastic form in children under 10 years of age and of the acute myeloblastic and chronic forms in the elderly.

Among older people, men are slightly more liable to the disease than women. The disease is rather commoner in the upper social grades than in the lower, but the difference is not pronounced.

Aetiology

The aetiology of leukaemia, like that of other types of cancer, is still obscure, though some information has been obtained from studies of the disease in man and in experimental animals. As with various other malignant growths, there are indications that transmissible virus-like agents, heredity and ionizing radiations may all play some part in the pathogenesis of the disease.

The *infective theory* dates from 1908, when Ellerman and Bang, studying a naturally-occurring leukaemia of fowls, were able to transmit the disease to normal fowls by inoculation not only with leukaemic cells but also with cell-free filtrates.[125] Since then, many attempts have been made to demonstrate a comparable filter-passing agent in the leukaemias of mammals. Although the results are still controversial, evidence has accumulated in recent years to give much support to the belief that a virus can induce leukaemia in an inbred strain of susceptible mice.[126] Attempts to transfer leukaemia from one person to another have failed. For instance, inoculation of blood, bone marrow and splenic pulp from patients with leukaemia into volunteers with inoperable cancer was not followed by the development of the disease in any of the recipients.[127] One of the volunteers received in all some 80 litres of blood, containing about 100×10^9 leukaemic cells per litre, by direct cross-transfusion: the normal blood picture was very soon re-established.[128] These negative results are inconclusive, for the incubation period of a virus-induced leukaemia might well exceed the survival time of these patients with cancer. A recent, important observation may be relevant to this argument.[129] A child with acute leukaemia was treated successfully by whole-body irradiation and a transplantation of bone marrow from her brother, whose HL-A tissue antigens were compatible with her tissues. The leukaemia eventually recurred, evidently affecting the donor cells. Such an occurrence may suggest the activity of a leukaemogenic agent.

It is well established that *hereditary factors* are important in the aetiology of murine and avian leukaemia. Some strains of inbred mice are so liable to leukaemia that 90 per cent of them die from the disease between the ages of six months and a year; other strains develop the disease infrequently. Little information is yet available about the familial incidence of the leukaemias in man: what is known comes mainly from studies of twins. If one of identical twins develops acute leukaemia it seems that there is a 20 per cent chance that the other twin will also develop acute leukaemia, usually within a few months:[130] this incidence is 12 times that observed in dizygotic twins.[131] It is interesting to find that a possible connexion between Down's syndrome, a condition known to be associated with a chromosomal abnormality, and acute leukaemia has been recognized (Fig. 8.27).[132] An increased incidence of leukaemia has been noted in other heritable disorders with known chromosomal changes: these include Fanconi's anaemia[133] (a familial form of aplastic anaemia with multiple congenital abnormalities), Bloom's syndrome[134] (telangiectatic erythema, photosensitivity and dwarfism) and ataxia-telangiectasia (Louis-Bar's syndrome[135]).[136, 137]

Ionizing radiations are recognized to be potent agents in the induction of leukaemia in man. Evidence for this has come from three sources. First, radiologists who were heavily exposed to X-rays before the introduction of adequate precautions have been found to have a significantly raised mortality from the disease.[138] Second, patients who have been treated over long periods by X-irradiation of the spine for the relief of pain from spondylitis have an increased incidence of leukaemia, its frequency rising with the extent of the irradiation.[139] Third, some years after the Hiroshima atomic bomb explosion, the incidence of leukaemia, mainly of acute or chronic myeloid type, began to rise in the survivors, especially in those who had been nearest to the hypo-centre of the explosion and therefore exposed to heavy irradiation.[140]

An earlier belief that leukaemia develops more frequently in children whose mothers have been exposed to X-rays during pregnancy is now generally questioned.[141]

Classification

Leukaemias may arise from any of the stem cells of the leucopoietic series. The three most frequent types may be classified as myeloid, lymphoid and monocytic, according to the type of cell concerned. Each of these three types of the disease may be subdivided into acute and chronic forms. The latter are comparatively rare before middle life, while the former are much more uniformly distributed throughout all age groups. In a German series, 173 out of a total of 191 cases of leukaemia in children were of the acute type.[142] The proportion of cases of acute leukaemia among children in Britain seems to be even greater.

There are significant differences in the treatment and in the prognosis of the three types of acute leukaemia—myeloid, lymphoid and monocytic. Therefore, although it may be difficult to make the distinction between them it is of practical importance to do so, using the various criteria that are available.[143]

The chronic forms of leukaemia are much more easily distinguished, for the cells in the blood are generally maturer. In the great majority of cases of chronic myeloid leukaemia, the neoplastic leucocytes belong to the neutrophil series, though very occasionally cases of eosinophil and basiphil leukaemia are seen. It is of interest that in cases of myeloid leukaemia the histamine content of the blood runs parallel to the basiphil count.[144]

Megakaryocytic leukaemia and plasma cell leukaemia are rare forms of the disease. Plasma cell leukaemia is almost always associated with myelomatosis and accompanied by paraproteinaemia (see page 488).

Acute Leukaemia

In acute leukaemia the neoplastic cells correspond to an early stage in leucopoiesis. If untreated, the disease progresses rapidly and is usually fatal within a few weeks. Its onset, which is often sudden, may be associated with fever, joint pains and sore throat, haemorrhagic manifestations and progressive anaemia. At this stage, the blood picture may already be diagnostic, or it may show little abnormality if few leukaemic cells have escaped from the marrow into the blood (the so-called *aleukaemic form of leukaemia*). About one third of all cases pass through an aleukaemic phase, and at this period the diagnosis can only be confirmed by examination of marrow.

Clinical Picture.—The clinical diagnosis may be difficult at first, but soon the typical features of leukaemia appear. Swelling and ulceration of the gums (Fig. 8.28) and fauces develop and haemorrhages appear in any of the mucous membranes (Fig. 8.29). Infiltration of the skin may be a prominent feature (Fig. 8.30). Grave liability to infection, especially with Gram-negative bacteria and fungi, is a feature of the disease and is largely

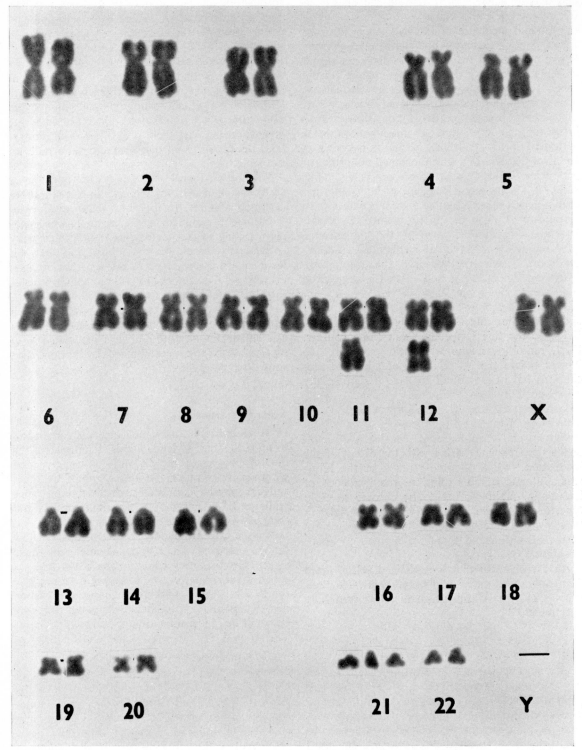

Fig. 8.27.§ Bone marrow cell culture in a case of acute lymphoblastic leukaemia in a child with Down's syndrome. Karyotype 49/XX,21+,C+. In addition to the characteristic trisomy D, there are two extra acquired C chromosomes associated with the leukaemic transformation.

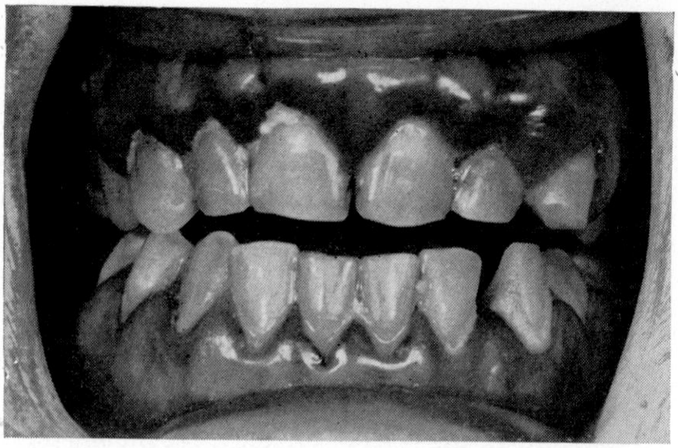

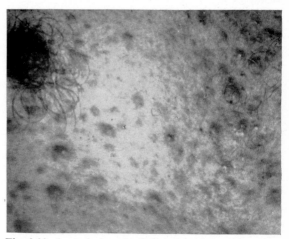

poiesis and in the formation of megakaryocytes accounts for the rapidly increasing anaemia and for the haemorrhages that result from thrombocytopenia. During the later stages of the disease, the liver and spleen, and sometimes the lymph nodes (Fig. 8.31), may become enlarged. There may be serious leukaemic involvement of the brain and spinal cord (see Chapter 34).

Fig. 8.28. Acute leukaemia. Swollen, infiltrated gums in acute monocytic leukaemia.

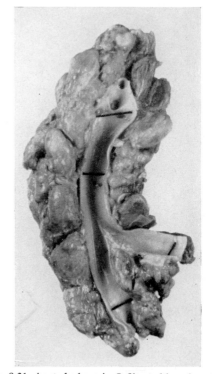

Fig. 8.30. Acute leukaemia. Infiltration of the skin of the chest.

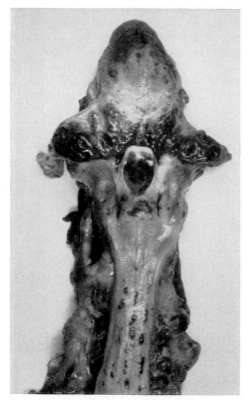

Fig. 8.29. Acute leukaemia. Haemorrhagic lesions in the tonsillar region and oesophagus in acute monocytic leukaemia.

due to the scarcity of functionally mature neutrophils; it is increased by the resistance-lowering side effects of the available therapeutic agents. The great overgrowth of the leukaemic blast cells in the marrow (Fig. 8.36D) leads to a marked and often serious fall in the production of normal leucocytes. A corresponding reduction in erythro-

Fig. 8.31. Acute leukaemia. Infiltrated lymph nodes.

Blood Picture.—Once any initial aleukaemic phase has passed, the white cells of the blood may increase greatly in number, though they seldom exceed $50 \times 10^9/l$ (Figs 8.34C, 8.35C and D). There may be marked fluctuations in the count. Severe thrombocytopenia, bleeding from ulcers in the alimentary tract (Fig. 8.32) and the extent of the replacement of the marrow by leukaemic cells result in the development of severe anaemia, the haemoglobin level commonly falling to about 4 g/dl. Normoblasts are seen in the blood films and there is polychromasia of many of the red cells.

The identification of the various types of blast cells as seen in Romanowsky-stained blood films is difficult and may not be possible. Staining with Sudan black usually distinguishes *myeloblasts* by showing the granules in their cytoplasm. The periodic-acid/Schiff reaction may show coarse, positive-reacting granules in the cytoplasm of *lymphoblasts*; these are not found in myeloblasts (Fig. 8.4C, page 450). Small forms of leukaemic myeloblasts—sometimes known as microblasts—may be mistaken for lymphocytes; similarly, the reniform outline of the nucleus of abnormal myelo-blasts may lead to their mistaken identification as monocytes.

The presence in the cytoplasm of blast cells of the structures that are known as Auer's rods indicates that the cells are myeloblasts. These structures are believed to be derived from altered cytoplasmic granules. They have characteristic appearances on light microscopy and electron microscopy (Fig. 8.33).

Myelomonocytic Leukaemia.—The term myelomonocytic leukaemia is applied to the not infrequent cases in which the cells of an acute leukaemia have features that are intermediate between myeloblasts and monoblasts.

Acute Monocytic Leukaemia.—In a smaller proportion of cases the cells—in spite of the acute nature of the disease—appear to be well-formed monocytes. Chronic forms of monocytic leukaemia are rarely encountered. The demonstration of an increased amount of muramidase (lysozyme) in the serum favours the diagnosis of monocytic leukaemia.[145]

Stem-Cell Leukaemia.—In some 5 to 10 per cent of cases of acute leukaemia the blast cells contain few or no granules and cannot be classified with the help of the usual range of cytochemical stains.[146] Because of this lack of evident differentiation these cells have been described as 'stem cells' and the leukaemia in which they are the cell type is referred to as stem-cell leukaemia.

Post-Mortem Findings.—At necropsy, the pale leukaemic marrow is seen to have spread down the shaft of the long bones at the expense both of the normal haemopoietic tissues and of the fatty marrow.

Occasionally, tumour masses develop beneath the periosteum: they may appear light green when first exposed, and they are composed of primitive marrow cells containing large amounts of myeloperoxidase. These tumours are known as *chloromas*; they are notably liable to grow in the orbit, where they can cause blindness from the effects of pressure and infiltration.[147]

Gross enlargement of the liver and spleen, such as is common in the chronic forms of leukaemia, is unusual in cases of acute leukaemia. The lymph nodes are seldom more than moderately enlarged. Again in contrast to chronic leukaemia, widespread infiltration of the tissue spaces of the major organs by leukaemic cells is unusual in acute leukaemia.

Haemorrhages are common. Acute bacterial and

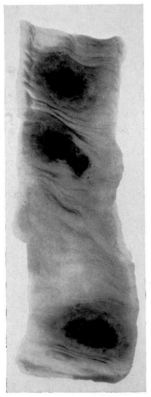

Fig. 8.32. Acute leukaemia. Ulceration of the intestine.

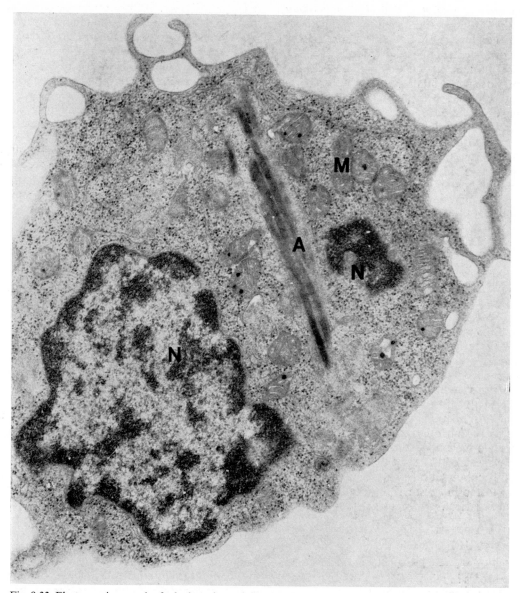

Fig. 8.33. Electron micrograph of a leukaemic myeloblast sectioned across an indentation between two nuclear lobes (N,N). Several Auer rods (A) are present. There are numerous mitochondria in the cytoplasm (M). × 30 000.

fungal infections, often with septicaemia, are frequent terminal complications.

It is important to recognize that, especially in those cases in which death occurs rapidly, there are often no specific macroscopical changes to indicate the diagnosis. Moreover, post-mortem autolytic changes vitiate the value of microscopical examination of the marrow. Cases that are not detected during life may therefore remain undiagnosed; if the presence of acute leukaemia is dis-closed by the post-mortem findings, it is very unlikely that the type of cell involved will be identifiable.

Prognosis and Treatment.—In the past the prognosis in cases of acute leukaemia was uniformly hopeless, with death from haemorrhage or infection, usually within a few weeks and at most within a few months. With the treatment now available, some 50 per cent of patients with myeloblastic, myelomonocytic and stem cell leukaemia show a good initial response; although the mean survival is still less than a year, a few patients live considerably longer. In cases of lymphoblastic leukaemia the outlook is better, particularly in children, more than 50 per cent of whom survive for a long period: indeed, the outcome may even be regarded as a cure in a significant proportion.[148]

Various therapeutic measures have their part in the attempt to control the course of the disease. Among the drugs that are used are purine antagonists such as mercaptopurine and thioguanine, mitotic inhibitors such as vincristine and other alkaloids of *Vinca rosea* (one of the dog-banes), antineoplastic antibiotics such as daunorubicin, the folic acid antagonist methotrexate, pyrimidine antagonists such as cytarabine (cytosine arabinoside), a specific amino acid antagonist (colaspase, or asparaginase), the alkylating agent cyclophosphamide, and corticosteroids and their synthetic analogues. All of these drugs interfere with cell division, but in different ways and at different phases of the mitotic cycle. Combinations of drugs have therefore been devised in order to produce the greatest synergistic action with as few side effects as possible. Transfusion of blood and of platelets plays an important role, particularly in the initial stages of treatment of acute myeloblastic leukaemia. Irradiation of the brain with X-rays and the prophylactic intrathecal administration of methotrexate have helped to reduce the incidence of involvement of the central nervous system in cases of lymphoblastic leukaemia and have been a major factor in improving the affected child's chances of survival.

Chronic Myeloid Leukaemia

Clinical Picture. — Chronic myeloid leukaemia usually appears in middle age and, if appropriately treated, runs a course of three to five years. Untreated, it usually leads to death in about two years. Its onset is insidious, with fatigue and loss of weight, abdominal discomfort and swelling, and attacks of pain in the left hypochondrium associated with enlargement of the spleen. Pain in the bones and joints is common, as a result of their infiltration with leukaemic cells. The skin, too, may be infiltrated, and the resulting symptom of pruritus can be distressing. In the later stages, bleeding—which may occur particularly in the brain, retina, middle and inner ear, gastrointestinal tract and urinary tract—is common; the immediate cause of death is often cerebral haemorrhage.[149]

Cytological Aspects.—In chronic myeloid leukaemia the neoplastic transformation almost always takes place primarily in the precursor cells of the neutrophil series, and much less often, perhaps because of the smaller numbers, in those of the eosinophil and basiphil series. The erythropoietic elements and, in the later stages of the disease, the megakaryocytes are crowded out by the proliferating myelocytes. The great increase in the number of these cells is generally evident in samples obtained by marrow puncture; their presence accounts for the fleshy, pinkish-grey appearance of the marrow when seen at necropsy (Fig. 8.23B, page 467). In the long bones, the neoplastic leucopoietic cells progressively replace the adipose tissue and even the bone trabeculae of the medullary cavity. When examined microscopically, at biopsy or necropsy, leukaemic marrow is seen to consist of masses of primitive white cells in various stages of maturation, with scattered surviving foci of erythropoiesis among them. Many of the myelocytes ultimately develop into neutrophils, but large numbers enter the blood stream while they are still immature.

By appropriate staining (Figs 8.4A and B, page 450) it can be shown that leukaemic neutrophils lack alkaline phosphatase.[150] This is almost a characteristic feature, although a deficiency also occurs in cases of acute myeloblastic leukaemia and of paroxysmal nocturnal haemoglobinuria.

Chromosome studies, using marrow cultures, show a specific deletion of one of the group G chromosomes. Chromosome-binding techniques have shown this small chromosome—known as the Philadelphia chromosome—to be one of pair 22 and to represent a translocation to a chromosome 9.[151]

Blood Picture.—In most cases of chronic myeloid leukaemia there is a very great rise in the white cell count—a figure of $200 \times 10^9/l$ is common, and counts of over $1000 \times 10^9/l$ are not rare. Differential counts show that almost all these cells belong to the granulocyte series (Figs 8.34B and 8.35B). The relative proportions of mature granulocytes, myelocytes and myeloblasts may vary widely—the more numerous the very primitive cells, the worse is the prognosis. This condition must be distinguished from *promyelocytic leukaemia*, which behaves as an acute leukaemia: in promyelocytic leukaemia the blood and marrow are overrun with distorted early promyelocytes that contain prominent cytoplasmic granules; a remarkable feature of this type of acute leukaemia is the frequency of its association with intravascular coagulation (see page

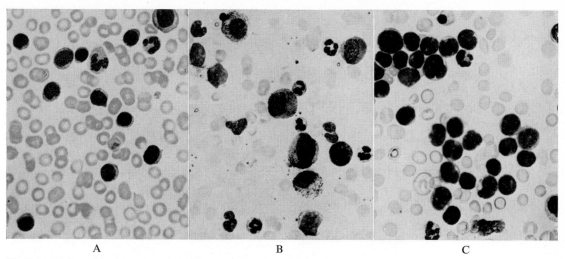

A   B   C

Fig. 8.34. Leukaemia—the peripheral blood. *Jenner–Giemsa stain.* × 500.

A. Chronic lymphocytic leukaemia. Many small lymphocytes in the peripheral blood.
B. Chronic myeloid leukaemia. Many myelocytes and young neutrophils in the peripheral blood.
C. Acute leukaemia. Numerous distorted 'blast' cells in the peripheral blood. A normoblast is seen at the top of the field.

497). In a significant proportion of cases of chronic myeloid leukaemia there is a gradual increase in the number of myeloblasts in the circulation and the disease ends with an acute leukaemic phase.

Since many of the circulating white cells in cases of chronic myeloid leukaemia show little lobation of their nucleus, films made from the peripheral blood resemble those prepared from marrow. Although most of the mature white cells can generally be seen from their granules to be neutrophils, the numbers of eosinophils and basiphils, especially the latter, are usually increased. In the early stages of the disease there may be evidence of polycythaemia, because the erythropoietic elements in the marrow are stimulated to increased multiplication before they become displaced by the proliferating neoplastic leucopoietic cells.[152] It seems that the erythropoietic cells may be involved in the neoplastic process and may have the Philadelphia chromosome.

In patients in whom anaemia has become severe, studies with radioactive iron and surface counting have indicated that some compensatory extra-medullary erythropoiesis may develop in the liver, spleen and lymph nodes.

The increase in the number of platelets in the blood may predispose to thrombosis; however, if these elements are defective in function haemorrhage may result. The eventual fall in the number of circulating platelets is partly responsible for the frequency of serious haemorrhage as the terminal event in this disease.

Pathology.—Once the neoplastic myeloid cells have entered the circulating blood, they may colonize any of the organs and tissues, giving rise to extravascular infiltrates. These infiltrates enlarge through the addition of further immigrant cells and by multiplication of the more primitive cells that have already settled in the area and retained the capacity to undergo mitotic division. Indeed, in many organs the infiltrates closely mimic the appearances found in the bone marrow.

Of the various organs, the spleen is the one that is usually most markedly affected. It is generally very greatly enlarged, though it tends to retain its usual shape and notched margin. At necropsy, it may extend far across the abdomen, even to the right iliac fossa, displacing the other viscera. It often weighs as much as 3000 g, and on occasion even more. Sometimes, large, pale depressed areas are visible through the capsule: on being cut across, these prove to be infarcts that extend deeply into the splenic substance. It is over these lesions that fibrous adhesions tend to form, binding the spleen to nearby structures. The cut surface of the splenic pulp is firm and uniformly greyish-red; the fibrous trabeculae persist, but there is little or no trace of the Malpighian follicles. Microscopical examination reveals the presence of enormous numbers of neutrophils, myelocytes and myeloblasts which have crowded out the splenic pulp and encroached upon or obliterated the lymphoid tissue.

The liver is always enlarged, although seldom greatly; it is pale, and whitish. Nodular masses of

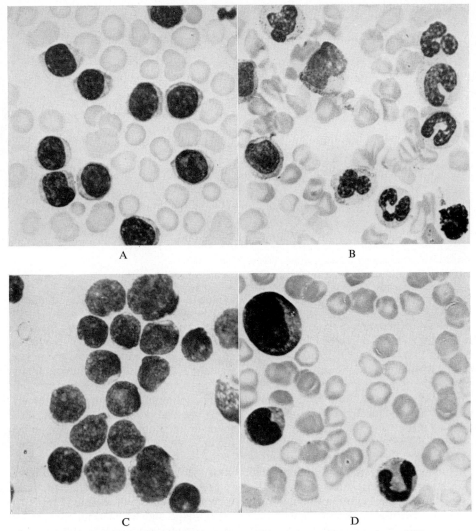

Fig. 8.35. Leukaemia—detail of the cells in peripheral blood. *Jenner–Giemsa stain.* × 1000.

A. Chronic lymphocytic leukaemia: small lymphocytes.
B. Chronic myeloid leukaemia: myelocytes and young neutrophils.
C. Acute myeloblastic leukaemia: myeloblasts.
D. Aleukaemic leukaemia: one primitive cell is seen at the top of the field.

infiltrate are seen on its capsular and cut surfaces. Microscopically, the portal tracts contain many leukaemic cells in all stages of development; these cells also infiltrate widely into the surrounding lobules, between the columns of hepatic parenchymatous cells.

In contrast to chronic lymphocytic leukaemia, the lymph nodes are rarely much enlarged in chronic myeloid leukaemia, although on microscopical examination their follicular pattern may be obscured by the infiltration of leukaemic cells.

Almost all the organs may show gross or micro-scopical infiltration by leukaemic cells. The kidneys are usually enlarged, and there are pale, often ill-defined, areas beneath the capsule and on the cut surface: these are foci of particularly heavy infiltration by leukaemic cells. The heart and lungs are particularly often involved. Nodular foci of infiltration are often found in the skin, especially near the anus.

Metabolic Disturbances. — The metabolism of patients with chronic myeloid leukaemia is often markedly altered, probably in consequence of the biochemical needs of the rapidly proliferating leucoblastic elements. It seems likely that it is the rapid turn-over of relatively short-lived cells in this disease that is responsible for the excretion of large amounts of the products of nucleic acid degradation (uric acid, and the purine bases, xanthine and guanine).[153]

Response to Infection.—In view of the importance of neutrophils in the defence of the tissues against infection, the cellular responses to inflammation in leukaemic patients have attracted some attention. It has been found in chronic myeloid and chronic lymphocytic forms of leukaemia that the leucocytes participating in the inflammatory reaction excited by invading bacteria differ little in appearance from those seen in normal people under similar conditions; this ensures a reasonably unimpaired defence. This is in contrast with acute leukaemia, in which the hazard of infection is much increased in consequence of the small number of circulating mature leucocytes.[154, 155]

Prognosis and Treatment. — Untreated chronic myeloid leukaemia usually results in death about two years after diagnosis. Treatment with busulphan prolongs life by about a year only, but the quality of life is much better than in the absence of treatment: most patients are without symptoms throughout most of the time.[156] Splenectomy may be advantageous, preventing the eventual occurrence of hypersplenism (see page 441), and—possibly— enabling the dose of busulphan to be kept to a smaller total so that the cumulative toxic effects of the drug, which include thrombocytopenia, wasting and cutaneous pigmentation, and—rarely—pulmonary fibrosis (see page 378), are delayed.

Chronic Lymphocytic Leukaemia

In this form of leukaemia, the neoplastic transformation affects the precursors of the lymphocytes. Its frequency has risen in recent years; in Britain it is now a common form of leukaemia. It occurs almost exclusively among the elderly, and mainly among men. Its onset is gradual, with vague pains, lassitude, loss of weight and enlargement of lymph nodes. The lymph node involvement is often accompanied by symptoms due to pressure on adjacent structures, such as stridor and other effects of enlargement of intrathoracic nodes. The symptoms and signs may be very diverse during the early stages of the disease: localized nodules or diffuse infiltrates in the skin, enlargement of cervical lymph nodes, tonsillar enlargement and infection, and pain in the sternum and other bones may be the initial features. In the later stages of the disease, haemorrhages may be conspicuous, and profuse bleeding may take place from ulcerated leukaemic foci in the alimentary tract or the skin. Patients with chronic lymphocytic leukaemia may live longer than those with chronic myeloid leukaemia, but very few survive more than 10 years after the diagnosis has been made.

Differential Diagnosis.—In its early stages, chronic lymphocytic leukaemia may be confused with infectious mononucleosis (Fig. 8.26C, page 477). The Paul–Bunnell test and the difference in the ages at which the two diseases usually appear assist in distinguishing them.

The clinical picture of Hodgkin's disease may be identical with that of chronic lymphocytic leukaemia: biopsy of a lymph node, together with a study of films made from blood and marrow, should help to give the correct diagnosis. The relative resistance of leukaemic lymphocytes to undergo transformation when incubated with phytohaemagglutinin helps to distinguish them from non-neoplastic lymphocytes (see page 522).

It may be noted that it is not always easy to distinguish between chronic lymphocytic leukaemia and those cases of lymphosarcoma in which there are many tumour cells circulating in the blood (see page 840).

In chronic lymphocytic leukaemia the number of white cells in the blood is greatly increased—counts of $50 \times 10^9/l$ to $100 \times 10^9/l$ are typical of the disease (Figs 8.34A and 8.35A). The increase is almost wholly in the number of small lymphocytes, which may make up 90 per cent or more of the circulating white cells; many of the lymphocytes are degenerate, and 'smudge' forms may predominate. The cells usually have the characteristics of B lymphocytes (see page 519).[157] Terminally, larger (less mature) cells of the lymphocyte series may appear in the blood.

Anaemia does not appear as early as in chronic myeloid leukaemia, in which the marrow is involved from the start, but it becomes increasingly evident. It is partly the result of the progressive replacement of the marrow by infiltrating lymphocytes (Fig. 8.36C), and partly, at least in some patients, an autoimmune reaction mediated by antibodies that give a positive direct antiglobulin reaction and that cause lysis of the patient's red cells. Autoimmune haemolytic anaemia is sometimes the presenting manifestation of the disease.

Pathology.—The structural changes in the major organs in chronic lymphocytic leukaemia differ materially from those in chronic myeloid leukaemia. In the latter, it is the precursor cells in the marrow that have undergone neoplastic transformation, while in the former it is those in the lymphoid structures. Indeed, it is the progressive enlargement of the lymph nodes and spleen through the neoplastic proliferation of lymphocytes that is often the presenting sign of chronic lymphocytic leukaemia. The enlarged nodes are usually painless, discrete, firm in texture, and pinkish. Microscopically, little remains of the normal structure of the nodes, which is replaced by a more or less uniform accumulation of small lymphocytes. A similar loss of normal structure occurs in all the foci in which lymphoid tissue is ordinarily found, such as the tonsils and Peyer's patches. The site of the infiltration in the liver differs from that of chronic myeloid leukaemia in being mainly in the portal tracts instead of diffuse.[158]

Since the main cellular proliferation in chronic lymphocytic leukaemia takes place outside the marrow, the haemopoietic elements there are less immediately affected. Consequently, at least in the early stages of the disease, the formation of granulocytes and red cells is not seriously affected. Ultimately, however, the leukaemic infiltration of the marrow displaces the normal haemopoietic and adipose tissues, and the marrow cavity becomes occupied by a firm, greyish-pink tissue that to the naked eye is not unlike that seen in chronic myeloid leukaemia. In so far as splenic enlargement and the infiltration of parenchymatous organs are concerned, the two forms of chronic leukaemia present many similarities. Such differences as are found terminally are mainly microscopical, and dependent on the identity of the white cell series that is involved.

Myelomatosis

This malignant disease of the plasma cells and their precursors in the marrow is closely related to leukaemia. Probably the commonest form is 'diffuse' myelomatosis, with widespread marrow involvement causing progressive anaemia but little formation of discrete tumours. In other cases, definite tumours arise within a generalized infiltration, giving the picture described as multiple myeloma (Fig. 8.23C, page 467; see also Chapter 37). Rarely, there is a single tumour arising within a bone, a solitary myeloma (plasmacytoma).

The disease is relatively rare. It is found in adults with a frequency of about 12 cases per million of the population.[159] Myelomatosis involves principally those parts of the skeleton in which haemopoiesis normally persists in adult life: the skull, vertebrae, ribs and pelvic bones, and the upper end of the humeri and femora. The nodules of growth may be microscopical in size, or they may enlarge to form dark red, soft tumours that cause much erosion and softening of the surrounding bone. The larger masses produce a typical X-ray appearance of 'punched out' areas of rarefaction without surrounding osteosclerosis. Spontaneous fractures readily occur.

Sometimes myelomas form masses in the viscera, notably in the kidneys and intestine. The extramedullary tumours occur particularly in those cases in which the cells are of the type that produce class D immunoglobulin (IgD) (see below).[160] Their histological structure is essentially the same as that of the tumours in the marrow.[161, 162]

The cells in myelomatosis may resemble mature plasma cells. Oftener, their appearance is that of an earlier, nucleolate form of plasma cell, with abundant basiphile cytoplasm (Fig. 8.36B).[163] In the tumour masses these cells lie close together, with little or no stroma. Although it is possible for the aspiration needle to miss the tumours themselves, the myeloma cells are commonly distributed diffusely and are usually to be found in aspirated samples. In advanced cases, the tumour cells may replace so much of the haemopoietic tissues that anaemia, leucopenia and thrombocytopenia become pronounced and the blood picture is that of leucoerythroblastic anaemia (see page 462).

Rarely, the myeloma cells escape into the peripheral blood (*plasma cell leukaemia*).

Protein Synthesis by Myeloma Cells.—The myeloma cells, like normal plasma cells, are generally able to synthetize immunoglobulins. As the tumour cells originate from a single cell, they are monoclonal and therefore the abnormal protein that they produce is, in general, of one specific type. The production of normal gammaglobulin is usually markedly diminished in cases of myelomatosis. On electrophoresis, the abnormal protein migrates as a dense, discrete band, usually in the gammaglobulin region but in some cases in the alphaglobulin or betaglobulin region (Fig. 8.37). The abnormal proteins formed by myeloma cells are known as *paraproteins*. Immunoelectrophoresis (see page 445), using antisera specific to the heavy

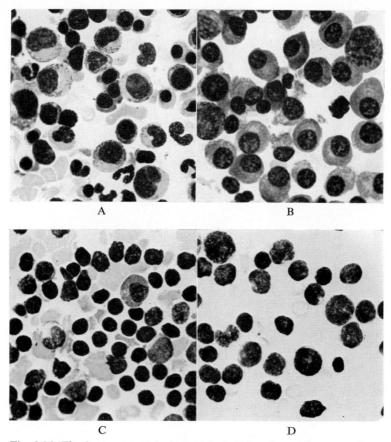

Fig. 8.36. The bone marrow in haematological disorders. *Film preparations: Jenner–Giemsa stain.* × 700.

A. Haemolytic anaemia. There is an increased proportion of normoblasts (compare with the changes in myelomatosis and leukaemia).

B. Myelomatosis. Some of the numerous plasma cells show primitive features, such as the presence of a nucleolus, that indicate that they are myeloma cells.

C. Chronic lymphocytic leukaemia. The marrow is infiltrated by many lymphocytes.

D. Acute leukaemia. The marrow is overrun by 'blast' cells.

chain fraction of the molecules, enables the paraproteins to be distinguished as IgG, IgA, IgD, IgM and IgE, the frequency of their occurrence being in that order (Fig. 8.38). Each of these immunoglobulins can be further subdivided into kappa and lambda types, according to the antigenic specificity of its light chains.[164, 165] Most of the paraproteins, which may constitute as much as 70 per cent of the total protein content of the plasma in cases of myelomatosis, appear to have no useful immunological activity.[166, 167]

The high concentration of paraprotein is responsible for the rouleau formation and the background staining seen in blood films and also for the greatly increased erythrocyte sedimentation rate charac-

teristic of myelomatosis. The paraprotein may also interfere with the coagulation mechanism.

A distinctive feature of myelomatosis is the excretion in the urine of a protein that is known after one of its discoverers as Bence Jones protein (see Chapter 24). This protein has a molecular weight about half that of plasma albumin, and it is, therefore, so readily excreted by the kidneys that it rarely reaches any significant concentration in the plasma. It is composed entirely of the 'light' polypeptide chains of immunoglobulins with either kappa or lambda structure (see page 445). Bence Jones protein possesses the distinctive property of being least soluble in urine at a temperature of about 60°C, so that on heating a specimen a

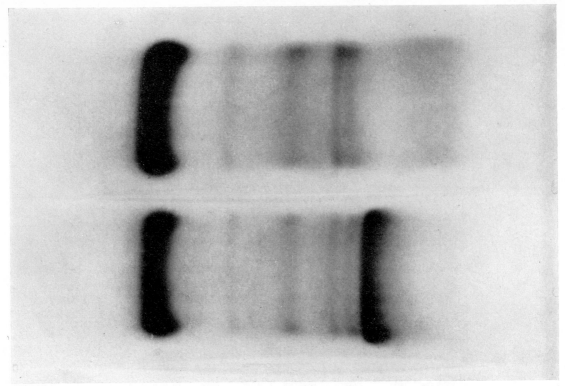

Fig. 8.37. Electrophoresis of serum on cellulose acetate. Normal serum above; serum of a patient with myelomatosis below. There is a heavy band of myeloma globulin in the latter; the amount of normal gammaglobulin is reduced. The bands, from left to right, are—albumin; α_1 globulin; α_2 globulin; β_1 globulin; β_2 globulin; γ globulin.

precipitate forms at about this temperature and redissolves as boiling point is approached. This simple test is positive in more than half the cases of myelomatosis; in those cases in which the heating test is negative, specific immunological tests on concentrates of urine, which are more sensitive, have shown that some Bence Jones protein is generally present.

Complications.—Five complications may dominate the later stages of myelomatosis: *pathological fractures* in any of the affected bones; *disturbances in renal function*, due either to infiltration of the kidneys by myeloma cells or to the peculiar condition known as 'myeloma kidney' (see Chapter 24), in which the tubules become blocked by protein casts that evoke a giant cell reaction in the surrounding tissue, ultimately leading to extensive glomerular atrophy and renal failure; the development of *amyloidosis*, which is apparently related to deposition of the abnormal plasma proteins in the tissues; *infections*, particularly in the lungs, following the leucopenia and the fall in the amount of normal gammaglobulins in the plasma;[168, 169]

and *bleeding*, especially from the gastrointestinal tract, due to paucity of circulating platelets and to disturbances in the plasma proteins.

Prognosis and Treatment.—The prognosis of myeloma remains bad, in spite of treatment with X-rays or cytotoxic drugs such as melphalan and cyclophosphamide. For a time these measures may have a remarkable effect in relieving the patient, and there may be a considerable fall in the production of paraprotein. Unfortunately, treatment usually does no more than delay the progress of the disease. The interval between diagnosis and death is, on average, two to three years.

DISORDERS THAT AFFECT THE PLATELETS, AND PURPURA

The number of platelets in the circulating blood is normally about $300 \times 10^9/l$. A pathological increase in the number of circulating platelets is known as thrombocytosis, or thrombocythaemia. A fall below

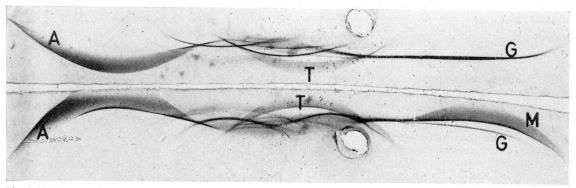

Fig. 8.38. Immunoelectrophoresis of serum protein. Control serum (above) shows normal IgG, for comparison with the myeloma IgG in the serum from a patient with myelomatosis (below). The arc formed by the myeloma protein (M) forks away from the normal IgG, which is reduced in amount. A, albumin; G, immunoglobulin G; T, transferrin.

the normal range is known as thrombocytopenia. The functions of the platelets may be affected by qualitative changes.

Thrombocytosis (Thrombocythaemia)

A temporary increase in the number of platelets usually follows any severe trauma and most major surgical operations, and tends to reach its maximum about the tenth day. This rise, together with vascular stasis, changes in the activity of the plasma coagulation and fibrinolytic systems, and an abnormal adhesiveness of freshly formed platelets, may account for the high frequency of postoperative venous thrombosis.[170] It is likely that these changes are initiated at the time of the operation.[171]

The number of circulating platelets is increased in cases of polycythaemia and of chronic myeloid leukaemia, and also rarely as a primary condition. Sometimes thrombocytosis occurs when the marrow is invaded by tumour cells; more frequently, such infiltration results in thrombocytopenia.

Thrombocytopenia[172]

The platelet count may be depressed in a wide range of conditions (see Table 8.10). The production of platelets may be affected in certain inherited diseases, or when the haemopoietic tissues are injured by ionizing radiation or by toxic chemicals or are replaced by neoplastic cells. Thrombocytopenia is occasionally a manifestation of 'hypersplenism' (see page 441). Again, platelets may be removed from the blood in excessive numbers, mainly by the spleen, or they may be destroyed by some immunological reaction. A feature that is common to all cases of severe thrombocytopenia is

purpura, a condition in which small, discrete haemorrhages appear in the skin (Fig. 8.39) and mucous membranes. Purpuric haemorrhages, of course, are not necessarily indicative of thrombocytopenia, for they can appear in a number of conditions in which abnormalities of platelet function, of the capillary endothelium or of the plasma proteins are responsible (see Table 8.10). The tendency to purpura, irrespective of its pathogenesis, may be demonstrated by the bleeding time.* This test assesses both platelet and capillary function and is independent of the coagulation mechanism.

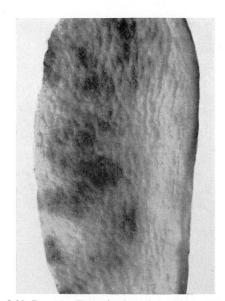

Fig. 8.39. Purpura. Extensive intradermal haemorrhages.

* The 'bleeding time' is the time for which a standard prick wound of the skin continues to bleed.

Table 8.10. *Classification of the Types and Causes of Purpura*

A. Thrombocytopenic Purpura
  1. Failure of platelet production (*amegakaryocytic thrombocytopenia*)
    (a) Congenital:
      i. Constitutional pancytopenia (Fanconi's anaemia)
      ii. Hereditary thrombocytopenias
      iii. Neonatal infections
    (b) Acquired:
      i. Aplastic anaemia
      ii. Infiltration of marrow by neoplastic cells
      iii. Myelosuppressive agents
      iv. Deficiency of vitamin B_{12} or of folic acid
      v. Certain viral infections
  2. Increased destruction, sequestration or loss of platelets (*megakaryocytic thrombocytopenia*)
    (a) Congenital:
      i. Infection
      ii. Immunological disturbance:
        drug sensitivity
        transfer of maternal antibody
    (b) Acquired:
      i. Infection
      ii. Disseminated intravascular coagulation
      iii. Immunological disturbance:
        idiopathic thrombocytopenic purpura
        drug sensitivity
      iv. Hypersplenism
      v. Haemorrhage
      vi. Massive blood transfusion
      vii. Haemolytic-uraemic syndrome
      viii. Thrombotic thrombocytopenic purpura (Moschcowitz's disease)

B. Non-Thrombocytopenic Purpura
  1. Defects of platelet function
    (a) Congenital:
      i. Thrombasthenia
      ii. Thrombocytopathy
    (b) Acquired:
      i. Uraemia
      ii. Myeloproliferative disorders
      iii. Macroglobulinaemia
  2. Vascular disorders
    (a) Hereditary:
      i. Hereditary capillary fragility
      ii. Hereditary haemorrhagic telangiectasia (Rendu–Osler–Weber disease)
    (b) Symptomatic:
      i. Infections
      ii. Scurvy
      iii. Dysproteinaemic purpura
      iv. Mechanical, hypoxic and degenerative forms of vascular purpura: including—
        senile purpura
        orthostatic purpura
        cachectic purpura
        mechanical purpura

Idiopathic Thrombocytopenic Purpura

The term idiopathic thrombocytopenic purpura has been given to two distinct diseases. One is an acute form of purpura, seen most frequently in children, usually from two to six years of age; the other is a more chronic disease, occurring in adults, particularly women. The acute form may follow a specific viral infection, such as varicella and rubella; more commonly, it follows a non-specific infection of the upper respiratory tract or lungs. There is usually no history of infection in cases of the chronic form of idiopathic thrombocytopenic purpura.

In both forms, the disease usually manifests itself with small purpuric spots in the skin, or by an abnormal tendency to bruising. Sometimes the haemorrhages, especially from mucous surfaces, may be severe and lead to much loss of blood. Bleeding into the gastrointestinal or genitourinary tracts may also occur. Involvement of the central nervous system is the most serious effect and may range from multiple petechiae, causing meningismus, to a large haemorrhage causing hemiplegia or death. Although the tendency to bleed varies inversely with the platelet count the correlation is not absolute. Curiously, only a small proportion of women affected while pregnant have post-partum haemorrhage.

The aetiology and pathogenesis of the disease are obscure. In some patients the condition appears to be inherited. More commonly, it is acquired and seems to be associated with an autoimmune reaction to the platelets, resulting in their premature destruction.[173] Such an immunological disturbance with the formation of an antiplatelet antibody, indicates a parallel between this form of thrombocytopenia and some forms of haemolytic anaemia (see page 465). The existence of an antiplatelet antibody is supported by the observation that a transfusion of plasma from a patient suffering from this disease into a normal person leads to a profound fall in the recipient's platelet count which can last for several days.[174]

The main change in the blood is the low platelet count. The various factors in the plasma that are responsible for coagulation are unaffected. Marrow films disclose little disturbance in erythropoiesis or leucopoiesis, unless there has been severe haemorrhage. The megakaryocytes are usually increased in number. They are immature, their nucleus lacking lobation and their cytoplasm being less abundant than is normal and lacking granules (Fig. 8.18B, page 458). The spleen is seldom palpable, but its participation in the destruction of platelets seems likely from the fact that their number in the blood generally rises after splenectomy. This participation may, however, be only secondary—the accelerated removal of the platelets by the reticuloendothelial cells of the spleen may depend upon sensitization of the platelets by a circulating autoimmune antibody, in the formation of which the spleen may play a part.

An unusually instructive variety of thrombocytopenia, although fortunately rare, is *purpura of the newborn*. This is observed soon after birth in the children of thrombocytopenic or normal mothers. It is presumed to be due to the passage of platelet antibodies across the placenta. In the cases in which the mother is not affected with thrombocytopenia it is possible that she has produced isoantibodies to her child's platelets, in a manner similar to the formation of red cell antibodies in erythroblastosis fetalis (see page 464).

Drug Purpura

The administration of certain drugs may lead to the development of thrombocytopenic purpura. Some, such as organic arsenical compounds and mustine (nitrogen mustard, mechlorethamine), bring this about through intoxication of the platelet-forming cells in the marrow. Others lead to an immune reaction in which large numbers of platelets are rapidly destroyed: the classic example in this group is the thrombocytopenia that occasionally followed administration of Sedormid (apronal, allylisopropylacetylurea). This drug becomes attached to the surface of the platelets, and forms there a complex that acts as an antigen, exciting the production of a specific antibody.[175] When Sedormid was given to a patient who had become sensitized by earlier use of the drug, the antibody reacted with the freshly-formed Sedormid–platelet complex and led to rapid destruction of the platelets.

Thrombotic Thrombocytopenic Purpura (Moschcowitz's Disease[175a, 175b])

Thrombotic thrombocytopenic purpura is an acute, rapidly fatal disease of unknown causation. It occurs at any age and is most frequent in young adults. It is characterized by thrombocytopenic purpura, haemolytic anaemia and curiously fluctuating neurological signs that result from the sequence of temporary occlusion of the smallest blood vessels in the central nervous system by platelet thrombi and the early re-establishment of local blood flow as the thrombi shrink.[176, 177] The fall in the number of platelets in the circulating blood is probably due, at least in part, to their incorporation in the thrombi that form throughout the body (see below) and that are so con-

C*

spicuous and characteristic a histological feature at necropsy (Fig. 8.40) and sometimes in biopsy specimens.[178] The unequivocal histological demonstration of these thrombi is essential to the diagnosis of thrombotic thrombocytopenic purpura, which cannot be accepted in their absence.[178a] Care must be taken not to mistake other vascular lesions for them, particularly in diagnostic biopsy specimens (and in the spleen, when this is sectioned after removal as part of a therapeutic regimen).

In a few cases there is distortion of some of the red cells, apparently as a result of mechanical damage while circulating past the microthrombi: the picture in the blood films in these instances is identical with that accompanying the haemolytic-uraemic syndrome, of which it is characteristic (see below). The haemolytic anaemia accompanying thrombotic thrombocytopenic purpura is only exceptionally associated with such morphological evidence of damage to the red cells, and in most cases its pathogenesis is unknown; the presence of autoantibodies has been demonstrated, but only in a very small proportion of cases.

The thrombocytopenia of thrombotic thrombocytopenic purpura has been attributed to the withdrawal of the platelets from the circulation as the great number of platelet thrombi form in the small arterioles and capillaries. A similar phenomenon is sometimes observed in rare cases of large haemangiomas (*Kasabach–Merritt syndrome*[179]) and angiolipomas in which, for some unexplained reason, extensive thrombosis occurs, sometimes quite suddenly, with accompanying thrombocytopenic purpura.[180, 181]

Haemolytic-Uraemic Syndrome

The haemolytic-uraemic syndrome, which is seen most frequently in the first year of life, is characterized by progressive haemolytic anaemia, jaundice, purpura and renal failure.[182] Burr cells (see Fig. 8.9F, page 450), helmet-shaped cells and other distorted forms of red cells give the blood picture a striking appearance. It is usually assumed that the distortion of the cells results from mechanical damage somehow sustained through obstruction to their passage by deposits of fibrin in the glomerular vasculature. The cause of the associated thrombocytopenia is uncertain.

There is evidence that at least some cases of the haemolytic-uraemic syndrome are a manifestation of immune-complex-mediated changes in the renal glomeruli resulting from a preceding viral infection (see Chapter 24).

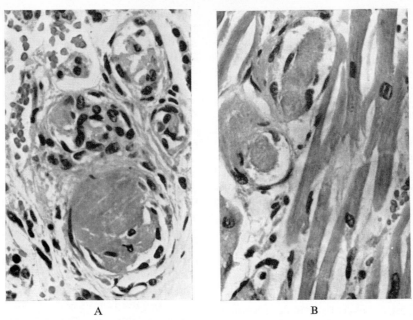

A   B

Fig. 8.40. Thrombotic thrombocytopenic purpura (Moschcowitz's disease). *Haema-toxylin–eosin.* × 200.

A. Typical thrombotic lesions in dilated capillaries of the adrenal cortex.
B. Thrombi and endothelial proliferation in capillaries in the heart muscle.

There is an observation of cardinal importance in distinguishing thrombotic thrombocytopenic purpura from the haemolytic-uraemic syndrome: the characteristically bulky, finely granular, early platelet thrombi of the former, and the accompanying aneurysmal dilatation of the small vessels, which occurs particularly at the arteriolocapillary junction area, are not features of the histological picture of the latter.[183]

Other Causes of Thrombocytopenia

Amegakaryocytic thrombocytopenia (that is, thrombocytopenia associated with deficiency or failure of platelet production) may be secondary to leukaemia, aplastic anaemia, myelomatosis and other disorders of the marrow, and to viral infections, particularly the exanthematous fevers of childhood. In contrast, a reduction in the life span of the platelets—usually associated with increased megakaryocytic activity ('megakaryocytic thrombocytopenia')—may accompany severe infections, especially septicaemia caused by Gram-negative bacteria, malaria, plague, typhoid and typhus fevers, and leptospirosis. Any of these conditions may initiate disseminated intravascular coagulation and thus lead to increased consumption of platelets (see page 497). An apparent shortening of their life span can also result from excessive sequestration of platelets in any condition that causes splenomegaly, including Hodgkin's disease.

A miscellaneous group of conditions associated with thrombocytopenic purpura includes large haemangiomas (see page 493), inherited disorders such as Aldrich's syndrome and the May–Hegglin neutrophil anomaly (see page 476), and the administration of large amounts of stored blood.

Prognosis of Thrombocytopenic Purpura

The prognosis of purpura depends upon its cause. In those forms that are due to thrombocytopenia, the state of the megakaryocytes gives some indication of the outlook. If they are numerous, there is some chance of recovery—if scanty and immature, the prognosis is correspondingly poorer.

From what has been stated above it should be clear that a first step in the management of purpura is to stop all drugs that might affect the formation or survival of platelets. Transfusion of platelets, concentrated from fresh blood, effects a transient improvement, and helps in the preparation of a patient for splenectomy, which may be curative in idiopathic thrombocytopenic purpura. Corticosteroids are of value in suppressing any immune reactions and reducing capillary fragility.

Non-Thrombocytopenic Purpura

Non-thrombocytopenic purpura comprises a confused group of conditions in which capillary defects, disorders of clotting factors and defects in platelet function are intermingled. In *von Willebrand's disease*[184] (Willebrand–Jürgens syndrome, constitutional thrombopathy, hereditary haemorrhagic thrombasthenia) there is a functional defect of the platelets and of the capillaries (see page 496). At the same time there is a lack of factor VIII in the plasma (see page 446): in contrast to haemophilia this appears to be due to a deficiency of some precursory factor, for it may be corrected by giving either normal or haemophiliac plasma.[185]

In another group of conditions, including the type of purpura known as *Glanzmann's disease*,[186] the platelets are abnormal in function and tend also to be abnormally large.

A classification of such platelet disorders under the headings *thrombocytopathy*, in which platelet participation in the clotting mechanism is defective, and *thrombasthenia*, in which the defect interferes with the ability of the platelets to form adhesive clumps, has been suggested (see Table 8.10, page 492). Occasionally, purpura occurs in association with thrombocythaemia: in such cases the platelets, although excessively numerous, are functionally defective. Platelet dysfunction may also complicate such conditions as macroglobulinaemia and uraemia.

Vascular Purpura

Vascular purpura may be congenital or acquired. An example of the former is *hereditary haemorrhagic telangiectasia* (Rendu–Osler–Weber disease)[187–189] in which numerous small foci of dilated capillaries are scattered throughout the skin and mucous membranes. This condition is inherited as a simple dominant. Bleeding, sometimes very severe, occurs from minor trauma and when the lesions are in the respiratory or gastrointestinal tract this can be particularly dangerous.

Acquired vascular purpura of the *Schönlein–Henoch type*[190, 191] causes visceral or joint symptoms in addition to skin lesions (see Chapter 39). An allergic reaction to a streptococcal infection or to some item of food is probably the usual cause. This type of purpura is usually accompanied by a local serous effusion, causing swelling of the affected tissues. Severe abdominal colic and vomiting may precede the appearance of the purpura. The joint manifestations tend to be mistaken for rheumatism,

especially as there is often a rise in temperature. Occasionally the disease runs a fulminating course, leading to death from renal failure within a few days.

Vascular purpura may be secondary to infections. A particular manifestation is the *Waterhouse–Friderichsen syndrome* of severe shock due to bilateral adrenal haemorrhage in meningococcal septicaemia (see Chapter 30). The same syndrome is sometimes seen in cases of septicaemia caused by other bacteria.

Drugs, including phenacetin and quinine, and *animal toxins*, such as snake venoms, may cause purpura. Purpura may be the main manifestation of *scurvy*. Occasionally, it is a feature of chronic diseases, especially renal disease with uraemia.

Purpura can also result from fragility of the vessels in old age (*senile purpura*) or in cachexia. It may also be caused by mechanical strain on the walls of the capillaries, especially hydrostatic pressure in the feet and legs accompanying prolonged standing.

DISORDERS OF THE COAGULATION MECHANISM[192]

The disorders that affect haemostasis in small blood vessels can be divided into those that are characterized by purpura, and associated with an abnormally long bleeding time (see footnote on page 491), and those in which bleeding is generally severer and more persistent, and attributable to some derangement of the coagulation mechanism (see pages 446–448).* The purpuras have been discussed above; the disorders of the coagulation mechanism are considered here.

Severe disorders of the clotting mechanism that may entail prolonged, and sometimes uncontrollable, haemorrhage, even from trivial wounds, usually manifest themselves in infancy. The less marked defects may come to light only after trauma, or following such minor operations as tonsillectomy and dental extractions. The bleeding may be

---

* In instances of very severe derangement of the clotting mechanism, coagulation of the blood *in vitro* at 37°C will be delayed. More refined tests are provided by the prothrombin time and the kaolin partial thromboplastin time. The *prothrombin time* tests the extrinsic pathway, which is activated by adding tissue factor (thromboplastin) to citrated plasma (see page 447). The *kaolin partial thromboplastin time* tests the whole of the intrinsic pathway: factors XI and XII are activated by contact with kaolin, and a substitute for platelet phospholipid is added to enhance the reaction (see page 446). Modifications of these tests using specifically deficient plasmas have been devised to assay the levels of particular clotting factors.

external, or it may take place into the tissues, with the formation of a large haematoma. Characteristically, in true haemophilia (factor VIII deficiency) and in Christmas disease (factor IX deficiency), the bleeding occurs into a joint cavity (haemarthrosis—see Chapter 38): the subsequent disability from intra-articular or periarticular fibrosis may be very great.

Most of the disorders of clotting are due to deficiency, either partial or complete, of one or other of the clotting factors (Fig. 8.8, page 447). In other cases, in which the defect is an acquired condition, substances may be present that interfere with the operation of these factors.

Congenital Deficiencies of the Coagulation Mechanism

Deficiency of factor VIII is by far the commonest of the inherited defects of coagulation. It occurs in two forms, classic haemophilia (haemophilia A) and von Willebrand's disease. There are about 3000 cases of haemophilia A in Britain and an unknown number of cases of von Willebrand's disease, the diagnostic criteria of which are not as clearly defined. Christmas disease (haemophilia B —factor IX deficiency) is next in frequency: some 300 cases are known in Britain. Congenital deficiencies of all the other known clotting factors have been described but are very rare.

Haemophilia A and Haemophilia B

Haemophilia A and haemophilia B are manifested as sex-linked recessive disorders—the responsible gene is located on the X chromosome and the abnormality is transmitted by the female and expressed in the male. Only in exceptionally rare instances are females overt haemophiliacs: this can arise when the patient is homozygous for the responsible gene, or lacks an X chromosome in the XO form of Turner's syndrome (see Chapter 26), or has the XY chromosome structure of testicular feminization (see Chapter 26). In a few instances the tendency to bleeding has been observed in heterozygous females;[193] occasionally, a haemophilia-like condition with an autosomal dominant inheritance has been found.[194]

The severity of the disease varies in any series of patients but tends to be fairly constant within each family. Usually only those individuals who have less than 1 per cent of the normal amount of factor VIII or factor IX activity suffer from spontaneous haemorrhage. The bleeding involves joints and

large groups of muscles, most frequently the knees and elbows and the muscles of the thighs. Spontaneous haemorrhage is unusual when the activity of factor VIII or factor IX is between 1 and 50 per cent of normal: in these cases the disease may be regarded as of moderate or mild degree.

Congenital Deficiency of Other Coagulation Factors

Congenital deficiency of other coagulation factors may cause disorders of clotting that are similar to the haemophilias but not sex-linked. For example, the *congenital form of fibrinogen deficiency* is inherited as an autosomal recessive character that affects the sexes equally. Spontaneous haemorrhages occur, but the bleeding is not as damaging as in haemophilia: as there can be no formation of fibrin a haemarthrosis resolves completely and the joint returns to its normal state.

Lack of factor XII (Hageman factor) hinders clotting of the blood *in vitro*, but does not appear to cause a bleeding disorder.

Von Willebrand's Disease

Von Willebrand's disease (see also page 495) is inherited as an autosomal dominant. In its severest form the plasma activity of factor VIII is low or absent and spontaneous haemarthrosis occurs. Irrespective of the severity of the disease, the bleeding time is prolonged and haemorrhage from mucous membranes is a conspicuous feature. It is possible that there is a link between the pathogenesis of von Willebrand's disease and that of classic haemophilia:[195] investigations with heterologous antibody to factor VIII show that the plasma of almost all patients with classic haemophilia contains a normal or increased amount of protein that is antigenically identical with factor VIII although functionally inert. In von Willebrand's disease the amount of this protein in the plasma is directly proportional to the factor VIII activity of the plasma. Even in its inert form this protein appears to be necessary for normal platelet and capillary function: its deficiency in von Willebrand's disease probably explains the prolongation of capillary bleeding in this condition (see page 495). The hypothesis is advanced that both normally functioning autosomes and the X chromosome are required for synthesis of active factor VIII. In von Willebrand's disease it is the autosomally determined substrate protein that is defective; in classic haemophilia this protein is produced normally but cannot be activated because of the abnormality of the X chromosome.

Treatment of Congenital Coagulation Deficiencies

These disorders can be treated effectively by the administration of fresh-frozen plasma or of a concentrated preparation of the clotting factor that is specifically deficient. Treatment should be begun as soon as possible after a haemorrhage develops. Factor VIII is the most difficult to supply in concentrated form, for it has a short life in the body, disappears quickly once blood has been shed, and is difficult to prepare as a freeze-dried concentrate.[196] Concentrates are still in relatively short supply, and a cryoprecipitate prepared from fresh-frozen plasma and rich in factor VIII and fibrinogen is the mainstay of treatment for classic haemophilia and for congenital (and acquired) deficiency of fibrinogen.

Most of the disability—particularly the crippling arthrosis—that formerly was so characteristic of these diseases can now be prevented by such treatment as is outlined above. Unfortunately, some 5 per cent of the patients develop inhibitors that rapidly neutralize infused factor VIII and factor IX; these inhibitors often make further substitution treatment ineffective, at least until a period of two months or so has passed. Rarely, a similar inhibitor or 'anticoagulant' may develop spontaneously following pregnancy, or as an accompaniment of rheumatoid arthritis, amyloidosis and possibly other conditions with an immunopathological basis.

Acquired Deficiencies of the Coagulation Mechanism

Coagulation factors II, V, VII, IX and X and fibrinogen are proteins formed in the parenchymal cells of the liver. The synthesis of some or all of them may be reduced in cases of liver disease.

Vitamin K Deficiency

Vitamin K is required for the production of the active forms of factors II, VII, IX and X. It is absorbed from the intestine, in part coming from the diet—especially green vegetables—and in part being synthetized by intestinal bacteria. Deficiency of vitamin K may account for a haemorrhagic tendency in association with malabsorption syndromes. In the newborn it may be induced by lack of the appropriate organisms in the intestinal flora.

Effects of Dicoumarol and Related Drugs

The orally administered anticoagulant drugs of the coumarin group block the action of vitamin K in the liver by competitive inhibition and thereby reduce the synthesis of factors II, VII, IX and X. Many drugs modify the anticoagulant action of the coumarin derivatives by affecting absorption of vitamin K, or by displacing the anticoagulant from its binding site on the serum albumin molecule, or by enhancing its metabolism by microsomal enzymes in the liver cells. If the anticoagulant action is excessive it can be reversed most rapidly by an infusion of fresh-frozen plasma. The administration of vitamin K is also effective but it takes up to 24 hours for the condition to be brought under control by this means.

Defibrination Syndromes and Excessive Fibrinolysis[197, 198]

Under physiological conditions the plasma coagulation and fibrinolytic systems are in equilibrium, fibrin being formed continuously and broken down continuously. A generalized acceleration of coagulation, often with secondary activation of fibrinolysis, is responsible for thrombotic and haemorrhagic manifestations in a wide variety of diseases. In its acute form this process is readily recognizable in the laboratory by the demonstration of a severe defect of coagulation, with a very low level of fibrinogen in the plasma (under 0·5 g/l: the normal range is 1·5 to 4 g/l). There may also be a marked reduction in the number of circulating platelets and in the level of many of the other coagulation factors in the blood. In such circumstances the outstanding clinical feature may be a haemorrhagic diathesis.

In the more chronic forms of these syndromes the body may be able to compensate fully for the increased consumption of the coagulation factors: their levels in the plasma, including that of fibrinogen, may then be normal or even increased. Clinical manifestations of failure of visceral function may result from the deposition of fibrin and active thrombosis in the vasculature of the kidneys, lungs or brain in cases of chronic disseminated intravascular coagulation.[199]

Acute defibrination may be initiated by such conditions as amniotic fluid embolism, severe intrapartum and post-partum uterine haemorrhage, septicaemia caused by Gram-negative bacteria, and incompatible blood transfusion. Chronic forms of defibrination occur in association with eclampsia, disseminated cancer, promyelocytic leukaemia (see page 484) and the respiratory distress syndrome of the newborn (hyaline membrane disease—see page 288).

Fibrinolysis.—A pathological degree of fibrinolysis is almost always secondary to intravascular fibrin deposition (disseminated intravascular coagulation —see above). The plasminogen that is absorbed in the widely dispersed fibrin is readily accessible to activating agents, and lysis follows. This has a beneficial effect in maintaining blood flow: ordinarily, therefore, no attempt should be made to inhibit the reaction. Rarely, excessive fibrinolysis follows intravascular coagulation. Occasionally, fibrinolysis is the primary process. Haemorrhage from this cause has been reported in cases of metastasizing prostatic carcinoma and of cirrhosis of the liver; it has also developed as a complication of operations that involve manipulation of the lungs. If the amount of plasmin formed exceeds the neutralizing capacity of the natural inhibitors that are ordinarily present in plasma, the excess will rapidly split and inactivate fibrinogen and many other proteins, including factor V and factor VIII. The effects of the loss of these coagulation factors are enhanced by the capacity of the split products of fibrinogen and fibrin to act as anticoagulants by blocking the conversion of fibrinogen to fibrin or by delaying polymerization of fibrin. In this situation, aminocaproic acid and other haemostatic drugs that directly or indirectly inhibit fibrinolysis may be helpful in controlling haemorrhage.

ABNORMALITIES OF THE PLASMA PROTEINS

Modern methods for the separation, characterization and analysis of the plasma proteins have demonstrated their great diversity. Many of them exist in more than one genetically determined form, or may be congenitally deficient—for instance, albumins, haptoglobulins, transferrins, lipoproteins and immunoglobulins.[200] The acquired changes in the plasma proteins in cases of myelomatosis have already been noted (see page 488). This section is concerned only with a consideration of other abnormalities of the immunoglobulins.

Macroglobulinaemia

Primary Macroglobulinaemia (Waldenström's Disease)

The clinical features of primary macroglobulinaemia, as originally described by Waldenström,[201]

whose name is now generally given to the condition, are lassitude, loss of weight, liability to infection, slight enlargement of the spleen and lymph nodes, and a very high erythrocyte sedimentation rate. Raynaud's phenomenon, a bleeding tendency and various bizarre neurological changes are among further clinical manifestations.

The disease is uncommon. It usually presents in the older age groups. The sexes are affected equally. The plasma may contain 30 to 100 grams of IgM macroglobulin per litre, an amount far in excess of the normal concentration, which is about 1·0 g/l. The protein is a polymer formed from five molecules of IgM monomer; its molecular weight is about 900 000. It may be identified specifically by ultracentrifugal analysis, immunoelectrophoresis and gel filtration. If a drop of serum containing excess IgM macroglobulin is added to distilled water, a heavy precipitate may form (Sia test): a positive result suggests the presence of abnormal protein but is not specific. The macroglobulin migrates very slowly during zonal electrophoresis; if it is present in a high concentration it may form a dense precipitate at the point of application.

Rouleau formation is a very marked feature in stained blood films and is accompanied by elevation of the erythrocyte sedimentation rate. The number of lymphocytes in the bone marrow is increased and cells that more or less closely resemble plasma cells are also present. The abnormal protein may interfere with the coagulation mechanism, with a consequential bleeding tendency.

Secondary Macroglobulinaemia

An increase in the amount of IgM macroglobulin in the serum may occur as a secondary phenomenon in cases of systemic lupus erythematosus, kala-azar, various liver diseases and toxoplasmosis. It is occasionally associated with neoplastic diseases, particularly lymphocytic lymphomas; the protein present in excess in these cases is not always a true IgM macroglobulin.

Occasionally, IgM monomer is synthetized in these cases rather than, or as well as, the polymer. Although antigenically similar to the polymer, monomeric IgM is of comparatively small molecular size and diffuses more rapidly through agar gels. As a result, estimation of IgM macroglobulin by immunodiffusion may give falsely high results if the monomer is present in significant amounts.

'Heavy Chain Disease'[202]

Several types of abnormal immunoglobulin molecule have been found in association with malignant disorders arising in the lymphoid tissues. In many instances these proteins have been demonstrated in the serum or urine and have proved to be immunoglobulin fragments that are antigenically related to the alpha, gamma or mu heavy chains of normal antibodies.

Alpha Heavy Chain Disease

The condition that is described as alpha heavy chain disease is probably the commonest of these three forms of paraproteinaemia. It is most frequently associated with the presence of a malignant lymphoma in the intestine; it may similarly be observed in association with a lymphoma of the respiratory tract or lungs.

Gamma Heavy Chain Disease

The lymphomas associated with gamma heavy chain disease usually present with lymphadenopathy, fever and anaemia. Hepatosplenomegaly develops during the course of the illness.

Mu Heavy Chain Disease

Abnormal protein related to mu heavy chains has been detected in the serum of a minority of patients with chronic lymphocytic leukaemia.

Cryoglobulinaemia[203]

The cryoglobulins are globulins that precipitate or gel when the plasma that contains them is cooled. Their composition and concentration vary widely from case to case. The most important types incorporate one or more immunoglobulins. Cryoglobulinaemia may be associated with macroglobulinaemia or occur independently. Sometimes it accompanies the disturbances of protein metabolism that characterize myelomatosis and the neoplastic diseases of the leucopoietic and lymphoreticular tissues. The concentration of the cryoglobulins in the plasma may vary from several milligrams to 50 grams or more per litre. The temperature at which they come out of solution differs considerably from case to case.

The main clinical interest of this form of paraprotein lies in the sensitivity of the patient to cold. If the blood is chilled by circulating through the hands and feet when these are cold, the cryoglobulin may gel within the finer vessels and obstruct them. As a result, ischaemia occurs: this takes the form of Raynaud's phenomenon, and may be associated with purpura of the affected parts. In the severest cases ulceration of the skin, and even gangrene, with the loss of fingers and toes, may result. The symptoms may occur even when the concentration of the abnormal protein in the plasma is as little as 0·3 g/l. Apart from the difference in the clinical picture, this condition may usually be distinguished from other forms of peripheral ischaemia by the observation of precipitation or gelation of the cryoglobulin when a specimen of plasma is cooled *in vitro*.

Hypogammaglobulinaemia[204]

Normally, plasma contains from 10 to 20 g of gammaglobulin per litre. Hypogammaglobulinaemia has been arbitrarily defined as a concentration of 2 g or less of gammaglobulin per litre—that is, a level of severe deficiency of IgG. Since the IgG fraction includes many important antibodies, patients with hypogammaglobulinaemia are liable to recurrent, severe infections, and these may at any time prove fatal. Usually, there is also a decrease in the amount of IgM and IgA in the plasma. The ABO isoagglutinins may be deficient or absent. Sometimes a relative increase in the IgM fraction may mask the deficiency of IgG.

Swiss Type of Hypogammaglobulinaemia[205]

Babies with the so-called Swiss type of hypogammaglobulinaemia lack immunoglobulins, are deficient in lymphocytes and plasma cells, and have impaired humoral and cellular immunity. They usually die of infection before reaching the age of two years; many die within a few weeks of birth. The condition is inherited as an autosomal recessive characteristic (see page 900).

Bruton Type of Hypogammaglobulinaemia[206]

This condition, which occurs only in males, is a form of congenital hypogammaglobulinaemia that usually becomes apparent at about the age of six months when the immunoglobulins that the baby acquired from his mother are exhausted. Humoral immunity is deficient, germinal centres and plasma cells being lacking; cellular immunity, mediated by T lymphocytes, is normal: in contrast to the Swiss type of hypogammaglobulinaemia, the thymus is not defective. There is a serious liability to infec-

106. Gray, C. H., in *Biochemical Disorders in Human Disease*, 3rd edn, edited by R. H. S. Thompson and I. D. P. Wootton, chap. 8. London, 1970.

107. Günther, H., *Dtsch. Arch. klin. Med.*, 1912, **105**, 89.

108. Magnus, I. A., Jarrett, A., Prankerd, T. A. J., Rimington, C., *Lancet*, 1961, **2**, 448.

109. Clark, K. G. A., Nicholson, D. C., *Clin. Sci.*, 1971, **41**, 363.

110. Heilmeyer, L., Clotten, R., *Dtsch. med. Wschr.*, 1964, **89**, 649.

111. Dameshek, W., Schwartz, S. O., Gross, S., *Amer. J. med. Sci.*, 1938, **196**, 769.

112. Tiggert, W. D., Duncan, C. N., *Amer. J. med. Sci.*, 1940, **200**, 173.

113. Caffey, J., *Amer. J. Roentgenol.*, 1951, **65**, 547.

114. Wiland, O. K., Smith, E. B., *Amer. J. clin. Path.*, 1956, **26**, 619.

115. Vaquez, L. H., *C.R. Soc. Biol. (Paris)*, 1892, **44**, 384.

116. Osler, W., *Amer. J. med. Sci.*, 1903, **126**, 187.

117. Guglielmo, G. di, *Boll. Soc. med.-chir.*, 1926, **1**, 665.

118. Brannon, E. S., Merrill, A. J., Warren, J. V., Stead, E. V., *J. clin. Invest.*, 1945, **24**, 232.

119. Lawrence, J. S., *Medicine (Baltimore)*, 1953, **32**, 323.

DISORDERS THAT AFFECT THE WHITE CELLS

120. Davidson, W. M., *Brit. med. Bull.*, 1961, **17**, 190.

121. Dameshek, W., Gunz, F., *Leukaemia*, 2nd edn. New York, 1964.

122. *Semin. Hemat.*, 1974, **11**, numbers 1 and 2.

123. Bennett, J. H., *Edinb. med. J.*, 1845, **64**, 413.

123a. Virchow, R., *Frorieps Notizen*, 1845, **36**, 151.

124. Hewitt, D., *Brit. J. prev. soc. Med.*, 1955, **9**, 81.

125. Englebreth-Holm, J., *Spontaneous and Experimental Leukaemias in Animals*. Edinburgh, 1942.

126. Gross, L., *Brit. med. J.*, 1958, **2**, 1.

127. Thiersch, J. B., *Cancer Res.*, 1946, **6**, 695.

128. Lanman, J. T., Bierman, H. R., Byron, R. L., *Blood*, 1950, **5**, 1099.

129. Fialkow, P. J., Thomas, E. D., Bryant, J. I., Neiman, P. E., *Lancet*, 1971, **1**, 251.

130. Macmahon, B., Levey, M. A., *New Engl. J. Med.*, 1964, **270**, 1082.

131. Zuelzer, W. W., Cox, D. E., *Semin. Hemat.*, 1969, **6**, 228.

132. Merrit, D. H., Harris, J. S., *A.M.A. J. Dis. Child.*, 1956, **92**, 41.

133. Fanconi, G., *Jb. Kinderheilk.*, 1927, **117**, 257.

134. Bloom, D., *A.M.A. Amer. J. Dis. Child.*, 1954, **88**, 754.

135. Louis-Bar, D., *Confin. neurol. (Basel)*, 1941–42, **4**, 32.

136. *Textbook of Paediatrics*, edited by J. O. Forfar and G. C. Arneil, page 899. Edinburgh and London, 1973.

137. Williams, W. J., Beutler, E., Erslev, A. J., Rundles, R. W., *Hematology*, page 708. New York, 1972.

138. March, H. C., *Amer. J. med. Sci.*, 1950, **220**, 282.

139. Court Brown, W. M., Doll, R., *Spec. Rep. Ser. med. Res. Coun. (Lond.)*, No. 295, 1957.

140. Oughterson, A. W., Warren, S., *Medical Effects of the Atomic Bomb in Japan*, page 279. New York, 1956.

141. Court Brown, W. M., Doll, R., *Proc. roy. Soc. Med.*, 1960, **53**, 761.

142. Oehme, J., Janssen, W., Hagitte, C., *Leukämie im Kindesalter*. Leipzig, 1958.

143. Hayhoe, F. G. J., Quaglino, D., Doll, R., *Spec. Rep. Ser. med. Res. Coun. (Lond.)*, No. 304, 1964.

144. Valentine, W. N., Lawrence, J. S., Pearce, M. L., Beck, W. S., *Blood*, 1960, **10**, 154.

145. Catovsky, D., Galton, D. A. G., Griffin, C., *Brit. J. Haemat.*, 1971, **21**, 661.

146. Hayhoe, F. G. J., Flemans, R. J., *An Atlas of Haematological Cytology*. London, 1969.

147. Wiernik, P. H., Serpick, A. A., *Blood*, 1970, **35**, 361.

148. Simone, J., *Semin. Hemat.*, 1974, **11**, 25.

149. Leidler, F., Russell, W. O., *Arch. Path. (Chic.)*, 1945, **40**, 14.

150. Hayhoe, F. G. J., *Leukaemia*, page 88. London, 1960.

151. Rowley, J. D., *Nature (Lond.)*, 1973, **243**, 290.

152. Elmlinger, P. J., Huff, R. L., Tobias, C. A., Lawrence, J. H., *Acta haemat. (Basel)*, 1953, **9**, 73.

153. Sandberg, A. A., Cartwright, G. E., Wintrobe, M. M., *Blood*, 1956, **11**, 154.

154. Jaffe, R. H., *Arch. Path. (Chic.)*, 1932, **14**, 117.

155. Braude, A. I., Feltes, J., Brooks, M., *J. clin. Invest.*, 1954, **33**, 1036.

156. Medical Research Council Working Party, *Brit. med. J.*, 1968, **1**, 201.

157. Catovsky, D., Galetto, J., Okos, A., Miliani, E., Galton, D. A. G., *J. clin. Path.*, 1974, **27**, 767.

158. Whitby, L. E. H., Britton, C. J. C., *Disorders of the Blood*, 9th edn, page 544. London, 1963.

159. Innes, J., Newall, J., *Proc. roy. Soc. Med.*, 1963, **56**, 648.

160. Hobbs, J. R., Corbett, A. A., *Brit. med. J.*, 1969, **1**, 412.

161. Putnam, F. W., *New Engl. J. Med.*, 1959, **261**, 902.

162. Osserman, E. F., *New Engl. J. Med.*, 1959, **261**, 952, 1006.

163. Evans, R. W., *Histological Appearances of Tumours*, 2nd edn, chap. 10. Edinburgh and London, 1966.

164. Gray, C. H., *Clinical Chemical Pathology*, 7th edn, chap. 6. London, 1974.

165. Solomon, A., McLaughlin, C. L., *Semin. Hemat.*, 1973, **10**, 3.

166. Martin, N. H., *Proc. roy. Soc. Med.*, 1964, **57**, 752.

167. Seligmann, M., Brouet, J. C., *Semin. Hemat.*, 1973, **10**, 163.

168. Crosbie, W. A., Lewis, M. L., Ramsay, I. D., Doyle, D., *Thorax*, 1972, **27**, 625.

169. Good, R. A., Bridges, R. A., Condie, R. N., *Bact. Rev.*, 1960, **24**, 115.

DISORDERS THAT AFFECT THE PLATELETS AND PURPURA

170. Wright, H. Payling, *J. Path. Bact.*, 1942, **54**, 461.

171. Flute, P. T., Kakkar, V. V., Renney, J. T. G., Nicolaides, A. N., in *Thromboembolism: Diagnosis and Treatment*, edited by V. V. Kakkar and A. J. Jouhar, page 2. Edinburgh and London, 1972.

172. Williams, W. J., Beutler, E., Erslev, A. J., Rundles, R. W., *Hematology*, part 4, sect. 10. New York, 1972.

173. Evans, R. S., Takahashi, K., Duane, R. T., Payne, R., Liu, C. K., *A.M.A. Arch. intern. Med.*, 1951, **87**, 48.

174. Harrington, W. J., Minnich, V., Hollingsworth, N. W., Moore, C. V., *J. Lab. clin. Med.*, 1951, **38**, 1.

175. Ackroyd, J. F., *Clin. Sci.*, 1954, **13**, 409.

175a. Moschcowitz, E., *Proc. N.Y. path. Soc.*, 1924, **24**, 21.

175b. Moschcowitz, E., *Arch. intern. Med.*, 1925, **36**, 89.

176. Symmers, W. St C., *Brain*, 1956, **79**, 511.

177. Bornstein, B., Bose, J. H., Casper, J., Behar, M., *J. clin. Path.*, 1960, **13**, 124.

178. Symmers, W. St C., *Lancet*, 1956, **1**, 592.
178a. Symmers, W. St C., in *XIV International Congress of Hematology, São Paulo, 1972—Lectures*, page 62. São Paulo, 1972.
179. Kasabach, H. H., Merritt, K. K., *Amer. J. Dis. Child.*, 1940, **59**, 1063.
180. Beller, F. K., Ruhrmann, G., *Klin. Wschr.*, 1959, **37**, 1078.
181. Inceman, S., Tangün, Y., *Amer. J. Med.*, 1969, **46**, 997.
182. Brain, M. C., *Semin. Hemat.*, 1969, **6**, 162.
183. Symmers, W. St C., *Brit. med. J.*, 1973, **2**, 614.
184. Willebrand, E. A. von, Jürgens, R., *Dtsch. Arch. klin. Med.*, 1933, **175**, 453.
185. Rizza, C. R., in *Human Blood Coagulation, Haemostasis and Thrombosis*, edited by R. Biggs, page 220. Oxford, London, Edinburgh and Melbourne, 1972.
186. Glanzmann, E., *Jb. Kinderheilk.*, 1918, **88**, 1.
187. Rendu, *Gaz. Hôp. (Paris)*, 1896, **69**, 1322.
188. Osler, W., *Johns Hopk. Hosp. Bull.*, 1901, **12**, 333.
189. Weber, F. P., *Lancet*, 1907, **2**, 160.
190. Schönlein, J. L., *Allgemeine und specielle Pathologie und Therapie*, vol. 2, page 48. Würzburg, 1832.
191. Henoch, E. H., *Berl. klin. Wschr.*, 1887, **24**, 8.

DISORDERS OF THE COAGULATION MECHANISM
192. *Human Blood Coagulation, Haemostasis and Thrombosis*, edited by R. Biggs. Oxford, London, Edinburgh and Melbourne, 1972.

193. Clark, K. G. A., *Lancet*, 1973, **1**, 1388.
194. Henson, A., Mattern, M. J., Loeliger, E. A., *Thrombos. Diathes. haemorrh. (Stuttg.)*, 1965, **14**, 341.
195. Bennett, B., Douglas, A. S., *Clin. Hemat.*, 1973, **2**, 14.
196. Wallace, J., *Clin. Hemat.*, 1973, **2**, 129.
197. McKay, D. G., *Proc. roy. Soc. Med.*, 1968, **61**, 1129.
198. Flute, P. T., *Progr. Surg. (Basel)*, 1971, **9**, 44.
199. Simpson, J. G., Stalker, A. L., *Clin. Hemat.*, 1973, **2**, 189.

ABNORMALITIES OF THE PLASMA PROTEINS
200. Giblett, E. R., *Genetic Markers in Human Blood*. Oxford and Edinburgh, 1969.
201. Waldenström, J., *Acta med. scand.*, 1944, **117**, 216.
202. Frangione, B., Franklin, E. C., *Semin. Hemat.*, 1973, **10**, 53.
203. Ritzman, S. E., Levin, W. C., *Arch. intern. Med.*, 1961, **107**, 754.
204. Seligmann, M., Fudenberg, H. H., Good, R. A., *Amer. J. Med.*, 1968, **45**, 817.
205. Glanzmann, E., Riniker, P., *Ann. paediat. (Basel)*, 1950, **175**, 1.
206. Bruton, O. C., *Pediatrics*, 1952, **9**, 722.
207. Gitlin, D., Janeway, C. A., Apt, L., Craig, J. M., in *Cellular and Humoral Aspects of the Hypersensitive State*, edited by H. S. Lawrence, page 375. New York, 1959.

ACKNOWLEDGEMENTS FOR ILLUSTRATIONS

Figs 8.12, 13. Reproduced by permission of the editor, Dr F. G. J. Hayhoe, and publishers, Cambridge University Press, from: Davidson, W. M., in *Lectures in Haematology*; Cambridge, 1960.

Fig. 8.17. Photomicrographs were provided by Professor H. A. Magnus, King's College Hospital Medical School, London.

Fig. 8.19. Preparation provided by Professor P. M. Daniel, Institute of Psychiatry and the Maudsley Hospital, London.

Fig. 8.27. Preparation by Dr L. Knight, Department of Haematology (Cytogenetics), King's College Hospital Medical School, London.

9: *The Lymphoreticular System*

by W. St C. Symmers

CONTENTS

9: *The Lymphoreticular System*

by W. St C. Symmers

INTRODUCTION

The *lymphoreticular system* consists of the lymphoid and reticuloendothelial tissues. These components of the lymphoreticular system are sometimes considered under separate headings as the lymphoid system and the reticuloendothelial system. This practice had some justification while the structural and functional criteria according to which the two systems were defined seemed so clearly different as to support the distinction. The anatomical definition of the lymphoid system reflected the view that most of its components could be regarded as organized in topographically distinct structures—lymph nodes, spleen, tonsils and lymphoid follicles of the alimentary mucosa. The characteristic distribution of the lesions of some important and frequent diseases that affect these lymphoid organs (particularly lymphomas, and involvement in the spread of tumours and infections) encouraged acceptance of the concept of the lymphoid tissues as constituting a well-defined system that did not include the reticuloendothelial cells. The latter were considered to form a system in their own right and the fact that elements of this system are situated within the tissues and organs of the lymphoid system was regarded as no more remarkable than the fact that elements of the reticuloendothelial system are found in the liver and many other situations apart from the lymphoid organs.

More recently, recognition of the interaction and interdependence of lymphoid and reticulo-endothelial cells in the essential immunological responses of the body has underlined the fact that the structural and functional congruity of the lymphoid and reticuloendothelial systems indicate that they form together an integral and inseparable system, the lymphoreticular system. The lymphoid and reticuloendothelial components of the lymphoreticular system have shared functions and comple-mentary functions, and functions that are peculiar to one or other component: understanding of the functional associations and of the independent functions (such as the role of the reticuloendothelial system in iron metabolism and in lipid metabolism) is an important key to understanding the pathology of the lymphoreticular system and of its component systems. Provided that it is recognized that the lymphoid and reticuloendothelial systems are integrated parts of a single system, it is useful to be able to distinguish them by these names.

The concept of the lymphoreticular system in the sense outlined here has been extended by some authorities to include the connective tissues of the body and the entire haemopoietic system, under the general designation *lymphomyeloid complex*.[1] This chapter is concerned mainly with the diseases that affect the lymphoid and reticuloendothelial tissues.

The *lymphoid system* consists of all the tissues that normally are composed predominantly of lymphocytes: its main parts are the lymph nodes, tonsillar tissue, intestinal lymphoid tissue, and the lymphoid tissue of the spleen and thymus gland. The *reticulo-endothelial system* is a much more widely dispersed system of large mononuclear cells that, among others, include the reticulum cells of the spleen, lymph nodes and bone marrow, and certain phagocytic endothelial cells in the sinuses of the lymph nodes and spleen and in the sinusoids of, for example, the liver. Reticuloendothelial cells, therefore, are an essential part of the structural organization of lymphoid tissue, wherever it occurs, and, although considerably less conspicuous, they are as important a constituent of it as the lymphocytes themselves. This histological intermingling of the lymphoid and reticuloendothelial systems is reflected

References to Other Chapters: A list of the chapters in each of the five volumes is on page v at the front of this volume.

506

in the large extent to which the two systems are functionally interdependent.

No other system is the subject of such misunderstanding and confusion as the lymphoreticular system. Its study in health and in disease continues to be obscured by lack of agreement on such fundamental matters as the terminology and definition of its component tissues and cells, the nature of its functions, and the classification of the diseases that affect it.

There have been great advances in knowledge of the cytology and functions of the lymphoreticular system since the corresponding chapter was written for the first edition of this book, more than a decade ago. These advances (see page 520) are largely due to the development and application of sophisticated immunological and cytological methods. They have led to notably better understanding of many forms of disease that arise in or otherwise involve the lymphoreticular system. During the same period—and complementary to, rather than directly following from, the progress in knowledge of normal structure and function—there has been much discussion of the natural history and classification of some of the diseases of the lymphoreticular system, notably the lymphomas (see page 777). The most carefully considered of these classifications may provide, perhaps for the first time, a reasonably reliable basis for clinical prognostication and possibly for therapeutic management. They have evolved during a time that has also brought further aetiologically important information—and some speculation—that perhaps can take us perceptibly closer to identifying the essential causes of some of these diseases.

The most fundamental advance has been the confirmation that lymphocytes are the key to the body's immune responses, a possibility that was suggested by Murphy, among others, as long ago as 1926[2] (see page 520). It has also become clear that lymphocytes are not at the end of a line of differentiating precursor cells but are themselves capable of further structural and functional differentiation. The former distinction between 'large' and 'small' lymphocytes has been reconsidered: new technical procedures have indicated that such simple morphological differences are not regularly related to differences in function or in cytogenesis, and that there are two morphologically congruous but functionally different varieties of lymphocyte, the T (thymus-dependent) lymphocytes and the B ('bursal') lymphocytes (see page 519).[3] Correspondingly, there is now much greater understanding of the nature and variety of immune response and of the

effects of deficiences in the functions that underlie the reactions involved (see Chapter 10, page 900).

LYMPHOID SYSTEM

Lymphoid tissue is remarkably labile, even in health, and there are considerable variations in its degree of development and evident activity at different ages and in different individuals. It reaches its greatest development early in the second decade and then regresses considerably, until—by the end of that decade—it has shrunk to its average adult extent; after middle age it undergoes further progressive atrophy, and in the elderly it is usually sparse. The lymphoid tissue throughout the body, together with the lymphocytes in the interstitial tissues, has been estimated to amount to about 1 per cent of the body weight of the healthy young adult.[4]

Until quite recently, lymphoid tissue has generally been regarded as occurring mainly in three or four situations. Three of these have been universally accepted—the lymph nodes, certain mucous membranes (particularly, the nasopharynx, the fauces and the back of the tongue, and the small intestine) and the spleen. The fourth situation is, of course, the thymus: in view of the almost unanimous agreement nowadays that lymphoid tissue is an essential component of the thymus (see page 899), it is interesting to recall the arguments that were still current only a decade or two ago about the identity of the cells in that gland that are now recognized to be lymphocytes. The lymphocytes in the thymus are still often referred to as thymocytes, a name much used in the past to indicate that they were thought to be peculiar to thymic tissue, although they were generally agreed not to be distinguishable from lymphocytes in appearance.

There is now recognized to be a fifth important topographical site of lymphoid tissue—the haemopoietic bone marrow. Bone marrow hitherto has tended to be considered as of relatively little importance in terms of its content of lymphoid tissue, the reason being that its haemopoietic activity, as the source of erythrocytes and of polymorphonuclear leucocytes, is so much more manifest than its role as a lymphoid organ. Now, however, it is generally agreed that the marrow is the source of the cells that eventually constitute both the T cell series and the B cell series of lymphocytes;[5] indeed, it seems that considerable numbers of lymphocytes are formed in bone marrow throughout life, although many of them are not released to migrate to other parts but die *in situ*, and so may be regarded, on present evidence, as 'ineffective'.

Lymphoid tissue, distributed among the situations just mentioned, may be separated into two categories—the primary (or central) lymphoid organs and the secondary (or peripheral) lymphoid organs (see below).[6] The essential functions of each of these categories of lymphoid organs are immunological, and the activity of each complements that of the other, with only a limited functional overlap.

Thymus-Dependent and Thymus-Independent ('Bursa-Equivalent'-Dependent) Immune Systems

Cell-mediated immunity accounts for delayed hypersensitivity reactions, resistance to infection by certain types of micro-organism, rejection of grafts, graft-against-host reactions, and manifestations of autoimmunity and of immunity to tumours: it is a function of the *cell-bound antibodies* that are attached to the surface of the T lymphocytes (see pages 520 and 521). The T lymphocytes (that is, the thymus-dependent lymphocytes) are categorically distinct from the B lymphocytes (the 'bursa-equivalent'-dependent lymphocytes), and the two varieties of lymphocyte reflect the functional differences between complementary but demonstrably distinct immune systems—the thymus-dependent system and the awkwardly named 'bursa-equivalent'-dependent (or 'bursa'-dependent, or thymus-independent) immune system. The 'bursa-equivalent'-dependent system is responsible for the synthesis of immunoglobulins and controls the formation of antibodies that circulate, free of cells, in the blood and tissue fluids (*humoral antibodies*).

Primary Lymphoid Organs (Central Lymphoid Organs)

The primary lymphoid organs are those in which lymphocyte precursors are prepared for the immunological function that will be imposed on them elsewhere in the body, particularly in the secondary lymphoid organs. The division of the lymphoid system into primary and secondary lymphoid organs and into thymus-dependent and thymus-independent systems is much more clearly defined in birds than in mammals. In the chicken, the primary lymphoid organs are the thymus gland and the cloacal bursa (bursa of Fabricius):[7] in man, as in other mammals, the primary lymphoid organs have not been defined with certainty, but they are probably the thymus and whatever may prove to be the equivalent of the bursal lymphoid tissue of birds. The cloacal bursa,

which is peculiar to birds, has no evident anatomical homologue in mammals: its equivalent, in man, may be the lymphoid tissue of the gastrointestinal mucosa (the so-called 'gut-associated' lymphoid tissue) or that of the bone marrow (see below).

The primary lymphoid organs have several distinct characteristics. They appear early during embryonic development and they involute as adult life approaches. Their cells are derived from stem cells that have reached them from elsewhere (see page 434). They are an important source of lymphocytes, and their output of these cells is controlled by an intrinsic lymphopoietic mechanism. They also control lymphopoiesis in the secondary lymphoid organs (see below). They show little or no evidence—such as the presence of plasma cells and the formation of germinal centres—that they are themselves the site of any immune response. However, their extirpation or aplasia results in specific immunological defects in consequence of lack of the humoral (hormonal) factors that normally they produce.

Thymus

The thymus (see Chapter 10) is the major primary lymphoid organ in mammals. While it is likely that much still remains to be discovered about its other functions, there is at last general agreement that it is a lymphoid organ as well. Superseded views, and uncertainty about functional interpretation, have a memento in the still common practice of referring to the lymphocytes in the thymus as thymocytes (see above).

Lymphocytes are first seen in the human thymus in the ninth week of embryonic development; this is in contrast to the observation that they do not appear in the lymph nodes and spleen until the twelfth week.[8] The thymic lymphocytes are now believed to develop from stem cells that have migrated to the gland from bone marrow,[9] differentiating among the thymic epithelial cells (but not arising from these cells,[10] as formerly was thought). The thymus continues to be the most active site of lymphopoiesis in the body for some time after birth, the mitotic rate of its lymphoid cells being up to ten times that in the peripheral lymphoid tissues:[11] this activity seems to depend on some function of the thymic epithelium and not to be related to an immunological stimulus.[12] Most of the lymphocytes that are formed in the thymus have a short life span[13] and die in the gland;[14] the long-lived minority provides most of the cells that migrate to the secondary (peripheral) lymphoid organs during fetal and early postnatal life, and possibly over a longer period.[15] It is important to note that not all lymphocytes that are thymus-dependent are derived from the thymus: thymus-dependent cells may originate in other lymphoid tissues, while sharing with thymus-derived cells the exposure to thymic influence.

The lymphocytes that are produced in the thymus, and those that are formed elsewhere from lymphoid cells derived from the thymus, are the T lymphocytes. They are concerned in cell-mediated immunity mainly, but they also collaborate with B lympho-cytes in the development of humoral antibody to certain antigens. The cell-bound antibody of the T lymphocytes characterizes cell-mediated immunity; their selective clonal expansion, induced by antigen,[16] and possible qualitative changes that result from priming with antigen, reflect the 'memory' function of these cells and their eventual specific responsiveness to a repeated exposure of the body to an antigen that has already sensitized it.

Bone Marrow

Lymphocytes are present in large numbers in bone marrow, mainly in those parts where there is active haemopoiesis. They are distributed both singly and in small follicular aggregates. Their production appears to be independent of the activity of the thymus and of the lymph nodes and to require no antigenic stimulus. The proportion of the lympho-cytes produced in bone marrow that die there is very large, and lymphopoiesis in the marrow is to this extent ineffective (see page 507); the survivors migrate, settling in the spleen and lymph nodes, in the fauciopharyngeal and intestinal lymphoid aggregates, and in the thymus. When chromosom-ally marked lymphoid cells from bone marrow are injected into mice that have been deprived of their own lymphoid cells by irradiation, the marked cells colonize and grow in the thymus as well as in the secondary lymphoid organs; in contrast, if the marked cells are from the thymus or lymph nodes, or from lymph obtained from the thoracic duct, they can be demonstrated in the thymus only rarely, although they readily colonize the lymph nodes and spleen.[10] This indicates that lymphoid cells from bone marrow, but not other lymphoid cells, are the precursors of the thymus-dependent lymphocytes (T cells). The thymus-independent lymphocytes (B cells) probably also originate in bone marrow: experimental evidence for this has been provided by reconstituting the lymphoid cell complement of irradiated animals with marked cells of thymic origin and of marrow origin, when it is found that the thymus-independent antibody-forming cells (B cells) are all of marrow origin.[17]

There is good reason for considering the bone marrow to be a primary lymphoid organ as defined above. Whether it is the equivalent of the bursa of Fabricius of birds is still far from clear (see below).

The Bursa of Fabricius and Its Possible Analogues

The cloacal bursa, or bursa of Fabricius, is an anatomical structure peculiar to birds. Embryo-logically, it is the second lymphoid organ to appear, its development beginning shortly after that of the thymus: like the latter, it is a primary lymphoid organ (see above). The lymphoid cells that differen-tiate within its epithelial follicles are now recognized to develop from immigrant stem cells, probably of yolk sac origin, and not from the epithelial ele-ments.[18, 19]

The bursal lymphocytes are independent of thymic control. They are responsible for the development of the humoral antibody system and they have no part in cell-mediated immunity, which is dependent on lymphocytes of thymic origin. In contrast to thymic lymphocytes, bursal lympho-cytes do not migrate to the secondary (peripheral) lymphoid organs.

There is controversy about the mammalian equivalents of the bursal lymphoid tissue of birds. It is pertinent to the question whether there is a bursal analogue in man that cloacal bursectomy in chickens causes a disturbance of immune response characterized by practically total absence of immunoglobulin from the serum while cell-mediated immune function remains intact: this disorder corresponds to the Bruton-type of hypogamma-globulinaemia in man (see page 902). The observa-tion that the production of humoral antibody is impaired in rabbits from which the entire alimentary lymphoid tissue has been removed suggested that this 'gut-associated' lymphoid tissue is the analogue of the bursal lymphoid tissue.[20] This and similar[21] experimental findings encouraged a belief that the gastrointestinal lymphoid tissue of other mammals, including man, may be the equivalent of the bursal lymphoid tissue of birds. However, there are observations that discredit this view, indicating that the gastrointestinal lymphoid tissue of mammals has the characteristics of a secondary lymphoid organ (see above): these include, for instance, the lack of pronounced development of the intestinal lymphoid tissue at birth, its positive response to antigenic stimulation, and the fact that when labelled lymphocytes are infused into the blood stream they accumulate in Peyer's patches as they do in lymph nodes and other indisputably 'secondary' lymphoid organs.[22] It is possible that the lymphoid tissue of the alimentary tract is not homogeneous in derivation and function but associates characteristics of both primary and secondary lymphoid organs in an anatomically indivisible complex (see page 1054). An alternative bursal equivalent is the lymphoid tissue of bone marrow, which, as has been noted above, behaves as a primary lymphoid organ.

It is a terminological misfortune that the B lymphocytes (see page 519) have come to be generally so named in mammals, as in birds, although the 'B' that signifies that these cells in birds are derived from (or dependent on) the lymphoid tissue of the bursa of Fabricius is less than appropriate in the context of mammalian biology.

Secondary Lymphoid Organs (Peripheral Lymphoid Organs)

The secondary lymphoid organs—also known, ambiguously, as the peripheral lymphoid organs—are the lymph nodes and spleen, the lymphoid tissue of the fauciopharyngeal ring, including the tonsils, the lymphoid tissue of the mucosa of the stomach and intestines (the so-called 'gut-associated' lymphoid tissue), and some subsidiary foci. It must be noted that the gastrointestinal lymphoid tissue is regarded by some as one of the primary lymphoid organs, by others as sharing functions that elsewhere are confined to either primary or secondary lymphoid organs, and by still others as a purely secondary lymphoid organ (see above). Such differences in interpretation illustrate again the uncertainty about the functions of the various anatomical divisions of the lymphoid tissues in different species, and particularly in man.

Aschoff,[23] and later Ehrich,[24] pointed out the significant differences in the lymphatic connexions of the lymphoid tissue in the structures that now are regarded as the secondary lymphoid organs. The *lymph nodes* are distributed, usually in groups, as filters on the lymphatic pathways between the tissue spaces and the blood stream, and they are provided with afferent and efferent lymphatic vessels. Some lymph nodes are bypassed by lymphatics that course directly to proximal groups. The *splenic lymphoid tissue*, in contrast, while in intimate contact with the blood circulating through the splenic vasculature into the pulp (see page 720), has no lymphatic connexions: indeed, there is no evidence that there are any lymphatics in the pulp of the spleen in man, although there may be some in the trabeculae and capsule. *Mucosal lymphoid tissue*, specifically that of the pharynx and alimentary tract, is drained by lymphatics but has no afferent vessels, being unencapsulate and in free contact with the fluid in the interstitial tissue spaces of the mucous membrane and of the submucosal planes.

Subsidiary foci of lymphoid tissue occur in many parts of the body. They may be no more than aggregates of lymphocytes, without follicle formation, or follicles may be conspicuous. It is debatable whether such foci may be regarded as normal, for a sharp line cannot be drawn between what is normal and what is a pathological degree of lymphocytic aggregation and follicle development. For instance, while lymphocytes are a normal, and important, constituent of healthy haemopoietic marrow (see above), it is doubtful whether lymphoid follicles are ever present in marrow except in pathological states.[25] The same is true of various other tissues, including the stomach, the bronchi and peribronchial connective tissue, and the thyroid gland.

Some functional characteristics of the main secondary lymphoid organs are considered in the following paragraphs.

Lymph Nodes

Until quite recently, the conventional anatomical view of the structure of the lymph nodes presented them simply as filters interrupting the lines of lymph drainage. This interpretation, supported by certain types of pathological change in nodes, such as their infiltration by carcinoma and the development in them of infective lesions following invasion by micro-organisms carried in the afferent lymphatics, led too often to their function being likened simply to that of any inert filter, without regard to the vital activities of their constituent cells. The nodes were seen as encapsulate structures interrupting the lymph flow at anatomically convenient sites, entered through their capsular surface by afferent lymphatics and drained through their hilum by efferent lymphatics. Their substance was recognized to be divided into a cortical region and a medullary region (Fig. 9.1). The cortex was characterized by the presence of lymphoid follicles, usually with germinal centres, and these were considered to be the source of lymphocytes; the medulla was defined as devoid of follicles, consisting instead of uniformly distributed, closely packed lymphocytes that occupy the centre of the node, including the hilar region, and that extend outward to merge with the lymphocytes situated between the cortical follicles. The lymph sinuses in the node, immediately deep to its capsule and extending everywhere between the lymphoid tissue and the radially disposed fibrous trabeculae

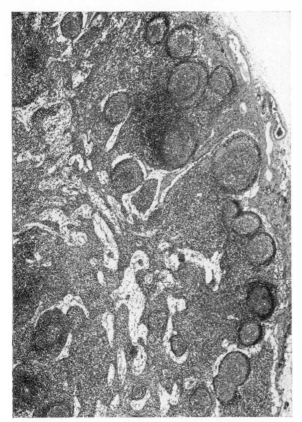

Fig. 9.1. 'Normal' mesenteric lymph node. The node was included in tissue excised during an emergency laparotomy in the case of a previously healthy man, aged 30 years, who had received an accidental penetrating wound of the small bowel one hour earlier, necessitating resection of a length of bowel with its mesenteric attachment. The sinuses in the central part of the node are wide. The follicles occupy a relatively small part of the organ. They vary in size and consist of a pale centre and narrow, dark, mantle zone that is more or less sharply defined from the adjoining tissues. In this specimen the mantle consists of small, deeply stained lymphocytes. The plane of the section includes several follicles from the region of the cortex on the other side of the node (below, left) as well as those under the capsule at the right. The circumstances in which the specimen was obtained suggest that the picture is consistent with 'normal' structure. See also Figs 9.2, 9.3 and 9.33. *Haematoxylin–eosin.* × 25.

from various advances in knowledge. There is now an understanding of the functional association between certain anatomical regions in the nodes and the primary lymphoid organs (specifically, the thymus gland and the 'bursa-equivalent' lymphoid tissue). A further factor that has clarified the role of lymph nodes is recognition of the immunological functions of lymphoid tissue and, in particular, the significance in this context of the formation of germinal centres in lymphoid follicles (see below). Thus, the cortex of lymph nodes is now considered to comprise two zones, a 'bursa-equivalent'-dependent superficial zone (the 'superficial cortex') and a thymus-dependent deeper zone (the paracortical region, paracortex or 'deep cortex').[26] Further, the development of lymphoid follicles, which topographically are related to both zones of the cortex of lymph nodes, is now believed to follow antigenic stimulation, for these distinctive aggregates of lymphoid tissue are absent or, at most, rudimentary in animals raised under microbiologically sterile and otherwise antigen-free conditions.[27]

The paracortical region of the lymph nodes is provided with specialized postcapillary venules that are lined by tall endothelial cells. Lymphocytes in the blood are believed to pass into the substance of the nodes mainly through the wall of these venules, insinuating themselves between the tall endothelial cells. Once past this vascular boundary, the lymphocytes migrate selectively to the thymus-dependent and 'bursa-equivalent'-dependent parts of the node, according to their identity as T cells and B cells respectively.

Some of these observations may be referred to in more detail: broadly topographical aspects will be considered now, the cytological aspects being discussed later (page 516).

Thymus-Dependent Region of Lymph Nodes.—It has been shown experimentally that certain parts of the lymph nodes are dependent on the presence of the thymus gland. These parts become depleted of lymphocytes after thymectomy; their lymphocyte content is then restored following an open thymic graft or implantation of thymic tissue enclosed in a diffusion chamber that is impermeable to cells, an observation indicating that the production of the lymphocytes that migrate to such thymus-dependent regions requires some diffusible substance that normally is elaborated in the thymus.[28] The cells involved in this sequence of depletion and restoration are T lymphocytes (see page 519). The thymus-dependent region of the lymph nodes forms the 'deep cortex', or paracortical region.[29] The corres-

that traverse the organ from capsule to hilum, were noted to be richly provided with reticuloendothelial cells: these, however, were seen merely as phagocytes, there for the purpose of extracting potentially harmful material, animate or inanimate, from the passing lymph, but not yet recognized to have an important role in the development of immunity.

The current change in the interpretation of the structure and functions of lymph nodes has resulted

ponding region of the spleen is the periarteriolar sheath (see page 515) and that of the gastrointestinal lymphoid tissue is the interfollicular zone (see page 516).

'Bursa-Equivalent'-Dependent (Thymus-Independent) Regions of Lymph Nodes.—The parts of the lymphoid tissue that are not thymus-dependent, in the sense outlined in the previous paragraph, are described as thymus-independent or, alternatively, as 'bursa-dependent' or 'bursa-equivalent'-dependent (the latter being preferable, as the primary site, or sites, of maturation of B lymphocytes, corresponding to the cloacal bursa of Fabricius in birds, has not been identified in mammals). The 'bursa-equivalent'-dependent parts of the lymph nodes comprise the superficial zone of the cortex, the medullary tissue ('medullary cords') and the follicles. The lymphocytes that constitute these parts are characteristically B cells (see page 519). Some T cells are identifiable also, particularly in the germinal centres:[30] this is one of several indications that the different types of lymphoid tissue merge and overlap within the limits of single lymphoid organs, and, indeed, in the lymphoid system in general. It must be recognized that the thymus-dependent and 'bursa-equivalent'-dependent parts do not have defined boundaries, and that the cells proper to either compartment are migrant in character and commonly traverse both compartments.

Lymphoid Follicles.—The fully developed lymphoid follicle consists of the germinal centre (Flemming centre) and one or more, more or less distinct, mantle zones, usually merging through a definable periphery with the adjoining lymphoid tissue (Figs 9.2 and 9.3). The cellular constitution of the germinal centre is quite different from that of the mantle (see below). The presence of lymphoid follicles is morphological evidence of antigenic stimulation and the consequent immune reaction. This is so whether the follicles are in lymphoid tissue proper or have formed in other tissues in the course of longstanding inflammation. Most protein antigens induce lymphoblastic transformation of lymphocytes in the paracortical region of the lymph nodes (see page 522), and this is followed by an increase in mitotic activity. In this context it is important to note that the designation lymphoblast is ambiguous, in that this term has commonly been applied in the past to a lymphoid cell, larger than the mature lymphocyte, and supposedly the precursor of the latter: the term is still widely used in this sense in relation to the tumour cells of acute lymphoid

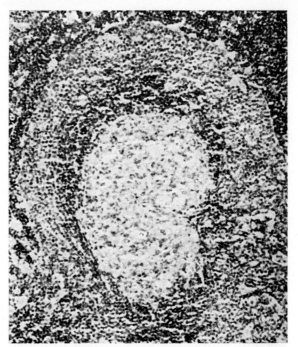

Fig. 9.2. Lymphoid follicle in a lymph node. The pale germinal centre (Flemming centre) consists of four types of cell: lymphocytes with cloven nucleus (see Fig. 9.5), immunoblasts (see Fig. 9.6), macrophages (see Fig. 9.4) and dendritic reticular cells (see text). It is surrounded by a zone of small lymphocytes that merges into an outer zone of larger, paler lymphocytes. These two zones form the mantles of the follicle; they are thicker on the aspect nearer the capsule of the node. Outside the mantles are the small lymphocytes of the interfollicular lymphoid tissue of the node. See also Fig. 9.3. *Haematoxylin–eosin.* × 150.

leukaemia and of some lymphomas (see footnote on page 522). *'Lymphoblastic transformation' (immunoblastic transformation)* in response to antigenic stimulation is a change in the character of the lymphocytes, both T cells[31] and B cells,[32] related to the production of antibodies and characterized by enlargement of the cells and pyroninophilia of their cytoplasm (see page 522): some of the transformed cells migrate into the medulla of the node in which they are situated and eventually reach the efferent lymph stream. The formation of follicles is a somewhat later event.

Mitotic activity is conspicuous in the germinal centres, but this represents a lymphopoiesis that is largely ineffectual, most of the new cells dying *in situ*. The proliferative activity and the short survival of the resulting cells account for the abundance of nuclear debris in the form of intensely haematoxyphile particles (Flemming's *'stainable bodies'*) in

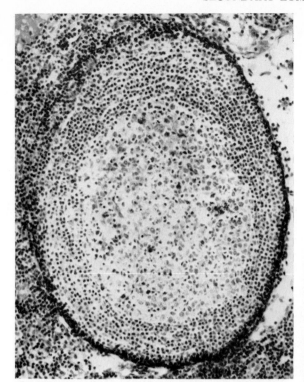

Fig. 9.3. Lymphoid follicle in a lymph node (compare with Fig. 9.2). This follicle shows a different normal pattern. The inner mantle in this instance consists of large lymphocytes with a considerable admixture of small lymphocytes, and the outer mantle is narrow, sharply outlined and formed of small lymphocytes. *Haematoxylin–eosin.* × 150.

the cytoplasm of macrophages in the follicles, particularly in the germinal centres themselves (Fig. 9.4). This evidence of the death and disintegration of lymphocytes in the central part of the follicles accounts for the view, now seldom accepted, that this region is a 'reaction centre',[33] a site for destruction of cells, rather than a 'germinal centre', as Flemming saw it,[34] where lymphopoiesis is also active.

The large lymphocytes of the germinal centres differ from lymphocytes of comparable size elsewhere—for instance, in the blood—in having a notched, or cloven ('cleaved'), nucleus (see page 517) (Fig. 9.5). They are believed to be precursors of the larger cells of the germinal centres, which are similar to, and probably identical with, the pyroninophile lymphoblasts (immunoblasts) mentioned above, and which, like the latter, produce antibodies.[35] The immunoblasts have a rounded, uncloven nucleus that contains one or more distinct nucleoli, and they have more cytoplasm than the cells with cloven nucleus (Figs 9.6A, 9.6B and 9.6.C).

The lymphocytes of the outer zone, or mantle, of the follicles proliferate more slowly than those of the germinal centres and are no longer regarded as derived from the centres;[36] like the lymphocytes of the germinal centres they are B lymphocytes, and they may be precursors of the plasma cells that elaborate humoral antibodies—for instance, as the response to immune stimulation by polysaccharide antigens (see page 522). [22, 37] The plasma cells that have this function are found in the medulla of the nodes during the period of reaction to the antigens.[38] In contrast to the humoral antibodies, the antibodies that are involved in cell-mediated immune reactions —for example, delayed hypersensitivity reactions

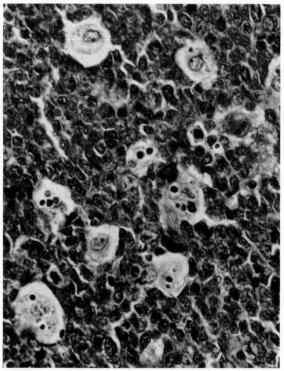

Fig. 9.4. Part of a large germinal centre in a lymphoid follicle in a lymph node. Flemming's 'stainable bodies' (*tingible Körperchen*) are seen in several of the macrophages (the large, pale cells). They are small, round or ovoid structures in the cytoplasm, most of them intensely haematoxyphile and some apparently surrounded by a narrow, pale halo (the halo may be a fixation artefact). Their appearances may lead them to be mistaken for intracellular parasites, particularly histoplasmas and leishmaniae (see Figs 9.94, 9.121B and 9.123): the possibility of such confusion is increased by the facts that Flemming's bodies are often Gram-positive and that their periodic-acid/Schiff reaction may be positive. They give an intense Feulgen reaction for deoxyribonucleic acid, and this helps to distinguish them from the parasites. They are believed to be debris of the nuclei of dead cells. *Haematoxylin–eosin.* × 500.

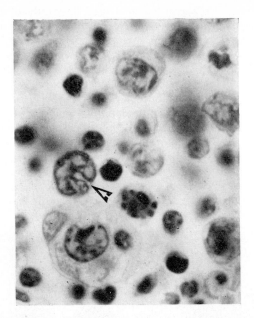

them from other reticulum cells and invalidates their designation as macrophages. Their role is evidently to take up antigen on their surface ('antigen-retaining reticular cell' is yet another of their synonyms). They are in intimate contact with lymphocytes and with the immunoblast derivatives of lymphocytes: these become enmeshed among their dendritic processes, and speculation suggests that the association is concerned with sensitization of lymphocytes, with their maturation in relation to specific antigenic stimuli, and possibly with the development of 'memory' cells (see page 520). In spite of the view that they are not phagocytic, the 'dendritic reticular cells' are generally considered to be a specialized line of cells that, while distinct from the macrophages, belong to the same cell system.

Fig. 9.5. Part of a germinal centre in a lymph node that showed well-marked simple follicular hyperplasia (see page 553). The arrow points along the line of a cleft in the nucleus of a large lymphocyte of the type that is peculiar to germinal centres (the cloven nucleus lymphocyte, or 'cleaved nucleus' cell). These cells are difficult to demonstrate photographically: use of the fine magnification adjustment showed that two of the other four cells of comparable size in this field also showed notching (cleaving) of the nucleus, although this is not evident in the plane of focus illustrated. The other large cells have conspicuous nucleoli and proportionately more cytoplasm, and their nucleus is uncloven: they are immunoblasts. The field also includes some cells in mitosis, macrophages containing indistinctly focused Flemming bodies (see Fig. 9.4), and a number of small lymphocytes (some of which have a notched nucleus, although this is not apparent in the photograph). *Haematoxylin–eosin.* × 1200.

(see page 521)—are formed by T lymphocytes, mainly in the thymus-dependent (paracortical) region of the nodes.

The association of lymphoid cells and reticuloendothelial cells is an essential in the course of the reaction to antigens. It is now recognized that the fully developed lymphoid follicle includes a zone on one aspect of the germinal centre in which there is a concentration of large mononuclear cells (reticulum cells) that are characterized by numerous, well-developed, dendriform, cytoplasmic extensions that intermesh with the corresponding processes of adjacent cells of the same type.[39-41] These cells have acquired many names—'*dendritic reticular cell*' is the term that currently is most frequently used (they are also known as dendritic macrophages and dendritic reticulum cells). They are commonly said not to be phagocytic: if this is so it distinguishes

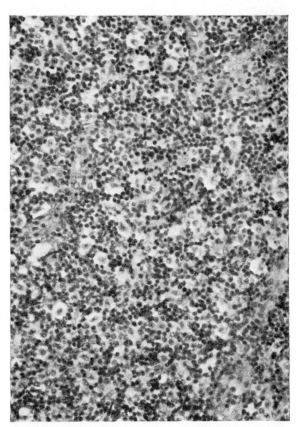

Fig. 9.6A. 'Immunoblasts' (transformed lymphocytes)—the large, pale cells among the small lymphocytes. In this instance, a case of 'immunoblastic lymphadenopathy' (see Fig. 9.153, page 704), the immunoblasts are distributed evenly and for the most part lie singly. Formerly, they would have been regarded as reticulum cells or as histiocytes. See also Figs 9.6B and 9.6C. *Haematoxylin–eosin.* × 160.

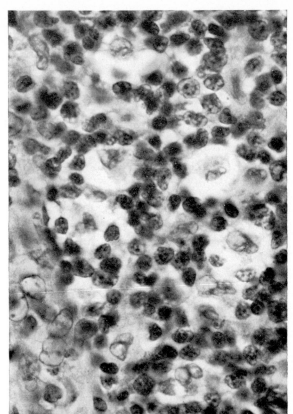

Fig. 9.6B. Higher magnification of a part of the field illustrated in Fig. 9.6A. Fixation artefact often results in shrinkage of the cytoplasm of immunoblasts, so that the nucleus appears to be enclosed by only a little, indistinct cytoplasm, a clear space of variable extent separating the latter from the cells in the vicinity. Similarly, the nucleus itself is liable to be distorted. Other immunoblasts in the same field may, as here, retain their characteristically opaque cytoplasm, which, in Unna–Pappenheim preparations, would show more or less marked pyroninophilia, because of their content of ribonucleic acid. *Haematoxylin–eosin.* × 630.

Spleen

The structure of the spleen is considered on page 719. The organ-dependence and functions of splenic lymphoid tissue are comparable to those of lymph nodes (see above). This tissue is disposed as a cellular sheath round the splenic arterioles (periarteriolar lymphoid sheath); numerous follicular aggregates (the splenic follicles, or Malpighian bodies) abut on and are in continuity with the sheath. The periarteriolar sheath is the thymus-dependent part of the splenic lymphoid tissue; the germinal centres and the lymphocytes surrounding them are essentially 'bursa-equivalent'-dependent. The immune reaction to most antigens, particularly protein antigens, is accompanied by proliferation of the lympho-

cytes in the periarteriolar sheath; its occurrence requires the presence of immunocompetent lymphocytes (see page 520), which reach the spleen in the blood and enter its pulp through the wall of the arterioles.[42] As in lymphoid tissue elsewhere, the dendritic reticular cells of the germinal centres (see above) are involved in the development of immune reactions.

Fauciopharyngeal Lymphoid Tissue

The important aggregates of lymphoid tissue in the mucosa and submucosa of the pharynx that collectively are known as Waldeyer's ring (see pages 238 and 990) are generally regarded as constituting one of the secondary lymphoid organs. Some authorities include this tissue, of which the palatine tonsils (faucial tonsils) are the largest part, with the gastrointestinal lymphoid tissue under the heading

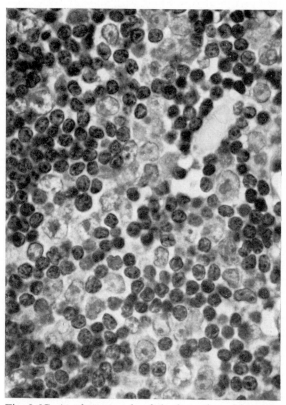

Fig. 9.6C. Another example of the formation of immunoblasts. In this instance, a case of persistent lymphadenitis following vaccination against smallpox, the immunoblasts are clustered and have been less affected by histological artefact (compare with Fig. 9.6B). Their cytoplasm was markedly pyroninophile. See also Figs 9.112A and 9.112B, pages 645 and 646. *Haematoxylin–eosin.* × 630.

of lymphoid tissue of the alimentary tract, or 'gut-associated' lymphoid tissue (see below).

Gastrointestinal Lymphoid Tissue ('Gut-Associated' Lymphoid Tissue)

The stomach normally has only a small component of lymphoid tissue: this includes a few solitary follicles, like those of the intestine, and a sparse scattering of lymphocytes elsewhere in the mucous membrane. In contrast, the intestines have abundant, well-developed lymphoid tissue: this comprises the macroscopically evident solitary lymphoid follicles* and aggregated follicles* (Peyer's patches) and the large concentration of lymphoid tissue that is a characteristic of the vermiform appendix. In addition, there is the much more variable component formed by the lymphocytes that lie free in the interstitial space of the lamina propria of the intestinal mucosa. The interfollicular lymphocytes in the macroscopical collections of lymphoid tissue and the free-lying lymphocytes in the mucosa are thymus-dependent; the lymphocytes of the follicles themselves, like those in lymphoid follicles elsewhere in the body, are 'bursa-equivalent'-dependent.

Particular interest has centred on the gastrointestinal lymphoid tissue as a result of speculation whether it, or, rather, part of it, such as Peyer's patches, is a primary lymphoid organ and, in fact, the mammalian equivalent of the lymphoid tissue of the cloacal bursa of birds (see page 509). The current view seems to be that it is not the equivalent of the bursal lymphoid tissue, because, for example, the depression of antibody response following extensive removal of the intestinal lymphoid tissue in mammals is slight, and not at all comparable to that in birds after bursectomy. Further, direct exposure of the intestinal lymphoid tissue to antigens causes germinal centres to form, with much accompanying mitotic activity, whereas exposure of primary lymphoid organs, such as the cloacal bursa and the thymus, to antigen has no such consequences.[43] More cogent still, because it demonstrates a response that is uniformly distributed, not confined to parts only of the widespread and topographically heterogeneous lymphoid tissue of the small intestine, is that lymphocytes that have been collected by cannulation of the thoracic duct, and then specifically marked, and injected into the blood stream, accumulate in Peyer's patches as they do in the lymph nodes and vermiform appendix.[22]

* The so-called 'lymphatic' follicles of the International Anatomical Nomenclature Committee (*Nomina Anatomica*, 1966).

Lymphocytes[44, 45]

Lymphocytes, because there is no manifestation of their function that is strikingly evident to the microscopist (in contrast to the readily visible presence of bacteria in the cytoplasm that indicates the phagocytic activity of neutrophile polymorphonuclear leucocytes), remained of only conjectural importance until the development of sophisticated immunological methods of investigation began to disclose their essential role. These advances have been made largely since the recognition, as recently as 1945, that lymphocytes are involved in immune responses,[27] and the definition, in 1958, of 'immunological competence'—the capacity to react to antigens—as the most significant lymphocytic function.[46] Lymphocytes are now regarded as the key component of the body's immune system, responsible for both cell-mediated and humoral immune responses. At the same time, it has been recognized that they are not 'end-cells' but capable of proliferation and of differentiation: lymphocytes from animals sensitive to a wide range of antigens proliferate *in vitro* when exposed to these antigens;[47] and lymphocytes may be stimulated by non-specific mitogens—classically, the phytohaemagglutinin obtained from the red kidney bean—both to proliferate and to differentiate into large 'blast' cells (immunoblasts, lymphoblasts—see page 522)[48] and sometimes into plasma cells.[22] The various types of lymphocytes, the derivative 'blast' cells and the plasma cells are commonly referred to as the 'lymphoid cells'.

Morphology

The former practice of distinguishing 'large' and 'small' lymphocytes had no real significance while there was no understanding of the function of this series of cells. Moreover, the distinction took no account of the fact that the variation in size from the smallest lymphocytes to the largest was continuous: attempts to categorize the cells on the basis of their size were arbitrary and, so long as a functional correlation was lacking, correspondingly pointless. It is now recognized that the size of lymphocytes—for instance, in blood—is related to certain other characteristics, particularly their life span. In general, however, it has become evident, as the functions of lymphocytes have become known, that morphological differences that are determinable by light microscopy, dimensional differences particularly, are a very inadequate index of functional differences. The latter relate mainly to types of immune activity that differ according to the organ-dependence of the lymphocytes (T cells and B cells—see below). The cells that subserve the fundamentally divergent, but complementary, immune functions can be distinguished by many features, but not by their size or by other aspects of their appearance under the light microscope. The distinguishing features include the presence or absence of cell-specific surface antigens,[49] complement receptors[50] and immunoglobulin receptors,[51] and differences in the capacity of the cells to adhere to glass and various other materials,[52] in their relative motility on free-flow electrophoresis,[53] and in their relative sensitivity to the inhibitory or cytopathic effects of various agents, including antilymphocyte serum,[54] corticosteroids and their synthetic and other analogues,[55, 56] cytotoxic drugs, such as cyclophosphamide,[57] other immunosuppressants, particularly azathioprine,[58, 59] and X-irradiation.[60]

Light Microscopy

The classic distinction between 'large lymphocytes' (8 to 16 μm in diameter, with clearly recognizable cytoplasm) and 'small lymphocytes' (7 to 9 μm in diameter, with no more than a fine rim of cytoplasm) in stained films of blood has proved to reflect a notable difference in the life span of the cells. The large lymphocytes have a life span of less than a day; the small lymphocytes may persist for many weeks, and some of them even for several years (see page 519).

Small Lymphocytes.—In conventional histological preparations (paraffin wax sections) of formalin-fixed tissue, stained with haematoxylin and eosin, the typical *small lymphocyte* measures about 5 to 7 μm in diameter (Fig. 9.7). Its cytoplasm is so scanty that shrinkage during processing of the specimen often gives the impression that the cell consists of nucleus alone. The nucleus of the small lymphocyte is practically round.

Small or larger lymphocytes with a notched (cloven,* or 'cleaved') nucleus are found in the germinal centres of lymphoid follicles (see page 513) and are known variously as 'cleaved' cells,[61] haematogones[62] and germinocytes:[63] they are regarded as precursors of larger lymphocytes with cytoplasm that is rich in ribonucleic acid and therefore pyroninophile: these are the so-called immunoblasts (see opposite and page 522), 'lymphoblasts' or

* It is good to have independent support for the use in English texts of 'cloven' rather than 'cleaved' (Lennox, B., *Lancet*, 1976, **2**, 1140).

D

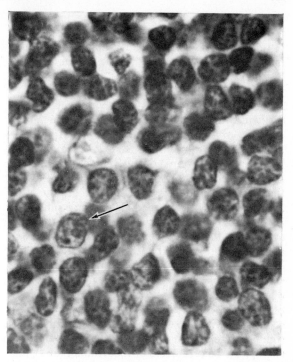

Fig. 9.7. Lymphocytes at the zone of junction between a follicle and the interfollicular tissue in a lymph node. Most of the cells are small lymphocytes; one of the larger lymphocytes is arrowed. *Haematoxylin–eosin.* × 1200.

'germinoblasts'[63] of contemporary parlance. The immunoblasts undergo repeated mitosis: as they differentiate further, some of their progeny acquire the appearance of small lymphocytes and others become plasma cells. The small lymphocytes with notched nucleus and the lymphocytes of intermediate size are frequently seen to be in contact with the cytoplasmic processes of the 'dendritic reticular cells' (see page 514),[39] which trap antigen on bulky cytoplasmic extensions.[40] The chromatin of small lymphocytes is in the form of numerous coarse clumps, so closely packed that the resulting intensity of nuclear staining allows little detail to be made out, while the nucleolus, which ordinarily is inconspicuous even in ideal preparations, is often completely obscured.

The small lymphocyte is the cell most commonly denoted by the histologist's reference to a 'round cell infiltrate' in chronically inflamed tissues and various other pathological states. Such infiltrates usually include other cells also, such as large lymphocytes, plasma cells and macrophages. There is a tendency nowadays to prefer the non-committal term 'mononuclear cells' for the constituent cells of such an infiltrate, on the grounds that electron microscopy may show that in some instances a proportion—even a large proportion—of the cells have the characteristics of macrophages, although indistinguishable from lymphocytes in conventional histological preparations.

Large Lymphocytes.—The large lymphocyte is less easily identified in paraffin wax sections than in films of blood or bone marrow and in imprint preparations from freshly cut, unfixed lymphoid tissue; however, the clumps of nuclear chromatin are neither so coarse nor so closely packed as those in the small lymphocyte, and the nucleus therefore appears less densely stained. The large lymphocyte has a more conspicuous nucleolus and, usually, more cytoplasm than the small lymphocyte, and its nucleus may be ovoid rather than circular. The distinction between large and small lymphocytes is most readily made in sections when the cells form distinct zones round the germinal centres of lymphoid follicles. Under certain conditions, the germinal centre—which consists mainly of lymphoblasts (immunoblasts), lymphocytes with a cloven nucleus (thought to be precursors of the lymphoblasts), and a scattering of macrophages—is surrounded by two zones, each several layers of cells in thickness (Figs 9.2 and 9.3). One zone—it may be the outer or the inner—is darker and consists of small lymphocytes; the other zone is paler and consists of large lymphocytes. The difference in the staining intensity of the two zones is due partly to the fact that the nucleus of the small lymphocyte normally stains more intensely and partly to the scantiness of its cytoplasm: the nuclei of adjacent cells are therefore close to one another and the tissue appears correspondingly dark. The large lymphocyte has a larger amount of cytoplasm and its nucleus usually is rather less haematoxyphile than that of the small lymphocyte: the result is that even when large lymphocytes are closely packed their nuclei are more widely spaced than those in the zone of small lymphocytes, and the tissue appears correspondingly paler. Elsewhere in the tissues it is generally impossible to identify large lymphocytes individually by conventional histological means; in most circumstances they appear to be much less numerous than small lymphocytes.

It is appropriate to note again that the appearance of the lymphocytes in histological preparations gives no information about their function. It may also be noted that lymphocytes are generally considered not to be phagocytes. Certainly, light microscopy shows no evidence of phagocytic activity, even in living cell cultures. Lysosomes are scarce or absent: as these organelles have many functions unrelated to phagocytosis, their occasional demonstration in electron micrographs of lymphocytes should not be interpreted as evidence that these cells are potentially capable of phagocytosis. It may be noted that descriptions of phagocytes that morphologically resemble small lymphocytes are now generally believed to relate in fact to cells that are not lymphocytes but derived either from macrophages or from cells of the granulocyte series.[64, 65] The pseudopodial activity of lymphocytes *in vitro* is not associated with ingestion of particulate matter but with the motility of the cells, as was finely illustrated in the pioneer cinephotomicrographic studies by R. J. V. Pulvertaft, at Westminster Medical School, London.

Origin of Lymphocytes

It is now considered that all the lymphocytes throughout the human body, whatever their functions and wherever they are situated, are descended from stem cells that are present in haemopoietic tissue, particularly bone marrow, during the development of the embryo.[66, 67] The cells that originate from these stem cells differentiate along one of two paths, depending on which of the two primary lymphoid organs acts on them (see page 508): the cells that are influenced by the thymus become the thymus-dependent lymphocytes (T cells) and those that are influenced by the equivalent of the lymphoid tissue of the avian cloacal bursa become the 'bursa-equivalent'-dependent lymphocytes (B cells) (see below).

It is no longer believed that lymphocytes may differentiate from reticulum cells (see page 525) or that thymic epithelium may, during embryonic life, be the source of some of the thymic lymphocytes (see page 508).

Distribution of Lymphocytes

Lymphocytes are the essential and predominant cells of the lymphoid tissues. They are numerous and closely packed in the lymph nodes, spleen, Waldeyer's ring of fauciopharyngeal lymphoid tissue, the thymus, and the solitary and aggregated lymphoid follicles of the intestine, and, in birds, the cloacal bursa. They are more loosely scattered among the haemopoietic cells in bone marrow and, apart from the lymphoid follicles themselves, among the connective tissue elements of the intestinal mucosa. From 20 to 45 per cent of the leucocytes circulating in the blood, and virtually all the cells in lymph, including the chyle in the major lymph ducts, are lymphocytes.

Organ Dependence

Thymus-Dependent Lymphocytes (T Lymphocytes).—The distinction between T lymphocytes and B lymphocytes was defined by Roitt and his colleagues in 1969.[68] The T lymphocytes are so named with the intention of indicating that they are 'thymus-dependent'; the term is sometimes interpreted as meaning that these cells are 'thymus-derived'—that is, formed in the thymus by proliferation of precursors situated there, the precursor cells themselves being derived from the stem cells in the marrow (see above)—but, in fact, by no means all thymus-dependent lymphocytes are derived from cells in the thymus. Some authorities prefer to use the expression 'thymus-processed', which perhaps indicates more explicitly the relation of these cells to the thymus.

The functions of the T cells are considered on the next page.

'Bursa-Equivalent'-Dependent Lymphocytes (B Lymphocytes).—The designation B lymphocyte was introduced to indicate that these cells, in birds, are dependent on the lymphoid organ of the cloacal bursa. In mammals, the term is interpreted as indicating that the cells are dependent on the bursa equivalent (whatever that may prove to be—see page 509: those who regard the bone marrow as the site of the bursa-equivalent lymphoid tissue enjoy the advantage of finding the abbreviation 'B lymphocyte' still appropriate). The B lymphocytes are also sometimes referred to as thymus-independent or 'bursa-equivalent'-derived or bone-marrow-derived lymphocytes: the last of these terms is so ambiguous, in view of current views of the origin of all lymphocytes from stem cells in the marrow, that it should not be retained.

The functions of the B cells are considered on page 522.

Circulation of Lymphocytes

The blood can be depleted experimentally of most of its lymphocytes if the thoracic duct is cannulated and drained. If labelled lymphocytes are then infused into a vein they will appear in the thoracic duct,[69] thus demonstrating that the cells circulate from blood to lymph and back to blood. About half the lymphocytes in the body circulate constantly between the blood and lymph compartments. The transfer from blood to lymph occurs in the thymus-dependent areas of lymph nodes (see page 511), the lymphocytes passing between the tall endothelial cells of the distinctive postcapillary venules and then migrating through the paracortical zone of the node (see page 511), eventually leaving the node by its efferent lymphatics and reaching the thoracic duct to regain the blood stream. Transfer from the blood to the lymph compartment takes place also across the periarteriolar lymphoid sheaths in the spleen (see page 720).

Most of the recirculating lymphocytes are T cells and it is notable that they are confined to the thymus-dependent parts of the secondary lymphoid organs (see page 510): for instance, in addition to the paracortical zone of lymph nodes and the periarteriolar sheaths in the spleen, they are to be found in the medullary lymph sinuses of the nodes, but not in the germinal centres. The bone marrow and thymus are outside the recirculation pathways.

Some B lymphocytes have been shown to recirculate also. Their notably greater affinity for tritiated thymidine distinguishes them from T lymphocytes and facilitates their specific recognition. They are found in the outer mantle of the germinal centres.[22]

Life Span of Lymphocytes

Lymphocytes may be short-lived or long-lived. It is estimated that about 20 per cent of lymphocytes in man have a mean survival of 3 to 4 days; the rest survive for 100 to 200 days (but see below).[70] Their site of destruction is uncertain; it is probably significant that all lymphoid tissues, and especially the thymus and the germinal centres of lymphoid follicles, contain numerous macrophages that enclose Flemming's stainable bodies in their cytoplasm, presumptive evidence of the destruction of cells—presumably lymphocytes—and of the breakdown of their nuclear substance (see page 512). Some lymphocytes may also be shed into the lumen of the intestine and there destroyed.

Nearly all the lymphocytes in the thoracic duct are long-lived; nearly all those in bone marrow are short-lived; 90 per cent of those in the thymus are short-lived; and 30 to 70 per cent of those in blood are short-lived. Most lymphocytes in the thymus-dependent areas of lymph nodes and spleen are long-lived; most of those in thymus-independent areas are short-lived.[71]

Much longer periods of lymphocyte survival have been indicated by experiments with the lymphocytes of patients who, many years earlier, had had radiotherapy. If these cells are induced to divide *in vitro* by exposure to plant mitogens, such as phyto-haemagglutinin (see page 522), the presence of visible chromosomal damage—the result of the irradiation—identifies cells that are undergoing mitosis for the first time since the radiotherapy. The results of such studies have been interpreted as suggesting that the mean life span of the lymphocyte may be as much as 4·4 years[72] and that there is a wide range of survival, even up to 20 years.[73]

Control of Lymphopoiesis

The means by which the production of lymphocytes is regulated are largely unknown. Antigens stimulate lymphoid tissues to produce lymphocytes and release them into the circulation; many of these cells have the morphological characteristics of lymphoblasts ('immunoblasts'), as mentioned on page 512.[74] Contrastingly, 'stress', through augmenting the output of adrenal cortical hormones, particularly cortisol, tends to cause lymphopenia, with involution of all lymphoid tissues, including the thymus.[75]

Functions of Lymphocytes

The known functions of lymphocytes are essentially immunological, and most of the research that has been undertaken in recent years in clarifying their role in the body's organization has consolidated and elaborated this concept of their activities. Other functions, not of an immunological nature, have from time to time been ascribed to these cells, but without adding significantly to what is now the well-established knowledge of their roles: they have been regarded as multipotential stem cells,[76] as cells that mediate nutritional needs of tissues (the so-called 'trephocytic' or 'feeder' function)[77, 78] and as regulators of tissue growth.[79] As regulation of other tissues is, in theory, dependent on specific recognition—by receptors on the lymphocytes—of tissue-specific components of the surface of other cells, these functions might also be classed as 'immunological': this concept has a parallel in the similar hypothesis that it is a function of lymphocytes to recognize and eliminate abnormal (that is, malignant) autologous cells.[80] In the following account, it is the immunological functions of lymphocytes that are mainly considered.

Immunocompetence.—Lymphocytes are described as immunocompetent when they are capable of reacting to antigens with the consequent formation of antibodies. Immunocompetence is a characteristic that they acquire as a result of their particular organ-dependence, which may be thymus-dependence or 'bursa-equivalent'-dependence (see above). Lympho-cytes that are immunocompetent are known also as 'antigen-reactive' lymphocytes and 'antigen-sensitive' lymphocytes. They belong among the recirculating lymphocytes (see page 519), and following challenge by antigen they become sequestered in the appropriately situated lymph nodes; this accounts for the conspicuous infiltration of the wall of postcapillary venules of lymph nodes during the course of an immune response. Several days after immunization there is a sharp rise in the number of lymphocytes in the efferent lymphatics of the nodes involved in the reaction: many of these cells have the characteristics of immunoblasts.

Functions of T Lymphocytes

The thymus-dependent lymphocytes (T lymphocytes) are associated with cell-mediated immunological mechanisms. These include the mechanisms that are concerned in delayed hypersensitivity (for example, the positive reaction to a tuberculin skin test) and in resistance to infection by certain types of micro-organisms (a classic instance of protective immunity). They also include the mechanisms that bring about the immune response to transplantation of tissues or organs (allograft rejection and graft-against-host disease) and to autologous tumours and other autologous tissues and tissue components (autoimmunity). These mechanisms depend basically on the special function of antigen recognition, which in turn depends on the presence of specific antigen receptors that are fixed on the surface of the lymphocytes, whether these are already sensitized (immune) through exposure to antigen [81, 82] or unsensitized (non-immune).[83–85] The surface receptors on the 'immune' cells are apparently immunoglobulins (antibody), although whether identical with circulating immunoglobulins or not is as yet uncertain: for instance, they may—at least in some circumstances—lack the polypeptide light chains that ordinarily are characteristic of immunoglobulins.[86]

Contact between antigen and surface receptors of T lymphocytes results in transformation of the lymphocytes into 'blast' cells (see below). The latter proliferate and differentiate to form at least three varieties of derivative lymphocytes: *effector cells* (sometimes called 'killer' cells, or k cells), which produce a range of biologically active 'mediator' substances and are involved in delayed hypersensitivity reactions and in transplant and tumour immunity and in autoimmunity; *'memory' cells* (primed antigen-sensitive cells) that, because of their long life span and development as a clone, provide persistent immunological 'memory' of previous exposure to the specific antigen concerned; and *'helper' cells*, which work with B lymphocytes in the production of humoral antibodies.

Macrophages and Immunity.—It is likely that macrophages have an important part in the development of immunity (see pages 514 and 517). Antigens may become immunogenic as a consequence of contact with the surface of macrophages,[87] which probably have surface receptors.[88] However, there is evidence that substances that are weakly immunogenic are taken up by macrophages only in small amounts, if at all, and are not retained on their surface in any high concentration.[89] Thus, it seems to be the case that not all antigens must be processed by macrophages before they are able to stimulate antigen-sensitive cells. The so-called 'killer' cells (see preceding paragraph) are thought by some to be a specialized line of macrophages[90] rather than specialized lymphocytes.[91]

Delayed Hypersensitivity.—Delayed hypersensitivity is a manifestation of cell-mediated immunity, which may be defined as an increase in reactivity to specific antigens that is a function of the reacting cells themselves and not related to the presence of antibody that is apart from cells. Delayed hypersensitivity is demonstrated in the local reaction that follows the intradermal inoculation of antigen such as tuberculin, histoplasmin and similar substances into the individual who has become sensitized in the course of infection by the organism from which the antigen is obtained. It is involved also in contact sensitivity[29] (in which the antigen is usually a comparatively simple compound of low molecular weight), in autoimmunity,[68, 92] in immunity to tumours,[93] and in reactions associated with transplants (see Chapter 24), both in the form of graft rejection (host-against-graft reaction)[94] and in that of graft-against-host reaction.[95]

Delayed hypersensitivity is a cellular event, evoked by contact of antigen with reactive lymphocytes, which then proliferate, becoming immunoblasts (see below), while at the same time mediator substances with a range of functions are released from the activated lymphocytes (see next paragraph). Macrophages accumulate locally in the region involved; they are mainly monocytes from the blood.

The type of reactivity to given antigens that characterizes the development of delayed hypersensitivity can be transferred passively from sensitized individuals to those who are not sensitive to the antigen. This transfer can be effected by intact lymphocytes or by extracts of lymphocytes, which therefore may be presumed to elaborate a 'transfer factor'. This factor confers on the uncommitted lymphocytes of the unsensitized recipient the capacity to react to the specific antigen.[96] Other mediators that are released from sensitized lymphocytes, after contact with the antigen that they are sensitive to, include a migration-inhibiting factor,[97] which enhances accumulation of macrophages at the site of the reaction by preventing their movement away from it, a chemotactic factor,[98] which attracts macrophages, a macrophage-activating factor,[99] which increases membrane activity and stickiness of macrophages, and a lymphotoxic factor.[100] These and several other biologically active substances are known sometimes as lymphokines. They are elaborated not only when sensitized lymphocytes are stimulated by contact with the specific antigen but also when lymphocytes are stimulated by non-specific mitogens (see below).

Resistance to Infection.—If it may be accepted that pathogenic micro-organisms are the cause of only three main forms of infection[101]—acute (and ordinarily brief) illness, chronic illness accompanying facultative intracellular parasitism by the causative organisms, and persistent or latent infection—it may be accepted that cell-mediated immunity is the basis of resistance to those organisms that cause chronic disease. In these diseases, which may be caused by certain bacteria (for instance, the mycobacteria), fungi (typically, *Histoplasma capsulatum*), protozoa (typically, the leishmaniae) and viruses, antigen-sensitive T lymphocytes are involved, bringing about activation of macrophages.[102] The latter not only are the cells mainly subjected to parasitism in these infections, they are also the cells that eventually may terminate the infection by inhibiting the further growth of the infecting organisms and so overcoming the disease. Both histiocytosis (proliferation of macrophages in the infected tissues) and granuloma formation (epithelioid metamorphosis of macrophages, with or without the development of multinucleate forms) are features, in varying degree, of such infections, which thus are characterized by true cellular immunity as well as by cell-mediated immunity.

In the case of viral infections, both cell-mediated immunity and cellular immunity contribute to defence, as well as such other mechanisms as the development of circulating specific antibodies and non-specific factors, including interferon. Macrophages are particularly important in combating the spread of viruses, particularly virulent strains of viruses, in the body.[103] Some viruses have been found to require immunoblastic transformation of lymphocytes before they can undergo replication.[104] It is becoming evident that reaction to many forms of infection, and the successful termination of infection (or its conversion into a tolerable mode of harmless persistence—for instance, infection by measles virus), may be regarded as the outcome of interaction of various defence mechanisms, among which those that involve lymphocytes and macrophages have important, interdependent functions.

Functions of B Lymphocytes

The 'bursa-equivalent'-dependent lymphocytes (B lymphocytes) are involved mainly in the humoral antibody response. One of the key questions relevant to this type of immune response is that of the relation of B lymphocytes to plasma cells. Most, if not all, circulating antibodies are elaborated by plasma cells. There is experimental evidence that small lymphocytes are the precursors of the cells that synthetize specific antibodies.[22, 105, 106] Contact with antigen that evokes the production of humoral antibody evidently causes differentiation of the small lymphocyte to form 'plasmablasts' and then mature plasma cells, which secrete specific immunoglobulin antibodies.

Although the cells that form humoral antibodies are the B lymphocytes (or their plasma cell derivatives), and although 'strong' antigens evidently are able to induce the B lymphocytes to produce humoral antibodies, even in the absence of T lymphocytes,[107] it has become clear that other antigens initiate an immune response by B lymphocytes only when T lymphocytes are present. As the latter circulate more widely and readily, they may prime antigen so that it is presented to the B lymphocytes in a form that the latter can respond to.[108]

A relatively small proportion of recirculating lymphocytes (see page 519) are B cells. Some of these are 'memory' cells (see page 520), and these are assumed to have been formed in the germinal centres of lymph nodes and of the spleen after initial immunization.

Lymphocyte Transformation

Normal lymphocytes, obtained from peripheral blood, can be stimulated in vitro, in various ways, to undergo transformation into immunoblasts (the so-called 'blast' cells*—see page 517). These are large cells with basiphile, pyroninophile cytoplasm and conspicuous nucleoli (see Figs 9.6A, 9.6B, 9.6C and 9.112B, pages 514, 515 and 646). They synthetize deoxyribonucleic acid and exhibit marked mitotic activity (hence their frequent use in the study of human chromosomes). Because of the pyroninophilia of their cytoplasm they are sometimes known also as pyroninophile cells, but this is a term that can as appropriately be applied to plasma cells. 'Immunoblastic transformation' ('blast transformation', 'lymphoblastic transformation') is induced by various specific and non-specific mitogens. The T lymphocytes and the B lymphocytes respond in different degree to different mitogens: for instance, phytohaemagglutinin[48]—a lectin or plant mitogen (phytomitogen) obtained from the common red kidney bean, Phaseolus vulgaris—acts selectively on T lymphocytes.[109]

Cells that are believed to be immunoblasts may be seen in lymphoid tissue in certain types of infection, including vaccinial lymphadenitis (see page 644) and infectious mononucleosis (see page 650).

Plasma Cells

Plasma cells are ovoid or, sometimes, round cells, from 7 to 15 μm in longest dimension; they have characteristic nuclear and cytoplasmic appearances (Fig. 9.8). The nucleus is traditionally likened to a clock face or cart wheel because of the more or less regular disposition of smallish masses of chromatin on the nuclear membrane, with threads of chromatin radiating to them from one or two centrally placed chromatinic foci. Typically, the nucleus is eccentrically placed close to the surface of the cell at its broader pole. The cytoplasm has a peculiar purplish colour in haematoxylin–eosin preparations; that part of it that abuts on the nucleus, in the central area of the cell, is paler and more eosinophile. There is abundant ribonucleic acid in the cytoplasm, which consequently is markedly pyroninophile. The high content of ribonucleic acid reflects the activity of these cells in synthetizing protein, specifically immunoglobulin, of which they are the major source: they are unquestionably responsible for producing most circulating antibody.

It is now generally accepted that the plasma cell is derived from the B lymphocyte (see above). After

---

* The use of the term 'blast' cell for these transformed lymphocytes has caused some confusion because the same term has been applied in cases of acute leukaemia to immature cells that cannot be precisely identified as related to the myeloid or monocytic or lymphoid series of cells.

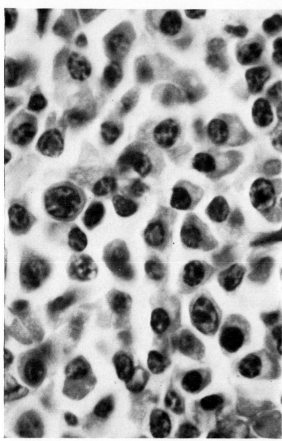

a syphilitic lesion or, in some situations, other specific infective diseases (for instance, scleroma—see page 204). Some authorities state that plasma cells are never found in healthy tissues, and attribute their virtually invariable presence in situations such as the lamina propria of the intestinal mucous membrane to the antigenic stimulus of micro-organisms or to other potentially damaging extrinsic influences resulting from the alimentary functions of the bowel. Corresponding arguments have been put forward in explanation of the finding of plasma cells in seemingly normal lymph nodes and in bone marrow. These views seem to depend on an unrealistically rigid interpretation of what is normal, and they do not take into account that, in order to survive under natural conditions, the body must react to stimuli arising outside itself, and that to an indefinable extent such reactions and their manifestations are not only natural but normal.

Fig. 9.8. Plasma cells and some plasma cell precursors in the interfollicular tissue of a lymph node in a case of brucella infection. The less mature cells have a large nucleus and relatively little cytoplasm; there are variations in the extent to which their chromatin has the distribution characteristic of the nucleus of the typical plasma cell, and there may or may not be a readily distinguishable nucleolus. The mature plasma cells show the eccentric placing of the nucleus and the relatively clear cytoplasmic zone abutting on it. *Haematoxylin–eosin.* × 1200.

THE RETICULOENDOTHELIAL SYSTEM[110, 111]

The reticuloendothelial system has long been regarded as distinct from the lymphoid system, although topographically closely associated with the latter in that reticuloendothelial cells are present in the lymphoid tissues even more conspicuously than in organs of unrelated systems, such as the liver (see page 526). The concept that these two systems are separable is artificial, and their close functional interdependence and anatomical overlap are now well recognized and, in essence, undisputed. Their complementary interaction in immunity is one of several means through which these complexly organized and multifunctional systems work together in the defence of the body against certain types of potentially harmful influences in the external environment (for instance, infection) and certain potentially harmful anomalies that arise in the body (for instance, neoplastic disease). These interactions depend on the contiguity of the cells—lymphoid cells and reticuloendothelial cells—that conventionally are described as the specific cells respectively of the lymphoid and reticuloendothelial systems. Lymphoid tissue exists nowhere without an intimate association with reticuloendothelial cells. The facts that reticuloendothelial cells are more widely distributed than lymphoid tissue, and that they have functions unrelated to those of lymphoid tissue (for instance, the various metabolic functions subserved by their enzyme systems), are sometimes thought to indicate that the two systems are distinct

contact with antigen the small lymphocyte is believed to undergo eventual transformation into a 'plasmablast', a relatively large cell that is intermediate in appearance between the lymphocyte and the plasma cell (see Fig. 9.8) and that matures into the latter as antibody production develops. Several stages of cell multiplication and differentiation intervene between the two events.

Plasma cells are particularly numerous in chronically inflamed tissues, but by no means all chronic inflammatory lesions are characterized by their presence. Their participation has no specific diagnostic significance, contrary to beliefs that still are expressed sometimes, such as that they indicate

and should be considered separately. On the contrary, the convenience and, more important, the propriety and necessity of considering the pathology of the two systems together are underlined by the need also to define conditions, such as storage diseases, that have their origin in disturbances of reticuloendothelial functions that are quite independent of any cellular activity of the lymphoid system. It is in such respects that the case for relating the two systems together as the *lymphoreticular system* (see page 506) comes into its own.

It is not always possible to be sure that particular cells that seem, on the grounds of their appearance, to be part of one of these systems are not in fact elements of the other. This point has been touched on in relation to certain lymphocyte-like phagocytes that are now generally identified as macrophages of modified appearance (see page 518). On another plane, some authorities believe the 'dendritic reticular cells', which have so important a part in the immunological maturation of some lymphocytes, to be modified lymphocytes themselves rather than reticuloendothelial cells. Such conflicts of opinion seem to be pointless in comparison with the importance of recognizing the functional associations of different cells; whether they develop as part of one system or the other is not necessarily as important as the purpose that they serve.

Definition of the Reticuloendothelial System

The definition of the reticuloendothelial system was owed to two particular circumstances, the recognition of phagocytosis (see page 530), which was one of the contributions of Ilya Ilyich Mechnikov (Elie Metchnikoff) to the study of inflammation,[112] and the observation by Paul Ehrlich of the phenomenon of vital staining[113, 114] and his encouragement of his associates, notably E. E. Goldmann,[115, 116] to investigate the biological significance of this phenomenon. Metchnikoff[112] distinguished the mononuclear phagocytes, which he observed to ingest large particles (erythrocytes, for instance) and which he therefore named *macrophages*, from the *microphages*, as he called the neutrophile polymorphonuclear leucocytes, which ingested only much smaller particles, such as bacteria. Ehrlich, in the course of his work on the staining of the myelin sheath of living nerves with methylene blue,[114] noted that the introduction into living tissues of certain of the then recently developed synthetic dyestuffs, in the form of colloidal suspensions, was followed by staining of the cytoplasm of some cells.

Vital Staining

Ribbert was among the first to publish significant observations on the results of vital staining,[117] using the dye lithium carmine. Many other non-toxic synthetic dyes are equally effective as 'vital stains', including brilliant vital red, trypan blue and Evans blue. Only those dyes that can pass through the lining of capillary blood vessels to reach the interstitial space are able to reach the extravascular phagocytes: some of the dyes, such as Evans blue,[118] rapidly become bound to plasma albumin and therefore are more suitable for determining plasma volume than for the vital staining of extravascular cells; in contrast, those dyes, like trypan blue,[119] that have a less avid affinity for albumin, escape from the blood unchanged and eventually combine with albumin in the tissue spaces to form complexes that the macrophages engulf.

The access of suitable dyes to the tissues, by intramuscular inoculation or by injection into the peritoneal cavity or directly into the blood stream, is followed by selective staining of certain cells.[115, 120] Selective staining is not seen when the same dyes are applied to dead tissue, for its occurrence is a manifestation of the vital function of *phagocytosis* by which the living cells engulf particulate matter, including particles in colloidal suspension, such as dyestuffs and carbon (for instance, in the form of India ink), which, in consequence, accumulate in their cytoplasm. It is these cells that constitute the reticuloendothelial system, as defined and named by Ludwig Aschoff and his school.[121–123] It is important to note that many types of cell are able to take up small amounts of dyes and other finely particulate matter, particularly if in the form of a colloidal suspension, by the process of pinocytosis. *Pinocytosis* is an ingestive function of living cytoplasm that is quite distinct from phagocytosis, although related to it; the two mechanisms are sometimes grouped under the term *endocytosis*.[124] Pinocytosis is generally considered to effect the absorption into the cytoplasm only of extracellular fluid and substances dissolved in it, but in fact very small particles suspended in the fluid can sometimes be identified in 'pinocytosis vacuoles'. The cells of the reticuloendothelial system take up material from their environment both by phagocytosis and by pinocytosis; in contrast, many other types of cell absorb by pinocytosis although they are incapable of phagocytosis of particulate matter. Pinocytosis probably accounts for the fact that traces of particulate dye may be found in the cytoplasm of some cells that lack the capability of taking up the very heavy load of dye that is characteristic of the vitally stained reticuloendothelial cell. Such traces of vital staining are seen in some endothelial cells of capillaries and other blood vessels and of lymphatics, and in occasional mesothelial cells, fibroblasts and even smooth muscle cells.

There are, of course, other mechanisms by which living cells may be stained—osmosis and simple diffusion. They apply to staining only by those dyes that are able to remain in true solution in body fluids. Such dyes persist in the cells only if the local chemical or physicochemical conditions tend to bind them to intracellular constituents: to this extent the staining may be selective, but such selective staining by readily diffusible dyes does not relate to reticuloendothelial cells in any systematic manner.

Reticuloendothelial Cells

Most types of cell throughout the body are incapable of ingesting particulate matter of macromolecular size and above, and therefore can neither be stained vitally by dyes injected in colloidal form nor recognized through the presence in their cytoplasm of stores of ingested particulate material. The cells that, by phagocytosis, can take up such substantial quantities of dye particles that their cytoplasm is conspicuously coloured constitute the *reticuloendothelial system* as defined by Aschoff.[123] This classic term is still the most widely used and generally understood of the names that have been applied to the system. It has been criticized on various grounds, and particularly because 'reticuloendothelial' is liable to be interpreted as excluding all but 'reticulum cells' and 'endothelial cells': in fact, several types of cell are generally regarded as part of the reticuloendothelial system (see below), and while most authorities include reticulum cells in the system, the majority of cells that are described as endothelial do not belong to the system, lacking both the phagocytic activity that is a cardinal functional characteristic of reticuloendothelial cells and the metallophilia that is another of their identifying features (see below). Those who continue to find the concept of the reticuloendothelial system realistic and useful, and they are in the majority, generally include the following among its cells.

Reticulum Cells (Reticular Cells).*—The reticulum cells are large mononuclear cells, some 12 to 18 μm

---

* Reticulum cells are sometimes misnamed reticulocytes, even by those who ought to know better. Reticulocytes are, of course, young erythrocytes (see page 432): they have nothing in common with reticulum cells.

D*

in their longest dimension (Fig. 9.9). Their cytoplasm has an irregular outline and tapering processes that join those of adjacent reticulum cells. In haematoxylin–eosin preparations the cytoplasm is faintly eosinophile and may have a ground-glass-like appearance; it and its processes are metallophile. The nucleus is oval, about 10 by 7 μm, and bounded by a fine but distinct nuclear membrane; the pale, clear nucleoplasm is traversed by scanty, fine threads of chromatin—the appearance is often described as vesicular, although the clear areas are not sharply outlined. One or two prominent, rounded nucleoli are present; they are about 3 to 4 μm in diameter, and they commonly have an eosinophile tint.

Reticulum cells are associated with the argyrophile connective tissue fibres (reticulin stroma) of lymphoid tissue. The argyrophile stroma is sometimes known as the *reticulum*, and it is from this name that the reticulum cells acquired their usual designation. The cytoplasmic processes of the cells are intimately applied to the fibres. Some authorities distinguish

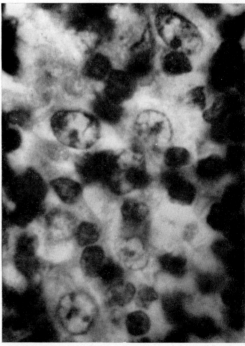

Fig. 9.9. Reticulum cells in the medulla of a lymph node. They are large, pale cells, with ill-defined cytoplasm that is relatively abundant and only slightly to moderately opaque. The nucleus is oval, but appears round when cut across its longer axis. Its delicate membrane encloses clear nucleoplasm traversed by a few fine chromatin threads. One or two eosinophile or somewhat haematoxyphile nucleoli are readily seen. *Haematoxylin–eosin.* × 1200.

between reticulum cells and the 'dendritic reticular cells' that have important functions in immunogenesis (see page 514); others regard these cells as virtually identical. The propensity of the cytoplasmic processes of the dendritic cells to bind antigens led to their synonym, 'antigen-retaining reticular cells'.

Because reticulum cells have relatively little phagocytic capacity in comparison with the free tissue macrophages (histiocytes—see below), some writers doubt the appropriateness of including them in a cell system that is defined in terms of the active phagocytosis that its constituent cells display.[125]

Endothelial Macrophages (Littoral Cells).—The name endothelial macrophage is a somewhat clumsy term applied to the syncytial phagocytes that line (or form the greater part of the lining of) lymph sinuses. The name is also given to the comparable mononuclear phagocytes that are distributed among the simple endothelial cells of blood sinuses (sinusoids) in certain organs, particularly the spleen, liver, pituitary and adrenals. In the liver these are the cells known as von Kupffer's cells, or *Kupffer cells*.[126] The endothelial macrophages often appear spindle-shaped in ordinary histological preparations; in thicker sections, and particularly when impregnated with silver, their radiating processes may be seen and their asteroid outline is then apparent. The syncytial cells of the sinuses of lymph nodes not only line these channels but also form a cell meshwork in the lumen, joined by their cytoplasmic processes and constituting a particularly efficient phagocytic filter through which the lymph must pass.

Endothelial macrophages have appreciably more phagocytic activity than reticulum cells, although with considerable differences from organ to organ. The phagocytic cells in the sinusoids of the pituitary and adrenals show little such activity in comparison with those in the liver and, particularly, in the lymph nodes and spleen.

Histiocytes.—Although the term histiocyte is often used either as a generic name for any macrophage (as in this book) or, more specifically, to describe any mononuclear phagocyte that can be so identified by reason of the presence of ingested material within its cytoplasm, it is also used in the narrower sense of the amoeboid macrophages that are present, and 'free', throughout the connective tissues of the body, including the stroma of the viscera. These are probably the most numerous, and undoubtedly the most widespread, of the reticuloendothelial cells. They are irregularly rounded and some 15 to 25 μm in

their longest dimension. When active, their cytoplasm is more abundant than when they are in the resting state, and they are therefore more readily seen. The cytoplasm is opaque and eosinophile, and sometimes has a rather granular appearance; it may contain scanty vacuoles, and these are usually small (4 to 5 μm in their longer dimension), ovoid and quite sharply outlined, with the consequence that they may be mistaken for intracellular parasites, such as leishmaniae and histoplasmas. The cytoplasmic outline of histiocytes is indistinct and becomes especially so when the cells undergo epithelioid (endothelioid) metamorphosis—for instance, during the development of a tuberculoid granulomatous reaction. In such conditions adjacent cells often come to be conspicuously united by their cytoplasmic processes.

The nucleus of the histiocyte is pale, and ovoid or kidney-shaped. It resembles the nucleus of the reticulum cell except that it is smaller (about 7 by 5 μm) and generally has more abundant chromatin, which is in the form of clumps and threads. If a nucleolus is apparent at all it is inconspicuous. When histiocytes are proliferating actively, nuclear division sometimes occurs without the cytoplasm dividing, binucleate forms resulting. A similar process may result in the formation of multinucleate giant cells, such as the Langhans cell of the tuberculous reaction and the so-called foreign body giant cells.

Various names have been given to the histiocytes. They have been called *clasmatocytes* (because of the fragmentary appearance of the margin of the cytoplasm) and *adventitial cells* (because of their occurrence in or adjacent to the adventitial coat of the blood vessels). Sometimes they are given special names when they are laden with some distinctive material that they have ingested or produced in notable amount through catabolic activity: *melanophages* ('melanophores'), *siderophages* and *lipophages* are among these terms. Sometimes histiocytes that have become greatly enlarged through storage of metabolites in excess are referred to as thesaurocytes.*

The *alveolar macrophages* of the lungs and the *peritoneal macrophages* and macrophages of other serosal cavities may be considered under the general designation of histiocytes.

Osteoclasts.—It has been suggested that the osteoclasts, which may be regarded as multinucleate

---

* The name thesaurocyte has also been given to a form of plasma cell (the Mott cell) that has been regarded as the source of the peculiar, hyaline, eosinophile globules known as Russell bodies (see Chapter 4, page 206).

phagocytes in bone, also belong to the reticulo-endothelial system, if—as has been assumed—they form through fusion of mononuclear phagocytes.[127]

Microglial Cells.—The microglial cells of the central nervous system (Hortega cells) are now generally accepted to be part of the reticuloendothelial sytem. They are most familiar in their actively phagocytic form, when they assume the appearance that earned them the name 'compound granular corpuscles' (see Chapter 34).

Monocytes.—Finally, and of particular importance because they maintain the numerical strength of the reticuloendothelial system throughout the body, the monocytes that circulate in the blood are cells of the reticuloendothelial system. Current views of the cytogenesis of reticuloendothelial cells derive all of them, under normal conditions, from precursor cells in bone marrow, the *promonocytes*. The promono-cytes give origin to the circulating *monocytes*, and the monocytes in their turn make their way to the various other organs and tissues where the fixed and wandering macrophages are found. Thus, the monocytes are not merely macrophages circulating in the blood, and therefore readily available when required to congregate in foci where this type of 'inflammatory' response is called for: they are also constantly in transit from their tissue of origin—bone marrow—to make good the physiological loss of effete reticuloendothelial cells in all situations.[128] Only when the need for macrophages is exceptionally increased, as in response to pathological conditions, is the haematogenous supply of new reticuloendo-thelial cells supplemented by proliferation of the cells already present locally in the tissues.

The Concept of the 'Mononuclear Phagocyte System'[125]

This may be a pertinent juncture at which to inter-polate a note on the revision of our views of the reticuloendothelial system that is called for by the continuing extension of our knowledge and under-standing of the cells, and their functions, that hitherto have been considered almost solely on the basis of the concepts that originated with Aschoff's deductions from observations on vital staining and phagocytosis.

Where, before, the criterion of a reticuloendo-thelial cell was simply that it could be stained vitally, there are now various additional characteristics that seem to confirm that the reticuloendothelial system includes cells that are not notably phagocytic, as well as the macrophages that are its essential consti-tuents. Thus, the property of metallophilia (see page 528) clearly relates the macrophages to cells that are not phagocytes but that show an identical or at least closely similar pattern of cytoplasmic impregnation by certain metal salts *in vitro*.[129]

The concept of the reticuloendothelial system has been attacked often, both on terminological grounds[130] and, more important, because of doubts as to its physiological and structural validity.[131] No satisfactory alternative concept has been produced. Alternative names have been proposed: one that has had some following is *reticulohistiocytic system*, which originally was intended to denote the consti-tuent cells unambiguously[132] and later was applied to an expanded concept of the histiocyte that embodied functional metamorphosis of many other types of cells—including, for instance, muscle cells and epithelial cells—that were thought to be capable of acquiring, irreversibly, the phagocytic and meta-bolic capacity and the motility that characterize true histiocytes.[131]

An authoritative recent view disposes of some of the causes of the present confusion by considering all the highly phagocytic mononuclear cells of the body as a comprehensive group of basically similar cells that together form the *mononuclear phagocyte system*.[111, 125] All morphologically similar but non-phagocytic cells, and cells with only slight phago-cytic activity, are excluded. The mononuclear phagocytes are more reliably identified by direct evidence of phagocytosis of particles than by the classic procedure of vital staining, which, as a result of pinocytosis, may label some cells that are not phagocytes. Another criterion of the mononuclear phagocytes is a peculiar roughening, or 'ruffling', of the surface of the cell, shown by phase contrast microscopy and especially well by electron micro-scopy;[133] this appears to be related to continuous pinocytic activity. A further distinctive characteristic of these cells is their firm adherence to a glass surface, a phenomenon that may be a manifestation of the processes involved in phagocytosis. It has to be noted that a great part of the work that has been done in identifying these cells and defining a mono-nuclear phagocyte system has been concerned with the cells of small laboratory animals, and that its applicability to man is in large part only deductive and conjectural. Nonetheless, there seems to be good correspondence between what is known of the reticuloendothelial cells in general—and of the macrophages (mononuclear phagocytes) in par-ticular—as they appear and function under labora-tory conditions, and what is known of their origin, distribution and behaviour in man.

Life Span of Reticuloendothelial Cells[128]

Less is known of the life span of the non-phagocytic precursor cells of the reticuloendothelial system (see page 527) than of the life span of the macrophages themselves. The identity of the earliest precursor cells, those that give origin to the promonocytes in bone marrow, is undetermined. The promonocytes are known to be multiplicative cells, in contrast to the monocytes, which are their progeny and which do not divide. Each promonocyte is believed to undergo a single division and so to have two daughter cells only. The monocytes enter the circulation within 2 hours or so of formation and then continue to circulate for about 32 hours before taking their place in the tissues and elsewhere (see page 527). Once they become fixed it seems that the macrophages do not return to the blood stream.[134] Their life span in the tissues is probably from several weeks to several months.

Phagocytic Activity of Reticuloendothelial Cells

The cells that are demonstrable by vital staining (see page 524) differ in the degree of their phagocytic activity and so in the intensity of their staining.[120] This variation is reflected in differences of anatomical situation, and probably in differences in other functions of the cells. Some cells, particularly fibroblasts and the endothelial cells of blood vessels and lymphatics, may ingest and store traces of dye: this is most evident among immature, proliferating fibroblasts and endothelial cells, such as are found in granulation tissue, an observation that has been explained on the basis that these cells and macrophages have a common stem cell and so may be expected to retain some functional characteristics in common until their differentiation is completed. An alternative explanation is that the metabolically active, immature cells may be more avidly pinocytic. The relatively very slight phagocytic activity of fibroblasts and of ordinary vascular endothelial cells, and their lack of metallophilia (see below) are generally considered to exclude these cells from the reticuloendothelial system: the cells proper to the latter ingest large, if variable, amounts of dye when stained vitally, and therefore tend to be intensely coloured. Among these true reticuloendothelial cells, the greatest phagocytic activity is shown by the free histiocytes in the tissues and organs and by the monocytes of the blood; the endothelial macrophages of the sinuses of lymph nodes and of blood sinusoids, including the Kupffer cells, are next in phagocytic activity and the reticulum cells are the least active.

Identification of Reticuloendothelial Cells in Man

The reticuloendothelial system was defined from observations of the distribution of vitally stained cells in animals. While it was obvious that a comparable system of cells is to be found in man, the identification of human reticuloendothelial cells had necessarily to depend partly on studies of the distribution of cells that ingest pathological particulate matter, such as malarial pigment, haemosiderin and certain types of parasites (leishmaniae and histoplasmas, for instance), and partly on the supposed identity of morphologically similar animal and human cells and tissues. Morphological identification of cell types, and of their precursors and derivatives, by light microscopy can be a great deal less precise than sometimes is appreciated: this has often led to confusion in attempts to relate various normal and pathological cells, particularly tumour cells, to the reticuloendothelial system. Electron microscopy and, to some extent, the methods of immunology have brought considerable clarification to this field; they have also uncovered fresh problems that could not have been foreseen before the ultrastructural and immunological characteristics of reticuloendothelial and related cells began to be defined. Other procedures have also helped in identifying the reticuloendothelial cells in man: vital staining being inapplicable, and the distribution of particulate matter that has been ingested by cells in the course of physiological or pathological conditions being of equivocal significance, other characteristics of the cells have been sought as a means to their identification. One of the more informative of these has been the affinity of the cytoplasm of reticuloendothelial cells for metal salts (metallophilia).

Metallophilia

In the course of investigating the nature of neuroglia, del Río Hortega observed that the microglial cells (Hortega cells[135]) of the central nervous system could be shown by impregnation with silver carbonate to have argyrophile cytoplasmic processes. As these cells were recognized to be the origin of the characteristic phagocytes of the central nervous system—the so-called compound granular corpuscles (see Chapter 34)—Hortega and his associate Jimenez de Asúa applied the same technical procedure to other tissues and found that the cytoplasm of their phagocytic cells was similarly characterized by argyrophile processes.[136, 137] Subsequent workers extended these studies and it is now known that silver impregnation specifically displays a system of cells that includes not only the reticulo-endothelial cells as defined by Aschoff[123] but also a series of cells that are not selectively demonstrated by vital staining. Salts of gold and of iron and some other metals can be used in place of silver salts in appropriately modified procedures, and show the same cells in the same fashion. The cytoplasm of these cells has such an affinity for these metal salts (metallophilia) that they have been called *metallophile cells* (Fig. 9.10).[129] If the techniques of vital staining and metallic impregnation are applied successively, it can be shown that cells that ingest and store the injected dye are also metallophile; in contrast, by no means all metallophile cells prove to have been stained vitally in such experiments.

Studies on the metallophile cells explained a number of discrepancies in the results of vital staining of the reticuloendothelial system. They also helped to clarify some terminological difficulties. For instance, Maximow described two varieties of cell that occur in close association with the reticulin stroma in lymph nodes, bone marrow and elsewhere: one variety he referred to as the *reticular cell*, and, because of its phagocytic activity and affinity

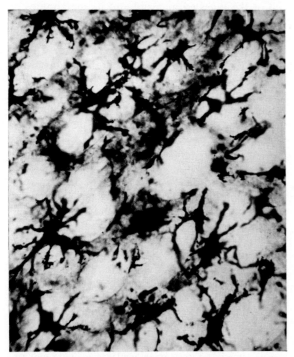

Fig. 9.10.§ Fixed metallophile cells in normal bone marrow of a rabbit. The cell bodies and cytoplasmic processes are impregnated with silver and appear jet black. *Weil–Davenport method of silver impregnation.* × 330.

§ See *Acknowledgements*, page 890.

for vital stains, he classed it as a histiocyte, the name by which he designated the cells of Aschoff's reticuloendothelial system; the other variety of cell Maximow regarded as part of an undifferentiated syncytium that he described as sheathing the reticulin fibres, and this variety he found to be without phagocytic activity, and therefore unable to store vital stains, but capable of transformation into 'reticular cells' or into lymphocytes.[138] In some of his writings, however, Maximow used the name reticular cell to refer to the syncytial cells. To add to the confusion, others have used the names reticulum cell and reticular cell, which should be synonyms, as if they were different in application. Some use the name reticulum cell as a general term for macrophages, wherever they occur; more recently, others have tried to avoid the term altogether, arguing that it is most familiar to pathologists in the designation of certain lymphomas as 'reticulum cell sarcomas' and that the tumours that have been so described are not tumours of reticulum cells at all but tumours of lymphocytic character. Confusion has been increased by differing usage of the word 'reticulum' itself: some use it to mean the meshwork ('network') of reticulin fibres that forms the framework of the lymph nodes, spleen and other lymphoid organs and tissues; others regard it as a collective term for whichever type of cell they consider to be identifiable by the name 'reticulum cell'; and still others have used it as a synonym of 'reticuloendothelial system'.

Silver impregnation has confirmed the existence of two varieties of cell, corresponding to those described by Maximow as associated with the reticulin fibres of the lymphoid tissues: the phagocytic variety is metallophile and the primitive, undifferentiated, variety is not metallophile. However, Maximow's view that the phagocytic reticulum cells are individual units and that the primitive cells form a syncytium is no longer accepted: cells of both types may have syncytial connexions with their fellows, but syncytium formation seems in fact to be inconspicuous among both. Aschoff's description of the reticulum cells as phagocytes, demonstrable by vital staining, has been supported by the more sophisticated technological studies of recent years, while the presence among these phagocytes of comparatively primitive cells that are not capable of phagocytosis has been confirmed. The non-phagocytic cells can be assumed on the grounds of ultrastructural and other studies to be so closely related to the phagocytic mononuclear cells that form the conventional reticuloendothelial system that they must be associated with the latter in any realistic assessment: the demonstration of phagocytic activity by vital staining is no longer a sufficient criterion for placing cells within or outside the reticuloendothelial system.

For the purposes of the present account of the lymphoreticular system and its diseases, it seems desirable to use the term reticuloendothelial system to encompass not only the system of cells demonstrable by vital staining, as defined by Aschoff and his associates, but also the wider system that includes the metallophile cells (among which the vitally stainable cells are numbered) and also the non-metallophile primitive cells that are found among the others and that appear to be 'reserve' cells and the precursors of the maturer members of the system.

Functions of the Reticuloendothelial System

The activities of the reticuloendothelial system fall into three major categories—phagocytosis, immunity, and metabolism. These are primitive activities of the reticuloendothelial cells: they may be regarded as originally closely related, although they eventually—and to a variable extent—became distinct and independent, yet complementary in certain important roles.

Phagocytosis

Phagocytosis subserves what is essentially a clearing or cleansing function, flushing out unwanted endogenous or exogenous materials and disposing of them, either by migratory shedding of particle-laden cells from the body (for instance, through the surface epithelium of the intestine into its lumen, and from the pulmonary alveoli) or by carrying them to particular foci where they slowly accumulate (for instance, in the aggregates of lymphoreticular tissue in the lungs) before eventual clearance through the lymphatics, a process that may never be completely effected. The disposal of haemosiderin formed in the lungs from the breakdown of erythrocytes in infarcts or as an accompaniment of chronic passive congestion is a classic example of this reticuloendothelial function. Another is the disposal of soot and coal dust which may be inhaled during a lifetime in an amount that is by a factor of many hundreds greater than the mass of carbon quantitatively demonstrable in the lungs after death.[139]

Reticuloendothelial phagocytosis of parasites, such as mycobacteria, certain fungi (for example, *Histoplasma capsulatum*) and certain protozoa (for example, *Leishmania donovani*), is a feature of the infections caused by these organisms. Similarly, parasitization of reticuloendothelial cells is characteristic of many viral infections. Epithelioid (endothelioid) metamorphosis of macrophages is a familiar characteristic of the tissue reaction in a wide range of granulomatous diseases. Particular forms of epithelioid cell are found in tuberculosis and other mycobacterioses, in sarcoidosis, in treponemal infections (particularly syphilis), in the blastomycoses and some other fungal infections, in Wegener's disease and in rheumatic and rheumatoid granulomas: their recognition, and their interpretation in relation to other histological characteristics, may be of great help in differential histological diagnosis. Giant cell metamorphosis—the development of multinucleate forms of macrophage—is another familiar feature of granulomas: the multinucleate cells may vary in form in granulomas of differing causation, and recognition of this variation may help sometimes in diagnosis. These variant forms of macrophage, both mononuclear and multinucleate, reflect variations in the interaction of the pathogenic stimulus (the infecting microorganism, for instance) with the cells: the interaction, at least in infective states, is the outcome of phagocytosis and of the consequent effects on the cell of the ingested material and its metabolites or breakdown products.

Phagocytosis of micro-organisms is not in itself a complete defence against persistence and progression of the infection. If the engulfed organisms are killed by enzymes or other agents evolved in the cytoplasm of the phagocytes the infection may be stemmed. If the organisms can survive and multiply within the phagocytes they may kill these cells and escape into the tissues, not only in increased numbers but possibly with their virulence enhanced through acquisition of additional resistance to the protection ordinarily afforded by the cells of the reticuloendothelial system; alternatively, a long-lasting state of intracellular parasitism may result, phagocyte and micro-organisms maintaining a condition of equilibrium that may be disturbed by any serious deterioration in the host's immunological defences.

In general, the phagocytic activity of the reticuloendothelial system in relation to bacteria is complementary to that of the neutrophile polymorphonuclear leucocytes. The latter ingest particularly those bacteria that are responsible for acute, progressive infections (for example, staphylococci, streptococci and neisseriae, and *Escherichia coli* and some other Gram-negative bacilli): these organisms are rarely, or never, demonstrable in macrophages, even when the infection that they cause becomes chronic. Some bacteria, such as *Mycobacterium tuberculosis*, and some fungi, such as *Blastomyces dermatitidis*, may provoke a cellular response that initially is characterized by accumulation of neutrophils and later by participation of macrophages: the histological picture may then become a complex of both types of phagocyte (for example, the 'suppurating pseudotubercle' of blastomycosis—see page 359) or, as occurs early in the course of the initial reaction to tuberculous infection, the neutrophils disappear and macrophages alone contribute to the developing granulomatous response, although often with an access of lymphocytes and plasma cells, in varying proportions, as the immunological defences mediated by these cells come into action.

Measurement of Phagocytic Activity.—Until comparatively recently there were no practical means of measuring the phagocytic activity of the reticuloendothelial system. The development of such means has made it possible to study the stimulant or depressant effects of various physiological, pharmacological and pathological conditions and agents on phagocytosis.[140, 141] The methods depend on the intravenous administration of pure, sterile, nontoxic, stable, colloidal suspensions, of uniform particle size, that are taken up by the cells of the reticuloendothelial system alone, and that are easily and accurately measurable in blood and in tissues. In experimental work on animals, pure colloidal suspensions of carbon, prepared electrolytically and stabilized with gelatin, are now commonly used as the test material in measuring the phagocytic function of the reticuloendothelial system. When such investigations are carried out in man it is obviously not possible to use carbon preparations, because of the visible persistence of the particles, and various other substances have been thought less objectionable: some of these may not meet the most stringent standards of safety as regards freedom from short-term or long-term dangers. Preparations of human serum albumin, labelled with radioactive iodine (^{131}I) and denatured by heating, have been much used, without published reports of serious side effects.* The rate of decline of radioactivity in the blood is a measure of the phagocytic activity of the reticuloendothelial system as its cells remove the labelled albumin particles from the circulation; soon afterwards, catabolism of the iodine-albumin complex in the cytoplasm of the reticuloendothelial cells results in the release of free radioactive iodine

* In an unpublished instance, immediate and almost fatal anaphylactic shock occurred in a medical student who had previously received an injection of a similar preparation in the course of an experimental study.

into the circulation and provides an index of the proteolytic activity of the phagocytes. It is a relatively simple physicochemical procedure to distinguish between the injected iodine-albumin complex and the free ^{131}I released from the cells.

Depression of the Reticuloendothelial System.— Procedures such as those described in the preceding paragraph disclose that the activity of the reticuloendothelial cells is depressed by certain factors and stimulated by others. Depression of phagocytic activity results from blockade of the cells with particulate matter: however, the depression particularly affects phagocytosis of the substance used to blockade the system and there may be little or no reduction in the capacity to ingest different particles. This specificity of blockade has been interpreted as evidence that there are different kinds of macrophages, each with particular selectivity of phagocytic activity.[142] Similar deductions had been made from the histological observation that the simultaneous injection of distinctive particles, such as carmine and colloidal silver, resulted in the accumulation of one of these substances in some Kupffer cells and of the other in other Kupffer cells.[143] It seems likely that the surface properties of ingested particles determine the effect of blockade on subsequent phagocytic potential: for example, reticuloendothelial blockade with colloidal carbon ordinarily has no depressant effect on phagocytosis of a colloidal suspension of, say, chromium phosphate, but if the carbon suspension has been stabilized with gelatin the blockade produced by this preparation will retard phagocytosis of the chromium phosphate suspension if the latter also has been stabilized with gelatin.[144]

Depression of the phagocytic activity of the reticuloendothelial system is caused by large doses (or sustained administration of smaller doses) of cortisone[145] and of cortisol (hydrocortisone) and of various synthetic analogues of these adrenal cortical hormones. Small doses have been observed to enhance phagocytosis.[146] Clinical experience suggests that impaired immunity to certain types of infection, possibly as an effect of diminished phagocytosis by macrophages, may result both from deficiency of corticosteroids (as in the chronic adrenal cortical insufficiency of Addison's disease) and from their excessive production (as in Cushing's syndrome).

A notable depression of the reticuloendothelial system is a specific effect of the lower alkyl esters of certain fatty acids, particularly oleates, palmitates and stearates. This has been attributed to a cyto-

control various forms of cancer. These drugs are cytotoxic and most of them act either by arresting cell division or by killing non-dividing cells (Fig. 9.11). They include alkylating agents (for instance, busulphan, chlorambucil, cyclophosphamide and mustine), which stop mitosis by effecting the cross-linkage of guanine bases in deoxyribonucleic acid, and the antimetabolites (for instance, azathioprine, mercaptopurine and methotrexate), which compete with physiological metabolites for intracellular enzymes and so prevent the normal metabolic functions of the cells. In addition, there are the so-called antineoplastic antibiotics (for instance, the actinomycins and daunorubicin), the vinca alkaloids (such as vinblastine), urethane, and a variety of other substances that have the same therapeutic potential. Considering the wide clinical use of these 'immuno-suppressant' and cytotoxic drugs, remarkably little is known in detail of their effects on normal and pathological cells and tissues. Most of the drugs that are used as immunosuppressants act at several points in the complex system of immune responsiveness, affecting not only lymphocytes but also the relatively less sensitive reticuloendothelial cells and neutrophils. It seems likely that B lymphocytes are usually more sensitive to immunosuppressants than T lymphocytes;[167] in some circumstances the opposite may be true.[168]

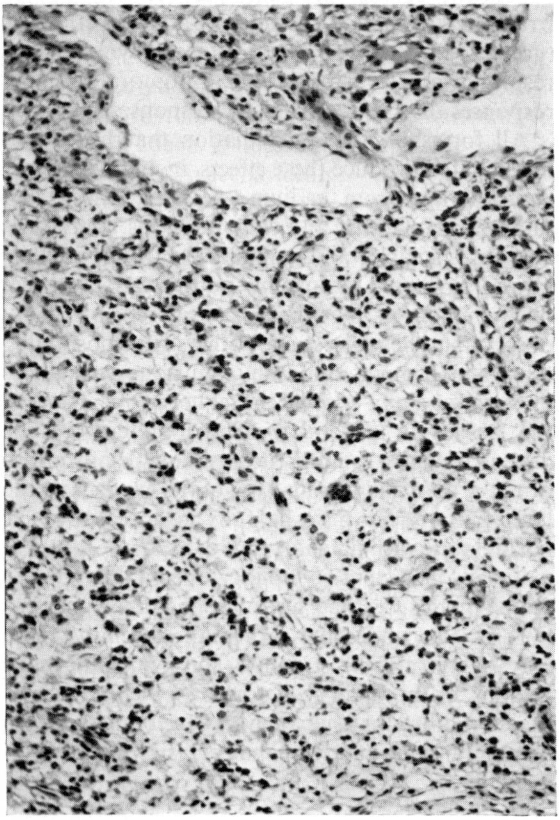

The immunosuppressant activity of these drugs, and of other therapeutic agents that interfere with immune responses, such as X-rays, corticosteroids and antilymphocyte serum, has the important practical side effect of predisposing to a wide range of different types of infection, including the so-called 'opportunistic' infections (see page 362). There is, consequently, a great danger of death from such infections when any of these agents is used in treatment, whether specifically to suppress immune responses or to combat malignant disease.

Fig. 9.11. Almost total disappearance of lymphoid cells from a lymph node as a result of a 10-fold error in calculating the dosage of cytotoxic drugs in the treatment of leukaemia by inexperienced doctors working without access to laboratory control. *Haematoxylin–eosin.* × 160.

Hormonal Influences

Adrenal Cortex.—The corticosteroids are described as 'lympholytic', by which is meant that their administration leads to a decrease in the number of lymphocytes in the tissues; in consequence of this loss of lymphocytes there is a corresponding suppression of immune responses, particularly of cell-mediated immunity. There are notable species differences in the extent to which these effects develop;[169] man, like the guinea-pig, is less sensitive by far than rats, mice and rabbits, in which the production of circulating antibodies is also inhibited.[170]

The gross insufficiency of adrenal cortical hormones that characterizes Addison's disease (see Chapter 30) is accompanied by a well-marked lymphocytosis in the blood in most cases, and there may be many large lymphoid follicles in the bone marrow,[171] which in the normal person is seldom, if ever, found to contain such foci. In some cases there is such an increase in the number of lymphocytes in the lymphoid tissues of patients with Addison's disease that a lymphoma may be simulated; an erroneous diagnosis of chronic lymphocytic leukaemia may be suggested by the extent of the interstitial accumulation of these cells in other tissues and organs.[172] These findings are thought to be due to release of the lymphoid tissues from the restraining effect normally exercised by the adrenal cortex.

Regression and eventual atrophy of the lymphoid tissues, comparable to the effects of adrenal cortical hormones, are also caused by corticotrophin, pre-

appeared, it seemed in order to write, 'The nomenclature of the true neoplasms of the lymphoreticular system is less muddled', with the implication that there was a reasonable measure of agreement on the terminology of the comparatively small number of tumours that were recognized to arise in these tissues. Since then, and partly as an outcome of the realization of the practical importance of diagnostic precision in relation to prognosis and to the choice of treatment from the expanding range of chemotherapeutic, radiotherapeutic and surgical measures, there has been intensive study of these tumours in many centres throughout the world. This study has greatly advanced knowledge of their cytology and of their cytogenesis: at the same time, its rapid progress has been expressed in the introduction of various new histological classifications and methods of staging the diseases, and these, perhaps unavoidably, are associated with the use by different groups of workers of differing and sometimes conflicting nomenclature. In consequence, the ordinary pathologist and clinician often find it difficult to comprehend the significance of the advances that are being made.

Historically, the first variety of lymphoreticular neoplasm to be recognized was the *lymphosarcoma*, which Virchow described in 1863,[195] thirty years before the classic account by Kundrat[196] that led to its general recognition. The occurrence of tumours derived from reticulum cells was suggested by James Ewing[197] in 1913, and the concept of *reticulum cell sarcoma* was soon recognized. In 1928 Oberling introduced the name *reticulosarcoma* as a generic term for all neoplasms of the lymphoreticular system,[198] and since then varieties such as lymphocytic and lymphoblastic reticulosarcomas, reticulum-cell reticulosarcoma, pleomorphic or anaplastic reticulosarcomas, and sundry more disputable cytological types have been catalogued in attempts to classify these growths. The name *Retothelsarkom* is sometimes used in German[199] and has much the same meaning as reticulosarcoma in English, although some writers in the latter language have used the term 'retothelial sarcoma' as though it referred to a distinct new variety of tumour.* American authors adopted lymphoma and lymphoblastoma as generic names for tumours of

* The word *Retothel* ('retothelium') was used by Rössle and Roulet as a convenient term for the network (*rete*) of interconnected cells that are intimately associated with the reticulin fibres of the lymph nodes and other lymphoreticular organs. It is still in occasional use as a generic name for these cells (reticulum cells—see page 525). The term *Retothelsarkom* was evidently introduced by Rössle (Rössle, R., cited in: Roulet, F., *Virchows Arch. path. Anat.*, 1930, **277**, 15).

the lymphoreticular system, and the former has now become the universally accepted term (see page 767).

The unequivocal view that Hodgkin's disease is neoplastic, and is to be classed among the lymphomas, and the suggestion that most 'reticulum cell' sarcomas are not tumours of reticulum cells at all but particular varieties of lymphocytic or histiocytic tumours, are innovations that mark the continuing progress of the history of the tumours of the lymphoreticular system (see page 849).

Generic Terms for the Diseases of the Lymphoreticular System

Many classifications of the diseases of the lymphoreticular system have been proposed, and a large number of synonyms has been used. Terminological ambiguity and confusion are found even among the best contributions to the vast literature; it is sometimes quite impossible to be certain of the identity of the diseases under discussion, and, consequently, attempts to make practical use of published figures, concepts and interpretations are often fruitless or misleading. It is not proposed to adopt any synthetic classification in this chapter: instead, the diseases of the component organs and tissues of the lymphoreticular system and the systemic diseases of the system as a whole will be dealt with singly or in such groups as they fall into naturally. It is necessary, however, to note some points concerning some of the generic terms that have been particularly liable to abuse or misunderstanding.

'*The Lymphadenopathies*'.—Some workers have considered all diseases of the lymphoreticular system under the general heading of *primary lymphadenopathies* or, simply, *the lymphadenopathies*. This has encouraged a misconception that these diseases are essentially diseases of lymph nodes: in consequence, the importance of involvement of other organs has sometimes been overlooked, while Hodgkin's disease and the like have been confused and, in a sense, identified with diseases of different nature, importance and prognosis—such as sarcoidosis—merely because lymph node involvement is common to them all.

'*The Reticuloses*'.—The term *reticulosis* was introduced by Letterer as a synonym for reticuloendotheliosis, by which he understood a disease characterized histologically by a systematized reticulum cell proliferation.[194] Some years later Letterer laid stress on the need to use the term only as originally intended, to describe a systematized proliferation of reticulum cells *without differentiation*.[200] Meantime, however, 'reticulosis' had been used by others in a wider sense,[201] and, following this trend, Robb-Smith drew up a complex classification of 'reticuloses' according to the cytology and the topography of the microscopical changes in lymph nodes.[202, 203] He classified a diverse collection of non-specific and specific inflammatory diseases, lipidoses, Hodgkin's disease, follicular lymphoma and leukaemias among other 'reticuloses'; he divorced these conditions from the unequivocal sarcomas of the lymphoreticular system, for which he introduced a separate cytological classification under a general heading, 'the reticulosarcomas'. The complicated subdivisions of the classifications of 'reticuloses' depend upon specialized and often subjective histological and cytological interpretations, and they have not been readily intelligible in practice or adaptable to day-to-day diagnostic work. Even the most complex of these classifications, some of which list as many as 25 and more varieties, fail to cover all the variant microscopical appearances that may be presented by the reactions of the lymphoreticular system in disease: this observation is fundamental, for the very diversity of the histological findings suggests that we may be dealing not with a correspondingly large number of entities but with a relatively small number, individual cases of which may differ in the detail of the tissue reaction, just as individual cases of tuberculosis or of other well-defined entities may show striking histological differences from other cases of the same disease.

In practice, difficulty was often experienced in identifying some of the varieties of 'reticulosis' that had been described: this encouraged a tendency to use the name reticulosis as if it were an adequate diagnosis in itself, thereby avoiding the problem of defining the histological picture precisely. In this wide sense, in fact, the term embraced conditions that range from the simplest of transient reactive changes to such mortal diseases as Hodgkin's disease. In view of this, the onus is clearly upon any pathologist who still uses this term to remember that it may be interpreted at the bedside as indicating the behaviour of the most familiar disease that the clinician knows to have been so called—Hodgkin's disease. Few authoritative publications by specialists in the field of lymphoreticular diseases nowadays perpetuate use of the term reticulosis, except perhaps as a synonym referring specifically to a very few, quite well-defined diseases that may be regarded as entities, such as some forms of malignant histiocytosis. If these specialists have succeeded in avoiding this term in their own current discussions and publications, the same is not true, yet, of medical practitioners in general, including many pathologists and many clinical specialists. A considerable experience of sharing the diagnostic problems of practising pathologists and of radiotherapists and other clinicians has not yet shown that the term reticulosis is obsolete: on the contrary, it still, although less frequently, leads to occasional misunderstanding, and therefore to inappropriate clinical action, and this risk will last until unambiguous diagnostic nomenclature is universally used.

THE LYMPH NODES[204-206]

INTRODUCTION

The lymph nodes combine the role of lymph filter with the immunogenic activity of their lymphoid tissue and reticuloendothelial cells and with other functions that are dependent on the phagocytic and metabolic activity of the latter component. All of these functions expose the nodes to pathogenic influences. The lymph that filters through them exposes them to infection and to damage by toxins and other harmful substances, and also to seeding with tumour cells. The vulnerability of lymph nodes to lymph-borne pathogenic stimuli of all sorts is paralleled by their comparable vulnerability to potentially harmful agents carried to them with their blood supply. Excessive or abnormal reaction to antigenic stimuli may cause significant changes in both the lymphoid and the reticuloendothelial components of the nodes. The phagocytic activity of the reticuloendothelial cells, and defects in their metabolic functions, may likewise lead to a variety of distinctive pathological pictures. Tumours may arise from any of the cells of the nodes, and the whole range of lymphomas is included among these.

In general, diseases of lymph nodes that result from their role as lymph filters are confined to the groups of nodes that drain the source of the disease-causing factor, which usually is a local infection or a primary tumour in the drainage area of the affected nodes. Blood-borne pathogenic stimuli tend to cause changes in the nodes throughout the body, and such changes are often accompanied by corresponding changes in other parts of the lymphoreticular system, such as the spleen.

The classic 'barrier theory' of defence by the lymph nodes dates from observations by Virchow.[207] Its validity was supported by recognition of the highly developed structural adaptation of the lymph nodes to act as filters of the lymph stream. Later, recognition of the reticuloendothelial system (see page 523), with its phagocytic and metabolic activities, indicated the functioning cytological complement of the structural filter, and, most recently, the many discoveries relating to the role of the lymphoid and reticuloendothelial systems in the development of immunity (see page 520) have given point to the earlier anatomical observations. It is for such reasons that the concept of the lymphoid system and the reticuloendothelial system as an anatomical and functional whole—the lymphoreticular system (see page 506)—is considered to be so well justified.

The barrier theory, applicable as it is to lymph nodes as filters, did not explain the purpose of lymphoid tissue in other situations, where the absence of afferent lymphatic connexions precludes a simple filter action: the theory had, therefore, to be elaborated. Hellman[208] suggested that the reticuloendothelial cells in lymphoid tissue, and particularly those in the central part of lymphoid follicles (what he called the 'reaction centre' of the follicles), filtered harmful material from the circulating blood. Thus, he considered that the lymphoid follicles, and particularly those in the spleen, have a filtering action on blood comparable to that of lymph nodes on lymph. While this could well be so in the spleen, in which the blood passes through the substance of the follicles on its way into the pulp, it is unlikely to be possible in, for example, the tonsillar or intestinal lymphoid tissue. It is now recognized that the functions of the follicles essentially relate to the development of the immune reaction to antigenic stimulation (see pages 512 to 514).

Because of the unusual lability of the lymphoid tissues, a wide range of appearances may be seen in lymph nodes under what are essentially physiological conditions. Similarly, the activity of the reticuloendothelial elements in the nodes varies considerably and the cellularity of the lymph sinuses may differ markedly without exceeding the range of normality (see page 559). Such variations must be taken into account when interpreting histological preparations: often, their assessment as normal or pathological is subjective and based on the observer's individual experience.

STRUCTURAL ANOMALIES

Epithelial Inclusions in Lymph Nodes

Benign epithelial inclusions have been described in lymph nodes from various parts of the body, and particularly in nodes in the vicinity of the major salivary glands or of the thyroid gland, and in the pelvis and axillae. They usually take the form of isolated acinar or tubular structures, lined by columnar, cuboidal or flat epithelial cells (Fig. 9.12). Occasionally they are small cysts. The acinar and cystic structures may contain proteinaceous or mucous material. Their origin is always debatable[209] and would seem to differ in the different sites.

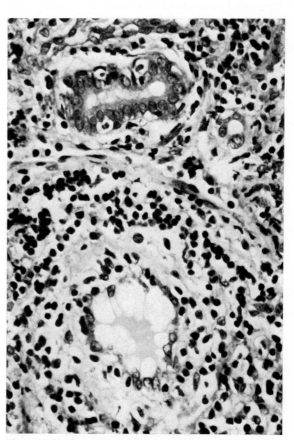

Fig. 9.12. Benign epithelial inclusion in a lymph node of an inferior deep cervical group in a young woman who had no symptoms other than slight enlargement of the cervical nodes, which proved to be due to toxoplasmosis (see page 652). The biopsy specimen contained several similar epithelial structures. All were lined by low columnar epithelial cells with opaque cytoplasm. The clear cells between these and the basement membrane may be myoepithelial. There was no abnormality of the breasts or salivary glands. The blood vessel in the photograph provides a comparison with the epithelial tubule (compare with Fig. 9.64, page 589). *Haematoxylin–eosin.* × 400.

Inclusions of Salivary Gland Tissue.—In lymph nodes adjacent to the parotid and submandibular salivary glands, and more rarely in other cervical nodes, ductules like those of the salivary glands, and occasionally even solitary acini or small clusters of acini, may be found (*Neisse–Nicholson inclusions*) (Fig. 9.13).[210] Lymph nodes with inclusions of salivary gland tissue have to be distinguished from lobules of salivary gland in which the parenchyma has undergone marked atrophy while abundant lymphoid tissue, characteristically with well-formed follicles, has developed in the stroma: these lobules, which resemble lymph nodes quite closely, still contain scattered, and often numerous, ductules and occasional acini of salivary tissue. Such an appearance is often seen in cases of the so-called 'benign lymphoepithelial lesion' (Sjögren's syndrome—see page 952): the absence of the characteristic trabecular framework and of the subcapsular and other lymph sinuses is useful in distinguishing these transformed lobules from lymph nodes.

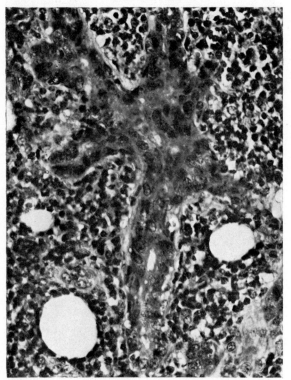

Fig. 9.13. The cellular structure with the radiating outline is an incompletely developed system of ductules of salivary gland type included in an otherwise normal lymph node of the superior deep cervical groups—it is one variety of Neisse–Nicholson inclusion. The three rounded spaces are fat cells, which are occasionally found in lymph nodes, particularly in older people (see page 548). *Haematoxylin–eosin.* × 325.

Inclusions of Thyroid Tissue.—There are important differences of opinion about the occurrence of inclusions of non-neoplastic thyroid tissue in lymph nodes. The view with the most ominous implications is that thyroid tissue in lymph nodes is always a manifestation of the metastasis of a primary carcinoma of the thyroid gland: the argument and its significance are comparable to those relating to the occurrence of 'lateral aberrant thyroid tissue' in the neck, at a distance from the thyroid gland itself (see Chapter 31). It is now generally accepted that the finding of papillary thyroid tissue in a lymph node must be regarded as evidence of metastasis of a primary thyroid carcinoma until this possibility has been excluded by the most thorough pathological examination of the entire thyroid gland. In contrast, the finding of colloid-containing thyroid follicles, totally devoid of papillary epithelial ingrowths, and lined by cuboidal or flattened epithelial cells that show no nuclear abnormalities sufficient to suggest the possibility of malignancy, is accepted by some experienced histopathologists as a benign manifestation,[211] and the opposite interpretation appears not to have been substantiated. The explanation of the presence of thyroid follicles in lymph nodes, as a benign condition, is debatable. The fact that such follicles are usually in the subcapsular lymph sinuses, although sometimes with further clusters of follicles within the lymphoid tissue itself and in the connective tissue immediately external to the capsule of the node, has been interpreted as support for the view that normal thyroid tissue may be carried in lymph from the thyroid gland to cervical lymph nodes (the so-called 'benign metastasis' of normal tissue) (see Chapter 31).[211, 212]

Thyroid follicles that conform to the characteristics described above as benign are said to be demonstrable in one cervical lymph node in about 3000 examined in the course of thorough dissections of the neck.[211, 213]

Inclusions of Endometriform and Endometrial Tissue.—Epithelial tubules that resemble non-secretory endometrial glands are a very occasional finding in lymph nodes of the iliac, sacral and inguinal groups.[214] These endometriform foci are not considered to be a manifestation of the usual forms of endometriosis (see Chapter 27); indeed, there is doubt whether their cells are of endometrial character. The origin of these foci is obscure. They may be metaplastic or developmental (heterotopic), but neither possibility has been supported by acceptable evidence.

Instances of unequivocal endometriosis of lymph

nodes are rarer. The affected nodes belong usually to the iliac groups and sometimes to the inguinal groups. It is the presence of clusters or cuffs of small, deeply stained, spindle-shaped cells, resembling the cells of resting endometrial stroma, in association with tubules, that suggests the endometrial nature of such foci. The absence of evidence of bleeding, fresh or old, and of fibrosis has been thought to disqualify this suggestion; however, experience of true endometriosis elsewhere indicates that it may exist without the occurrence of bleeding or other evidence of response to cyclical hormonal changes.

Endometriosis might develop in lymph nodes as a result of metaplasia, or of carriage of endometrial fragments in lymph, or of extension of the disease directly from deposits in adjoining tissues. Of these possibilities, metaplasia is an entirely conjectural explanation, and it is difficult to conceive of grounds for regarding the pelvic lymph nodes as liable to a metaplastic change that lymph nodes elsewhere do not undergo. The second possibility, that of 'benign metastasis' of endometrial tissue by way of lymphatics,[215] has not been demonstrated unequivocally: the occasional finding of fragments of endometrium in lymphatics—for instance, in the wall of the uterus or in the mesosalpinx or mesovarium—is probably explicable as an artefact, caused during dissection of the specimen.[216] Nevertheless, the lymphogenous implantation of viable endometrium in the sinuses of the nodes is the likeliest explanation of those cases in which the endometrial foci are wholly within the normal confines of the nodes. The third explanation of endometriosis of lymph nodes—their involvement by direct extension of the disease from adjoining foci—is certainly true of some examples of the condition, both in the pelvis and in the inguinal regions. Endometriosis of inguinal nodes is particularly rare; it has been observed as an accompaniment of endometriosis in the inguinal prolongation of the saccus vaginalis of the peritoneum (canal of Nuck)[217] when this structure has persisted after fetal life, so providing a route by which endometrial fragments can reach the inguinal region from the general peritoneal cavity. The involvement of lymph nodes in the vicinity is not attributable to any invasive tendency of the endometrial tissue but results during the course of the inflammatory reaction in the affected tissues: this extends into the nodes and encourages incorporation of endometrial structures within them (Fig. 9.14).

It is unusual for the endometrial foci in lymph nodes to show clear evidence of the effects of the ovarian hormones (Fig. 9.15). In an exceptional case, which presented with recent onset of painful

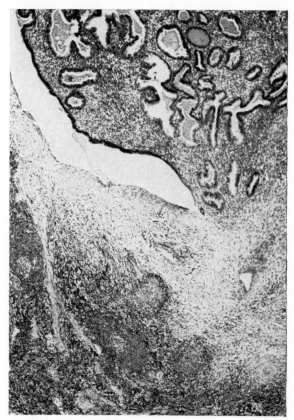

Fig. 9.14.§ Endometriosis associated with the saccus vaginalis of the peritoneum (canal of Nuck). The endometrial focus (above) protrudes into the blind end of the canal and forms the lining of its wall on one aspect. Part of a lymph node is seen below, its structure merging into the fibrotic tissue associated with the endometriotic condition. *Haematoxylin–eosin.* × 40.

enlargement of an inguinal node, there was marked secretory activity and distension of the endometrial glands and the stroma showed changes typical of a decidual reaction.[216] These findings led to consideration of the possibility that the patient, who had had a uterine curettage a month earlier, might have an ectopic pregnancy. The surgeon did not consider the histological evidence sufficiently convincing to justify laparotomy; the patient died a week later from rupture of a gravid uterine tube.

Significance of Benign Epithelial Inclusions in Lymph Nodes.—The importance of distinguishing these benign inclusions from carcinomatous deposits in lymph nodes is obvious. With the exception of endometriosis, which may cause pain during menstruation and be associated with bleeding into the foci, the inclusions are, in general, harmless. There is a theoretical possibility of malignant change

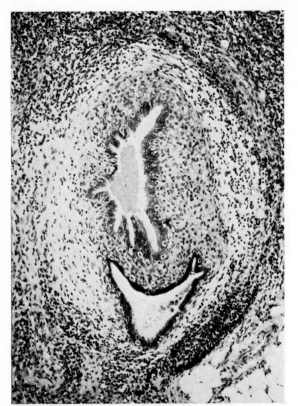

Fig. 9.15. Endometriosis of a partly atrophic inguinal lymph node (fatty infiltration is seen on the right, below). One of the endometrial cysts is lined by pale, somewhat hyperplastic epithelium; the stroma surrounding it shows a well-marked predecidual change (see Chapter 27). The other cyst is lined by relatively atrophic and inactive epithelium that is deeply stained. *Haematoxylin–eosin.* × 85.

occurring in any epithelial inclusion; the development of a carcinoma in an endometrial focus in a pelvic node has been reported.[218]

Provided the possibility of their occurrence is remembered, the real nature of the various types of benign inclusion can usually be recognized. This is so even when they are found in lymph nodes removed in the course of radical surgery for cancer, for the benign inclusions are fully differentiated, mature-looking structures and are unlikely to resemble closely any carcinoma with which they may be associated coincidentally. Obviously, it can be very important not to misinterpret them as secondary deposits: to do so may lead to mistakes in staging and prognostication, and even to inappropriate treatment.

So-Called Naevus Cells in Lymph Nodes[219, 220]

The benign presence in lymph nodes of clusters of cells that have been variously interpreted as naevus cells (Fig. 9.16),[219] such as characterize the common pigmented naevi of the skin, and as glomus cells[220] is probably less rare than the small number of published cases—about 50 (24 of them in one report[219])—may suggest. The nature of these cells is uncertain, and electron microscopy has not led to their identification.[220] Melanin has been found in them only in exceptionally rare instances: in a case that I have seen the appearances of the clusters were unquestionably those ordinarily associated with benign dermal naevi (Fig. 9.17). In a few cases the disposition of the cells in relation to blood vessels, and the appearance of the cells themselves, have been notably reminiscent of a glomangiomatous hamartoma (see Chapter 39);[220] it is possible that such cases represent a distinct form of hamartoma or —possibly—of heterotopia (Fig. 9.18). Oftener, the

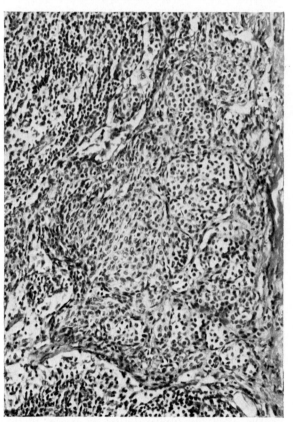

Fig. 9.16.§ Typical solid alveolar clusters of naevus cells just under the capsule of a superficial lymph node and abutting on its subcapsular sinus. The lateral limit of the focus is not well defined above, and there is a single cluster of naevus cells in a connective tissue septum in the sinus. These observations suggest that the condition was continuing to extend locally, but they do not indicate that it is malignant. There is no known instance of cancerous change in such foci. See also Fig. 9.17. *Haematoxylin–eosin.* × 160.

thought to indicate the characteristic adaptation to the connective tissue environment that may be a feature of dermal naevus cells.[219]

Naevus Cells in Lymph Nodes in Association with Blue Naevi of the Skin.—Pigmented cells are, rarely, found in lymph nodes draining the site of a cellular blue naevus (Jadassohn–Tièche naevus—see Chapter 39) of the dermis.[221] Usually these are simply macrophages that have ingested melanin carried to the node from the naevus in the skin, but in rare instances the pigmented cells have the characteristic appearance of the cells of the blue

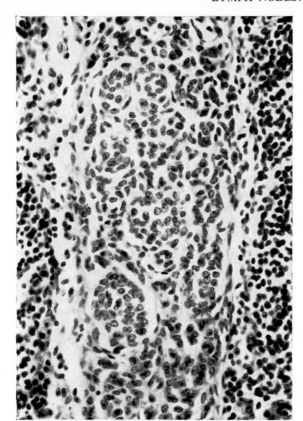

Fig. 9.17. Collection of solid alveoli of naevus cells in a trabecula of an axillary lymph node. A very small proportion of the alveoli included cells containing scanty brown pigment that gave the chemical reactions of melanin. The biopsy was part of the investigation in a case of illness that turned out to be infectious mononucleosis; the naevus cells were an incidental finding. *Haematoxylin–eosin.* × 300.

cells either have no particular arrangement, being clustered compactly in a rather uniform collection that is moulded to the adjoining structures of the node, or they are grouped in small, solid alveoli enclosed in a delicate connective tissue framework and resembling the cell clusters of certain forms of dermal naevus (see Chapter 39). The fact that the affected nodes have evidently all been from superficial groups, draining the skin, has been thought to strengthen the interpretation that the cells are in fact naevus cells, carried to the nodes in the lymph from the skin.

The cells are usually confined to the connective tissue of the nodes (capsule and trabeculae); rarely, they are in the wall of blood vessels or in a lymph sinus, or in the lymphoid parenchyma, but even in these situations they are in closest relation to connective tissue fibres, an observation that has been

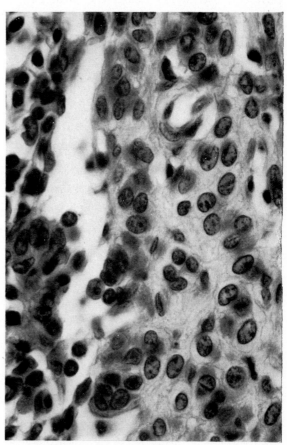

Fig. 9.18. This photograph of a cervical lymph node shows, from left to right, the pulp, the subcapsular sinus, and the capsule itself. The latter contains small cells of distinct outline, with a rounded or ovoid, sometimes indented, nucleus. Some of these cells are disposed in relation to blood vessels in the fashion of glomus cells. Although their nature is still undecided, these cells are commonly considered to be glomus cells and the appearances illustrated to represent a form of glomeral hamartia. The picture is liable to be confused with that of the clusters of naevus cells that may be found in the same situation in otherwise normal lymph nodes (see Figs 9.16 and 9.17). *Haematoxylin–eosin.* × 750.

naevus, with multiple, fine, branching cytoplasmic processes that are finely stippled with melanin (Fig. 9.19). In some instances there is such extensive growth of the naevus tissue in the nodes that only the absence of further spread and the long persistence of the condition without deterioration in the patient's general health justify the benign interpretation.

Significance of Naevus Cells in Lymph Nodes.— From the practical viewpoint, the importance of the presence of pigmented naevus cells in lymph nodes is that they may lead to a mistaken diagnosis of metastatic melanoma. Conversely, great care is

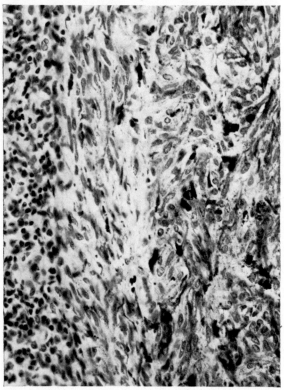

Fig. 9.19.§ Infiltration of the capsule and subcapsular sinus of a lymph node by spindle-shaped cells among which are numerous cells heavily laden with melanin. Some of the pigmented cells are macrophages; others are elongated and have long, fine cytoplasmic extensions that also contain melanin. The appearances are those typically seen in the so-called blue naevus of the skin (see Figs 39.77 and 39.78, Chapter 39). The patient had had a cutaneous blue naevus removed from a finger 5 years before the incidental finding of a 'black' lymph node in the corresponding axilla during dissection of a recurrent lesion of infiltrative fibromatosis of the shoulder region from which she also suffered. There has been no recurrence of the blue naevus during 10 years since the lymph node was discovered. *Haematoxylin–eosin.* × 250.

needed before the microscopist commits himself to identifying the cells as naevus cells and not as melanoma cells. The possibility that such naevus cells in a lymph node might become the starting point of a malignant melanoma is a theoretical one that, in the event, could only be sustained after the most rigorous exclusion of a primary melanoma in any other site.

The presence of naevus cells in lymph nodes could result from 'benign metastasis' of the cells of a dermal naevus[221a] or blue naevus.[221] An alternative suggestion, in those cases in which the cells are of the type characteristic of the dermal naevus, is that they were misplaced during migration from the neural crest in embryonic life.[222] In the latter case it would be expected that such cell clusters would be found in abdominal and thoracic nodes as well as in those superficially placed.

Finally, it must be noted that these clusters are occasionally misinterpreted as carcinomatous, particularly as secondary deposits of mammary carcinoma. Perhaps they are even oftener overlooked altogether, because of their likeness to lymphoid aggregates.

Giant Lymphoid Hamartoma ('Giant Lymph Node', 'Angiofollicular Lymph Node Hyperplasia' and Similar Conditions)[223, 224]

Occasionally, and then usually in adults, of either sex, a large, solitary, encapsulate mass of non-neoplastic lymphoid tissue is found in the mediastinum or elsewhere. It is liable to be mistaken, in the mediastinum, for a thymoma (see page 907), both radiologically and, with less reason, histologically. The histological appearances of these masses differ in detail in different specimens: one well-defined type predominates and is the subject of most of the following account. It is probable that a number of entities may present in this way; as they all have in common their benign course and non-neoplastic nature, this seems a convenient place to consider them.

Most specimens of these conditions have been chance findings—for example, on radiological examination of the chest. Some have presented with symptoms due to pressure on adjoining structures, or have been in a superficial situation and attracted attention because of their size. They usually occur in regions where lymph nodes are present normally: the commonest sites are the mediastinum (including its anterior and posterior parts, especially the latter, and the pulmonary hilum), the neck (especially the anterior triangle) and the abdomen (retroperitoneal tissue and mesenteries); other sites include the axillary and inguinal regions. More rarely, similar masses have been found in skeletal muscle and in some other parts where lymph nodes are not ordinarily present: it is probable that these lesions are inflammatory (see page 546).

Often on the assumption that all such solitary, encapsulate masses of lymphoid tissue are essentially of the same nature, they have been described by different investigators as hyperplastic lymph nodes,[225] hamartomas[226] and benign lymphomas.[227] The uncertainty about their nature is reflected in their many synonyms.[228] A tendency to refer to them as tumours—'benign lymphoma',[227] for instance, or eponymously as 'Castleman's lymphoma'[228] is unfortunate: all the reported cases appear to have had a benign course and there are no histological grounds for regarding any of the varieties as neoplastic. Certainly, they should not be described as lymphomas, since this term is now applied by so many clinicians only in the sense of malignant tumours that arise in the lymphoreticular tissues.* A widely used term is 'angiofollicular lymph node hyperplasia':[224, 229] 'angiofollicular hyperplasia' describes the histological picture of a large proportion of these masses, but whether they are properly regarded as lymph nodes is less certain (see below). The name 'giant lymphoid hamartoma', which does not relate the lesions specifically to lymph nodes, has been preferred in presenting this account of the condition.

Histopathology.—The classic histological picture of these encapsulate lymphoid masses is quite distinctive (Figs 9.20 to 9.22). The lesion is almost always solitary. It various considerably in size, ranging from a spheroidal mass some 4 cm in diameter to an ovoid measuring as much as $14 \times 9 \times 7$ cm and weighing 700 g. Microscopically,[224] the most striking feature is the large number of blood vessels traversing the lymphoid tissue, particularly between the lymphoid follicles (Fig. 9.21). The vessels are usually conspicuous because their wall is thick and cellular or hyaline. Each lymphoid follicle is entered by one or more vessels, their thick, palely staining wall contrasting with the darkly stained lymphocytes clustered round them (Fig. 9.22). The number and proximity of the follicles vary considerably, but their size is usually appreciably smaller than that of the

* I know of two cases of giant lymphoid hamartoma of the posterior part of the mediastinum needlessly referred for radiotherapy or chemotherapy because of misunderstanding of the significance of the histological diagnosis of respectively 'solitary lymphoma' and 'Castleman's lymphoma' that had been made after excision of the lesions.

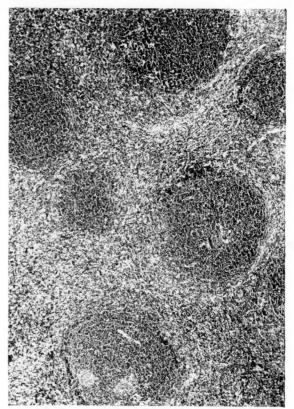

Fig. 9.20. Giant lymphoid hamartoma ('angiofollicular lymph node hyperplasia'). Several follicles are included in the field, some with blood vessels entering their substance. The follicle at the bottom of the picture has two small germinal centres. The tissue between the follicles is pale because it consists largely of a complex of small blood vessels, which are separated by lymphocytes. The entire extent of this specimen was of the same structure as illustrated. There were no lymph sinuses. The lesion was a chance radiological finding in the mediastinum. It measured $7 \cdot 5 \times 5 \times 4$ cm. See also Figs 9.21 and 9.22. *Haematoxylin–eosin.* $\times 35$.

average hyperplastic follicle in instances of simple follicular hyperplasia (see page 553). The follicles consist of mature lymphocytes, often arranged in a more or less concentric pattern; sometimes there are a few large pale cells, possibly histiocytes, immediately adjoining the blood vessels. Germinal centres are present only in a minority of specimens: the follicles that contain them are large and, in general, resemble those of simple follicular hyperplasia. It is significant that the cases in which germinal centres are found are those in which there are general symptoms (see below).

Lymph sinuses are lacking in the classic form of giant lymphoid hamartoma. They are present in the rare variant in which the mass seems to be an aggregate of incompletely formed lymph nodes:

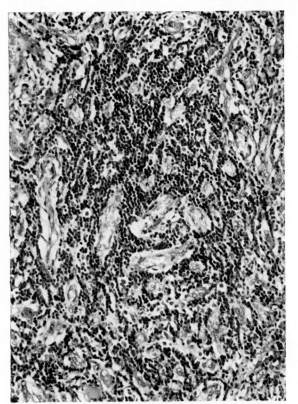

Fig. 9.21. Giant lymphoid hamartoma. Another specimen. Field of interfollicular lymphoid tissue showing a large number of small but conspicuous blood vessels lined by large, pale endothelial cells. *Haematoxylin–eosin.* × 150.

distinct traces of the trabecular framework of the nodes persist in this variant, and the trabecular and subcapsular sinuses can be identified in parts of their course. The usual type of lymphoid hamartoma, in contrast, lacks regular trabeculae as well as sinuses, and in its organization resembles tonsillar or intestinal lymphoid tissue rather than lymph nodes, although it is to the latter that it is usually likened. The absence of sinuses, which are so essentially a feature of normal lymph nodes, throws doubt on the suggestion that the giant lymphoid hamartoma is basically a lymph node and supports the view that it is a hamartoma of lymphoid tissue rather than a hamartomatous lymph node.

Varieties.—The variety that seems to consist of incompletely separated lymph nodes has been mentioned in the preceding paragraph. Another variety consists of splenic tissue and is found in the retroperitoneal tissue, particularly in the vicinity of the body and tail of the pancreas: its structure mainly is that of the white pulp of the spleen, but

typical red pulp is sometimes present also. It may be regarded as a retroperitoneal spleniculus (see page 726).

The solitary encapsulate masses of lymphoid tissue that are found from time to time in muscles, and other situations where lymphoid structures are not ordinarily seen, have been described in various publications as of the same nature as the lesions referred to here as giant lymphoid hamartomas. The few that I have seen have been quite different in structure, and have seemed rather to be inflammatory in nature or akin to the so-called lymphocytic granulomas of the skin (see Chapter 39). Although they are outlined by a definite fibrous zone, there is usually some extension of the lymphocytic accumulation outside this capsule-like limit. Germinal centres are often very conspicuous in the follicles,

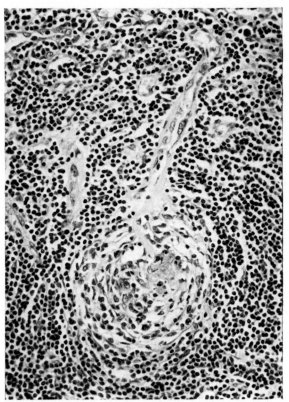

Fig. 9.22. Giant lymphoid hamartoma. Another specimen. A small blood vessel enters a lymphoid follicle from the upper part of the field and other vessels are also seen. The nature of the curious, concentrically patterned structure at the centre of the follicle is uncertain: in the instance illustrated it includes a small core of fibrinoid material, possibly of thrombotic origin. Similar structures may be seen in lymph nodes as germinal centres undergo regressive changes; germinal centres are not usually present at all in the giant lymphoid hamartomas. *Haematoxylin–eosin.* × 200.

and the curious vascularity of the giant lymphoid hamartoma is absent (Fig. 9.23).

General Symptoms Accompanying Giant Lymphoid Hamartoma and Similar Conditions.—In about 10 per cent of cases of these solitary encapsulate lymphoid masses, and most commonly in association with the mediastinal examples, the patient has general symptoms. The latter include malaise, fever, loss of weight and loss of energy, and they are accompanied by such findings as splenomegaly, hypochromic anaemia, leucocytosis, an abundance of plasma cells in the bone marrow, accelerated erythrocyte sedimentation, an increase in the amount of circulating immunoglobulins and of fibrinogen and a fall in the amount of albumin in the serum. All these manifestations quickly revert to normal after excision of the lesion.

Histological examination of the excised mass in these cases shows that the follicles have germinal centres. These centres may be multiple, and discrete or confluent, in a given follicle, and they are often of very irregular outline. In other respects the structure of the lesion is similar to that described above, including the presence of many small blood vessels between and in the follicles.

It is possible that the occurrence of this clinical syndrome indicates a functional accompaniment of the lymphoid hamartoma, presumably with an immunological basis, although the nature of the disturbance is not known. Alternatively, the giant lymphoid hamartoma without germinal centre formation and without symptoms may be an entity unrelated to the condition represented by the lymphoid mass with germinal centres and the associated syndrome. The symptoms and laboratory findings in the cases of this syndrome are similar to those that accompany an exceptionally rare type of pleomorphic, but evidently benign, mediastinal tumour of undetermined nature:[230] in one case, the histological pictures of giant lymphoid hamartoma, with germinal centres, and of the pleomorphic tumour were associated in different parts of an encapsulate mass situated just above the diaphragm in the costovertebral angle.[216]

A case is on record in which a giant lymphoid hamartoma in the mesentery of the small intestine was accompanied by the nephrotic syndrome; the

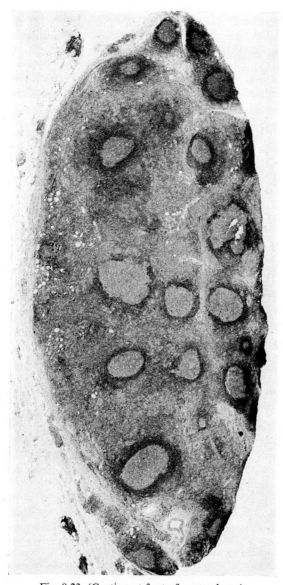

Fig. 9.23. (Caption at foot of next column).

Fig. 9.23. This ovoid, encapsulate mass of lymphoid tissue was excised from the adipose tissue immediately superficial to the epimysium of a deltoid muscle. The patient's history was of persistent pain and swelling at the site of injection of a combination of mixed gas-gangrene antitoxin and tetanus antitoxin one year before the mass was removed surgically. The lesion has a distinct resemblance to a lymph node, with conspicuous lymphoid follicles containing large germinal centres and cellular interfollicular tissue. The latter is in places fibrotic and elsewhere cellular, with small lymphocytes, immunoblasts, plasma cells and histiocytes in varying proportions. There is no trabecular framework or formation of sinuses. It is clear that in this instance the lesion is an inflammatory response to an identified stimulus. The well-developed germinal centres and the absence of any peculiar vascularity of the follicles and of the interfollicular tissue distinguish such lesions from the giant lymphoid hamartoma, with which they are liable to be confused (see Figs 9.20 to 9.22). *Haematoxylin–eosin.* × 15.

renal disturbance disappeared after removal of the hamartoma.[231]

Neoplastic Change.—There has been nothing in the histological picture of any of the recorded cases (134 up to 1971[224]) to suggest that the lesions under consideration in this section are neoplastic. A previously unreported case in which a giant lymphoid hamartoma and a pleomorphic, but presumptively benign, tumour were associated is noted in the preceding paragraph. In another instance, an otherwise typical giant lymphoid hamartoma in the posterior part of the mediastinum included several small foci of classic Hodgkin's disease; this was considered to represent involvement of the hamartoma by Hodgkin's disease in the course of its generalization throughout the tissues of the lymphoreticular system.[216] In the great majority of cases the giant lymphoid hamartoma may be regarded as a benign, non-neoplastic condition.

Fatty Infiltration

Isolated fat cells and small foci of adipose tissue are quite commonly found in lymph nodes, especially after childhood (see Figs 9.13 and 9.15). This is regarded as a normal finding and may be an accompaniment of the physiological regression of lymphoid tissues from early adult life onward.[232] In obese people it is not unusual for a considerable part of the substance of the lymph nodes to be replaced by well-developed adipose tissue, leaving only a peripheral, and often incomplete, zone of lymphoid tissue. Lymph nodes showing such fatty metamorphosis or, as it is better called, fatty infiltration are familiar to surgical pathologists accustomed to making detailed studies of, for example, the axillary tissues in radical mastectomy specimens from obese patients. Usually the affected nodes are no bigger than normal nodes, but in some cases they are greatly enlarged, measuring even up to 7 cm in their longest dimension. These very large fatty lymph nodes ('*lipolymph nodes*'[233]) are likelier to be found in the abdomen and pelvis than elsewhere; they may easily be mistaken for lipomas, and even microscopical examination may fail to disclose their true nature if the sections examined happen not to include remnants of identifiable lymphoid tissue. Comparably extensive replacement of lymphoid tissue by fat, but without enlargement of the nodes, is commonly seen as a manifestation of physiological atrophy in the elderly, even in the absence of obesity.

Haemal Nodes and Haemolymph Nodes

It is not generally accepted that the structures known as haemal nodes and haemolymph nodes occur in man. *Haemal nodes* resemble lymph nodes in most respects except that their sinuses are filled with blood and they have no afferent lymphatic connexions.[234] They are found in many animals, including cattle (Fig. 9.24), the rat (in which they have been studied particularly) and some small primates. They are usually smaller than lymph nodes in the same species; they are red, from their content of blood, and usually they are situated in front of the cervical and lumbar vertebral bodies. They are supposed to play a part in the disposal of effete red blood cells.

The name *haemolymph node* has been used variously, as a synonym of haemal node and to designate a structure that is intermediate between haemal node and lymph node, having both afferent and efferent lymphatics as well as blood-filled

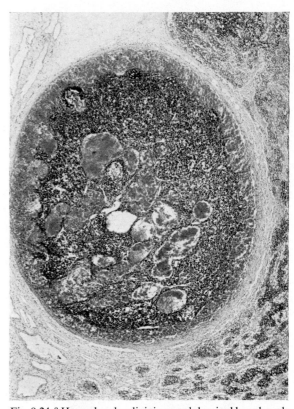

Fig. 9.24.§ Haemal node adjoining an abdominal lymph node in an ox. The two structures are quite distinct; they are separated by their fibrous capsules, which are in part fused. The haemal node includes a few small lymphoid follicles. Its peripheral and central sinuses are distended with blood. *Haematoxylin–eosin.* ×20.

sinuses. It is important to note that various circumstances can cause blood to appear in the sinuses of ordinary lymph nodes: for instance, when there has been bleeding in the tissues that they drain, and as a result of injury to the nodes themselves, such as may occur during surgery. In such cases there may be so much blood within the sinuses that they appear distended, and the node is uniformly red to the naked eye.

Haemic Influx and Lymph Sinus Vascularization.—A rare and interesting source of blood in the sinuses of lymph nodes may be seen in certain cases of obstruction to the venous return from the kidneys, whether from pressure by a tumour, or during surgery, or associated with thrombosis of major tributaries of the renal veins. In these circumstances it appears that there may be a flow of blood into the efferent lymphatics of nodes in the vicinity of the affected kidney: ordinarily, these lymphatics may drain directly into the renal veins—if the veins are obstructed beyond the entry of the lymphatics there may be retrograde flow of blood into the latter and so back to the nodes.[216] A similar phenomenon has been observed in rats.[235] When the condition in man is of long duration, the sinuses of the affected nodes undergo fibrosis in association with the development of a spongework of endothelium-lined spaces that may contain lymph or blood. The changes have been described as vascularization or vascular transformation of the lymph sinuses.[236] They have also been observed in abdominal lymph nodes of patients with vena caval obstruction in the mediastinum, [237] in axillary nodes following radical mastectomy[216, 237] and thrombosis of the subclavian vein,[216] and in popliteal nodes in a case of longstanding traumatic arteriovenous aneurysm of the femoral vessels.[216] It is clear that such findings in lymph nodes have nothing in common with the occurrence of haemolymph nodes as specific structures.

DEGENERATIVE AND OTHER MISCELLANEOUS
CONDITIONS

Fatty Infiltration

Fatty infiltration of lymph nodes is considered on the opposite page.

Hyalinization

Some degree of hyaline thickening of the fibrous framework, particularly the capsule and trabeculae,

E

is usual in the lymph nodes of older people. It is particularly frequent and extensive in the inguinal and iliac nodes, and longstanding, non-specific lymphadenitis of low-grade is the usual underlying cause. In some cases the greater part of the affected nodes is converted into a hyaline mass, only a small amount of atrophic lymphoid tissue surviving in the interstices here and there. A comparable picture is seen too in lymph nodes that are the site of burnt-out sarcoidosis: in such nodes it is usually possible to find an occasional cluster of epithelioid cells or an occasional Schaumann body to give a hint of the diagnosis (see page 748). Calcium salts may be laid down in the hyaline material in any case of hyalinization. The distribution of the deposits and the general pattern of the histological picture, particularly the absence of caseation or other types of necrosis, make it unlikely that there will be confusion with other

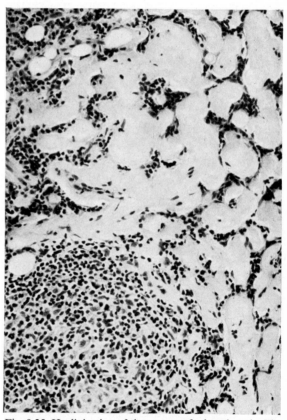

Fig. 9.25. Hyalinization of the stroma of a lymph node. The cause is unknown. The homogeneous hyaline material is eosinophile and can be distinguished from amyloid only by its lack of affinity for stains that demonstrate amyloid and by its strong coloration by acid fuchsin (Van Gieson's stain) and other stains for collagen. Compare with Fig. 9.26. *Haematoxylin–eosin.* × 190.

causes of calcification in lymph nodes, such as healing tuberculosis and histoplasmosis.

Sometimes hyalinization affects the reticulin framework of nodes rather than the coarser collagenous structures. The hyaline tissue and interposed narrow streams of surviving cells present a picture that can be confused with that of amyloidosis (compare Figs 9.25 and 9.26).

Amyloidosis

The lymph nodes may be affected in primary or secondary amyloidosis (Fig. 9.26). The amyloid deposit may be confined to the tissue immediately surrounding the blood vessels in the node, or it may cause much enlargement of the node, which may be almost wholly converted into a mass of amyloid. The diagnosis is one that has to be kept in mind if the true nature and significance of amorphous, hyaline material in lymph-node biopsy specimens is not to be overlooked.

In some cases of amyloidosis, both primary[238] and secondary,[239] amyloid lymphadenopathy may be the presenting manifestation.

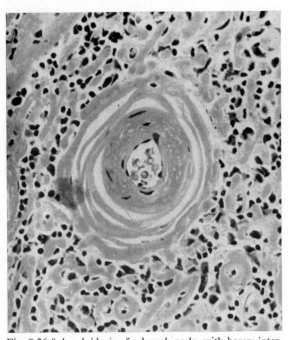

Fig. 9.26.§ Amyloidosis of a lymph node, with heavy intercellular deposition of amyloid and circumvascular rings of amyloid. The conspicuous involvement of the media of the arteriole is characteristic of 'primary' amyloidosis but may be seen also in some cases of secondary amyloidosis. Compare with Fig. 9.25. *Haematoxylin–eosin.* × 300.

Pigment in Lymph Nodes[240]

Various pigments may be found in lymph nodes. They may be formed *in situ* as a product of the metabolic activities of the macrophages, or they may be carried to the nodes in the lymph and taken up by these cells, maybe later to be deposited in the interstices of the node, particularly if fibrosis occurs.

Endogenous Pigments.—*Haemosiderin* is commonly seen in lymph nodes after haemorrhage into the tissues that they drain and is then usually confined to the macrophages in the sinuses. More marked and extensive haemosiderosis accompanies chronic haemolytic anaemia and haemochromatosis, and may follow often-repeated blood transfusion; in cases of haemochromatosis the abdominal nodes are particularly affected, and the deposits of pigment may lead to considerable fine fibrosis. The nodes draining haematomas may contain considerable amounts of bright orange-yellow *haematoidin* (unconjugated bilirubin) in addition to haemosiderin. In cases of obstructive jaundice there may be generalized pigmentation of the lymph nodes by *conjugated bilirubin*, and this is often strikingly marked in the nodes in the hilum of the liver. The bilirubin in the nodes in cases of obstructive jaundice usually appears greenish in histological sections.

Other endogenous pigments that may be found in lymph nodes include lipofuscins (among them perhaps the peculiar pigmented structures that are commonly referred to as Hamazaki–Wesenberg bodies, or ceroid bodies—see page 562), melanins (see below) and malarial pigment (see page 667).

Melanin in Lymph Nodes.—The finding of melanin in lymph nodes requires careful consideration. The occurrence of what are believed to be naevus cells in lymph nodes is referred to on page 542.

Melanin may be present in small amounts in scattered macrophages in nodes draining any area of the skin in which there is a lesion accompanied by overactivity of melanocytes: such lesions include recent sunburn, chronic ulcers, many varieties of dermatitis, and the pigmented tumours and tumour-like conditions. Conspicuous amounts of melanin are a feature of dermatopathic lymphadenitis (see page 687). It is particularly when melanin is present in nodes draining the site of tumours of the skin that its presence may cause errors in diagnostic interpretation. Even in cases of proven malignant melanoma of the skin the finding of melanin in the regional lymph nodes is not evidence that the tumour has spread to them: pigment released from tumour cells in the primary growth—for example, in areas of necrosis—may be carried in lymph to the nodes and there taken up by macrophages. This is a frequent cause of over-pessimistic prognostication in cases of melanoma. Similarly, the recognition of melanin in the regional nodes may encourage mistaking a benign tumour of the skin, such as a melanotic basal cell papilloma ('verruca senilis'—see Chapter 39), for a malignant melanoma. In this context it is pertinent to recall that the presence of haemosiderin in lymph nodes draining a dermatofibroma of the siderotic variety may similarly increase the liability of this benign lesion to be mistaken for a malignant melanoma (see Chapter 39).

In cases of melanosis of the mucous membrane of the colon (see page 1128) the melanin, or pseudomelanin, may be carried in lymph to the regional lymph nodes in such quantity that they are black to the naked eye (*melanosis of the abdominal lymph nodes*). Such marked pigmentation of the nodes is found in only a minority of cases of melanosis of the colon. Its observation at laparotomy can alarm the surgeon, and if he sends one of the nodes for immediate histological examination the microscopist may be misled by the pigment-laden macrophages into interpreting the condition as metastatic involvement by melanoma.

Exogenous Pigments.—The exogenous pigments that may be found in lymph nodes include carbon, siliceous dusts, cinnabar and other colouring matter from tattoos, silver in cases of argyrosis, iron (particularly after injection), and very many others. Some of these materials—silica, for example, and, in certain circumstances, carbon—cause extensive fibrosis of the nodes: whorled, hyaline nodules like those in the lungs may be found in the tracheobronchial lymph nodes in cases of *silicosis* in coalworkers and others (see page 381). Very rarely, heavy deposits of carbon, even when demonstrably free from accompanying silica, may cause extensive fibrosis of pulmonary hilar lymph nodes; in some instances this may be associated with necrosis of the core of the resulting fibrotic masses, as sometimes occurs in the pulmonary lesions in cases of progressive massive pulmonary fibrosis ('complicated pneumoconiosis') in coal miners (see page 380). *Necrosis of anthracotic nodes* may be complicated by their perforation into the trachea or a bronchus or into an adjoining blood vessel, usually a pulmonary vein;[241] it is likely that in most cases of this rare event the anthracosis has been accompanied by infection, particularly tuberculosis, but sometimes careful investigation, microbiological as well as histological, shows no evidence of an infective element.[242] Entry of the anthracotic material into the blood stream results in widespread phagocytosis of the carbon particles by the cells of the reticuloendothelial system: the pigment may be visible to the naked eye in the spleen and liver, and elsewhere.

Simple anthracosis of mediastinal lymph nodes is commonplace in town dwellers. It is characterized by conspicuous pigmentation of macrophages, and some proliferation of these cells, both within the sinuses and in the substance of the nodes, but there is no accompanying fibrosis unless as a consequence of some other condition, particularly infection.

Siderosis of lymph nodes may follow parenteral administration of iron in the treatment of anaemia. The inguinal nodes may be heavily pigmented following injections of iron dextran into the gluteal muscles, and there may be generalized siderosis of the lymph nodes, as well as of other parts of the reticuloendothelial system, when iron dextran has been administered intravenously (see page 696).

Circulatory Changes in Lymph Nodes

Disturbances of the circulation of the blood are not of great practical significance in relation to lymph nodes. There may be considerable swelling of the thoracic and abdominal nodes in cases of severe congestive heart failure. The nodes are soft, red and wet, and when incised much watery fluid may flow from the cut surface: although this state is generally described as oedema of the nodes it is probable that most of the fluid is lymph that has been dammed back in the sinuses and pulp because of the retardation of the lymph flow resulting from the raised venous pressure.

The influx of blood into the lymph sinuses of lymph nodes through their efferent lymphatics as a result of obstruction to the venous return from a kidney is referred to in the discussion of haemal nodes and haemolymph nodes on page 549.

Infarction of Lymph Nodes.—Lymph nodes ordinarily have an abundant arterial supply and venous drainage. The main vessels pass through the hilum but others provide a collateral circulation through the capsule over the convexity of the nodes. Experimental infarction can be produced by ligating the arteries and veins of lymph nodes in animals, particularly the popliteal node in the rabbit:[243] a thin rim of lymphoid tissue survives just deep to the capsule, and eventually the node may regenerate from this zone. Similar findings have been described in superficial lymph nodes in man (Fig. 9.27).[244]

Such lesions present with painful enlargement of the affected node, of sudden onset; in most cases the node has been in an axilla or groin.[244] Similar changes in an abdominal node have been the cause of acute pain, necessitating surgical exploration; the symptoms apparently result from irritation of the parietal or visceral peritoneum overlying the infarcted node.[245] In some cases infarction may be a result of vascular disturbances during the course of surgery in the vicinity, such as radical mastectomy; in others vascular obstruction is the outcome of degenerative changes in the wall of vessels, thrombosis resulting. Polyarteritis is an occasional cause (see page 693).

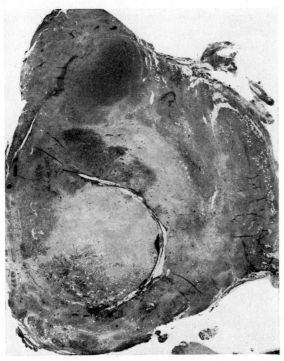

Fig. 9.27. Infarction of a pectoral lymph node. The patient, an undernourished man, had been treated for a fracture of a clavicle by strapping the arm to his body, with a padded mass of plaster of Paris placed in the axilla to keep the shoulder well out from the chest. Severe pain in the side of the chest developed soon afterwards and was found to be associated with a tender swelling under the pectoral muscles on the medial wall of the axilla. The mass was thought to be a foreign body and was removed. It proved to be the infarcted node illustrated. The central part of the node shows ischaemic necrosis with some adjoining haemorrhage. Parts of the peripheral zone are free from necrosis, presumably because of a blood supply across the capsule. The vessels in the hilum of the node were filled with thrombus. The likely cause is pressure of the external pad on the region of the node, which was situated superficial to a rib. *Haematoxylin–eosin.* ×9.

The histological changes are those of ischaemic infarction, the ghost-like remains of the original structure persisting, and the reticulin framework of the node appearing almost unaltered. There is a marked leucocytic infiltrate in the vicinity of the capsule, with survival of a recognizable but patchy zone of lymphoid tissue deep to the latter. Fresh or organizing thrombus is often to be seen in veins in the hilum or elsewhere outside the capsule, and occasionally in arteries. In older lesions there is organization of the infarcted tissue from the capsule inward, with more or less interstitial regeneration of lymphoid tissue and recanalization of both lymph sinuses and blood vessels. Sometimes an infarcted node seems to be totally replaced by a hyaline nodule of scar tissue.

From the practical point of view the most important consideration is to be sure that what appears to be an infarcted lymph node is not in fact a necrotic primary or secondary tumour. Almost total 'coagulative' necrosis of tumours in lymph nodes is by no means rare: it occurs most frequently in the lymphocytic and so-called immunoblastic lymphomas and in metastatic melanomas and small cell anaplastic bronchial carcinomas ('oat cell' carcinomas). The ghost pattern of the tumour is often too indeterminate to be diagnostic, and demonstration of a more or less normal reticulin framework can be misleading as rapidly growing tumours do not necessarily destroy or significantly disturb the pre-existing connective tissue fibres. The evidence of the real nature of the necrotic tumours is to be found in surviving foci of the growth (Fig. 9.28): these foci may elude anything less than a search of many sections, and care is needed to make sure that what looks like a cuff of pleomorphic tumour cells round a blood vessel is not in fact a collection of atypical, regenerating, non-neoplastic lymphoreticular cells in young granulation tissue.

Infarction of a lymph node is unlikely to be confused with a necrotic granulomatous lesion. Tuberculosis, syphilis, histoplasmosis, cryptococcosis and sporotrichosis have been known to mimic massive infarction: they can usually be correctly recognized by the traces of their characteristic histological picture or by demonstration of the organisms concerned, or by the history, associated laboratory findings and therapeutic response. It is important to remember that infection may predispose to infarction by involving the blood vessels in the hilum of a lymph node.

Extensive haemorrhagic necrosis is a feature of the lymphadenitis that accompanies severe diphtheria (see page 580)[246] and of some cases of acute

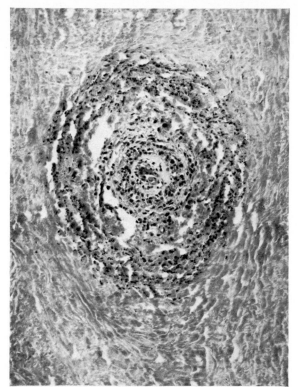

Fig. 9.28. The only clue to the nature of the change underlying the total necrosis of a lymph node was this persistent focus of haematoxyphile nuclear debris and a few surviving tumour cells round a small, still patent blood vessel. The rest of the node, up to the capsule, was converted into a uniformly eosinophile mass in which the outlines of cells and stromal fibres could be made out, but without certainty as to the nature of the dead cells. The few surviving cells round the vessel in the picture appeared to be undifferentiated tumour cells, and subsequent events proved that the patient had a pleomorphic undifferentiated lymphoma. See also Fig. 9.269, page 853. *Haematoxylin–eosin.* × 120.

streptococcal lymphadenitis, particularly in fatal cases of scarlatina.[242] It may occur also in anthrax lymphadenitis (see page 578)[247] and in the ileocolic lymph nodes in some cases of gangrenous appendicitis.[245] In any of these conditions the changes in the nodes may be misinterpreted as primarily ischaemic if the pathologist fails to consider the alternative, an oversight that is encouraged by the rarity of some of the causative infections in certain parts of the world nowadays. In each of these conditions there are usually clear indications of the true diagnosis: nevertheless, the recent increase in awareness of the occurrence of infarction of lymph nodes, following publications drawing attention to it, has resulted in an uncritical proclivity to make this diagnosis. Instances of all the conditions named in this para-

graph, except scarlatina, have been among material sent to my laboratory for confirmation of a diagnosis of infarction.

LYMPHADENITIS AND OTHER 'REACTIVE' CHANGES IN LYMPH NODES*

It is impossible to distinguish sharply between normal states of functional activity in lymph nodes and pathological changes. This is because it is a function of the lymph nodes, as part of the body's defences, to react to pathogenic influences—a normal lymph node, in the narrow sense of one unaffected by influences originating outside the body, is something unknown after the end of fetal life. The most straightforward reactive changes in lymph nodes are hyperplasia of the lymphoid follicles, proliferation of the endothelial macrophages of the lymph sinuses, and proliferation and histiocytic differentiation of reticulum cells. These three types of reaction may occur together in any combination, or any one of them may dominate the picture, or be present alone. It is helpful to consider these reactions under separate headings, but it must be stressed that they are not unrelated responses but integral parts of the functional reactivity of lymph nodes as part of a general system of defence.

Simple Follicular Hyperplasia
(Reactive Follicular Hyperplasia)

Hyperplasia of the lymphoid follicles is a striking and very frequent manifestation of inflammatory stimulation of lymph nodes (Fig. 9.29) and of lymphoid tissue elsewhere. It has many causes. The follicles are enlarged and may be increased in number, appearing in the medullary cords of the lymph nodes, where they are not ordinarily found. The most characteristic feature of the hyperplastic follicles, however, is the formation of the pale germinal centres (Flemming centres) (see page 512). The germinal centres are by no means constant in their cytological make-up and various classifications of the appearances have been suggested: in human

* The distinction between lymphadenitis, an expressly inflammatory state, and 'reactive' changes in this context is indefinable and has no justification or sanction other than established terminological practice. In this context, 'reactive' implies a definite cellular response to a stimulus: lymphadenitis itself is thus 'reactive', but convention does not as readily allow that simple follicular hyperplasia or sinus histiocytosis be described as 'lymphadenitis'.

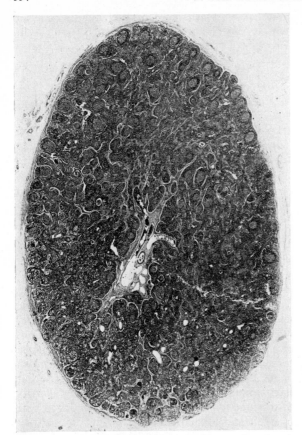

Fig. 9.29. Simple follicular hyperplasia in a tonsillar lymph node in a case of chronic non-specific tonsillitis. The multiplicity of lymphoid follicles and the presence of germinal centres (relatively pale) are seen. *Haematoxylin–eosin.* × 10.

lymphoid tissue the follicles generally show various combinations of these cytological features (Fig. 9.30), which need not be detailed. The most important practical consideration is to ensure that the hyperplastic follicles are not confused with those of follicular lymphomas (see page 836): the distinction can generally be made without difficulty, and this is particularly true when the 'starry sky' appearance is seen in the germinal centres—this appearance results from the scattering of large, pale macrophages among the rather darker, closely packed lymphoid cells (Fig. 9.4, page 513), and it is seen best under the lower powers of the microscope. Follicular hyperplasia is a feature of many forms of lymphadenitis. It also occurs in the lymphoid tissues generally, and particularly in the spleen and nodes, in cases of active *rheumatoid arthritis* in adults (Fig. 9.31) and in the related *Still's disease* (*Chauffard–Ramon–Still syndrome*) of childhood (see page 690).

Giant Follicle Hyperplasia*

Giant follicle hyperplasia is a particular variety of follicular hyperplasia (reactive follicular hyperplasia) as described in the preceding section. It is generally confined to one group of cervical lymph nodes: several nodes in the group may be affected, and the resulting mass may be very noticeable clinically, although the largest nodes seldom exceed about 3·5 cm in their longest dimension. The cause has not been identified.

Clinically, the condition may simulate follicular lymphoma (see page 836). Histologically, the large follicles resemble those of simple follicular hyperplasia: the same varieties of lymphocytes are present, and also macrophages containing Flemming's 'stainable bodies'. The follicles vary greatly in size and shape. The largest may measure up to a centi-

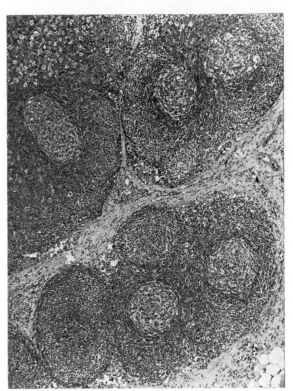

Fig. 9.30. Simple follicular hyperplasia in chronic non-specific lymphadenitis. There are differences in the size, cellular constitution and pattern of different follicles. The considerable fibrosis of the capsule and trabeculae of the node is a result of the chronic inflammatory state. *Haematoxylin–eosin.* × 60.

* The term 'giant follicle hyperplasia' must not be confused with 'giant follicular hypertrophy', the name by which Douglas Symmers (New York) described follicular lymphoma (see page 835).

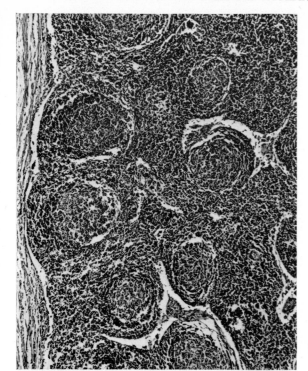

Fig. 9.31. Simple follicular hyperplasia in a lymph node in a case of rapidly progressive rheumatoid arthritis in an adult. The appearances in this specimen are atypical. Ordinarily, the lymphadenopathy that occurs in some cases of rheumatoid arthritis in adults and as part of the syndrome of the so-called Still's disease of childhood is characterized by very prominent development of germinal centres in the hyperplastic follicles. The variant picture illustrated here is unusual, and unless it is identified correctly it is liable to be mistaken for a follicular lymphoma because of the comparatively uniform cellular constitution of the follicles. The artefactual fissuring along part of the periphery of the follicles in this specimen was a further diagnostic pitfall, such fissuring being a frequent characteristic of follicular lymphoma (see page 837 and Figs 9.250 to 9.252). *Haematoxylin–eosin.* × 50.

metre in longest dimension and up to 2 mm in width. The cytological composition of the follicles and their uncommonly large size, irregular shape and tendency to confluence (Fig. 9.32) enable the important distinction from follicular lymphoma to be made.

Giant follicle hyperplasia may persist for many months before it subsides. It is benign.

'Reactive' Changes in the Sinuses of Lymph Nodes

Dilatation and Histiocytosis of the Lymph Sinuses

It is often particularly hard to draw the line between the physiological states of the lymph sinuses and

their abnormalities. Mesenteric lymph nodes commonly show a very considerable degree of dilatation of the sinuses (Fig. 9.33), with only sparse cells in the lumen and little or no enlargement of the endothelial macrophages: this appearance in nodes in this anatomical situation is frequent enough to rank as physiological, a view that may be supported by the observation that the dilatation is not accompanied by fibrosis.

Somewhat similar dilatation of the sinuses is seen as a frankly pathological state in axillary, inguinal and iliac lymph nodes when these are distal to obstructive lesions of the lymphatics that have resulted in lymphoedema. In such cases much—even almost all—of the lymphoid tissue in the affected

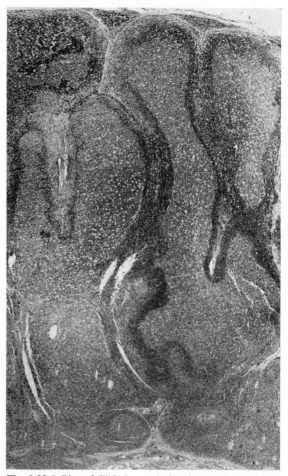

Fig. 9.32.§ Giant follicle hyperplasia of a lymph node. The very large size and irregular outline of the follicles, some of which extend across the whole thickness of the node, are evident. Macrophages scattered singly among the lymphoid cells of the massive germinal centres account for the 'starry sky' appearance of the hyperplastic tissue. *Haematoxylin–eosin.* × 17.

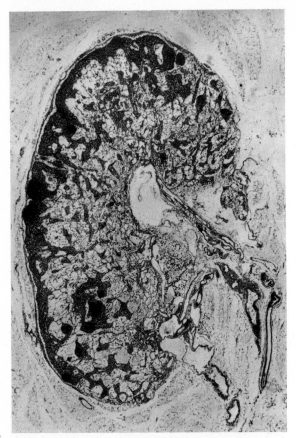

Fig. 9.33. A lymph node from the mesentery of the small intestine. The node has been sectioned longitudinally in the plane of its hilum. There is marked dilatation of the efferent lymphatics and of the sinuses throughout much of the node. The subcapsular sinus, although conspicuous, is not distended to a comparable degree. Some afferent lymphatics, just outside the capsule, are also dilated. There was no evidence that the condition of the node was in any way pathological: wide sinuses are regularly found in the nodes from the mesentery. See also Fig. 9.1, page 511. *Haematoxylin–eosin.* × 15.

nodes atrophies as the sinuses dilate, and the nodes become converted into lymph saccules traversed by the fibrotic remnants of the trabecular framework.

Whipple's Disease

In Whipple's disease ('intestinal lipodystrophy', or 'lipophagic intestinal granulomatosis'—see page 1083), the sinuses of the mesenteri cand, often, of the pre-aortic and lateral aortic lymph nodes become distended by the fatty material that accumulates there during the course of the disease. This leads eventually to replacement of the node by an encapsulate mass of pasty or putty-like material; lipid

crystals are often conspicuous in this material, leaving a characteristic pattern in paraffin wax sections, having been dissolved from the tissue in the course of histological preparation.

In the earlier stages of the disease there is a conspicuous histiocytic reaction in the sinuses (Figs 9.34 and 9.35), often with the development of multinucleate giant cells. The histiocytes are vacuolate, and they contain granular material that gives a positive periodic-acid/Schiff reaction and does not react with stains for lipids. Later, all traces of the cellular reaction may disappear. Electron microscopy shows the bacilliform bodies that have also been recognized in the phagocytes in the lamina propria of the bowel (see page 1084). The changes of Whipple's disease may be found also in lymph nodes outside the abdomen—for example, in the groins, axillae or neck. In these situations the

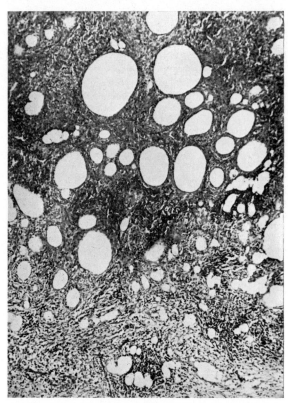

Fig. 9.34. Whipple's disease ('intestinal lipodystrophy'). A lymph node from the mesentery of the small intestine: the clear spaces contained lipid that had accumulated in the sinuses, setting up a granulomatous response (see also Fig. 9.35). Such appearances have to be distinguished from those resulting from lymphangiography (see Fig. 9.47, page 567) or from the presence of gas (see Fig. 9.36) or biliary material (see Fig. 9.37). *Haematoxylin–eosin.* × 50.

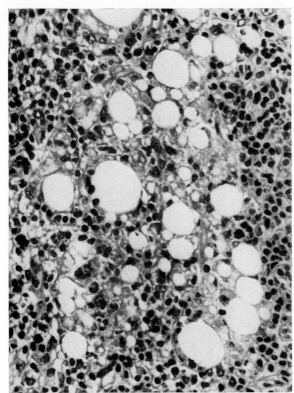

Fig. 9.35. Whipple's disease at a stage earlier than that illustrated in Fig. 9.34. An accumulation of macrophages obliterates the lumen of a sinus in a lymph node from the mesentery of the small intestine. The cytoplasm of these cells is vacuolate, due to the presence of lipid (which has been dissolved and lost during histological preparation). The same histological picture is seen in cases of chole-granulomatous lymphadenitis (see Fig. 9.37) and of the lymphadenopathy that follows lymphangiography (see Fig. 9.47, page 567): the feature that distinguishes the lymphadenopathy of Whipple's disease from the conditions that resemble it is the presence in the macrophages of abundant granular material that gives a positive periodic-acid/Schiff reaction. *Haematoxylin–eosin.* × 350.

diagnosis is elusive unless the possibility is remembered.[248, 249]

It is noteworthy that an appearance similar to that of the earlier stages in the development of Whipple's disease may be seen in lymph nodes following lymphangiography (see page 566).

Gas 'Cysts'

In cases of gas cyst formation (cystic pneumatosis) in the alimentary tract (see page 1087), bubbles of gas may collect within the sinuses of the mesenteric and retroperitoneal lymph nodes (Fig. 9.36). In the chronic variety of this condition, which occurs in

adults ('*adult pneumatosis*'), the presence of bubbles of gas in the sinuses causes a histiocytic reaction, often with the formation of multinucleate giant cells;[250] the histological picture is similar to that resulting from the presence of globules of fat. In the rarer acute type of intestinal pneumatosis, which occurs in infancy ('*infantile pneumatosis*'), there is little or no reaction to the gas in the sinuses of the nodes and in the associated lymphatic vessels;[251] this disease of infants may be due to the entry of gas-forming coliform bacteria into the lymphatics as an accompaniment of the changes in the intestinal contents that result from weaning.

In some instances of intestinal cystic pneumatosis, the characteristic lesions have been found not only in lymph nodes within the abdomen but also in nodes elsewhere, particularly in the inguinal region[248] and also in the mediastinum and neck.[252] The correct diagnosis may be overlooked when

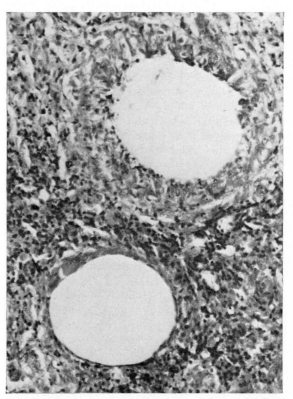

Fig. 9.36. Gas in a lymph node from the mesentery in a case of gas cyst formation in the small intestine ('cystic pneumatosis'). The two clear spaces are gas bubbles. It is not known why the presence of gas should be accompanied by a granulomatous reaction, as is seen here. The reaction is identical with that around fat globules, such as is found in the lymphadenopathy of Whipple's disease (see Figs 9.34 and 9.35). *Haematoxylin–eosin.* × 150.

biopsy specimens are being interpreted in such cases, unless the presence of the disease in the alimentary tract has already been recognized. Comparable appearances have been seen in inguinal lymph nodes as an accompaniment of the rare puerperal condition of *vaginal pneumatosis* (see Chapter 27).

Gas cysts that develop in lymph nodes in association with alimentary or vaginal pneumatosis may be confused with the changes that result from the presence of clostridia, particularly *Clostridium welchii* (*Clostridium perfringens*), which, carried in lymph from the bowel to the lymph nodes, colonize the latter in some dying patients, particularly those with ulcerative lesions of the large intestine. In these cases the gas formation is mostly a post-mortem occurrence, and there is advanced post-mortem disruption of the tissues; the organisms are readily seen in the sections, and misinterpretation of the changes should not occur. In cases of gas gangrene, the clostridia may be carried in the blood to lymph nodes as to other organs and tissues, giving rise to gas formation that continues after the patient's death (see page 1227).

Cholegranulomatous Lymphadenitis

Although this condition might be more appropriately considered among the granulomatous forms of lymphadenitis, it is comparatively rarely seen in the fully developed granulomatous state and its earlier manifestations are essentially the reaction of the cells lining the lymph sinuses. There is well-marked lipophagic vacuolation of the endothelial macrophages, often with the formation of multinucleate giant cells (Fig. 9.37). The condition occurs particularly in some cases of cholecystitis, especially when there is ulceration of the lining of the gall bladder; it may also accompany obstructive jaundice. The nodes involved are those of the hepatic group, and often particularly the cystic node. The cytoplasm of the altered macrophages is usually coloured by bile pigment, and in cases of chronic obstructive jaundice is often very heavily stained (see page 550). The reaction is considered to result from the presence of bile that has been absorbed through the lymphatics. At this stage, the picture may be mistaken for the early phase of the lymphadenopathy of Whipple's disease (see page 556); the site of the affected nodes, and the presence of bile staining, should be helpful in reaching the correct diagnosis.

A characteristic early extension of the reaction is the development of small clusters of epithelioid macrophages in the lymphoid tissue adjoining the affected sinuses. Except for the presence of bile

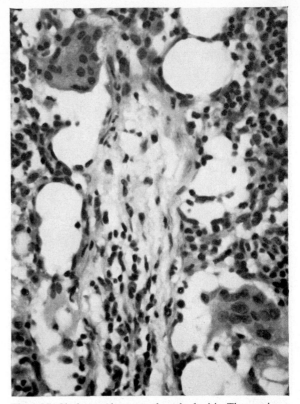

Fig. 9.37. Cholegranulomatous lymphadenitis. The specimen is the lymph node of the anterior border of the epiploic foramen, which, with the cystic node (node of the neck of the gall bladder) is most frequently the seat of this condition. The sinus on each side of the trabecula is traversed by fine or coarser septa that partly enclose globular spaces from which lipid has been dissolved. Multinucleate cells have formed as part of the reaction to the lipid material, which is presumed to be of biliary origin. In the original preparation it was possible to distinguish the presence of small amounts of bile pigment in the macrophages: this is helpful in distinguishing the picture from that of similar granulomas, such as those of the early stages of Whipple's disease (Figs 9.34 and 9.35) and those resulting from lymphangiography (Fig. 9.47, page 567). *Haematoxylin–eosin.* × 320.

pigment and lipophages in the sinuses (both may be sparse in a given node), the picture may be taken for that of early tuberculosis;[253] in this context it is relevant that acid-and-alcohol-fast substances such as ceroid lipofuscins may be present in these hepatic lymph nodes and, exceptionally, may be mistaken for mycobacteria. Other conditions that must be considered include toxoplasmosis and other forms of lymphadenitis that are characterized by the presence of many small clusters of large epithelioid macrophages (see page 656). In longstanding instances of cholegranulomatous lymphadenitis, discrete or confluent sarcoid-like granulomas form in the lymphoid tissue of the affected nodes. This condition is sometimes described as 'lipogranulomatous pseudosarcoid'.[254]

Apart from the presence of the bile pigment, the picture in the early stages does not differ from that resulting from absorption of various endogenous and exogenous oily substances (see page 566).

'Sinus Catarrh'

The commonest pathological change in the sinuses of lymph nodes is the condition known as 'desquamative sinus catarrh' or, simply, 'sinus catarrh'. It is characterized by dilatation of the sinuses, particularly the subcapsular sinus, which receives the afferent lymphatics as they penetrate the capsule of the node over its convexity. The dilatation is accompanied by proliferation of the endothelial macrophages (Figs 9.38A and 9.38B), which become enlarged and detach themselves from the wall to lie free in the lumen, where some of them may be seen

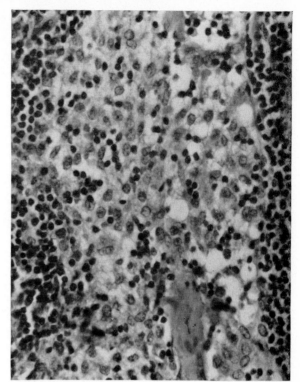

Fig. 9.38B. Same specimen as in Fig. 9.38A, to show detail of the cellular accumulation in the sinuses. *Haematoxylin–eosin.* × 325.

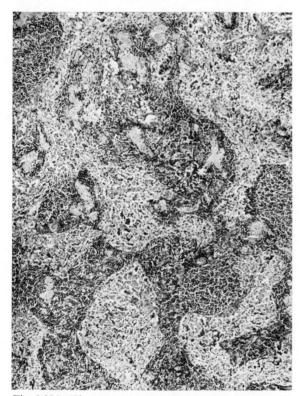

Fig. 9.38A. 'Sinus catarrh'. The sinuses of the lymph node are widened as a result of proliferation of the endothelial macrophages (littoral cells), which appear pale in the photograph. There is a scattering of lymphocytes among the macrophages. See also Figs 9.38B and 9.39. *Haematoxylin–eosin.* × 55.

to have engulfed red blood cells and, less often, lymphocytes (Fig. 9.39). Some polymorphonuclear leucocytes, lymphocytes and plasma cells may also accumulate in the sinuses, the types of cell that are present depending largely on the nature of the stimulus. Often, sinus catarrh appears to be no more than a response to the varied range of substances, including normal metabolites, that are carried to the nodes in the lymph. It differs from the condition described below as simple sinus histiocytosis only in the degree of cellularity of the sinuses and—less regularly—of their dilatation.

Sinus Histiocytosis

In addition to the rare condition that is known as 'sinus histiocytosis with massive lymphadenopathy' (see page 564), two morphologically differing conditions are currently described by the term 'sinus histiocytosis'. The two conditions may be referred to as 'simple sinus histiocytosis' and 'immature sinus histiocytosis': it is debatable whether they should be regarded as of different cellular origin, and therefore of different functional significance. It seems to be

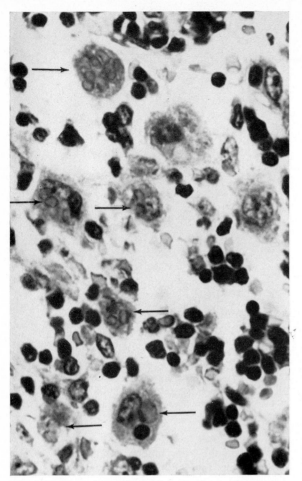

histological contrast between the dark lymphoid tissue of the node and the pale cellular mass within the widened sinuses is striking. There is little tendency for the histiocytes in the sinuses to encroach on the adjoining lymphoid tissue, and the sinuses and pulp therefore remain quite well demarcated (Fig. 9.40). The histiocytes are of remarkably uniform size and appearance. They are mononucleate. The nucleus, which may be indented, is large and oval, and has a delicate chromatin pattern; the nucleolus is rather small and may be duplicated. The uniformity of the cells and the absence of atypical nuclear features readily distinguish the picture from that of the comparatively rare condition of 'sinus histiocytosis with massive lymphadenopathy' (see page 564), which is an entity distinct from the varieties of sinus histiocytosis under dis-

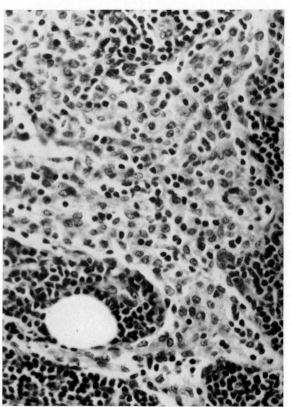

Fig. 9.39. 'Sinus catarrh'—another specimen. Free macrophages and lymphocytes are seen in the lumen of the sinus. In this case there had been local excision of a carcinoma of the breast 2 days before: the node illustrated was one of those that drained the operation site, where a large haematoma had formed. The node was included in the radical mastectomy specimen when the further operation followed diagnosis of the nature of the mammary disease. Several of the macrophages in the sinus have ingested red blood cells (arrowed), and at least two of them have ingested a lymphocyte also. *Haematoxylin–eosin.* × 850.

agreed that in both conditions the cells that are involved are macrophages and that the difference is in their maturity.

Simple Sinus Histiocytosis.—It is impossible to define a distinction between well-marked sinus catarrh (see above) and the earlier stages in the development of simple sinus histiocytosis. It is characteristic of the established state of simple sinus histiocytosis that the sinuses are completely, or practically completely, filled with histiocytes. The

Fig. 9.40. Simple sinus histiocytosis. The sharp demarcation between the sinus and the surrounding lymphoid tissue is characteristic, but is not always as clearly defined as in this instance. The picture illustrated can be confused with carcinomatous permeation of the sinuses of lymph nodes (see Fig. 9.41): mistakes are particularly likely to occur because simple sinus histiocytosis is seen most frequently in axillary nodes in cases of mammary carcinoma. *Haematoxylin–eosin.* × 345.

cussion here. As in all types of sinus histiocytosis, with the important exception of the 'immature' variety discussed below, the cells in the sinuses in cases of simple sinus histiocytosis may ingest red blood cells and, sometimes, lymphocytes and neutrophils.

The histiocytes accumulate in the sinuses as a result of active multiplication of endothelial macrophages. The condition is seen with special frequency in axillary nodes, and particularly in association with primary carcinoma of the breast of the same side. The affected nodes are firm and often rather larger than the average normal axillary node. Although they lack the induration that usually characterizes nodes extensively invaded by mammary carcinoma, they are sufficiently obtrusive to cause clinical concern. The condition has sometimes been interpreted as an attempt to hinder lymphatic dissemination of carcinoma. Alternatively, and likelier, the stimulus that causes the endothelial macrophages to proliferate has been thought to be some irritant, possibly of lipid nature, formed during breakdown of the tumour or of tissues invaded by it. It is noteworthy that the condition, although usually unilateral, is sometimes found to be equally marked in both axillae, even when there is a tumour in the breast on one side only.

The observation that simple sinus histiocytosis is seen most frequently as an accompaniment of carcinoma of the breast may reflect only the circumstance that it is the surgical treatment of this disease that provides the great majority of occasions to examine axillary lymph nodes microscopically. Similar changes are found sometimes in the local nodes in association with carcinoma of the stomach; they are seldom, if ever, seen in cases of carcinoma of other parts of the alimentary tract or arising in other systems. Some investigators have put forward evidence suggesting that the prognosis of cancer of the breast and stomach may be significantly better in those cases in which sinus histiocytosis occurs;[255, 256] this is debatable.

Care is necessary if the pitfall of mistaking the picture of simple sinus histiocytosis for that of infiltration of the sinuses by undifferentiated mammary carcinoma (Fig. 9.41) is to be avoided. Sometimes, too, sinus histiocytosis is confused with the epithelioid cell stage in the development of the tuberculoid reaction that may be found in the sinuses and pulp of nodes draining mammary, gastric and other cancers (Fig. 9.42). The two types of reaction—histiocytosis and the tuberculoid granuloma—appear to be quite distinct. The tuberculoid response is considered on page 682; it

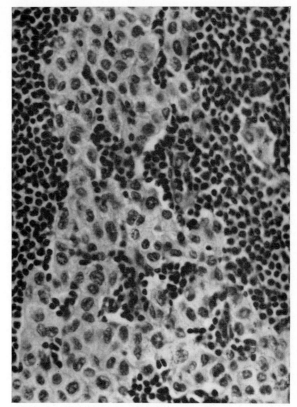

Fig. 9.41. Undifferentiated carcinoma of mammary origin permeating the sinuses of an axillary lymph node. Although the tumour cells have begun to grow into the lymphoid tissue adjoining the sinus, this feature is seldom helpful in distinguishing carcinoma from histiocytosis, in which the demarcation between the lymphoid pulp and the macrophages in the lumen is not always as distinct as in Fig. 9.40. *Haematoxylin–eosin.* × 345.

has no evident prognostic significance, and it is probably a reaction to lipid material from the tissues invaded and destroyed by the cancer or formed in breaking down tumour tissue.[257, 258] The granulomatous lesions have a patchy distribution, in contrast to the diffuse change throughout the sinuses that is typical of simple sinus histiocytosis; although they may be centred on sinuses they are seen much oftener in the pulp of the nodes.

'Immature Sinus Histiocytosis'.—The so-called immature form of sinus histiocytosis differs from the simple variety described above in the general appearance of the cells that fill the sinuses, in the extent of the involvement of the affected nodes and in the nature of the diseases that it is associated with.

The cells are uniform in character (Fig. 9.43). In

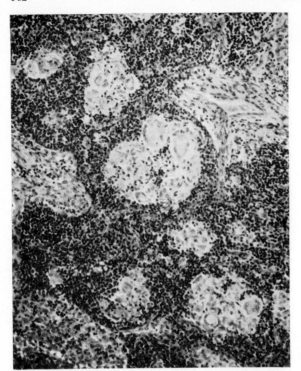

Fig. 9.42. Non-necrotizing tuberculoid granulomatosis in the pulp of an axillary lymph node draining a carcinomatous breast. There is also simple sinus histiocytosis. Multi-nucleate giant cells are conspicuous in the granulomatous foci in this instance, as usually is the case; occasionally, giant cells are scanty or absent. In some instances the tuberculoid reaction develops in the sinuses, and it is then that confusion with simple histiocytosis is likeliest to occur. See also Figs 9.137A and 9.137B, page 684. *Haematoxylin–eosin.* × 120.

comparison with the cells of simple sinus histiocytosis they are smaller and their single round or oval nucleus has a coarser chromatin pattern and contains a single, more haematoxyphile nucleolus. While the accumulation is predominantly within the widened sinuses, the demarcation between the latter and the pulp is less clear-cut than is the case in simple sinus histiocytosis, the cells tending to infiltrate slightly into the lymphoid tissue. There is no evidence of phagocytosis by these cells. They are said to be young, 'immature' histiocytes and not hyperplastic endothelial macrophages as in simple sinus histiocytosis; it has been suggested that they are not derived from the endothelial macrophages of the sinuses but from histiocytes or their precursors in the connective tissue of the capsule and trabeculae of the nodes. The functional immaturity of the cells led to the description of the condition as 'immature' (*unreife Sinushistiocytose*[258a]). In this context it

should be noted that the occasional endothelial macrophage that may be present in the sinuses among the immature histiocytes may ingest erythrocytes or other cells: this should not be thought to invalidate a diagnosis of immature sinus histiocytosis.

Immature sinus histiocytosis is seen most characteristically in toxoplasmosis (see page 654 and Fig. 9.116C) and infectious mononucleosis (see page 650 and Fig. 9.113). It may occur in some other infections also, particularly brucella infection (see page 591).

'Hamazaki–Wesenberg Bodies' ('Ceroid Bodies')[259]

The peculiar structures that, until their nature and significance are known with certainty, may perhaps

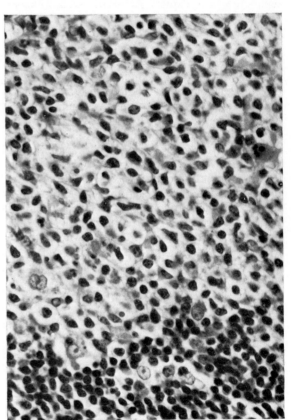

Fig. 9.43. 'Immature sinus histiocytosis' in a case of toxoplasmic lymphadenitis. The cells are smaller and more compactly arranged than in simple sinus histiocytosis (see Fig. 9.40), and they encroach more on the lymphoid pulp, the demarcation between sinus and pulp being less clear. The nucleus of the cells is smaller and has a denser chromatin pattern. See also Figs 9.113, 9.116C and 9.117 (pages 651, 655 and 656). *Haematoxylin–eosin.* × 400.

best be referred to eponymously, as Hamazaki–Wesenberg bodies,[260, 261] are a common finding in lymph nodes.[261a] They occur particularly in the sinuses, and particularly in the presence of sinus catarrh and of the more marked form of the latter that has been described above as simple sinus histiocytosis. In appearance they range from spherules of about 3 μm in diameter to ovoid and spindle-shaped bodies up to 20 μm in length and from 3 to 10 μm across (Figs 9.44A and 9.44B). They are found both within the cytoplasm of macrophages and free in the lumen of the sinuses;

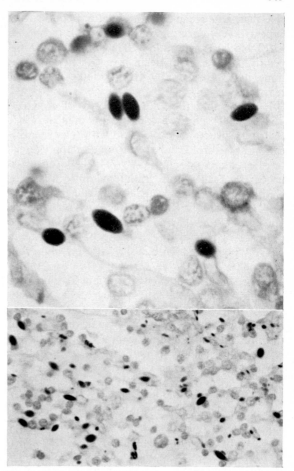

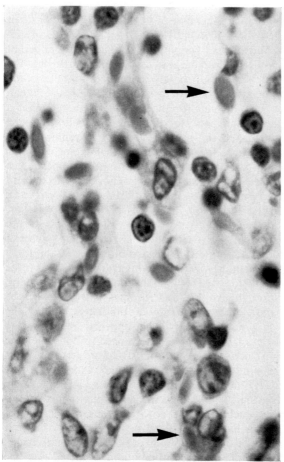

Fig. 9.44A. 'Hamazaki–Wesenberg bodies' ('ceroid bodies') in a sinus of a lymph node. The field includes at least 10 of these pigmented ovoid bodies. The arrowed example in the upper part of the field has a distinct, centrally placed, circular zone of relative pallor, liable to be mistaken for the internal structure of a parasite, such as a fungal cell might show. Other examples in the picture show comparable traces of a central pattern. The arrowed body at the foot of the picture appears to have a fine, halo-like peripheral zone, which is possibly a shrinkage artefact. See also Fig. 9.44B. *Haematoxylin–eosin.* × 1200.

Fig. 9.44B.§ 'Hamazaki–Wesenberg bodies'. These bodies are sometimes overlooked in haematoxylin–eosin preparations (Fig. 9.44A), especially if overstained with eosin, which tends to obliterate the contrast between their natural brown colour and the background of the section. They are often quite strongly Gram-positive, but in Gram preparations it is not easy to distinguish the details of the tissue, and their orientation to tissue structures and to cells is therefore obscured. Giemsa's stain shows them very well, usually as dark greenish blue bodies. An excellent means of confirming their presence and relating them to the topographical features of the node is to take advantage of their acid-fast staining capacity, as here. The photograph at the lower magnification gives an indication of how numerous they may be. *Ziehl–Neelsen stain; methylene blue counterstain.* Lower picture:§ × 375. Upper picture: × 1200.

less often, they are seen among the cells of the lymphoid tissue of the nodes. In their natural state their colour ranges from pale brownish yellow to deep greyish brown; the colour is unaffected by staining the sections with haematoxylin and eosin, although an excess of eosin reduces the contrast between the bodies and their surroundings and makes them less readily visible. They are strongly acid-fast, and because of their natural colour they appear a very dark purple, or brownish purple, in Ziehl–Neelsen preparations. They are often Gram-positive, they appear greenish in Giemsa preparations, and they give a positive periodic-acid/Schiff reaction.

It seems that they are composed of a ceroid lipofuscin.[259] Electron microscopy indicates that their ultrastructure is consistent with their identification as a ceroid and shows none of the characteristics of micro-organisms.[259, 262] Their occurrence in cases of the fatal granulomatous disease of childhood that is associated with deficient bactericidal activity of the neutrophils is noted on page 710 and is of interest in relation to the characteristic presence in that disease of macrophages that are heavily pigmented with a lipochrome or ceroid substance.

At present, their greatest importance seems to be in their nuisance value, for they are a frequent source of concern to diagnostic histologists who, observing them from time to time in the course of their practice, and finding them undescribed in the texts that are usually to hand, are repeatedly under pressure to decide whether they represent some uncommon form of parasite. For instance, their misinterpretation as possibly cells of a novel brown fungus, and the premature disclosure of this suggestion[263] following their observation in large numbers in the abdominal lymph nodes of a patient who had died of ulcerative colitis, led to a major hospital laboratory being overwhelmed with demands from the clinical staff for the search for fungi in the excreta of all the patients attending a very large gastroenterological clinic. The clinic was in charge of a physician whose dedication, in 1949, to finding the cause of ulcerative colitis was exceeded only by the unwariness of his mycologically inexperienced histopathological colleague.

Whatever the origin of Hamazaki–Wesenberg bodies may eventually prove to be, it seems clear now that they are not micro-organisms.

'Sinus Histiocytosis with Massive Lymphadenopathy'[264, 264a]

This awkwardly named condition was defined as an entity only comparatively recently,[264b, 264c] although it had been referred to by Robb-Smith, in 1947,[265] under the name 'giant cell sinus reticulosis in children'. It is characterized by great enlargement of lymph nodes, almost always in the neck, on both sides, with at most relatively minor involvement of other groups of nodes. Apart from some fever, the clinical condition of the patients has usually been good. In some cases the lymphadenopathy recedes fully after a period of from some months to several years; in other cases it has persisted, the patient's general health remaining good. The ultimate course of the disease cannot yet be confidently described as benign. In the only considerable series so far recorded, 34 cases,[264] there were two deaths: one patient died of pseudomonas pneumonia, apparently resulting from depression of immunity by radiotherapy and cytotoxic drugs; the other died 8 years after the onset of the lymphadenopathy, of renal amyloidosis that appeared 2 years before death. It is of interest that renal amyloidosis was the cause of death in another case, also 8 years after the onset of the lymphadenopathy.[266]

The affected lymph nodes are enlarged, adherent and firm. The enlargement is often so great that the clinical picture precisely reproduces that classically associated with advanced Hodgkin's disease: it can be very difficult for the clinician to accept that a lymphadenopathy of this extent is believed to be benign and self-healing, and not to require treatment. In a few instances the enlargement of the nodes is much more modest, and in some only a single node or a small group of nodes is affected and the resulting mass may not exceed 4 to 5 cm in its largest dimension.

Histology.—Even in the earliest stages the sinuses of the nodes are distended and already contain many conspicuously large macrophages (Fig. 9.45A); the lymphoid tissue between the sinuses is still abundant, although atrophic, and it contrasts starkly with the pallor of the contents of the latter. Later, the lymphoid tissue largely disappears as the sinuses undergo progressive distension. At all stages the most conspicuous and most characteristic cells in the sinuses are large macrophages with granular or foamy-looking cytoplasm and a large, usually vesicular, round or oval nucleus that has a prominent nucleolus (Fig. 9.45B). Some of the macrophages have markedly eosinophile cytoplasm, and many of these eosinophile cells have several nuclei, or a single hyperchromatic and distorted nucleus. Continuity of their cytoplasm may be conspicuous, giving the cells a syncytial character. Mitotic figures are infrequent or absent. There are also some lymphocytes, plasma cells and neutrophils free within the sinuses. Eosinophils are notably few and often cannot be found at all: this is sometimes helpful in differential diagnosis, particularly in making the distinction from some of the forms of malignant histiocytosis, which are commonly

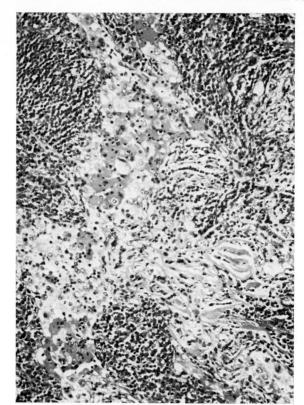

Fig. 9.45A. 'Sinus histiocytosis with massive lymphadeno-pathy'. The sinuses are distended and contain large macro-phages, some pale and some dark (see Fig. 9.45B). There are some lymphocytes among the macrophages but they are not particularly numerous. The outline of the sinuses is well maintained in places but elsewhere is obscured, particu-larly where fibrosis has occurred. *Haematoxylin–eosin.* × 150.

characterized by the presence of many eosinophils (see page 858).

It is a particular feature of the large macrophages of this type of sinus histiocytosis that many of them contain lymphocytes and often other cells, including plasma cells, neutrophils and erythrocytes, within their cytoplasm. The engulfed cells often lie within distinct vacuoles and they may be so numerous as almost totally to obscure the structure of the macro-phage. They often look remarkably normal under the light microscope, but electron microscopy shows that degenerative changes are usually present;[267] eventually they are completely broken down.

The remains of the lymphoid tissue of the nodes contain mature lymphocytes and often many plasma cells and plasma cell precursors, and there may be numerous Russell bodies. Lymphoid follicles are small and few, and eventually disappear. There is no necrosis or granuloma formation (but it may be

noted that this variety of histiocytosis has been observed in association with bacteriologically proved tuberculosis of the same nodes;[266] such presumably coincident infections inevitably modify the histological picture). The capsule of the nodes and the immediately surrounding tissues are often markedly fibrotic; fibrosis within the nodes is seldom a conspicuous feature, at least until the condition is undergoing regression (Fig. 9.46).

In a few reported cases the opportunity to examine other tissues has shown a comparable accumulation of macrophages of the same types in tonsils, orbital tissue, testis and skin.[264]

Aetiology.—The cause of this remarkable condition is quite unknown. It appears to be significantly commoner in black people than in those of other races, and to affect children in the first decade most frequently. Onset of the disease after the age of

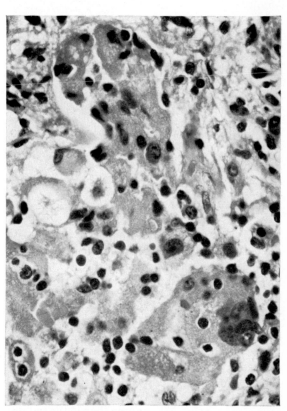

Fig. 9.45B. 'Sinus histiocytosis with massive lymphadeno-pathy'. The large macrophages contain ingested lymphocytes and erythrocytes. Their opaque cytoplasm is strongly eosin-ophile and their nuclei are clustered or scattered. In this field only a few of the macrophages have clear cytoplasm, but elsewhere in the nodes such cells may predominate (see Fig. 9.45A). *Haematoxylin–eosin.* × 540.

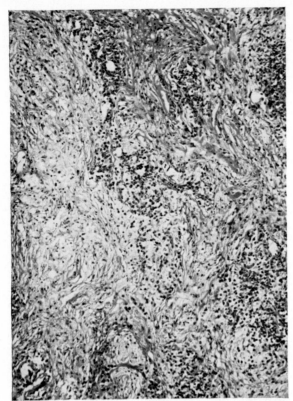

Fig. 9.46. 'Sinus histiocytosis with massive lymphadenopathy' —stage of regression. Loose-textured connective tissue occupies the sinuses and extends into the pulp. Plasma cells are numerous in the latter. Some vacuolate macrophages are scattered in the interstices of the young fibrous tissue, but they are inconspicuous. The bizarre cells with opaque cytoplasm, so characteristic of the earlier stages of the disease, are lacking (compare with Figs 9.45A and 9.45B). *Haematoxylin–eosin.* × 135.

20 years is rare. There is no significant difference in sex incidence. The geographical distribution of the recognized cases suggests that the disease may occur throughout the world. No micro-organisms have been found, and the electron microscopical appearances in the few cases investigated have given no indication of an infective cause.[267, 268] It has been suggested that infection by *Klebsiella rhinoscleromatis* might be the cause.[268, 269] Lymphadenitis seems to have been observed only rarely as an accompaniment of scleroma. In two examples that I have seen, the large, clear or vacuolate, macrophages were more numerous in the pulp than in the sinuses; the klebsiellae were demonstrable in a proportion of these cells in both situations, but particularly in the pulp of the node (see Figs 9.65A and 9.65B, page 590). Plasma cells are more abundant in the scleromatous node, both in the sinuses and in the lymphoid

tissue, than in sinus histiocytosis with massive lymphadenopathy, and Russell bodies are usually numerous. Although it seems unlikely, the possibility that there may be a relation between klebsiella infection and this peculiar lymphadenopathy has not been ruled out. It is relevant that persistently raised titres of antibodies to klebsiellae, with the highest levels related to *Klebsiella rhinoscleromatis* and *Klebsiella ozaenae*, were found in the case of a white child with the disease.[264a] The significance of this observation is uncertain. The same is true of the raised titre of antibodies against the Epstein–Barr virus noted in some cases.[264, 269a]

There is no evidence that sinus histiocytosis with massive lymphadenopathy is a manifestation of a disorder of immunity.

Differential Diagnosis.—Clinically, the massive enlargement of the cervical lymph nodes suggests the possibility of Hodgkin's disease or other lymphoma, including Burkitt's lymphoma. Histologically, the only conditions likely to be confused with this condition are other forms of sinus histiocytosis (see above), including lipidoses and other storage diseases (see page 757), malignant forms of histiocytosis (see page 858) and the rare disease of infancy known as 'familial haemophagocytic reticulosis', in which sinus histiocytosis with marked phagocytosis of erythrocytes and, to a smaller extent, of other cells is a feature (see page 862).

'Iatrogenic' and Related Sinus Lymphadenopathies

The best known of the lymphadenopathies that are caused by therapeutic or other medical procedures include the remarkable lymphoma-like changes that may occur during treatment with certain drugs, particularly hydantoin drugs (see page 697), and the infective lymphadenopathy caused by the bacillus Calmette–Guérin (BCG—see page 603). These conditions involve the nodes as a whole. There is also a series of conditions in which substances that have been administered for diagnostic or therapeutic purposes cause changes that affect the sinuses of the nodes predominantly, and only secondarily involve the lymphoid tissue itself. These may conveniently be considered here.

Lymphadenopathy Following Lymphangiography

Lymphangiography was introduced by Kinmonth,[270] in 1952; he used a water-soluble contrast medium in order to display the lymphatics radiologically in cases of lymphoedema. The subsequent development of low viscosity iodized oil contrast media, such as 'Lipiodol' Ultra-Fluid (Iodised Oil Fluid Injection, British Pharmacopoeia; Ethiodized Oil, United States Pharmacopeia), made more extensive radiological investigations of the lymphatics and lymph nodes possible. Lymphangiography is now used for a range of purposes, including the detection of primary and secondary tumours in nodes, staging various forms of cancer, and investigating the nature of intra-abdominal masses.[271] Ordinarily, the amount of medium injected in the case of an adult is from 4 to 15 ml, according to the site under investigation: a total of 15 ml is sufficient to show the lymphatics of both legs and fill the sinuses of the inguinal, iliac, pre-aortic and lateral aortic lymph nodes. The medium is retained in the nodes for a period that may range from a few weeks to several months, and traces have still been demonstrable radiologically in some normal people as long as 24 months after the injection and histologically even after 4 years.[266]

Histology.[272, 273]—The oily base of the contrast medium causes an oleogranulomatous reaction in the sinuses of the lymph nodes, particularly the subcapsular sinus. This accompanies some degree of distension of the sinuses by the oil, which can be demonstrated in frozen sections. The granulomatous response begins with enlargement and proliferation of the endothelial macrophages, many of which come to lie free in the lumen of the sinuses. Their cytoplasm may be finely or coarsely vacuolate, enclosing droplets of oil, or it may be opaque and eosinophile. Larger droplets of oil in the sinuses come to be surrounded by these cells, and the granulomatous response spreads to a variable extent into the adjacent lymphoid tissue, in which small clusters of vacuolate macrophages appear. Multinucleate macrophages may become a feature of the reaction (Fig. 9.47). Eosinophils are conspicuous among the macrophages in some specimens, particularly within the first few weeks after introduction of the oil. Neutrophils may be numerous during the few days following the injection but later are no longer a feature. Plasma cells are present in the affected sinuses and in the lymphoid tissue, and occasionally they are very numerous.

Similar changes are sometimes seen in the afferent lymphatics and their immediate vicinity, particularly just before they enter the capsule of the nodes. The efferent lymphatics are less often affected.

Not infrequently, when there is occasion to examine sections of the spleen and of other organs containing many reticuloendothelial cells it is found

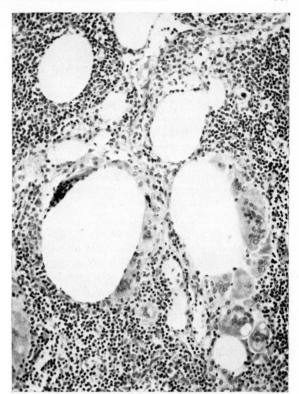

Fig. 9.47. Lymphadenopathy resulting from lymphangiography with iodized oil. The picture is that of an oleogranulomatous reaction, with multinucleate giant cells surrounding some of the larger globules (represented by the clear spaces, from which the oil was removed during histological preparation). Fine droplets of oil elsewhere in the sinuses account for the small vacuoles in other giant cells and the general increase in the number of macrophages. The reaction is comparable to that in Whipple's disease and other forms of lipid granuloma (see Figs 9.34, 9.35 and 9.37—pages 556 to 588). *Haematoxylin–eosin.* × 120.

that minute globules of oil are present in the macrophages. This is presumed to result from the eventual escape of some of the contrast medium into the blood (see page 741).

Differential Diagnosis.—The histological appearances are sometimes confused with those of the earlier stages of the lymphadenopathy of Whipple's disease (see page 556), but the macrophages do not contain the characteristic inclusions of periodic-acid/Schiff-positive material that distinguish the latter. In general, the picture is that of any oleogranulomatous lymphadenitis: a comparable picture may be seen in the nodes draining the sites of injection of drugs in an oily base (see below).[274] The changes in lymph nodes associated with the presence of gas cysts in the alimentary tract (cystic pneumatosis—

see page 557) may also closely resemble those following lymphangiography.

Lymphadenopathy Complicating Parenteral Depot Medication

Many substances have been used as vehicles in which active drugs may be suspended or dissolved so that, when administered by intramuscular or subcutaneous injection, the drug will be absorbed only slowly from the site of inoculation, thus providing sustained action over a period substantially longer than follows injection in aqueous or other simple media.

Lymphadenopathy Caused by Various Fixed Oils.— The fixed oils, particularly arachis oil (peanut oil), have been the most widely used of the 'depot vehicles'; they commonly cause sclerosing oleogranulomas at the site of injection and occasionally carriage of some of the oil to regional lymph nodes is followed by the development of comparable lesions in the sinuses and adjacent lymphoid tissue. Therapeutically much more satisfactory results were obtained, for instance with penicillin, once specific compounds, such as procaine penicillin, that are inherently less soluble, were produced, and the use of oily depot preparations of drugs has become infrequent except in the case of a range of agents that it is practical to administer only in oily suspension, and that require to be used in a slow-release, sustained-action manner. These agents include various hormonal preparations and a few other drugs, such as the chelating compound dimercaprol ('British anti-lewisite', BAL), which is injected in a mixture of arachis oil and benzyl benzoate. Among recently observed examples of depot medication causing local oleogranulomatous lymphadenitis have been the injection of vasopressin tannate in arachis oil in the treatment of diabetes insipidus,[274] deoxycortone acetate (desoxycorticosterone acetate) in a mixture of arachis oil and ethyl oleate in the treatment of chronic adrenal cortical insufficiency,[266] esters of oestradiol and testosterone in an undisclosed fixed oil solvent in the treatment of menopausal symptoms,[266] and dimercaprol in the treatment of acute arsenical and acute mercurial poisoning.[266]

Polyvinylpyrrolidone (Povidone) Lymphadenopathy.

—Substances other than fixed oils that have been used as depot vehicles for parenteral administration of therapeutic agents include polyvinylpyrrolidone (povidone). This substance may accumulate in con-

siderable amounts in the lymph nodes draining injection sites, and a great proliferation of endothelial macrophages in the sinuses and of the macrophages in the lymphoid tissue may result.[275, 276] The cytoplasm of the cells may appear clear or it may enclose opaque, homogeneous globules that are presumably derived from the polyvinylpyrrolidone (Fig. 9.48); these globules usually stain delicately with eosin, but sometimes they take up haematoxylin and show a pale azure tint.

Polyvinylpyrrolidone is produced also in a grade supposedly suitable for intravenous administration: it has been used in this form as a substitute for dextrans to restore or maintain the blood volume. This may result in its accumulation in the reticulo-endothelial cells throughout the body;[276, 277] lymph

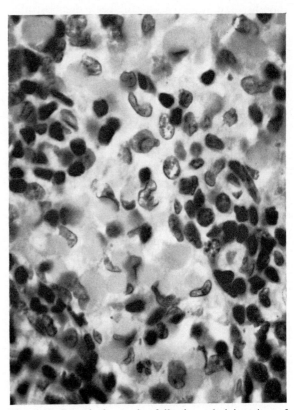

Fig. 9.48. Lymphadenopathy following administration of insulin in a solution of 'parenteral grade' polyvinylpyrrolidone (povidone) in order to delay absorption. Repeated injections were given over a period of several weeks, mainly into the buttocks. Enlargement of the inguinal lymph nodes resulted. Homogeneous globules are present in the cytoplasm of macrophages in the sinuses or free in the lumen. Their identification caused considerable perplexity until the history of the injections was elicited. Chemical analysis confirmed the nature of the material in the biopsy specimen. See also Fig. 9.49. *Haematoxylin–eosin.* × 850.

node involvement in such cases is incidental to the systemic storage (Fig. 9.49).

Silicone Lymphadenopathy

The polymeric organosilicon compounds (silicones) that are used in medicine, usually for prosthetic purposes and as an adjunct to plastic surgery, and also in cosmetic surgery, are said to be biologically inert and not to be absorbable. The development of granulomatous changes in tissues, such as the breasts (see Chapter 28), into which silicone fluid (liquid dimethylpolysiloxane, or dimethicone) of the grade intended for this purpose has been injected, may be due to adulteration of the fluid. Indeed, in the so-called Sakurai formula[278] fatty acids are added to the pure preparation so that fibrosis may be

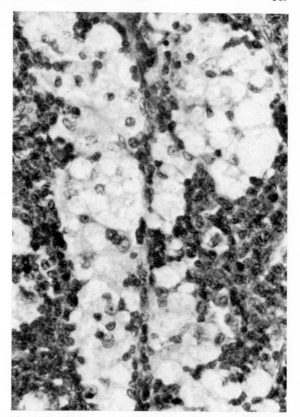

Fig. 9.50. Silicone lymphadenopathy. The accumulation of large, vacuolate macrophages in the sinuses and adjoining pulp of the node is strikingly defined by the contrast with the deeply stained lymphocytes. The patient had had a succession of injections of silicone fluid into the breasts in order to augment their size. Sclerosing mastitis and enlargement of the regional lymph nodes began to appear some 18 months after the first injections (Case 1 in Reference 280, page 869 of this chapter): Fig. 28.26A in Volume 4 illustrates the mammary changes in the same case. The close resemblance of the lymphadenopathy to that of lepromatous leprosy is remarkable (see Fig. 9.81, page 609). See also Figs 9.49, 9.51A and 9.51B. *Haematoxylin–eosin.* × 370.

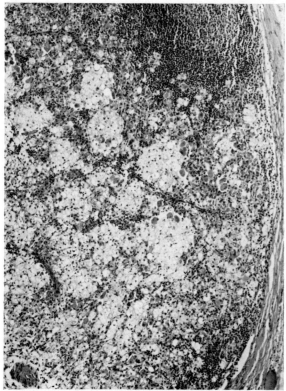

Fig. 9.49.§ Lymphadenopathy following administration of 'parenteral grade' polyvinylpyrrolidone (povidone) intravenously as a plasma substitute. There is a marked, multifocal proliferation of macrophages with copious, clear cytoplasm, mainly in the interfollicular tissue but also in the sinuses in some areas. The involvement of the lymph nodes was part of a general histiocytosis throughout the reticuloendothelial system, with phagocytosis of the injected material. Compare with silicone lymphadenopathy (Fig. 9.50) and lepromatous leprosy (Fig. 9.81, page 609). See also Fig. 9.48. *Haematoxylin–eosin.* × 65.

induced in the tissues with the intention of preventing the fluid from gravitating or otherwise escaping from the site where it is required. There seems to be no doubt that silicone fluid is sometimes absorbed and carried in lymph to regional lymph nodes, where a marked histiocytosis may develop in the distended sinuses and—sometimes predominantly—throughout the lymphoid tissue (Fig. 9.50).[279, 280] The picture in the lymph nodes, as seen in haematoxylin–eosin preparations, may closely resemble that of lepromatous leprosy (see Fig. 9.81, page 609): the presence of globi—the characteristic aggregates of leprosy bacilli, detectable in haematoxylin–eosin preparations and readily demonstrated when stained by an appropriate method for acid-fast organisms—confirms the diagnosis of the latter. The similarity of the changes to those in some cases of Hand–Schüller–Christian disease is also noteworthy (see page 763).

Lymphadenopathy Associated with Silicone Rubber Prostheses.—Certain types of silicone rubber, particularly the non-swelling fluorosilicone rubber of surgical quality, have proved to be valuable for the moulding of prosthetic joints as a replacement for those that have been greatly disabled through the effects of rheumatoid arthritis. Some rare instances have been observed in which regional lymph nodes have become enlarged some years after insertion of the prostheses.[266, 280a] The lymphadenopathy may be characterized by the formation of many discrete, rounded, multinucleate giant cells throughout the

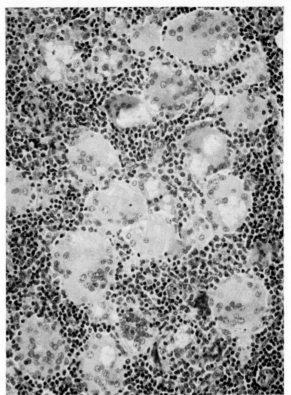

Fig. 9.51B. Lymphadenopathy associated with fluorosilicone rubber prosthetic joints. The higher magnification of the node illustrated in Fig. 9.51A shows that the macrophage reaction is exclusively giant-celled. The cytoplasm of many of the cells contains a cluster of vacuoles. The vacuoles contain clear, amorphous material; some of the material was seen to be moderately birefringent when examined in polarized light. Its identity has not been determined. Plasma cells are numerous among the background of lymphocytes. *Haematoxylin–eosin.* × 170.

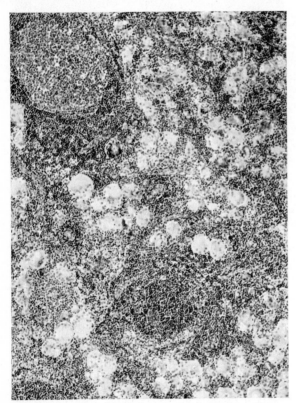

Fig. 9.51A. Lymphadenopathy associated with fluorosilicone rubber prosthetic joints. An extensive giant cell reaction has developed in the interfollicular tissue of the node. The picture is essentially the same as that of the pure giant-celled lymphadenitis of unknown causation referred to on page 684 of the text (see Fig. 9.138, page 685). The prosthetic joints were inserted in the patient's hand 4 years before slowly progressive enlargement of the axillary nodes began to develop on the same side. See Fig. 9.51B. *Haematoxylin–eosin.* × 65.

pulp of the affected nodes, and in proximity to the sinuses (Figs 9.51A and 9.51B). The giant cells appear opaque but may contain a well-defined vacuole in which there is amorphous, clear material that sometimes is doubly refractile. Except for the foreign material in the cytoplasm of the giant cells, the picture is the same as that of a rare form of lymphadenitis accompanying Crohn's disease (see page 682) and of the peculiar 'pure giant-celled lymphadenitis' described on page 684.

Lymphadenopathy Complicating the Introduction of Other Materials into the Tissues

Just as silicone fluid, used in various parts of the world today to augment the size of the breasts, may cause a regional lymphadenopathy, so might many agents that were used in earlier decades for the same purpose cause not only a sclerosing mastitis (see Chapter 28) but often an accompanying granulomatous lymphadenitis. Among these agents, the paraffin waxes were particularly notorious for the disfigurement that eventually followed their use in a high proportion of cases: in spite of the fact that the grades of wax chosen for injection were characterized—for obvious reasons—by a solidification point rather above the range of human body temperature, some of this material reached the lymph nodes draining the inoculation site and led to the development there of a paraffin wax granuloma ('paraffinoma'—see Chapter 28). Similarly, the once prevalent practice of packing the incised cavity of an abscess with medicated pastes, and the insertion of gauze packs impregnated with yellow soft paraffin (petrolatum) into surgical cavities, such as the perineal wound following excision of the rectum, was sometimes followed by painful enlargement of the regional lymph nodes that biopsy showed to be associated with the formation of an oleogranulomatous type of lymphadenitis.

'Reactive' Changes in the Interfollicular Lymphoid Tissue of Lymph Nodes

Lymphocytosis.—An increase in the number of lymphocytes in the interfollicular regions of lymph nodes accompanies the hyperplasia of the follicles that is a feature of various 'inflammatory' states. This lymphocytosis is part of the general immune reaction of the lymphoid tissues. It is difficult to assess its degree, because of the impracticability of determining what may be regarded as normal, and because accompanying hyperplasia of the follicles and changes in the lymph sinuses are likely to overshadow any interfollicular lymphocytosis that may be present.

Epithelioid Cell Clusters.—In contrast to the equivalent situation regarding lymphocytic hyperplasia (see above), hyperplasia of the mononuclear phagocytes—the reticuloendothelial cells—in the lymphoid tissue of the lymph nodes is readily apparent, and particularly so when they undergo epithelioid metamorphosis and form clusters or larger aggregates (Fig. 9.52). The epithelioid macrophages (epithelioid histiocytes) stand out clearly among the much smaller, deeply stained and closely packed lymphocytes.

These discrete clusters of epithelioid cells may form in response to various stimuli that affect lymph nodes and other lymphoid tissues. The stimuli are of so many types, and the reaction is so lacking in

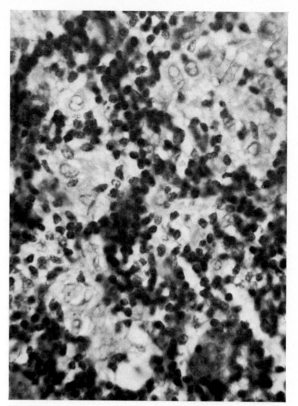

Fig. 9.52. Epithelioid cell clusters in the pulp of a lymph node. This type of proliferation and metamorphosis of macrophages is common to many varieties of lymphadenitis. See, for example, Figs 9.74 (page 601), 9.116A and 9.116B (page 654) and 9.206 (page 601). *Haematoxylin–eosin.* × 375.

specificity, that a confident histological diagnosis of the cause is not often possible. In some cases no specific cause is identified, the lymphadenopathy subsiding without its nature being discovered. In other cases, with essentially the same histological picture, the condition proves to be acquired toxoplasmosis—the commonest cause (see page 654)—or one of several other identifiable diseases that, at some stage in their development, may give rise to this type of reaction in the lymphoreticular tissues (see page 656). The particular diagnosis in individual instances is indicated by the results of specific laboratory investigations, sometimes with the further evidence of clinical response to appropriate treatment. Tuberculosis is one of few causes of this type of histological reaction in which the lesions tend to differ significantly from those of most of the other diseases that may be accompanied by the same basic picture: the difference is the presence of incipient caseation. Another infection that usually is recognized quite readily is leishmaniasis, the causative organism often being easily seen in the cytoplasm of the epithelioid cells forming the clusters (see Figs 9.121A and 9.121B, page 662).

It is important to note that a similar appearance may be seen in the early stages of some cases of Hodgkin's disease (see Fig. 9.206, page 801).

Infective Lymphadenitis

There are various bases for classifying lymphadenitis: according to cause, and whether acute or chronic; according to the character of the histological changes; according to the anatomical sites involved; according to associated clinical observations; and so on. Any of the changes in lymph nodes that have been described in the earlier pages of this section (page 533 onward) might, with justification, be regarded as forms of lymphadenitis; but it seemed useful to consider them separately, and in the following account to describe those diseases in which there is a clear association of the agent responsible for the lymphadenitis and the occurrence of histological changes that in most instances include some measure of destruction of the normal tissues and their local replacement by the product of of the inflammatory response.

The 'classification' used here is basically an aetiological one. The categories are—
   acute bacterial lymphadenitis (see below)
   subacute and chronic bacterial lymphadenitis (page 588)
   actinomycetous lymphadenitis (page 616)
   fungal lymphadenitis (page 617)
   algal lymphadenitis (page 631)
   rickettsial lymphadenitis (page 631)
   chlamydial lymphadenitis (page 634)
   viral lymphadenitis (page 640)
   protozoal lymphadenitis (page 652)
   metazoal lymphadenitis (page 669)
   lymphadenitis without animate cause (page 680).

Acute Bacterial Lymphadenitis

Anatomical Localization of Acute Bacterial Lymphadenitis

The commonest cause of acute lymphadenitis is an acute local septic infection—tonsillitis, an infected wound or burn of the skin, cellulitis, abscesses and visceral infection are among the conditions that are familiar causes of acute inflammation of regional lymph nodes.

Cervical, Axillary and Inguinal Lymphadenitis.— The lymph nodes of the neck, axillae and inguinal regions are those most frequently affected by acute inflammation. This reflects the frequency of infection in the corresponding drainage areas, which include the throat, skin and external genitalia.

*Retropharyngeal Lymphadenitis.—*Acute suppurative inflammation may develop in the retropharyngeal lymph nodes as a complication of acute streptococcal pharyngitis. These nodes are situated between the pharynx and the prevertebral fascia: if an abscess that has formed within one of them ruptures the infection may spread rapidly downward into the posterior part of the mediastinum.

*Iliac Lymphadenitis.—*The iliac groups of nodes may be involved in cases of suppurative inflammation of the skin or deeper tissues of the lower part of the trunk and of the leg of the corresponding side. There may be little or no evident involvement of the inguinal nodes in these cases, particularly in children,[281] in whom the manifestations of the iliac lymphadenitis may be mistaken for acute appendicitis or even acute arthritis of the hip.

*Mesenteric Lymphadenitis.—*Suppurative inflammation of the mesenteric lymph nodes, particularly those in the ileocaecal angle, may accompany acute appendicitis and staphylococcal enterocolitis. This condition is rare, and quite distinct from acute non-suppurative mesenteric lymphadenitis (see page 574).

*Local Lymphadenitis Accompanying Other Visceral Diseases.—*The *hepatic group of lymph nodes,* particularly the *cystic lymph node,* may be acutely inflamed as an accompaniment of acute cholecystitis. This condition is not to be confused with cholegranulomatous lymphadenitis (see page 558). Acute inflammation of the *bronchopulmonary and tracheobronchial lymph nodes* is a surprisingly infrequent accompaniment of acute pneumonia; it may be found in a proportion of cases of acute suppurative bronchopneumonia, and in some instances there is formation of abscesses in the nodes. The enlargement of these nodes in cases of lobar pneumonia is often most marked in the stage of resolution, and is then due mainly to the abundance of fluid absorbed in the lymphatics as the pneumonic exudate liquefies (see page 317). There is always some degree of infiltration by neutrophils, even at this stage.

As in other instances of acute inflammatory diseases of the viscera, the primary manifestations of the illness so dominate the clinical picture of, say, cholecystitis and pneumonia, that an accompanying lymphadenitis is seldom evident, although in a very few cases it may have serious complications. These include frank suppuration and the eruption of the ensuing abscess into structures adjoining the nodes, with the consequent development of, for example, suppurative mediastinitis or peritonitis.

Acute Suppurative Lymphadenitis

Streptococcal and Staphylococcal Lymphadenitis, and Lymphadenitis Caused by Other Pyogenic Bacteria

In keeping with the characteristic capacity of *Streptococcus pyogenes* to spread rapidly in infected tissues, whereas *Staphylococcus aureus* tends to remain localized, lymphadenitis occurs earlier in the course of infection by the former and, usually, is much severer and accompanied by more marked inflammation in the tissues round the nodes (periadenitis). In cases of staphylococcal lymphadenitis fewer nodes are involved and their enlargement is seldom more than moderate, even when there is abscess formation within them. Periadenitis is not a conspicuous feature of staphylococcal lymphadenitis unless an abscess extends from the substance of an infected node into the surrounding tissues. Lymphadenitis is less often a complication of staphylococcal infection than of streptococcal infection: for instance, it is comparatively rare to find a significant degree of lymphadenitis accompanying a boil or a carbuncle, and even in cases of acute osteomyelitis it is unusual to find evidence of severe involvement of the regional nodes.

The acutely inflamed lymph nodes are usually hyperaemic, tense, and more or less enlarged. Microscopical examination shows sinus catarrh with very many neutrophils in the sinuses and throughout the adjoining pulp, and—particularly in cases of staphylococcal infection—destruction of tissue and frank suppuration and abscess formation. The causative organisms are readily demonstrated in most cases, particularly in Gram-stained preparations. The lymphoid follicles are hyperplastic and often contain conspicuous germinal centres; like the rest of the lymphoid tissue of the nodes they are infiltrated by neutrophils.

Gonococcal Lymphadenitis.—Acute gonorrhoea may be accompanied by a rapidly developing and severe suppurative lymphadenitis, particularly in men. The nodes involved are usually those of the inguinal groups, and there is usually symmetrical involvement of both sides. The infection may spread to the iliac nodes on one or both sides, and in exceptional cases affects these predominantly, with symptoms that may be mistaken for those of other acute intra-abdominal or pelvic conditions. Lymphadenitis may also occur in the regional nodes draining other foci of gonococcal infection, but—with the occasional exception of abscess formation in the sacral and iliac nodes in cases of acute gonococcal proctitis—its severity is seldom marked.

Other Pyogenic Bacteria.—The lymphadenitis that accompanies infection by other pyogenic bacteria—such as infection of burns or wounds by *Pseudomonas aeruginosa* (*Pseudomonas pyocyanea*) and localized peritoneal and other abscesses caused by *Escherichia coli* or *Streptococcus faecalis*—is commonly of very moderate degree, and seldom characterized by abscess formation. An exception is sometimes seen in cases of rapidly spreading infection by *Pseudomonas aeruginosa*, particularly in patients whose resistance has been seriously lowered by disease or therapeutic procedures that interfere with immunity: in such cases suppurative lymphadenitis—and even extensive necrosis without frank suppuration—may be found, although usually only in the nodes that drain the site of the initial seat of the infection.

Chancroid.—The primary lesion of chancroid—the 'soft sore' or 'soft chancre'—on the genitalia is accompanied by the development of acute suppurative regional lymphadenitis due to the spread of the causative organism, *Haemophilus ducreyi*, through the lymphatics. Necrosis appears in numerous foci throughout the infected nodes and these foci soon become confluent abscesses as neutrophils accumulate.[282] The oedematous and inflamed capsule of the node may soon be perforated and the suppuration extends through the surrounding tissues to involve the skin and give rise to a sinus with spreading local ulceration. The organisms can sometimes be recognized in histological preparations.

It can be difficult to distinguish the lymphadenitis of chancroid from that of lymphogranuloma inguinale (see page 636): however, suppuration is generally more widespread in chancroid, which also lacks the epithelioid cell zone and the occasional multinucleate giant cells that characterize the necrotic foci of the chlamydial infection.

Rare Causes of Acute Suppurative Lymphadenitis.—Many types of bacterial infection are occasional causes of acute suppurative lymphadenitis. For instance, a pure suppurative reaction is seen in some cases of the rare type of infection by *Listeria monocytogenes* (see page 577) in which the disease appears to be confined to cervical nodes, which break down and discharge through the skin; in other cases of this clinical type the histological picture is that of the confluent necrotizing granuloma with epithelioid histiocytosis and suppuration described on page 636.[283]

Suppurative lymphadenitis may develop in the course of *glanders* in man, as in horses and other animals, forming the so-called 'farcy buds'. Usually it is a subacute or chronic lymphadenitis (see page 595), [284, 285] but in exceptional cases it is acute.

Acute Non-Suppurative Lymphadenitis

Acute Mesenteric Lymphadenitis

There is considerable confusion about the nature of acute mesenteric lymphadenitis, particularly in relation to its causation. Clinically, this term is used to describe a condition that occurs quite commonly in childhood and early adult life, presenting with symptoms that simulate acute or subacute appendicitis; it has been said to account for as many as 30 per cent of abdominal emergencies in the practice of some paediatric surgeons. In some cases the histological picture is that of an acute non-necrotizing lymphadenitis with no specific features; no specific infective cause has been identified in these cases. In other cases there are epithelioid cell clusters, without necrosis, or a more extensive, necrotizing epithelioid histiocytosis: in most of these instances the disease is believed to be caused by *Yersinia enterocolitica*[286] or, less often, by the closely related organism *Yersinia pseudotuberculosis* (*Pasteurella pseudotuberculosis*) (see page 584);[287] very rarely, the same histological picture is seen as a result of infection of the mesenteric nodes by *Francisella tularensis* (see page 586).

The evidence suggests that there are two main aetiological forms of the disease that is generally known to clinicians as acute mesenteric lymphadenitis: one form is a manifestation of yersinial infection (see page 584) and the other is of unknown causation. Various other infective agents may be responsible for comparable symptoms and surgical findings: the syndrome has been observed as a manifestation of lymphadenitis caused by species of actinobacilli (see page 616), or occurring in the course of measles (see page 641), rubella (see page 643), poliomyelitis (see page 643), infectious mononucleosis (see page 649) and—possibly—cat-scratch disease (see page 639), the last presenting the same histological picture as yersinial infection.

When no cause is recognized, and the histological picture is of the simple, non-granulomatous type, without necrosis, that is described below, the condi-

tion is commonly referred to as '*acute non-specific mesenteric lymphadenitis*'. This designation distinguishes it from lymphadenitis caused by yersiniae (see page 584) and salmonellae (see page 575) and from other well-defined infective lesions, such as the rare form of tuberculous mesenteric lymphadenitis that presents with an acute clinical illness (see page 599), and—formerly—the rare cases of lymphadenitis following oral administration of bacillus Calmette–Guérin (BCG—see page 606).

Macroscopical Findings.—Laparotomy shows the appendix to be normal, contrary to the usual clinical expectation, which reflects the closeness of the resemblance of the signs and symptoms to those of acute appendicitis. In a few cases there is hyperaemia of the serosa of the terminal part of the ileum, sometimes with a little local fibrinous exudate; the wall of the affected part of the bowel may be thickened by oedema ('acute terminal ileitis'—see page 1072). There is no extension of this inflammatory condition to the large intestine. In fact, in the great majority of cases the only abnormality is a considerable enlargement of the mesenteric lymph nodes, particularly—in most cases—those in the ileocaecal angle, but sometimes predominantly the nodes in the root of the mesentery of the small intestine. The affected nodes are hyperaemic and firm or tense.

Histology.—The histological changes in the nodes are those of an acute inflammatory reaction without specific features. The sinuses are distended by a massive accumulation of lymphocytes (Fig. 9.53), sometimes to such an extent that the distinction between sinuses and lymphoid pulp—ordinarily so conspicuous in mesenteric lymph nodes—may be obliterated: the picture may be mistaken for that of chronic lymphocytic leukaemia or a lymphocytic lymphoma, although the reticulin framework is preserved. The lymphoid follicles tend to be small, and germinal centres are inconspicuous or lacking. There are often many neutrophils, but the picture is not that of incipient suppuration. Eosinophils may be scattered throughout the affected nodes but are not strikingly numerous except in those cases, mainly in tropical lands, in which the patient coincidentally has a heavy infestation by metazoal parasites.[266] Histiocytes are a notable feature in some cases: they are not usually grouped but tend to lie singly among the lymphocytes (Fig. 9.53). Sometimes, before the sinuses become filled with lymphocytes, there is an obvious proliferation of the endothelial macrophages.

Examination of the *appendix*, which is usually

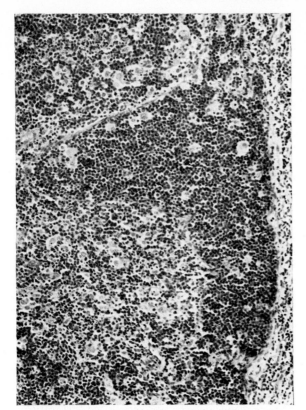

Fig. 9.53. Acute non-specific mesenteric lymphadenitis. The subcapsular sinus and its extensions alongside the trabecula are distended with lymphocytes among which there is an occasional large mononuclear cell. Histiocytes and immunoblasts are present in the adjoining pulp. *Haematoxylin–eosin.* ×120.

removed in these cases, rarely shows any abnormality. Such changes as are present are usually of the type associated with 'chronic non-specific appendicitis' (see page 1172) and may be regarded as coincidental. The clusters of epithelioid histiocytes or immunoblasts that are seen in a small proportion of appendices from patients with yersinial mesenteric lymphadenitis (see page 585) are not a recognized feature in cases of acute non-specific mesenteric lymphadenitis.

Differential Diagnosis.—Clinical and surgical findings indistinguishable from those just described may be caused by various other diseases that present more or less distinctive histological changes in the mesenteric lymph nodes. Most of these are indicated in the introductory paragraphs of this section (see above). The need to exclude lymphoma and leukaemia as the cause of the lymphadenopathy has also been mentioned above. Very rarely, immuno-

blastic lymphadenopathy presents with acute symptoms due to involvement of abdominal nodes (see page 703).

Salmonella Infections

Typhoid and Paratyphoid Fevers.—In both typhoid fever and the paratyphoid fevers the mesenteric lymph nodes are always severely affected, and there may be similar changes in the lymph nodes throughout the body.[288] The generalized nature of the lymphadenitis accompanying these diseases results from the septicaemic nature of the infections and the predilection of the causative organisms for the lymphoid tissues. The predominant cells in the lesions are discrete, pale or dark mononuclear cells that are distributed diffusely or in small—sometimes confluent—nodules throughout the nodes, particularly in and near the sinuses but also in the pulp, and then mainly in the close vicinity of the follicles (Fig. 9.54). These cells are believed to be derived directly from the reticulum cells of the nodes.[289] Another interpretation is that some of them are immunoblasts (see page 522). As the infection proceeds, some of the cells become increasingly large, with abundant, eosinophile cytoplasm, and show a tendency to ingest other cells, particularly lymphocytes and erythrocytes:[290] it is these large macrophages that are most properly called 'typhoid cells',* and they develop not only among the proliferating cells of the pulp of the lymphoid tissues but also from the endothelial macrophages of the sinuses of lymph nodes. Plasma cells are also numerous in the nodes in typhoid and paratyphoid fever. Focal necrosis is common in any lesion of typhoid or paratyphoid fever and is often conspicuous and extensive in the affected lymph nodes; clusters of the bacilli are sometimes demonstrable in the necrotic foci.

It is generally true to say that the lesions in the lymph nodes, as in the other affected organs and tissues, are severer in typhoid fever (infection by *Salmonella typhi*) than in paratyphoid fever (infection by *Salmonella paratyphi*, of which—in the Linnaean nomenclature—there are three species, *Salmonella*

* The fact that the disease that is known in English as *typhoid fever* (that is, 'typhus-like fever') is commonly known to German-trained doctors as *typhus abdominalis* once led to mistranslation of *Typhuszelle* as 'typhus cell', and, perhaps by extrapolation, to the misstatement that the same cell may be a feature of the histological picture in rickettsial infections. The disease that is known in English as *typhus fever* (rickettsial infection—specifically, louse-borne infection by *Rickettsia prowazekii*) is the *typhus exanthematicus* of many doctors on the European mainland.

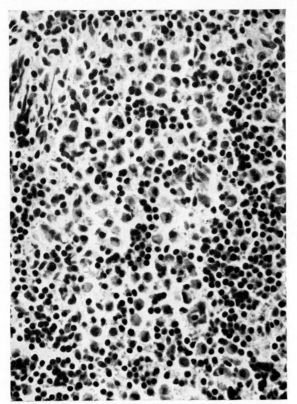

Fig. 9.54. Lymph node from the mesentery of the small intestine in a case of typhoid fever. The occurrence of multiple perforating ulcers in the terminal part of the ileum necessitated resection of part of the bowel; the node illustrated was included in the specimen. The typhoid cells have relatively abundant, pale cytoplasm and a small, darkly stained nucleus. Some of the cells are binucleate. A few have ingested a lymphocyte or other cell. *Haematoxylin–eosin.* × 330.

paratyphi A, *Salmonella paratyphi* B and *Salmonella paratyphi* C). However, there is considerable variation, and any of the paratyphoid organisms may cause very severe and widespread lesions.

Other Salmonella Infections (Salmonella 'Food Poisoning').—Salmonella 'food poisoning'—acute gastroenteritis from infection by salmonellae ingested with food (other than the salmonellae of typhoid and paratyphoid fevers)—is accompanied by regional lymphadenitis in at least some instances, although this can be verified only in those cases that are of such severity that the patient dies of the infection or presents equivocal clinical manifestations that require laparotomy for investigation of the possibility of a serious surgical emergency. In most of the recorded cases in which lymph node

involvement has been described the infecting organism was *Salmonella typhimurium*.[291] The nodes may be a little enlarged but seldom exceed 1·5 cm in their longest dimension. They may be oedematous and hyperaemic. Histologically, there is sinus catarrh, with proliferation of the endothelial macrophages, some of which have ingested red blood cells and lymphocytes. There is often some accumulation in the pulp of the nodes, particularly near the sinuses, of mononuclear cells that closely resemble those that are a characteristic feature of typhoid and paratyphoid lymphadenitis (see above): these cells are not conspicuously numerous in the nodes in cases of salmonella 'food poisoning'. In some cases of salmonella 'food poisoning', including cases in which *Salmonella typhimurium* is isolated in pure culture from abdominal lymph nodes at laparotomy or at necropsy,[292] neutrophils are quite numerous in the nodes, both in the sinuses and throughout the pulp; in other cases this may result from an accompanying infection by other organisms. Focal necrosis is very rarely seen in the nodes in cases of salmonella 'food poisoning'.

Listeria Infection (Listeriosis)[293–295]

Infection by the organism that is known now as *Listeria monocytogenes* was recognized first in 1926, as the cause of a progressive fatal disease in a laboratory colony of rabbits, in Cambridge.[296] A characteristic feature of the disease was the presence of a marked increase in the number of large mononuclear cells (monocytes) in the blood, and the lymph nodes were always enlarged. Later, this organism was identified as the cause of naturally occurring disease in many other types of domesticated and wild animals:[297] in rodents, 'mononucleosis' in the blood is a common accompaniment of the infection; in ruminants, meningitis and encephalitis are frequent and the disease is often of economic importance. In cattle, sheep and goats, transplacental infection leads to death of the fetus or premature birth; the dam usually recovers from the associated metritis but often develops persistent mastitis, excreting the listeriae in the milk for long periods.[298]

The association of monocytosis in the blood of animals infected by *Listeria monocytogenes* and the occasional isolation of this organism in cases of glandular fever (infectious mononucleosis, as it is now called) in man led to the suggestion that the latter is caused by the listeria. Although this is now recognized not usually to be the case (see page 648), the possibility that a disease with closely similar clinical and pathological findings is due to listeria infection cannot be dismissed (see below).

'Opportunistic' Listeria Infection.—In man, listeria infection is probably seen most frequently as an 'opportunistic' infection in patients whose resistance has been lowered by another disease, particularly a lymphoma, and the treatment given for it.[299] The usual manifestations in such cases are septicaemia and meningitis.[300] An increase in the number of large mononuclear cells in the blood is not usually a feature of these 'opportunistic' infections: it is possible that the absence of mononucleosis in these circumstances is due to the fact that in most such cases the predisposing illness has been treated with agents such as cytotoxic drugs, X-rays and corticosteroids, which might inhibit proliferation of these cells.

Listeria Infection in the Fetus.—Fatal septicaemic listeria infection in the fetus causes stillbirth or premature delivery and death early in infancy.[301] This condition, which is sometimes described as *'granulomatosis infantiseptica'*,[302] has been attributed to infection of the mother by drinking raw cow's milk. The mother's symptoms are those of a mild or moderately severe febrile illness, from which she recovers quickly.

Lymphadenitis Accompanying Listeria Infection.— Neither 'opportunistic' nor transplacental infection caused by listeria, nor the apparently milk-borne infection of the mothers of babies with listeria septicaemia, is accompanied by particularly conspicuous involvement of lymph nodes, although in any of these varieties of 'listeriosis' there may be an increase in the number of macrophages in the sinuses and pulp, and small foci of necrosis may develop. In contrast, changes in lymph nodes are a major feature of the clinical and pathological manifestations of two forms of disease that have been attributed to this organism: these will be described now.

Cervical Lymphadenitis without Other Local Lesions. —There is a rare form of infection by *Listeria monocytogenes* that is characterized by rapidly developing enlargement of the nodes on one or both sides of the neck; the nodes suppurate, and there is often sinus formation with the discharge of pus through the skin (see page 638).[283] The listeria can be isolated in cultures from the discharge or from the nodes

before they break down. There is no notable inflammation in the throat or elsewhere. In at least some cases the number of circulating monocytes is increased. In some instances of this cervical form of listeriosis the histological picture (Fig. 9.55) closely resembles that of the necrotizing granulomatous lymphadenitis, with epithelioid histiocytosis, that results from yersinial and similar infections (see page 584).[266]

'Anginose Listeriosis'.—The so-called anginose* or anginoseptic form of infection by *Listeria monocytogenes* is the one that has been confused with

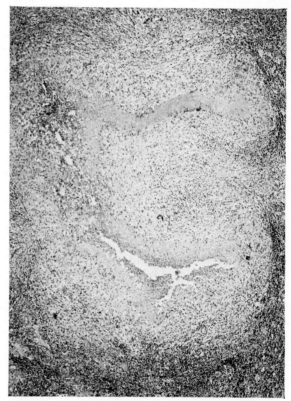

Fig. 9.55. Acute necrotizing cervical lymphadenitis caused by *Listeria monocytogenes*. A confluent epithelioid cell granuloma has undergone central liquefaction. An occasional multinucleate giant cell is seen. The picture is essentially the same as that of lymphogranuloma inguinale, cat-scratch disease and other infections that give rise to this pattern of epithelioid cell granulomatosis with confluence, necrosis and a tendency to form sinuses. See also Figs 9.106 and 9.109 (pages 637 and 640). *Haematoxylin–eosin.* × 35.

* 'Anginose' is used in the sense that relates to ulcerative pharyngitis, which formerly was referred to by the term *angina*, with its implication of suffocation or choking (see footnote on page 991).

infectious mononucleosis (see page 476). It precisely reproduces the clinical picture of infectious mononucleosis, with acute tonsillitis and pharyngitis (sometimes with membrane formation and ulceration), enlargement of the cervical lymph nodes, and a notable increase in the number of monocytes (or cells that are believed to be either abnormal monocytes or abnormal lymphocytes) in the peripheral blood.[303] Like the form of listeriosis that affects only the cervical lymph nodes (see above), it occurs mainly in adults, and oftener in those whose resistance to infection is lowered by conditions that impair cell-mediated immunity. Its histological picture is indistinguishable from that of infectious mononucleosis (see page 650), except in a small proportion of the cases, in which small discrete clusters of epithelioid histiocytes form in the sinuses and in the pulp.

Diagnosis of Listeria Infection.—The diagnosis is best made by isolation of *Listeria monocytogenes*. In cases of the anginose form the organism may be isolated from the cervical lymph nodes[304] and, sometimes, from the blood.[305] It may be noted that *Listeria monocytogenes* has been isolated in some instances of classic infectious mononucleosis,[306] with strongly positive heterophile antibody test (Paul–Bunnell reaction) and antibody absorption by ox erythrocytes and not by guinea-pig kidney, and—in some instances[266]—the appearance during the illness of antibodies to the Epstein–Barr virus. These may be cases of double infection; if so, it is uncertain whether both infections are causally related to the clinical illness.

Complement-fixing antibody and a rising titre of specific agglutinins against *Listeria monocytogenes* can be demonstrated in the serum of patients during the course of infection by this organism. The serological findings must be interpreted with great circumspection and are not alone diagnostic. The absence of demonstrable heterophile antibody (Paul–Bunnell test) in otherwise typical cases of infectious mononucleosis in which there is proven infection by *Listeria monocytogenes*, and particularly if there is a prompt response to antibiotic treatment, should suggest the possibility that the disease is a manifestation of listeria infection. Most authorities regard listeria as, at most, a very rare cause of infectious mononucleosis (or of an infectious-mononucleosis-like illness); some deny it this role. The evidence seems to favour the view that there is more than one aetiological type of infectious mononucleosis (see page 648, *Causation*).

Acute Necrotizing Non-Suppurative Non-Granulomatous Lymphadenitis

There are several aetiological varieties of acute necrotizing infective lymphadenitis in which neither suppuration nor a granulomatous element is part of the histological picture. As it is helpful to distinguish these conditions from the suppurative forms and from the granulomatous forms of acute necrotizing lymphadenitis, they are considered together here.

Anthrax

Lymphadenitis is a common accompaniment of anthrax. Involvement of the nodes draining the initial cutaneous lesion is usual,[307] and generalized lymphadenitis invariably develops in the course of anthrax septicaemia, although it may be evident only microscopically in fulminant cases. In cases of pulmonary anthrax the hilar and other mediastinal nodes are always severely affected.

Except in rapidly fatal cases of septicaemia, nodes that are involved in anthrax are enlarged and they may be greatly so. When the infection is severe, the nodes are dark red and the fluid that exudes from their cut surface resembles blood. The lesion is essentially an acute, necrotizing, haemorrhagic lymphadenitis, the main features of the inflammatory reaction corresponding to those characteristic of anthrax of the skin (see Chapter 39) and elsewhere. Similar changes are found in the tissues round the nodes.

Histology.[308, 308a]—Microscopically, the earlier stages of anthrax lymphadenitis are marked by dilatation of the sinuses, which contain protein-rich fluid, many free macrophages and large numbers of red blood cells, among which the bacilli are often numerous. Later, there is extensive haemorrhagic oedema, with widespread precipitation of fibrin, thrombosis of blood vessels and considerable destruction of the lymphoid tissue. The lymphoid follicles that remain often show central necrosis, and such foci may be infiltrated by neutrophils: apart from these lesions, neutrophils are not conspicuous in the reaction to infection by anthrax bacilli and generally they are said to be no more numerous in the haemorrhagic inflammatory exudate than in the circulating blood.

The causative organisms may be present in great numbers in the affected nodes (Fig. 9.56). Their characteristic appearance, and their arrangement in chains and—when they are abundant—in sweeping

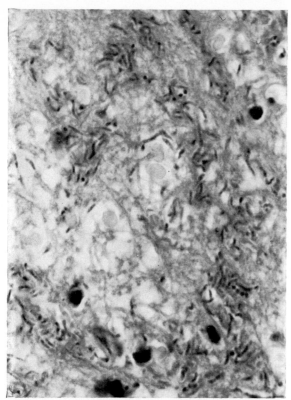

Fig. 9.56. Anthrax lymphadenitis. This field, from the subcapsular region of a cervical lymph node draining the site of a cutaneous lesion on the face, shows complete necrosis of the tissues, with haemorrhagic oedema and large numbers of anthrax bacilli. The disease had progressed to the stage of septicaemia and the patient died of rupture of the infected spleen (see Fig. 9.169, page 735). *Haematoxylin–eosin.* × 850.

fascicles, should make them readily identifiable, even in haematoxylin–eosin preparations; nevertheless, they are surprisingly often mistaken for threads of fibrin. It may be noted that the bacilli rapidly cease to be Gram-positive and begin to disintegrate when drugs to which they are sensitive have been used in treatment: such bacilli may escape recognition, both in the initial lesion—for instance, in the skin— and in lesions elsewhere in the body (see Chapter 39, Figs 39.167C and 39.167D).

Post-Mortem Diagnosis.—The autolytic changes that ordinarily take place in the body after death, and effects of saprophytic and other micro-organisms, are so inimical to *Bacillus anthracis* that it is itself rapidly destroyed after the patient's death. This demands that specimens for culture, films for staining and tissue for histological examination must be obtained as soon as possible: delay may make it impossible to prove the diagnosis of anthrax.

Pathogenesis of Anthrax.—In most cases of anthrax in man the infection starts in the skin (see Chapter 39); pulmonary anthrax (see page 321) has always been much rarer, and anthrax primarily involving the alimentary tract is exceptionally infrequent. In animals, in contrast, infection by the alimentary route, whether through the pharynx or, likelier, through the small intestine, is usual; pulmonary infection is much less frequent, and infection through the skin is a rarity. It is now known that as anthrax sets in, in animals, the bacilli spread from the portal of entry into the body by way of the lymph, causing lymphadenitis that develops successively in the groups of nodes that are situated along the lymphatic pathway between the portal and the inflow of the main lymph ducts into the great veins.[309] The same sequence may be recognized in at least some cases of anthrax in man: for instance, in the case of a microbiologist who accidentally inoculated the little finger of one hand with a pure culture of *Bacillus anthracis*, the resulting lesion in the skin was accompanied by massive haemorrhagic lymphadenitis of the supratrochlear node, marked but less severe haemorrhagic lymphadenitis of the lateral group of axillary nodes of the same side, and less marked—but still conspicuous—haemorrhagic lymphadenitis of the apical group of axillary nodes and of a few of the lower deep cervical nodes, again of the same side; the corresponding lymph nodes of the other side of the body, like the nodes elsewhere, showed a comparatively minor, and quite uniform, degree of lymphadenitis.[310] Such findings may be interpreted as marking the course of the infection from the site of inoculation by way of the lymphatics and lymph nodes to the blood; the resulting septicaemia, and phagocytosis of the circulating bacilli by reticuloendothelial cells, would account for the uniform, generalized involvement of the lymph nodes elsewhere than along the initial path of the infection.

It is possible that the haemorrhagic necrosis that is so characteristic of the lesions of anthrax is due to the action of a toxin produced by the bacilli. The remarkable intensity of the haemorrhagic oedematous reaction in the infected tissues suggests the occurrence of an acute local intoxication affecting the vasculature. Toxin extracted from cultures of *Bacillus anthracis* produces oedema by increasing vascular permeability[311] and causes thrombosis in capillary blood vessels.[312] Its significance in the pathogenesis of the naturally occurring disease is controversial.

Diphtheria[313]

In many cases of diphtheria the lymphadenitis in the region draining the infection is apparently no more than a simple acute inflammation without specific features. However, when the disease is severe, and caused by a highly toxigenic strain of *Corynebacterium diphtheriae*, massive lymph node enlargement is characteristically one of the striking clinical effects. This severe lymphadenitis results from the action of diphtheria toxin.[314] The toxin is absorbed from the site of infection, usually in the throat, and carried in the lymph to the regional nodes: it is very unusual for the corynebacterium itself to enter the tissues and reach the nodes, and most authorities deny that this ever occurs. In exceptional cases, other organisms, particularly *Streptococcus pyogenes*, may be isolated from the affected nodes in cases of proven diphtheria: these are cases of severe diphtheria, with extensive changes in the nodes as a result of the effects of diphtheria toxin, and these changes completely obscure any effects that may be caused by the streptococcal infection.

The enlarged lymph nodes of severe diphtheria are haemorrhagic and necrotic. There is much hyperaemia and oedema of the surrounding tissues, and both here and in the lymph nodes themselves there are conspicuous foci of fibrin precipitation. The necrotic areas of the nodes are partly firm and opaque and partly diffluent. In most cases the lymphadenitis involves the cervical nodes on both sides and, as a consequence of the extension of the mucosal infection into the trachea, the paratracheal and sometimes the tracheobronchial nodes.

Histology.—The nodes are markedly hyperaemic and there is thrombosis in many of the small arteries and veins. Fibrinoid necrosis of the arteries may be a feature.[315] Oedema, with characteristically extensive formation of threads and clumps of fibrin in the fluid exudate, and multifocal or massive haemorrhage are typical of the severely affected nodes, and there is widespread necrosis (Fig. 9.57). Necrosis may be centred on sinuses, extending into the adjoining pulp, and is often noticeably more marked in the regions where the afferent lymphatics enter the node through the capsule over its convexity. There is often necrosis in the lymphoid follicles also, associated with thrombosis of the related blood vessels and permeation of the interstices by fibrin

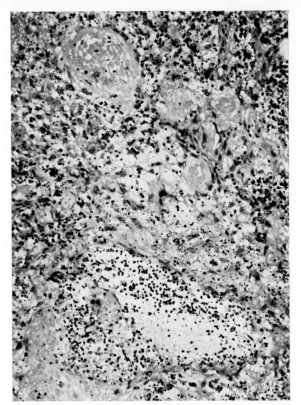

Fig. 9.57. Lymph node in diphtheria. There is acute necrosis, with oedema, precipitation of fibrin and much nuclear debris. Such changes accompanying diphtheria are the result of carriage of the toxin to the nodes in the lymph draining the site of infection. *Haematoxylin–eosin.* × 140.

deposits. Comparable focal necrosis may be seen in lymphoid follicles in lymph nodes throughout the body and in other lymphoid tissues, and is presumed to result from a direct action of toxin that has gained access to the general blood circulation. The severe oedema, widespread precipitation of fibrin, and haemorrhages, and the necrosis centred on the sinuses, are not seen in nodes other than those directly draining the site of the infection.

While the changes described are those ordinarily associated with infection of the throat by virulent, toxigenic strains of *Corynebacterium diphtheriae*, comparable but less severe changes may be seen in the regional lymph nodes in cases of infection of the skin. The cutaneous lesions, which usually are solitary, are caused by toxigenic strains, usually of *Corynebacterium diphtheriae mitis*. The observation of foci of necrosis in the follicles, with conspicuous formation of fibrin in their vicinity and in the dilated sinuses, on examination of an enlarged regional lymph node was the clue to the diphtherial nature of a persistent cutaneous ulcer in a student from North Africa who was working in Britain.[310]

As mentioned, the changes in the lymph nodes in diphtheria result from the action of the toxin produced by *Corynebacterium diphtheriae* at the site of infection in the throat or elsewhere, the organism itself not entering the tissues. In other words, the lymphadenitis of diphtheria is a manifestation not of infection of the nodes but of their intoxication. Other species of corynebacterium, in contrast, are occasional causes of true infective lymphadenitis (*Corynebacterium ulcerans* and *Corynebacterium ovis*, for instance): the histological picture is that of a chronic tuberculoid granulomatous lymphadenitis, and the condition is considered under this heading on page 610.

Plague

Lymphadenitis is a cardinal manifestation of infection by *Yersinia pestis* (*Pasteurella pestis*). It is the lesion that presents as the bubo, the characteristic enlargement of the nodes in the inguinal region of the side on which the flea bite, the source of the patient's infection, occurred. The bubo is the feature that gave the disease the name *bubonic plague*. In about a third of the cases of plague that present with enlargement of a group of lymph nodes the lymphadenitis is axillary or cervical; strictly speaking, swellings elsewhere than in the groin should not be called buboes, but it is convenient to accept this usage of the term. In a small proportion of cases the nodes in both groins, or those in both armpits, are enlarged. In many cases it is demonstrable that there is similar enlargement of the deeper nodes that drain those first involved: for instance, the iliac nodes are often palpably enlarged in association with a bubo in the inguinal region of the same side.

In classic cases the bubo forms a mass from 4 to 8 cm across. In the so-called abortive or ambulatory cases ('*pestis minor*'), which are a feature of all outbreaks of plague, the affected nodes are usually much less enlarged.

In *septicaemic plague*, lymphadenitis is generalized, but the nodes are usually only a little enlarged. In cases of *pneumonic plague* (see page 321), massive involvement of the mediastinal lymph nodes is the rule.

Histology.[316]—In the earliest stages of the infection there is dilatation of the sinuses and a notable proliferation of the endothelial macrophages. The cells are vacuolate and may contain red blood cells and neutrophils as well as yersiniae. The organisms spread rapidly throughout the substance of the node; many are ingested by macrophages and many more lie free, sometimes forming substantial collections. They are Gram-negative and difficult to see in Gram preparations. With care, they can be identified in haematoxylin–eosin preparations, but ordinarily it is desirable to stain sections with Giemsa's solution, which shows them admirably (Fig. 9.58).

Widespread necrosis develops in the nodes and there is often much bleeding into the necrotic tissue. The necrotic material contains great numbers of the organisms, many of which—evidently dead—appear red instead of blue in Giemsa preparations. It is uncertain whether the death of the tissue is due to

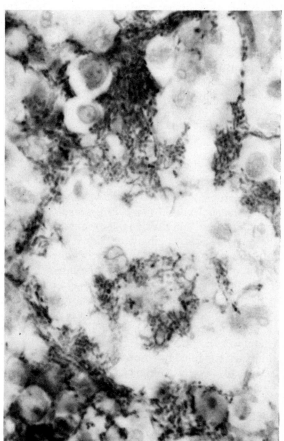

Fig. 9.58.§ Lymphadenitis of plague (bubonic plague). *Yersinia pestis* is present in great numbers between the cells and in the cytoplasm of macrophages, occupying even the cytoplasmic processes of the latter as they link with neighbouring cells in the sinus and adjoining pulp. A large part of the infected node was destroyed by necrosis. Neutrophils were frequent in the necrotic areas, although in general they showed less phagocytic activity toward the bacilli than the macrophages. *Giemsa.* ×1200.

F

ischaemia resulting from thrombosis of the blood vessels, which is often a conspicuous feature, or to the release of endotoxins from the dying organisms. The reticulin framework of the nodes persists in the necrotic zones except in those cases in which neutrophils accumulate and suppuration sets in.

There is inflammatory oedema and haemorrhage in the tissues round the affected lymph nodes, often with obvious necrosis. The cellular infiltrate in these tissues may consist mainly of macrophages with a small proportion of neutrophils, but the latter become preponderant in those cases in which suppuration develops. Even when the lymphadenitis is left to take its course, the necrosis spreading to the skin and a sinus or sinuses forming, suppuration is often lacking, and its presence may indicate secondary infection by pyogenic organisms. Once the bubo has formed, it is unlikely to be absorbed, however well the general condition responds to tetracycline or other appropriate treatment: if its contents are not aspirated the probability is that it will point through the skin. Eventual recovery tends to be complicated by the development of lymphoedema—for instance, of the related limb or of the genitalia—as a result of fibrosis round the nodes.

Vincent's Infection ('Fusoborreliosis'; 'Fusospirochaetosis')

The anaerobic symbionts—*Fusobacterium fusiforme* and *Borrelia vincentii* (*Treponema vincentii*)—that together cause Vincent's angina (see page 991) and the acute ulcerative gingivitis known as Vincent's infection (see page 981) occasionally spread to the lymph nodes draining the site of the initial lesions. The commonest source of this form of lymphadenitis is the throat (Vincent's angina); occasionally it is a complication of infection of the lungs (see page 313) or bronchi (see page 311), or of the genitalia (see Chapter 26). Vincent's gingivitis, although sometimes accompanied by a non-specific lymphadenitis, is notably rarely complicated by extension to lymph nodes of infection by the organisms responsible for the condition of the gums.

The infected lymph nodes are enlarged and tense. There is often very extensive necrosis, and the necrotic matter has the characteristically offensive smell associated with infection by these organisms. The organisms are easily demonstrated in films of the exudate from the nodes but are often surprisingly difficult to demonstrate in histological sections. Neutrophils may be numerous in the infected nodes, but usually there seems to be remarkably little cellular reaction.

Necrotizing Lymphadenitis in the Primary Stage of Syphilis

In the usual form of lymphadenitis in the primary stage of syphilis there is well-marked follicular hyperplasia, with conspicuous germinal centres, an abundant accumulation of plasma cells throughout the pulp, and occasional or numerous small clusters of epithelioid histiocytes, with or without the formation of multinucleate giant cells (see page 612). Fibrosing endarteritis and periarteritis, and corresponding changes in the veins, are present. The capsule and trabeculae show fibrous thickening. Perilymphadenitis is also found, and plasma cells and lymphocytes are present in variable numbers between the connective tissue fibres. Necrosis is not usually a feature, and when it is present it often results from infection by other organisms. However, there are exceptional cases in which the lymph nodes draining the site of a primary chancre, usually on the external genitalia, enlarge rapidly and undergo acute necrosis, without frank suppuration and without granuloma formation. The explanation of this occurrence is uncertain. The angitis that is always a feature of the lymphadenitis of the primary stage of the infection is uncommonly marked in at least some of these cases, and thrombosis is sometimes present. There is no evidence that the strain of *Treponema pallidum* causing the infection in these patients is exceptionally virulent or otherwise peculiar. In one case the patient had been treated for proven, serologically negative primary syphilis 5 years before again developing a chancre; no unusual lymph node changes had been noted clinically during her first infection and there was nothing unusual about the course of the chancre during the second infection, only the severity of the accompanying lymphadenitis being remarkable.

The occurrence of necrotizing regional lymphadenitis at the height of the development of the primary chancre is said to be commoner among people in communities that have not previously been exposed to syphilis. It is said to have occurred in parts of Africa and Polynesia and Micronesia during the world wars, when syphilis was introduced from countries where the disease had been endemic for centuries. However, the same destructive lymphadenitis may be seen in the indigenous population of sophisticated lands, although without the tendency to develop into a very severe, sometimes fatal, illness, as is said to have been observed in populations experiencing their introduction to syphilis.

In some cases the necrotizing lymphadenitis extends to involve the nodes draining the group that is primarily affected. When the iliac nodes are thus affected acute abdominal symptoms may result from involvement of the overlying peritoneum in the perilymphadenitis.[310]

Histology.—Apart from the presence of the treponemes, which can be shown only by the use of special techniques, there is nothing specific about the histological picture of this form of necrotizing syphilitic lymphadenitis. The usual appearances of the nodes in the primary stage of the infection (see above) are overlaid by extensive necrosis. The necrotic tissue is infiltrated by neutrophils and epithelioid histiocytes; there is neither frank suppuration nor any organization of the epithelioid cells into granulomatous foci (Fig. 9.59A). The changes in the blood vessels are mentioned above; their

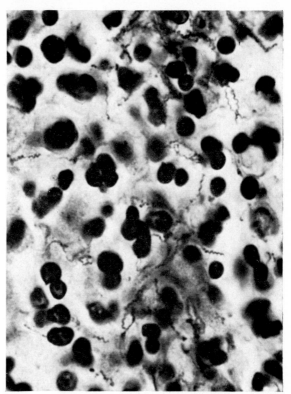

Fig. 9.59B. Same specimen as Fig. 9.59A, impregnated with silver to demonstrate the large number of treponemes among the inflammatory cells. The organisms were most abundant at the margins of the necrotic areas. *Warthin–Starry.* × 1500.

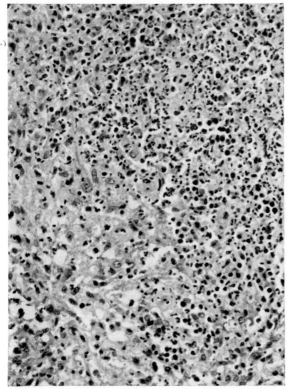

Fig. 9.59A. Acute necrotizing inguinal lymphadenitis in the primary stage of syphilis. Neutrophils predominate among the inflammatory cells. There are many plasma cells in the necrotic area (above and right); epithelioid histiocytes are more conspicuous in the rest of the field. This is an uncommonly severe and destructive lymphadenitis, in contrast to the typical lymphadenitis of this stage of syphilis (see Figs 9.83 and 9.84, page 613): such destructive inflammation in these circumstances is ordinarily due to an accompanying infection by *Haemophilus ducreyi* (the cause of chancroid, or soft sore) or by pyogenic bacteria, but none of these was found in this case. See Fig. 9.59B. *Haematoxylin–eosin.* × 170.

significance in the pathogenesis of the necrosis is uncertain. In some instances it is clearly evident that the necrosis has started in the sinuses and spread thence into the pulp of the nodes, without any topographical relation to the blood vessels.

Great numbers of treponemes can be demonstrated in silvered preparations (Fig. 9.59B).

Differential Diagnosis.—A necrotizing syphilitic bubo should be distinguishable from other swellings in the groins by the presence of a well-established primary chancre. If the latter escapes observation, usually through neglect to examine the patient sufficiently thoroughly, the clinical manifestations of the lymphadenitis may be misinterpreted: the condition has been taken for a strangulated hernia[310] and, as in a recent embarrassing instance, for bubonic plague (see page 581). In every case in which the diagnosis of acute necrotizing syphilitic lymphadenitis is considered, it is essential to investigate the possibility that there is a dual or even multiple infection: among the other infections that might be present are gonococcal lymphadenitis (see page 573), the lymphadenitis of chancroid (see page 573) and that of lymphogranuloma inguinale (see page 635).

Acute Necrotizing Granulomatous Lymphadenitis

While granulomatous conditions are classed, almost by definition, as chronic diseases, there are some cases in which the clinical onset and development are so rapid that the description 'acute' is valid. Acute necrotizing granulomatous lymphadenitis is a term applicable to a number of bacterial diseases, among them the rare acute form of tuberculous lymphadenitis (see page 599), some instances of listeria infection (see page 577), glanders (see page 595), melioidosis (see page 595), some cases of yersinial mesenteric lymphadenitis, and tularaemia. Only the last two of these will be considered in this section. Before doing so, it may be noted that, with the exception of the acute tuberculous infection, a clear histological distinction cannot be drawn between these conditions and the clinically acute, subacute and chronic forms of the variety of granulomatous lymphadenitis that is typified by the lymphadenitis of lymphogranuloma inguinale (see page 636). While lymphogranuloma inguinale itself, as a chlamydial infection, is outside the scope of this account of bacterial lymphadenitis, it must not be forgotten that there are bacterial infections that cause pathological changes in lymph nodes that are indistinguishable from those that it causes. This histological type of lymphadenitis is described in more detail elsewhere (see page 636): characteristically, there is extensive replacement of the normal structure of affected nodes by confluent epithelioid cell granulomas enclosing large foci of necrosis that is part caseous or colliquative and part suppurative. The nodes tend to break down and discharge through the skin. According to the rate of its evolution, such a lymphadenitis is liable to be mistaken clinically for acute suppurative lymphadenitis or for tuberculous lymphadenitis.

Yersinial Mesenteric Lymphadenitis (Pseudotuberculous Mesenteric Lymphadenitis; Masshoff's Disease[317])*

It has already been noted that the clinical syndrome of acute mesenteric lymphadenitis has a number of known causes (see page 574). In most cases the condition is either due to yersinial infection or has no recognized cause. Some of the yersinial cases

* Yersinial mesenteric lymphadenitis is sometimes known as 'abscessing reticulocytic lymphadenitis', which is a literal but insensate translation of *abscedierende reticulocytäre*

present a characteristic, but not pathognomonic, histological picture; the cases without recognized cause present the simple, non-granulomatous reaction, without necrosis, that is referred to as acute non-specific mesenteric lymphadenitis (see page 574).

In some cases it is not possible to distinguish the histological changes in mesenteric nodes that are infected by yersiniae[318] from those of certain other infections of lymph nodes, typified in lymphogranuloma inguinale (see page 636) (Fig. 9.60). In

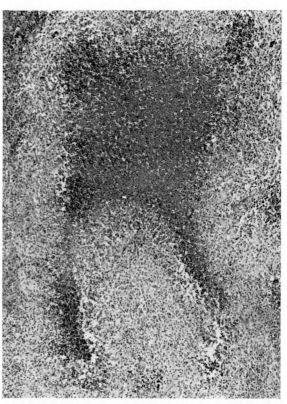

Fig. 9.60. Yersinial mesenteric lymphadenitis. Extensive epithelioid cell granulomatous reaction with central necrosis. The necrotic material is uniformly but rather lightly infiltrated by neutrophils, accounting for the stippled appearance of the dark core of the lesion. The picture does not differ significantly from that of the listerial lymphadenitis illustrated in Fig. 9.55 (page 577) or from the lymphadenitis of established lymphogranuloma inguinale (Fig. 9.106, page 637) and cat-scratch disease (Fig. 9.109, page 640). Compare with the example of yersinial lymphadenitis illustrated in Figs 9.61A and 9.61B. *Haematoxylin–eosin.* × 40.

Lymphadenitis, the name given to the condition in an early study (Masshoff, W., Dölle, W., *Virchows Arch. path. Anat.*, 1953, **323**, 664). The German is less inelegant than the English version and lacks the ambiguity of 'reticulocytic', which in this context, of course, relates not to reticulocytes but to reticulum cells (see footnote on page 525).

other cases the picture is identical with that described on page 574 as characteristic of acute non-specific mesenteric lymphadenitis (Figs 9.61A and 9.61B). The specific identity of the yersinia responsible is the subject of controversy: the present view seems to be that the organism concerned is usually *Yersinia enterocolitica*[286] and that this organism was responsible for many—but not all—of the cases in the past in which the isolates were thought to be *Yersinia pseudotuberculosis* (*Pasteurella pseudotuberculosis*).[287]

The clinical picture of yersinial mesenteric lymphadenitis is entirely comparable to that of

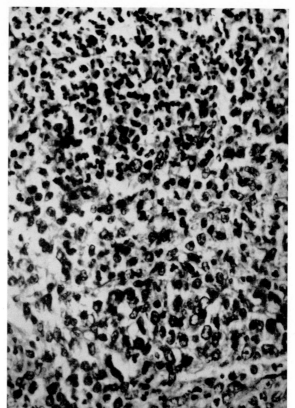

Fig. 9.61B. Higher magnification of the area of Fig. 9.61A that is enclosed in the rectangle. Neutrophils predominate in the upper half of the field; histiocytes are more abundant in the lower half, where there is also an admixture of lymphocytes. *Haematoxylin–eosin.* × 345.

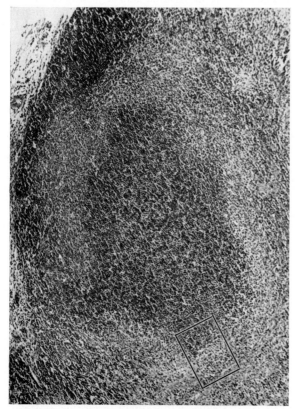

Fig. 9.61A. Yersinial mesenteric lymphadenitis. In this instance, when compared with Fig. 9.60, there is less extensive destruction of the node, the epithelioid cell response is less marked (and is more obscured by the infiltration of neutrophils), and the participation of neutrophils in the reaction is predominant. The same type of picture may be seen in cases of acute mesenteric lymphadenitis in which no causative organism can be identified (see page 574): in the case illustrated here, the organism isolated from the biopsy specimen was identified by culture and serological examination as *Pasteurella pseudotuberculosis* (now *Yersinia pseudotuberculosis*), but may have been *Yersinia enterocolitica*, which at that time was not clearly distinguished from the species named. The area of the field that is enclosed in the rectangle is shown in Fig. 9.61B. *Haematoxylin–eosin.* × 55.

acute non-specific mesenteric lymphadenitis, irrespective of the species of yersinia responsible. Laparotomy may show changes in the terminal ileum, exactly as in the non-specific cases (see page 574). As in the latter, the appendix is normal macroscopically, but histological examination is said to show occasional small clusters of cells that may be epithelioid histiocytes or 'immunoblasts' (transformed lymphocytes). These clusters occur in the mucous membrane and submucosa; those near the lumen may ulcerate although elsewhere necrosis is not a feature.[319] Eosinophils may accumulate in the vicinity of the cell clusters. These histological changes, which obviously are of the same nature as those in the lymph nodes, but less extensive and lacking the characteristic pattern of necrosis, are found in only a small proportion of cases; their demonstration may require a search of sections cut at several levels in each block of tissue from the base to the tip of the organ.

Prognosis.—Yersinia infection of the mesenteric lymph nodes, whether or not there is evident involvement of the ileum and appendix, ordinarily runs a benign course. Paralytic ileus caused death in one case.[320] Fatal yersinial peritonitis resulted from spontaneous rupture of massive involved nodes in the case of a child under treatment with actinomycin D (dactinomycin) and X-rays for nephroblastoma;[321] it is possible that the treatment had lowered resistance to the organism. In another case, death resulted from intestinal obstruction caused by adhesions at the site of the fibrotic remnants of mesenteric lymph nodes that had been shown histologically and bacteriologically to be infected with a yersinia at the time of the acute illness three years earlier.[322]

Relation of Yersinial and Acute Non-Specific Mesenteric Lymphadenitis.—The most striking feature that is common to the two main aetiological forms of acute mesenteric lymphadenitis (see page 574) is the occasional involvement of the terminal part of the ileum. Although the scanty information available seems to indicate that the histological changes in the terminal ileum, and in the appendix, differ between the non-specific cases and the yersinial cases in the presence in the latter of clusters of 'reticulum cells' or epithelioid histiocytes, the data are insufficient to justify an assumption that the two forms of lymphadenitis are distinct diseases. It is equally impossible to interpret the evidence as either supporting or disproving the concept that the seemingly non-specific cases are a histologically uncharacteristic manifestation of yersinial infection. The fact that several other types of infection may cause this syndrome (see above) rather supports the view that the non-specific cases are aetiologically unrelated to those due to infection by a yersinia.

Tularaemia

Tularaemia, caused by *Francisella tularensis*, a pasteurella-like organism, and first described as a plague-like disease of ground squirrels in Tulare County, in California, in 1911,[323, 324] was long thought to occur only in North America, where rabbits, hares and ground squirrels are the most frequently affected among the considerable range of animals in which the disease is known to occur naturally.[325] The first case to be diagnosed in man was recorded in 1914.[326] Since then, many thousands of human cases have been recognized. The disease has been seen with the greatest frequency in the United States of America and in the Soviet Union,

but occurs also in most other parts of North America and Europe,[327] and in Asia Minor and Japan. It was very prevalent among troops in eastern Europe during the second world war;[328] occasional cases were seen among German prisoners of war in camps in North Africa and in Britain,[329] the patients being men who had acquired the infection on the eastern fronts before transfer to other theatres of the war.

Indigenous cases in the British Isles appear to be exceptionally rare. A fatal case in Northern Ireland, in 1941, followed a bite by a tick (*Ixodes ricinus*).[330] Another patient, recently arrived in England from County Clare, in Ireland, had a history of being scratched by a cat and presented with a regional lymphadenitis that was considered to be typical, histologically, of cat-scratch disease:[331] the Frei test (lymphogranuloma inguinale antigen) and the corresponding skin test with antigen from known cases of cat-scratch fever were negative; an organism identified at the time as *Pasteurella tularensis* (that is, *Francisella tularensis*) was isolated in pure culture from the necrotic lymph nodes, and the patient's serum agglutinated *Francisella tularensis* at a titre of 1 in 5120 and *Brucella abortus* at a titre of 1 in 2560 (antibodies to these two organisms are known to give cross-reactions). In a recent case, diagnosed in England, the patient's infection was acquired while on the European mainland (Fig. 9.62).[332]

In peacetime, tularaemia is most frequently an occupational or domestic disease among people who come in contact with rodents or with dust or articles that have been contaminated by these animals or their excreta. In Europe, the rodent reservoir of the infection is most frequently a hare or a vole.[333] Farmers, fur ranchers, trappers and butchers are among those particularly at risk. The disease is also very readily acquired in laboratories where the organism is present in cultures or in inoculated animals.[334] During the second world war, soldiers on the eastern fronts were thought to become infected mainly from contaminated soil of dug-out shelters or of land harried by bombardment or the passage of tanks.

Francisella tularensis is commonly borne by ticks, such as the wood tick (*Dermacentor andersoni*) in North America, and by other arthropods, including biting flies, such as the American deer-fly (*Chrysops discalis*), the stable fly (*Stomoxys calcitrans*), and various mosquitoes and the bedbug (*Cimex lectularius*). It can also pass through intact or abraded skin. Infection can take place through the conjunctiva and by ingestion and inhalation of

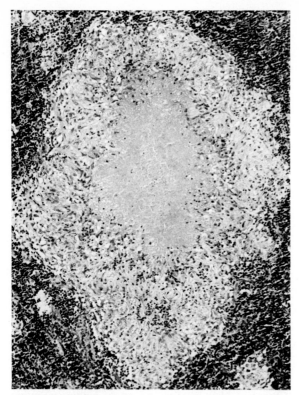

Fig. 9.62.§ Lymphadenitis of tularaemia. There is nothing about this lesion that distinguishes it from a tuberculous granuloma or from the lesions of any of the wide variety of conditions that may be characterized by the development of this type of necrotizing tuberculoid reaction. The diagnosis of tularaemia in this case was confirmed bacteriologically. The infection was acquired on the European mainland but the patient's illness developed while he was in England (Reference 332 on page 869). *Haematoxylin–eosin.* × 85.

infected material. The organism was assigned successively to the genera *Pasteurella*, *Brucella* and *Yersinia* before the genus *Francisella* was defined to accommodate it. The disease itself has various synonyms, among them deer-fly fever, Pahvant Valley fever (after the region in Utah where some of the first infections recognized in man were contracted), rabbit fever and pseudoplague of rodents. It is sometimes known in Scandinavia as lemming fever: this condition, long known in rural communities at the time of migration of the lemmings,[335] has been attributed, in Norway, to contamination of water by lemmings infected with tularaemia[336] and, in Swedish Lapland, to mosquito-borne infection from lemmings.[337] In Japan, the infection is sometimes known as Ohara's disease, after the doctor who first recognized its occurrence there.[338]

Tularaemia has several forms of clinical presentation. Lymphadenitis is an essential feature of most cases. Subclinical infection is common in areas where the disease is prevalent: it is said that more than 20 per cent of the population of parts of Sweden show serological evidence of past infection, and that a third of these people have had no overt illness attributable to the infection.[339] At the other clinical extreme are the comparatively very rare acute septicaemic and pneumonic forms that, in the absence of effective antibiotic treatment, have a high mortality. The great majority of cases fall into the categories of cutaneous tularaemia and ocular tularaemia.

Cutaneous Tularaemia ('Ulceroglandular Tularaemia').—Infection of the skin, whether by the bite of an infected insect or by contact with infective material, is followed within a few days by the development of a papule that soon becomes necrotic and ulcerates.[340] This lesion, which most frequently is on a hand, may be evanescent or it may persist for weeks; healing is accompanied by scarring. The patient is often quite ill during the initial stage of the disease. The lymph nodes draining the site of the subcutaneous lesion become painful and enlarged within a week to a month of the onset of the infection; they eventually break down and discharge through the skin, and healing may not be complete for many months.

Ocular Tularaemia ('Oculoglandular Tularaemia'). —The organism may enter one or both conjunctival sacs, setting up an acute conjunctivitis that rapidly progresses to superficial ulceration, usually affecting only the inner aspect of the eyelids but occasionally involving the bulbar conjunctiva. The infection spreads to the superficial and deep parotid lymph nodes on the same side, the submandibular nodes and sometimes the deep cervical nodes: the affected nodes enlarge, soften and eventually discharge, multiple sinuses occasionally resulting.

Oral and Abdominal Tularaemia.—Very rarely, and perhaps as the result of eating raw or undercooked meat from animals that were infected, the initial lesions are in the mucous membrane of the mouth or throat[341] and possibly of the small intestine. Regional lymphadenitis develops, as in the cutaneous and ocular forms, and peritonitis has been known to occur as a complication of necrosis of the mesenteric nodes.

Histology.[342]—The lymphadenitis of tularaemia is characterized by an epithelioid cell granulomatous reaction, often with extensive necrosis (Fig. 9.62).

The epithelioid cells may be arranged in a palisade-like fashion where they abut on the necrotic core of the granulomatous mass. Multinucleate giant cells of Langhans type are present in many instances. The necrotic material is liquefactive rather than caseous, and may contain the more or less identifiable remnants of cells, particulate nuclear debris and occasional well-preserved neutrophils and free histiocytes. The picture is comparable to that of lymphogranuloma inguinale (see page 636), yersinial lymphadenitis (see page 584) and the other members of the group of aetiologically heterogeneous infections that produce this pattern of necrotizing epithelioid histiocytosis. The earliest lesions may consist of clusters of epithelioid cells, without necrosis, tularaemia at this stage being one of the many conditions that more or less closely reproduce the histological picture of toxoplasmic lymphadenitis.

Tularaemia cannot be shown to be present by histological examination alone: bacteriological and serological confirmation is mandatory.

Generalized Lesions in Tularaemia.—In fatal cases of tularaemia it is usual to find necrotic epithelioid histiocytic granulomas of miliary size throughout the viscera, including the lymph nodes.[343, 344] The finding of such lesions in biopsy specimens from severely ill patients should suggest the possibility of tularaemia, among the many other possible causes; in cases in which tularaemia has been responsible, treatment with streptomycin or other appropriate antibiotics has been life-saving.

Subacute and Chronic Bacterial Lymphadenitis

Many types of lymphadenitis develop insidiously and run a chronic course. In other cases, chronic lymphadenitis is the outcome of acute lymphadenitis, and almost any variety of the latter may become chronic. Sometimes the onset, while not frankly acute, is characterized by quite rapid lymph node enlargement, possibly with considerable local discomfort or pain, and it is appropriate to describe the condition as subacute. Several of the diseases of lymph nodes that are described in the preceding section of this chapter may fit in such a category.

The histological picture of chronic lymphadenitis is often lacking in features that give a clue to its causation. Alternatively, there may be changes—a a tuberculoid reaction, for instance—that indicate a certain range of possible causes. However, precise identification of the cause of chronic lymphadenitis in a particular case is seldom possible by histological examination alone: other investigations—clinical, microbiological and immunological—are often necessary, and in a proportion of cases these also fail to explain the condition, which then usually resolves undiagnosed.

It is a maxim of diagnostic histology that the only truly specific histological pictures associated with infections are those in which the causative micro-organism can be seen and morphologically identified with certainty. This is the case, for example, with some fungal infections, such as cryptococcosis, and in those cases of syphilis in which *Treponema pallidum* can be demonstrated unequivocally. It is not always realized how few of the micro-organisms that can be demonstrated in tissue sections can be identified with absolute certainty on the grounds only of their morphology and staining reactions—even such organisms as mycobacteria and actinomycetes can be identified specifically only by culture and a range of other means, including careful appraisal in the light of the clinical picture. As lymph nodes are commonly involved in infections, the maxim cited has particular relevance to the problems of lymph node biopsy interpretation.

Chronic Non-Specific Lymphadenitis (Simple Chronic Lymphadenitis)

Chronic lymphadenitis without specific histological features may be seen in any group of lymph nodes, the site depending on local causal factors. These factors include chronic infections of the skin, repeated cuts and abrasions, chronic tracheobronchitis, chronic tonsillitis, dental sepsis, and so on. The affected nodes are generally only moderately enlarged, but they are firmer than usual and therefore often readily palpable. Microscopically, their capsule and trabeculae are thickened by fibrosis, and there is an increase in collagenous fibres in the medulla as a result of transformation of some of the reticulin. The small blood vessels are unusually conspicuous (Fig. 9.63), owing to thickening of their walls and enlargement of the endothelial cells (Fig. 9.64). Sinus catarrh and follicular hyperplasia (see pages 559 and 533) are commonly found; their relative extent varies from case to case.

Scleroma (Rhinoscleroma)

Enlargement of lymph nodes in the neck develops in a proportion of cases of scleroma, as an accompaniment of the infection in the nose and other parts of the upper respiratory tract (see page 204). The

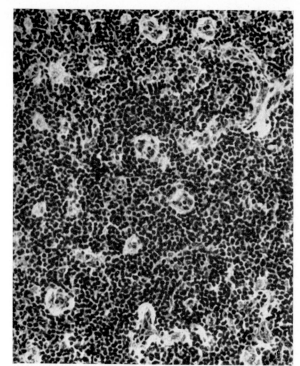

Fig. 9.63. Chronic non-specific lymphadenitis. Conspicuous thickening of small blood vessels throughout the field, due to an increase in the fibrous tissue of their wall and hypertrophy of the endothelial cells. Most of the vessels illustrated are cut across their length, and it is known for such a picture to be mistaken for the focal epithelioid cell granulomatosis of early sarcoidosis, toxoplasmosis and the like, or for early lesions of Hodgkin's disease. The true nature of the change is immediately evident when the section is examined at a higher magnification, and when attention is paid to the appearance of those vessels that are cut lengthwise (see upper right of the photograph). *Haematoxylin–eosin.* × 170.

enlargement was clinically apparent in only 3 of 11 patients with the disease whom I saw in southern Africa. In one of these three patients the lymphadenopathy was the presenting manifestation and the diagnosis was made on histological examination of one of the enlarged nodes (Figs 9.65A and 9.65B). The picture in this node was identical with that in lymph nodes from three other patients with the disease, seen in Europe. A general account of the disease is given in the chapter on the nose and nasal sinuses in Volume 1 (page 204). Only the histology of the involved lymph nodes will be considered here.

Scleromatous Lymphadenitis.—It may be mentioned at once that the term 'scleromatous lymphadenitis' has been applied, regrettably, to the changes in lymph nodes that are found in occasional cases of

systemic sclerosis (see page 693). The latter is a disease of the connective tissues and has nothing in common with scleroma, which is an infection, caused by *Klebsiella rhinoscleromatis.*

There are two main pathological features. First, the sinuses are dilated and contain numerous plasma cells and free-lying, finely vacuolate macrophages, many of which have ingested lymphocytes or red blood cells. Klebsiellae are found with difficulty in this situation, and only in some instances. Second, there is a heavy accumulation of plasma cells throughout the pulp of the node, with many Russell bodies; more important, there are more or less numerous macrophages among the plasma cells, and klebsiellae are readily seen in a substantial proportion of these characteristically large and vacuolate cells (Figs 9.65A and 9.65B). The changes in the

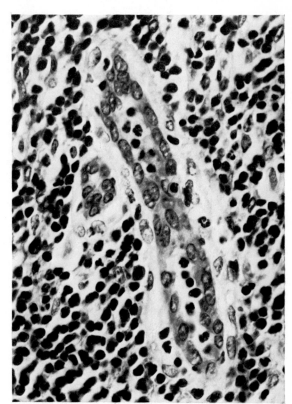

Fig. 9.64. Chronic non-specific lymphadenitis. There is a striking increase in the size and number of the endothelial cells in the two small blood vessels illustrated, one cut lengthwise and the other across. The explanation of this striking occasional finding is not known. A similar picture may be seen in some specific forms of lymphadenitis and, exceptionally, in immunoblastic lymphadenopathy (see Fig. 9.155A, page 705). Sometimes this change is mistaken for a carcinomatous tubule or for a benign epithelial inclusion (see Fig. 9.12, page 539). *Haematoxylin–eosin.* × 55.

F*

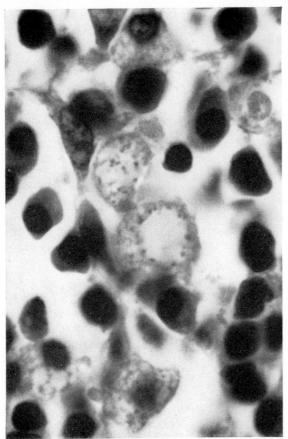

Fig. 9.65A. Scleromatous lymphadenitis. Numerous kleb-siellae are present in the cytoplasm of the two macrophages at the centre of the field. In one of the cells the organisms are at the periphery of a large vacuole, as often is the case; in the other they are dispersed more evenly in the cytoplasm. Elsewhere in the field are several macrophages with finely vacuolate, foamy-looking cytoplasm ('Mikulicz cells'); klebsiellae are demonstrable in only a minority of the cells in any case. Most of the other cells in the infected tissue are plasma cells. Russell bodies were abundant in other fields (see Fig. 4.5, page 206, volume 1). See also Fig. 9.65B. *Haematoxylin–eosin.* × 1500.

pulp are essentially the same as those in the infected tissue of the upper respiratory tract (see page 204).

The suggestion that the lymphadenitis of scleroma may reproduce the histological picture of 'sinus histiocytosis with massive lymphadenopathy', a view that does not tally with my experience of the two diseases, is mentioned on page 566.

The appearances of the infected macrophages are very like those of macrophages infected by *Donovania granulomatis*, the cause of granuloma inguinale (see page 593), as may be appreciated on comparing Figs 9.65A and 9.68.

Brucella Infection (Brucellosis; Undulant Fever)

Infection of lymph nodes draining the portal of entry of the brucellae—usually the small bowel—is a regular occurrence in cases of disease caused by these organisms: indeed, it is an essential feature in the pathogenesis of the illness. The early proliferation of the brucellae in these regional nodes is followed by extension of the infection to the blood stream. Clinical evidence of lymphadenopathy is usually found only in the subacute or chronic phase of the disease: the lymphadenitis is generalized in these cases and there is clinically detectable spleno-megaly in about 50 per cent of the patients. It is noteworthy that the classic picture of an undulant fever is by no means always present and that in a proportion of cases there is no fever at all.

The pathological picture is essentially the same whether the infection is caused by *Brucella abortus*,[345] *Brucella melitensis*[346] or *Brucella suis*.[347] Infection by *Brucella abortus* is usually acquired from cattle and is of worldwide distribution (it was first recognized in man in what was then Southern Rhodesia[348]); in cattle, *Brucella abortus* is the cause of one form—Bang's disease[349]—of contagious abortion, and this is often associated with persistent mastitis. Infection by *Brucella melitensis* is the cause of Malta fever (Mediterranean fever, or Bruce's disease[350]), which is usually acquired from goats; the disease in the latter is characterized by abortion (Zammit's disease[351]). Infection by *Brucella suis* is

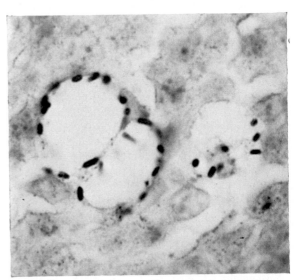

Fig. 9.65B. Same specimen as Fig. 9.65A. The klebsiellae are blackened by the deposition of silver. This facilitates their demonstration, but they can usually be found readily in haematoxylin–eosin preparations. *Warthin–Starry.* × 1500.

usually acquired from pigs; it is rarely seen outside the Americas.[347] All three species of brucella may infect domestic animals other than those with which they are classically associated (see above); infection of wild animals is sometimes recognized.

In Britain, *Brucella abortus* is the only indigenous species. However, infection by either of the other species may be seen, usually in patients who have acquired the disease abroad, but sometimes as a result of eating infected foodstuffs, such as imported cheese made from sheep's milk (*formaggio pecorino*) infected with *Brucella melitensis*.[352] Attempts to eradicate the infection from cattle in Britain are having considerable success.[352a]

Pathology

The lymph nodes are usually no more than moderately enlarged, seldom exceeding 2 cm in longest dimension.

Simple Form.—In some cases there is no abnormality of the lymph nodes other than follicular hyperplasia and sinus histiocytosis; the latter may be quite marked and is either of the simple type (see page 560) or of the so-called 'immature' type (see page 561). Plasma cells are sometimes found in considerable numbers in the pulp in these cases (Fig. 9.8, page 523), and there may be a proliferation of larger, pale cells throughout the lymphoid tissue between the follicles. These large cells were formerly described as reticulum cells: a possibility that they are immunoblasts (transformed lymphocytes—see page 522) has not yet been resolved. As the pale cells of this simple form of brucella lymphadenitis can be seen to give origin to the clusters of epithelioid cells that are characteristic of the granulomatous form (see below), it seems likelier that they are reticuloendothelial cells and that the original interpretation as reticulum cells is still reasonable.

Granulomatous Form.—Oftener, the picture is that of a granulomatous reaction.[345] This is characterized by a well-marked development of clusters of epithelioid cells; these clusters are commonly intermediate in size between tubercles and the cell clusters of toxoplasmosis, but they tend to become confluent and may then form large foci of irregular outline (Fig. 9.66). Langhans giant cells may be present, but usually are neither numerous nor particularly large. Sometimes, there is a tendency for the epithelioid cells in the smaller clusters to be disposed radially. Occasional eosinophils and plasma cells are seen in many cases. Fibrosis is inconspicuous or lacking,

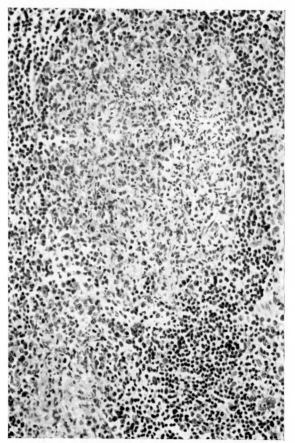

Fig. 9.66. Lymphadenitis associated with infection by *Brucella abortus*. Granulomatous form. A large focus of epithelioid cells and an adjoining smaller cluster (below, left) are seen. There is some infiltration of these lesions by neutrophils: traces of nuclear debris indicate a degree of necrobiosis, but there is no frank necrosis in this instance. Such lesions may be inconspicuous; sometimes they are mistaken for germinal centres of follicles. *Haematoxylin–eosin.* × 200.

and necrosis—apart from fibrinoid foci in the larger cell clusters in some cases—is not a usual feature, although small foci of caseation are seen in exceptional cases.

The granulomatous reaction is most marked in the pulp of the lymph nodes and may be confined to it. Sometimes a small cluster of epithelioid cells is seen within the germinal centre of a lymphoid follicle or in a lymph sinus, but this is a comparatively rare finding.

Relation to Hodgkin's Disease.—Considerable controversy was caused by some observers who described changes in cases of brucella infection that they considered to resemble those of the classic form of Hodgkin's disease (the form nowadays described as of 'mixed cellularity'—see page 800).[353] The main point of similarity was the presence of cells that more or less closely resemble the Sternberg–Reed cells of Hodgkin's disease.[354] Sometimes the resemblance was considered to be so close that the histological picture was regarded as typical of Hodgkin's disease.[355] Present opinion is that in most instances the similarity is not close (Fig. 9.67), and that the cells in question are not neoplastic but various forms of binucleate or small multinucleate cells of the immunoblast or plasma cell series or, possibly, reticulum cells.[356] The possibility that brucella infection may be a cause of Hodgkin's disease is no longer entertained. Cases of brucella infection in which the histological picture of Hodgkin's disease is seen are now interpreted as cases of Hodgkin's disease complicated by brucella infection; Hodgkin's disease is recognized to predispose to manifestations of brucella infection that may be severer than those usually seen in patients whose cell-mediated immune responses are not attenuated by a systemic disorder of the lymphoreticular system. Moreover, brucella infection is common enough for its chance coexistence to be anticipated in a proportion of patients with a lymphoma: where brucella infection is endemic such associations with other diseases, including lymphoma, is frequently observed.

Other Manifestations of Brucella Infection.—The complications of brucella infection include arthritis and bone abscess, bronchopneumonia, meningitis and encephalitis, endocarditis (see pages 33 and 99), orchitis and hepatitis (see page 1229).[357] A haemorrhagic tendency is sometimes seen, with bleeding from mucous membranes and into the skin. In general, these various manifestations of severe infection are commoner in cases of infection by *Brucella melitensis* and *Brucella suis* than in those due to *Brucella abortus*.

Diagnosis.[358]—Brucella infection may be suspected as a result of histological examination but the diagnosis can be confirmed only by other means. In many cases it is more difficult to establish the diagnosis than is generally recognized.[358a] Culture of the causative organisms from the blood, even using refined techniques and repeated at frequent intervals, is successful in only up to half the cases; it is particularly likely to be unsuccessful in cases of *Brucella abortus* infection. Serological tests are often less helpful than might be expected: although the agglutination reaction is often positive at a high titre in the acute stage of the disease, the titre falls rapidly during the transition to the chronic stage and may reach zero. Moreover, there may be cross-reactions in patients who have antibodies to yersiniae (particularly *Yersinia enterocolitica*) or to *Francisella tularensis*; the serum of some people who have been immunized against cholera may also agglutinate brucellae. The specific complement-fixation test may be positive in the chronic stage of brucella infections. Latent infections and previous subclinical infections may produce a low titre reaction in the agglutination test; in cases of latent infection the complement fixation test may be positive. The brucellin skin test is of limited value, again because of the high incidence of positive reactions among people whose occupation or residence has exposed them to a greater than average risk of infection in the past.[359]

In cases in which a well-based clinical suspicion that brucellosis is present cannot be unequivocally resolved by other means, it is worth considering

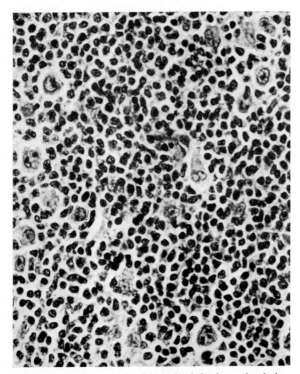

Fig. 9.67. Lymphadenitis of brucella infection—simulation of Hodgkin's disease. There is a scattering of atypical large mononuclear cells among the lymphocytes. Some of these cells are binucleate and some nuclei are hyperchromatic or contain multiple nucleoli. The picture is likely to be mistaken for Hodgkin's disease unless the possibility of brucella infection is considered and the appropriate investigations are carried out. *Haematoxylin–eosin.* × 360.

whether to undertake lymph node biopsy for the purpose of trying to isolate the organism. This has been successful in some instances of *Brucella abortus* infection in which other diagnostic measures were inconclusive.[360]

Chronic Suppurative Bacterial Lymphadenitis

Chronic suppurative lymphadenitis in the sense of inflammation characterized simply by a heavy infiltrate of neutrophile polymorphonuclear leucocytes, with more or less destruction of tissue and the formation of simple abscesses, is very uncommon. It is seen as a rare accompaniment of chronic staphylococcal infection—for instance, of the skin or of bones or joints: in most cases of such chronic staphylococcal disease the changes in the related lymph nodes are merely those of a chronic non-specific lymphadenitis (see page 588), perhaps with more neutrophils in the sinuses and pulp of the nodes than is usual, but short of sufficient to warrant description as suppuration. The same is true of the lymph nodes draining the site of other chronic abscesses, such as an appendix abscess or a dental abscess, a pleural empyema or a tubo-ovarian abscess, all of which are often the result of infection by pyogenic bacteria other than *Staphylococcus aureus*.

Lymphadenitis Accompanying Infection by Donovania granulomatis

Donovania granulomatis is a small, bacilliform, often encapsulate, Gram-negative intracellular organism that was recognized by Donovan, in 1905,[360a] 2 years after his account of the causative organism of leishmaniasis (see footnote on page 659). The donovania, which is sometimes referred to as the 'Donovan body' and therefore liable to be confused with the Leishman–Donovan body (see page 659), is the cause of the condition that is known as granuloma inguinale,* granuloma venereum,* 'ulcerating granuloma of the pudenda', 'serpiginous ulceration of the groin', the 'fourth venereal disease'† and donovaniosis. The disease is not very contagious, and there is doubt whether it is usually transmitted by sexual intercourse.[360b] However, its greater frequency in promiscuous people, parti-

cularly in temperate climates, where it is ordinarily a rare disease except among those in seaports and the like who associate with individuals who have acquired the infection in the tropics, and the usual involvement initially and severely of the genital organs indicate that a significant proportion of cases results from sexual transmission of the donovania. In contrast, it is quite uncommon for an infected person's sexual partner to develop evidence of the disease.

The disease is considered in Chapters 26, 27 and 39. Only the question of lymphadenitis is discussed here. In fact, it is generally stated quite categorically that the donovania does not set up a lymphadenitis, and that the presence of enlarged lymph nodes in an affected region indicates some other cause,[360c] such as coexistent syphilis, secondary infection spreading from the extensive cutaneous ulcers, or incidental tumour deposits. However, the lesion illustrated in Fig. 9.68 was unquestionably an instance of lymphadenitis caused by *Donovania granulomatis*: there was extensive enlargement of the nodes in both groins and in one axilla, the ulceration being confined to the external genital organs and the contiguous area of skin of both thighs and groins and part of the abdominal wall. The biopsy specimen was from the axilla, and 35 cm distant from the nearest margin of the ulcer. There was widespread suppuration in the node, amounting to small foci of frank abscess formation. Large, pale macrophages were conspicuously numerous throughout the affected tissue and contained large numbers of donovaniae.

The parasites are commonly distributed at the periphery of one or more large vacuoles in the cells, the appearances closely reproducing those seen in cases of scleroma (see page 589). They are readily seen in haematoxylin–eosin preparations, although more easily demonstrated in silvered preparations, the Warthin–Starry method being particularly convenient and effective.[360d]

Chronic Necrotizing Granulomatous Bacterial Lymphadenitis with Suppuration

The term chronic suppurative lymphadenitis is quite frequently applied to lesions that are not 'pure' abscesses but a combination of suppuration, characterized by accumulation of neutrophils, with a necrotizing granulomatous condition. This is the type of lesion that has been described as a '*suppurating granuloma*'. It is seen as a manifestation of several varieties of infection, some of them bacterial (see footnote on page 584), some chlamydial (see

---

* The terminological confusion of granuloma inguinale (granuloma venereum), which is due to infection by *Donovania granulomatis*, with lymphogranuloma inguinale, which is a chlamydial infection, is referred to in footnote [†] on page 635.

† But see also footnote [‡] on page 635.

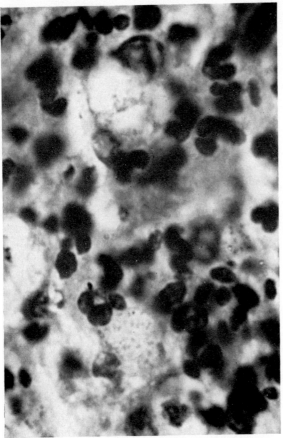

Fig. 9.68. Chronic suppurative lymphadenitis due to infection by *Donovania granulomatis*. Although the reaction is predominantly purulent, with a heavy infiltration of the node by neutrophils, the organisms are found almost exclusively within macrophages. Several parasitized cells are included in this field. The picture differs from that of scleroma (see Fig. 9.65A): predominance of plasma cells and lack of neutrophils typify the latter. *Haematoxylin–eosin.* × 1500.

page 634) and some of undetermined nature, and it is typified in lymphogranuloma inguinale (see page 636). The distinction between acute, subacute and chronic forms is only arbitrarily definable. 'Acute' necrotizing granulomatous lymphadenitis is referred to on page 584, with particular reference to yersinial mesenteric lymphadenitis (page 584) and tularaemia (page 586). Some instances of histologically comparable, but clinically subacute or chronic, infections by other bacteria may be noted briefly here.

Infection by Pasteurella septica

Pasteurella septica (*Pasteurella multocida*) has been recognized as the cause of rapidly fatal haemorrhagic septicaemia and of various forms of acute visceral infection in many types of domestic and wild animals.[361] It is comparatively rarely the cause of disease in man:[362] usually it appears to be a secondary invader of tissues or organs damaged by other conditions, but sometimes, and particularly as the result of a bite or a scratch by a cat or a dog, it is primarily responsible for infection. In cases of infection resulting from a bite or a scratch there is progressive enlargement of the lymph nodes that drain the site of inoculation of the organism. The nodes do not break down, and their enlargement gradually subsides.[363] The distinction from the lymphadenitis of cat-scratch disease (see page 638) has been based on the absence of any reaction to 'cat-scratch disease antigen' and—perhaps more significantly—on the observation that an intracutaneous inoculation of a filtrate of cultures of *Pasteurella septica* results in acute swelling of the affected lymph nodes, fever, and erythema of considerable extent at the site of the injection.[363]

Histology.—Histological examination seems not to have been undertaken in the published cases of this infection. In a bacteriologically proven case, in which submandibular lymphadenitis followed a cat bite on the nose, the histological picture was that of multiple, small, sometimes confluent, epithelioid cell granulomas with a palisade-like arrangement of the cells abutting on the necrotic core of the lesions.[364] The necrotic material consisted mainly of structureless debris, heavily infiltrated by neutrophils, with frank abscess formation in the larger foci (Fig. 9.69).

Relation to Infections by Other Bacteria.—As the bacteriological nomenclature has changed so considerably, it is pertinent to note that the organisms that were formerly known as *Pasteurella pestis* and *Pasteurella pseudotuberculosis* are now named *Yersinia pestis* (see page 581) and *Yersinia pseudotuberculosis* respectively, and that most of the cases of acute mesenteric lymphadenitis that were attributed to the latter are now known to be caused by the related species, *Yersinia enterocolitica* (see page 585). Similarly, *Pasteurella tularensis* has been renamed *Francisella tularensis* (see page 586).

The histological changes in lymph nodes infected by *Pasteurella septica* are, in general, comparable to those in nodes infected by *Yersinia enterocolitica*, *Yersinia pseudotuberculosis* or *Francisella tularensis*. The changes accompanying infection by the plague bacillus, *Yersinia pestis*, are of a much more acute nature, and lack the development of the epithelioid

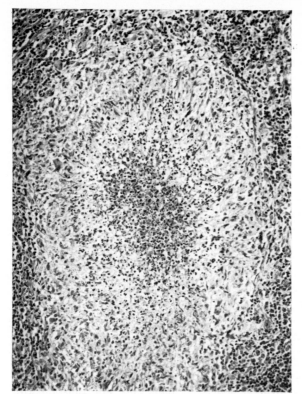

Fig. 9.69. Lymphadenitis caused by *Pasteurella septica*. Epithelioid cell granuloma with palisading of cells round the necrotic core. Neutrophils have accumulated in the core and indicate incipient suppuration. This condition developed in submandibular lymph nodes following a cat bite on the nose. The cutaneous lesion healed while the lymphadenitis was forming. The causative organism was isolated from the latter, and enabled the condition to be distinguished from the lymphadenitis of cat-scratch disease (see Fig. 9.109, page 640). *Haematoxylin–eosin.* × 120.

cell granulomatous element that is a feature of so many cases of infection by the other bacteria named (see page 581).

Glanders

Glanders has always been rare in man, even when the infection was common in horses.[365] There is comparatively little risk of contagion from naturally infected animals, even among those working most closely with them; in contrast, infection from dealing with cultures of the causative organism under laboratory conditions is very frequent.[285] Acute infection of the respiratory system has a high mortality, but is much rarer than infection of the skin, which usually runs a chronic course. Abscesses in the skin and subcutaneous tissue, in skeletal muscles and along the course of the subcutaneous

lymphatics are characteristic of chronic glanders in man: the lymphatic involvement corresponds to farcy in horses,[366] and the enlarged lymph nodes to the 'farcy buds'.

Histology.—The lymphadenitis of glanders in man is characterized by an epithelioid cell granulomatous reaction with central suppuration.[284, 285] The more acute the lesion, the more marked the necrosis and the less evident the granulomatous component. The picture is not in itself diagnostic of glanders; isolation of the organism is the only certain evidence of the nature of the infection.

The causative organism, variously known as *Bacillus mallei*, *Malleomyces mallei*, *Loefflerella mallei* and—now most usually—*Pseudomonas mallei*, occasionally forms small colonies in the purulent exudate in infected tissues, particularly in man. These colonies may become surrounded by a deposit of homogeneous eosinophile material (probably fibrin and immunoglobulins): when the colonies are very small the resulting appearance has been known somewhat to resemble the so-called asteroid of sporotrichosis (see Chapter 39 and Figs 39.179A and 39.179B). For this reason, glanders in man has occasionally been mistaken for sporotrichosis, an error that may be initiated by the fact that both infections give rise to ulcerative lesions at intervals along the course of the subcutaneous lymphatics. In other cases, larger colonies form (Fig. 9.70) and the picture may be confused with that of a nocardial mycetoma (see page 617).

Melioidosis

Clinically, melioidosis may resemble glanders.[367] Visceral infection, particularly pneumonia, which may be very extensive, and septicaemia, with the appearance of widespread necrotic or purulent foci, are the usual manifestations of the disease, which may be acute or chronic in its course. Lymphadenitis is an occasional presentation. The causative organism, which has many synonyms, is now most usually known as *Pseudomonas pseudomallei*, or Whitmore's bacillus. The disease is seen most frequently in south-eastern Asia. It is also indigenous in parts of Australia (Queensland and Northern Territory), Turkey and Central America. Chronic cases are sometimes seen elsewhere, among patients who have travelled from the areas where the infection is endemic (see below).

Melioidosis is enzootic in various wild and domestic animals in those parts of the world where it occurs in man. Human infection is believed to result

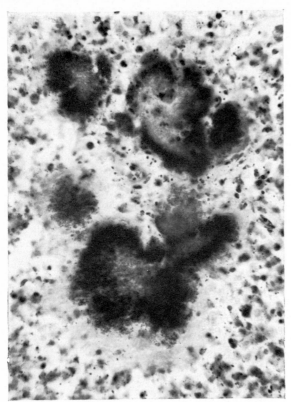

Fig. 9.70. Lymphadenitis in a case of glanders. The colonies of the glanders bacillus that are illustrated were present in the pus that occupied much of the core of the confluent granulomatous masses that destroyed most of the tissue of the infected nodes. There is a homogeneous precipitate of pale eosinophile material at the surface of the colonies, most apparent in relation to the colony in the lower part of the picture: this is an instance of the so-called Splendore–Hoeppli phenomenon (see page 750). Such colonies have to be distinguished from those of actinobacilli and certain actinomycetes that may grow in this manner in infected tissues (see Figs 9.88 to 9.91, pages 618 and 619). The initial histological diagnosis in this case was actinomycosis. The patient was a schoolgirl in England who spent most of her time working with horses; none of the animals showed evident infection. *Haematoxylin–eosin.* × 400.

from exposure to infected soil or surface water, and may take place through trivial breaches in the surface of the skin; sometimes the organisms are inhaled and pneumonia is the initial manifestation.[368]

Lymphadenitis has been known to follow immersion in muddy water. In many cases it has resulted from subcutaneous injection of drugs of addiction without sterilization of the water used as the solvent.

Histology.—The histological picture in lymph nodes infected with melioidosis is much the same as that

of glanders (see above). Colonial 'asteroids' are rarely seen, but in the more acute cases the bacilli are often so numerous in the infected tissues that they can be demonstrated readily. Bipolar staining of the organisms is often a conspicuous characteristic and has been known to lead pathologists to misidentify them as *Yersinia pestis*, with consequent misdiagnosis of the disease as plague. As in cases of glanders, a diagnosis of melioidosis requires to be confirmed by identification of the causative organism in cultures.

In a case of melioidosis recently seen in a visitor to Britain, the histological appearances in a lymph node biopsy specimen exactly reproduced the picture of cat-scratch disease (see page 640), a diagnosis favoured at first because the patient had been clawed by a kitten shortly after arriving in Europe from Malaysia. *Pseudomonas pseudomallei* was isolated from the node, and review of the history indicated that the lymphadenopathy had already begun to develop before the patient left Asia.

Chronic Granulomatous Lymphadenitis—Tuberculous and Tuberculoid Lymphadenitis

There are many causes of granulomatous lymphadenitis. Some of them are not infective (for instance, berylliosis, and the tuberculoid reaction that is an occasional accompaniment of a carcinoma in the area drained by the affected nodes—see pages 681 and 682 respectively); the nature of others is not known (for instance, sarcoidosis—see page 745). Of the infective causes, some regularly give rise to a granulomatous reaction, or do so in all but most exceptional circumstances (for instance, the tubercle bacillus—see page 600); others sometimes cause granuloma development and sometimes a simpler, non-granulomatous response (for instance, brucella infection and listeria infection—see pages 591 and 577 respectively).

This section is concerned mainly with tuberculous and other mycobacterial forms of lymphadenitis.

Tuberculous Lymphadenitis

Tuberculous lymphadenitis that is apparent clinically, or that attracts attention macroscopically, either at operation or at necropsy, is most characteristically seen only as part of the primary complex of tuberculosis (for example, Ranke's complex in cases of primary tuberculous infection in the lungs[369]—see pages 332–333). The heavy involvement of the regional lymph nodes draining the site of the initial tuberculous infection is the substance of Parrot's law (page 332).[370] That there is usually no such gross involvement of the regional nodes draining post-primary ('reinfection') tuberculous lesions—for example, chronic cavitation of the sub-apical part of the lungs—is in accordance with the phenomenon of hypersensitivity, as observed by Robert Koch in 1891:[371] when an animal that has already been infected with the tubercle bacillus is reinfected with this organism after an interval of at least a few weeks, there is both an accelerated necrotizing response of the tissues at the site of the reinfection inoculation and an absence of macro-scopically evident inflammation of the regional lymph nodes. However, microscopical examination of the nodes draining sites of post-primary tubercu-lous lesions in man often shows that there are scattered tuberculous foci: in most cases these are small caseating tubercles—the considerable enlarge-ment of the nodes, with extensive confluent casea-tion, that is characteristic of the lymphadenitis of the primary stage of the disease is usually lacking (see page 341). Occasional cases are seen, and they appear to be becoming less rare, in which post-primary tuberculosis presents with lymphadenitis, usually in the neck:[372] the source of the infection of the nodes in these cases is debatable. The rare condi-tion of generalized caseating tuberculous lymph-adenitis is considered on page 601.

Bacteriology of Tuberculous Lymphadenitis.—For-merly it was found that almost all cases of tubercu-lous lymphadenitis were caused either by *Myco-bacterium tuberculosis* (the 'human type of tubercle bacillus') or by the organism that is now known as *Mycobacterium bovis* (previously described as the 'bovine type of *Mycobacterium tuberculosis*'). Moreover, the latter was found to be the cause of most cases of cervical and mesenteric lymphadenitis, while the former was the cause of most cases of mediastinal lymphadenitis: this distribution of the two types of tubercle bacillus corresponded with the fact that infection with the bovine organism resulted from ingestion of milk, and consequently the portal of entry was the pharyngeal lymphoid tissue or the small intestine, whereas infection with the human type of organism resulted from inhalation of air-borne droplets into the lungs to establish the Ghon focus. Changing patterns of mycobacterial infection in man and in domestic animals, and the recognition of many additional species of mycobacteria that can cause tuberculosis-like diseases, have made it necessary to revise the former assessment of the types of organism responsible for 'tuberculous lymphadenitis'.

In 1975, the number of cases of mycobacterial lymphadenitis reported to the Epidemiological Research Laboratory of the Public Health Labora-tory Service in Britain was 76 (many other cases doubtless went unreported, and therefore this number may not be regarded as an indication of the frequency of the condition).[373] *Mycobacterium tuberculosis* was responsible for 57 cases: all these patients were adults, and about half of them were believed to be native to Britain; the infection was in cervical nodes in 49 of the patients, in axillary, thoracic or abdominal nodes in six and in an un-specified site in two. *Mycobacterium bovis* was responsible for six cases: the six patients were adults, and the infection was cervical in all of them. In one of the remaining 13 cases the organism was not identified specifically; in the other 12 it was said to belong to the 'avium–intracellulare' group of mycobacteria, which comprises the closely related species *Mycobacterium avium* and *Mycobacterium intracellulare*: all 12 patients were believed to be native-born British, the cervical nodes were affected in 11, and 10 of the patients were children up to 7 years of age.

Some rarer mycobacterial causes of lymph-adenitis are referred to on page 606.

Lymphadenitis of Primary Tuberculosis

The site of the primary infection determines whether the accompanying lymphadenitis is clinically con-spicuous.

Pulmonary and Mediastinal Tuberculous Lymph-adenitis.—The lymphadenitis accompanying a primary focus of tuberculosis in the lungs is rarely a cause of clinical manifestations. Bronchial obstruc-tion may lead to distensive panlobular emphysema and tracheal obstruction to stridor (see page 335). Erosion of a caseating node into the trachea or bronchi is a cause of tuberculous bronchopneumonia (see page 334). The infected nodes may become adherent to the blood vessels in the hilum of the lung: extension of the infection through the wall of the vessels gives rise to haematogenous dissemina-tion, either into the lung itself, because of invasion of a pulmonary artery, or—oftener—throughout the body, because of invasion of a pulmonary vein (see page 335). Healing of the lymphadenitis, with shrinkage of adhesions that have formed between the nodes and adjacent structures, is a cause of traction diverticulum of the oesophagus (see page 1001).

Cervical Tuberculous Lymphadenitis.—In contrast to the mediastinal lymphadenitis that develops as an accompaniment of a primary focus of tuberculosis in the lungs, tuberculous cervical lymphadenitis (Fig. 9.71)—usually associated with an initial infection of tonsillar tissue (see page 993)—is unlikely to escape notice, particularly when a sinus forms between a node and the surface of the skin.

Tuberculous Mesenteric Lymphadenitis.—Tuberculous infection of the mesenteric lymph nodes* is usually the accompaniment of a primary infection through the small intestine (Fig. 9.72). It occupies

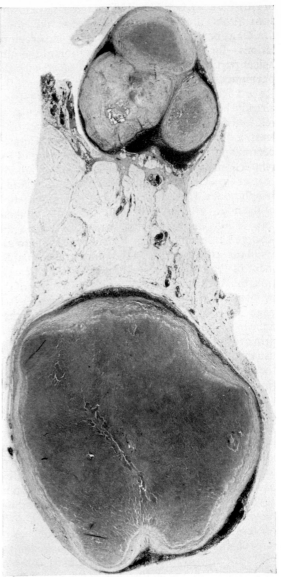

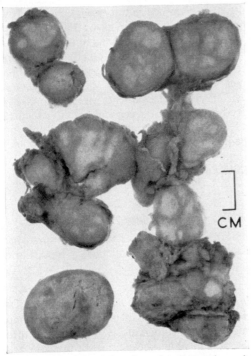

Fig. 9.71.§ Tuberculous lymph nodes dissected surgically from the neck in the days before the introduction of antibiotics and chemotherapy. The variegated appearance of the cut surface is explained by the different aspects of the caseous core and the darker surrounding granulomatous tissue (compare with Fig. 9.72). There is a tendency for the nodes to become matted through extension of the inflammatory reaction into the tissue between them, with subsequent fibrosis. It is not always possible to distinguish macroscopically between tuberculous and lymphomatous nodes (see Fig. 9.191, page 792). The latter comparatively rarely show necrosis, although they are often appreciably larger than tuberculous nodes; when they contain necrotic foci these seldom show the sharply defined 'geographical' outline and dry texture that characterize tuberculous caseation.

   * Tuberculous mesenteric lymphadenitis was formerly often referred to as *tabes mesenterica*, because of the wasting nature of the disease in overt cases. The word 'tabes' means wasting.

Fig. 9.72. Tuberculous lymph nodes in the mesentery of the small intestine. The larger node consists mainly of the caseous core, which is enclosed by a narrow zone of fibrotic tissue outside which there is an incomplete covering of lymphoid tissue (the lymphoid zone appears black in the photograph). The smaller node contains three discrete foci, connected together by fibrous tissue: the two smaller foci have a simple caseous core; the largest focus is almost wholly hyalinized but includes a group of sharply outlined clefts from which lipid crystals have been dissolved. Lipid crystals form occasionally in caseous matter. *Haematoxylin–eosin.* × 6.

an intermediate position in its liability to attract clinical attention. The anatomical relation of the infected nodes to the peritoneum may lead to irritation or even local infection of the latter, with consequent abdominal symptoms. During healing, adhesions may form between the nodes and adjacent structures: these are occasionally a cause of intestinal obstruction, which may occur many years after the infection subsided. In other cases, the infection does not remain confined to the involved nodes but extends through the surrounding tissues: this is one of the sources of generalized tuberculous peritonitis (see page 1183). If symptoms of lymphadenitis are lacking, or overlooked, the eventual recognition of the condition is generally incidental to laparotomy for some other reason, or to necropsy. Once the nodes have become calcified (see below) they may be found by chance during a radiological examination. Tuberculosis of mesenteric nodes is now much less frequent in Britain, as in many other parts of the world, than it was when tuberculosis was prevalent in cattle and unpasteurized milk a common medium of infection by *Mycobacterium bovis*.

Rarely, tuberculous mesenteric lymphadenitis presents as an acute clinical illness. This is associated with extensive necrosis of the nodes and a poorly developed epithelioid cell granulomatous reaction. Bacilli may be very numerous in these lesions. Clinically, the condition resembles—and must be distinguished from—acute non-specific mesenteric lymphadenitis (see page 574) and yersinial mesenteric lymphadenitis (see page 584). If it is not treated promptly, generalized tuberculous peritonitis may follow.

Lymphadenitis Accompanying Primary Cutaneous Tuberculosis.—In those exceptional but important cases in which the primary infection with tuberculosis results from entry of the organisms through the skin, the infection spreads to the corresponding regional lymph nodes, which become much enlarged, matted and caseous, eventually with the formation of one or more sinuses that open through the skin. These sinuses are liable to secondary infection by other bacteria. The inoculation site is most frequently on a hand or forearm, and according to the lymphatic pathway followed it is the supratrochlear or axillary nodes, or nodes in both situations, that are involved in these cases. Formerly, such infection was seen among butchers' apprentices and young employees in slaughter houses or on farms, and occasionally in pathologists and other members of the staff of medical and veterinary laboratories.* Contamination of cuts or scratches or

* The hazard to laboratory workers has not disappeared. Among patients whom I have known to acquire the disease in this way, in Europe, during the period from 1950 to 1975, have been two medical laboratory technicians infected

inoculation by splinters of bone or glass gives the bacillus access to the tissues. Tuberculosis acquired through the skin is often notably less severe when caused by *Mycobacterium bovis*[374] than when *Mycobacterium tuberculosis* is responsible, as is likelier to be the case when the infection is acquired in the course of work in medical laboratories.

Apart from such occupational hazards, primary cutaneous tuberculosis may result from other misadventures. Infrequently, but not rarely, it has been caused by direct infection of the wound during ritual circumcision by an operator who has active pulmonary tuberculosis.[375] The lymphadenitis in these cases is in the inguinal region and it may be bilateral. Comparably, contamination of the syringe used by a doctor with pulmonary tuberculosis when carrying out immunization of school children was the cause of over a hundred cases of primary cutaneous tuberculosis and accompanying regional lymphadenitis.[376]

Lymphatic Obstruction.—If the axillary or inguinal groups of lymph nodes are extensively involved by tuberculosis, obstruction to the flow of lymph may develop and lead to lymphoedema.[377] This has to be distinguished from filarial lymphoedema in the case of patients who have lived in regions where filariasis is endemic.[378]

Calcification of Tuberculous Lymph Nodes.—Dystrophic calcification eventually occurs in the caseous material in the infected lymph nodes of the primary tuberculous complex, particularly in cases of childhood infection and particularly in pulmonary and mediastinal nodes and in mesenteric nodes.*

* Calcification of caseous tissue is seen also in healing histoplasmic lymphadenitis, particularly in the mediastinum (see Figs 9.96A and 9.96B), and possibly in other types of mycotic lymphadenitis (blastomycotic, coccidioidal and cryptococcal)—see pages 627, 626 and 621. It must not be assumed that calcified lymph nodes are evidence of tuberculosis exclusively.

through cuts by broken culture bottles, a hospital's animal-house attendant infected while assisting at the post-mortem examination of an inoculated guinea-pig, and a medical student infected while assisting at the post-mortem examination of a patient with Hodgkin's disease, whose terminal disseminated tuberculosis, although known to the physicians, had not been noted in the clinical summary. None of these four patients had been examined for evidence of previous tuberculous infection at any time before the infection was acquired at work, and none of them had been immunized against tuberculosis. The medical student died following an operation for the relief of hydrocephalus resulting from tuberculous meningitis that had developed in the course of miliary tuberculosis, the result of eruption of a caseating axillary lymph node into the axillary vein.

The presence of calcium salts has been demonstrated histologically within 2 months of the onset of a known accidental infection; the deposit does not become heavy enough to show in clinical radiographs until 10 [379] to 18 months after infection. In the Lübeck catastrophe (see footnote on page 606), calcium was found in the mesenteric nodes at necropsy 58 days after the date of oral administration of virulent tubercle bacilli; in contrast, the shortest interval before calcification was demonstrable by radiological examination of the abdomen of the children who survived was 14 months.[380]

The occurrence of calcification does not indicate that the infection has been overcome. Indeed, tubercle bacilli have been isolated from lymph nodes that seemed to be wholly replaced by calcium salts, and in the absence of evidence of active infection.

In some cases the calcified material is replaced by bone, and the bone may develop a marrow cavity containing fat and, sometimes, haemopoietic tissue.

Histology.—The histological picture of tuberculous lymphadenitis is so familiar that it needs no description here. It is in the occasional case in which the picture is not typical (Fig. 9.73) that the disease is likeliest to be mistaken for some other condition. This may occur in those early cases in which the reaction consists simply of small epithelioid cell aggregates (Fig. 9.74), like those more familiar as the classic manifestation of toxoplasmosis (see page 654). Again, the picture of generalized 'non-reactive' tuberculosis may be misinterpreted (see page 602). Conversely, it is appropriate to note that many other conditions may present a picture that exactly corresponds to some aspect of the range of histological appearances that are associated with tuberculosis (see below).

Although tuberculosis may be suspected to be the cause of a particular lesion in a histological specimen, even the demonstration of morphologically typical acid-and-alcohol-fast bacilli in the lesion is not proof of the diagnosis, which requires confirmation by culture and identification of the organism. Lymphadenitis associated with infection by mycobacteria other than *Mycobacterium tuberculosis* and *Mycobacterium bovis* are considered below. Other infections—and some non-infective conditions—that may be mistaken for tuberculosis are referred to elsewhere in this chapter, as indicated in the following list—

yersinial mesenteric lymphadenitis (page 584)
tularaemia (page 586)
brucella infection (page 590)
glanders (page 595)

melioidosis (page 595)
Corynebacterium ovis infection (page 610)
syphilis (page 611)
some deep mycoses (pages 621 to 628)
lymphogranuloma inguinale (page 635)
cat-scratch disease (page 638)
toxoplasmosis (page 652)
some varieties of metazoal lymphadenitis (pages 670 to 680)
sarcoidosis (page 745)
berylliosis (page 681)
Crohn's disease (page 682)
cholegranulomatous lymphadenitis (page 558)
non-infective lymphadenitis accompanying neoplasia in the drainage area (page 682).

The Diagnostic Problem of Caseating Tuberculoid Lymphadenitis Accompanying Secondary Carcinoma.—The presence of certain metastatic tumour

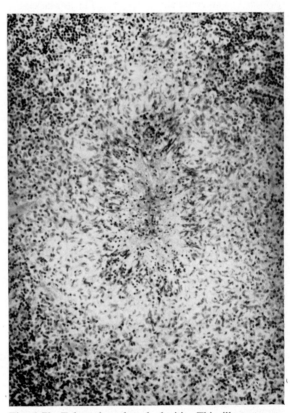

Fig. 9.73. Tuberculous lymphadenitis. This illustrates an unusual histological variant, with palisading of epithelioid cells round the central necrotic area, a broad and ill-defined zone of epithelioid cells at the periphery, and no giant cells. Mycobacteria were found in Ziehl–Neelsen preparations and *Mycobacterium tuberculosis* was cultured from the node. *Haematoxylin–eosin.* × 100.

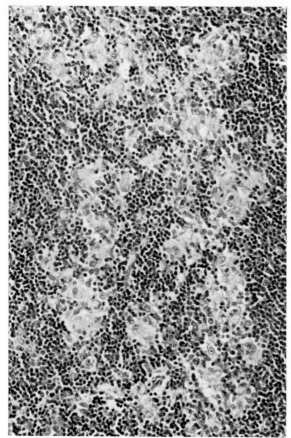

Fig. 9.74. Very early tuberculous lymphadenitis, histologically simulating toxoplasmosis (compare with Figs 9.116A and 9.116B, page 654). The clusters of epithelioid histiocytes tend to fuse. There is no trace of necrosis. Mycobacteria were demonstrable in small numbers in Ziehl–Neelsen preparations. The patient was a laboratory technician in training who cut her hand deeply with the broken glass of a bottle containing a culture of *Mycobacterium tuberculosis*. She was known not to have a positive tuberculin skin test but had not been offered immunization. Tenderness and slight swelling of the supratrochlear lymph node appeared 2 weeks later and the node was excised 18 days after the accident. *Haematoxylin–eosin.* × 160.

deposits in lymph nodes may lead to the development of a non-infective caseating tuberculoid lymphadenitis. A rare error that may be noted here is to misinterpret, as tuberculous, the caseating tuberculoid reaction that occurs in the cervical (and sometimes more distant) lymph nodes in a minority of the cases in which they are involved by metastasis of anaplastic carcinoma arising in the nasopharynx or oropharynx (the so-called 'lymphoepithelioma', or Regaud–Schmincke tumour—see page 241). This reaction, which perhaps is an uncommonly severe and extensive manifestation of the tuberculoid

granulomatosis that is occasionally seen in lymph nodes draining the site of any carcinoma (see page 682), may exactly simulate caseating tuberculosis except that there is identifiable tumour tissue in some part of the affected nodes. In some cases the presence of the tumour cells is overlooked, as they may blend with the tissue of the lymph nodes in a way that readily escapes recognition if examination is cursory. The metastatic tumour may appear long before the primary growth attracts attention directly, and in such cases an extensive caseating granulomatous reaction is particularly liable to be misinterpreted (Fig. 9.75).[381] The same problem is experienced in exceptional cases of some other forms of metastatic tumour in lymph nodes, including seminoma, anaplastic large cell carcinoma of the lungs and adrenal cortical carcinoma. An extensive caseating tuberculoid reaction is sometimes seen in lymph nodes invaded by a gastrointestinal or other adenocarcinoma: in these cases the tumour tissue is so evident that its presence is unlikely to be overlooked.

It must be noted in this context that lymph nodes that are already the seat of caseating tuberculosis may be invaded by metastatic tumour.

Generalized Caseating Tuberculous Lymphadenitis[382]

A serious and comparatively rare manifestation of tuberculosis of lymph nodes is a form that is characterized by the successive or simultaneous involvement of the nodes in many or all parts of the body in a histologically typical caseating tuberculosis. The nodes are enlarged and more or less completely replaced by the caseous granuloma, in which in some cases there is extensive calcification. When the condition successively involves different groups of nodes it tends to start in the cervical region, on one or both sides, and then to appear in the axillary, mediastinal, abdominal and inguinal groups. In such cases the degree of involvement of the nodes may be correspondingly severer the earlier they were affected in the course of the illness, which may extend over many months. In other cases, the illness may present rather suddenly, with fever and marked general malaise, and there is much the same degree of involvement in all the affected groups of nodes. The prognosis is grave and the response to treatment is sometimes very unsatisfactory.

Many, but not all, the patients with generalized caseating tuberculous lymphadenitis are in already poor general health when the infection manifests itself. Diabetes is a predisposing factor,[383] and malnutrition was blamed for the notable incidence

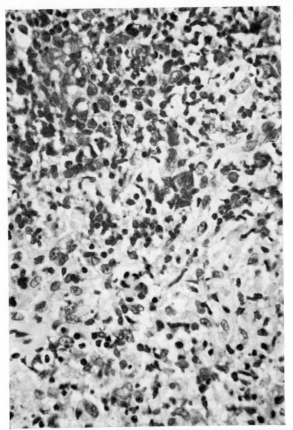

Fig. 9.75. The ill-defined area occupying the upper left corner of the photograph is the edge of a mass of anaplastic carcinomatous tissue infiltrating a cervical lymph node. Abutting on the tumour is a zone of epithelioid histiocytes at the margin of a large focus of caseous necrosis, the periphery of which forms the right margin of the field in the lower half of the picture. Both the tumour and the zone of epithelioid cells are infiltrated by neutrophils. The granuloma formed as an accompaniment of the developing tumour deposits; when the latter are small, and difficult to distinguish in the substance of the node, the true nature of the lesion is easily overlooked. This type of reaction to secondary carcinoma is rare. It is seen most characteristically and frequently in cases of anaplastic carcinoma of nasopharyngeal origin (the so-called lymphoepithelioma). The section shown here is from the patient whose primary nasopharyngeal growth is illustrated in Figs 5.1 and 5.2 on page 241 (Volume 1). *Haematoxylin–eosin.* × 370.

of the disease in parts of Europe toward the end of the second world war and in the immediately succeeding years.[384] Young adults and those in middle age are most frequently affected. The condition is supposedly associated with generalized dissemination of the infection (presumably in the blood stream), localization in the nodes, and progression in this situation because of 'organ predisposition'

(which may mean that lymph nodes are specially liable to suffer in generalized tuberculosis because of their phagocytic activity as part of the reticulo-endothelial system). In fact, in a small proportion of these cases similar tuberculous lesions are present in the spleen and bone marrow and sometimes in the liver. In other cases, necropsy has shown that there are tuberculous foci in the organs or tissues drained by the affected groups of lymph nodes.[385]

Miliary Tuberculosis

Involvement of lymph nodes in cases of miliary tuberculosis is no more than incidental in the course of the generalized haematogenous dissemination. The role of tuberculous lymphadenitis in the pathogenesis of miliary tuberculosis has been mentioned elsewhere (see page 597).

Generalized Non-Reactive Tuberculosis ('Tuberculo-sepsis')[386]

The lymph nodes throughout the body may be heavily infected in cases of this rapidly fatal form of generalized haematogenous tuberculosis, in which discrete and confluent foci of necrotic tissue are present in all parts. The histological picture characteristically lacks both giant cell granulomas and any organized arrangement of epithelioid histiocytes (Fig. 9.76A). However, the more thorough the search, the larger the proportion of cases in which traces of an incipient tuberculous reaction are to be found (Fig. 9.77). In some cases there are numerous plasma cells in the surviving lymphoid tissue. Neutrophils are usually conspicuously absent. The necrotic foci commonly abut sharply on the uninvolved surrounding tissue.

In most cases the necrotic tissue is very heavily infected with tubercle bacilli (Fig. 9.76B), and sometimes to such a degree that areas of the Ziehl–Neelsen preparations are red to the naked eye. Occasionally, by contrast, the organisms are very difficult to find. The condition is seldom recognized before the patient's death, which may follow within a few days to a few weeks of the onset of the acute febrile illness. The danger to those attending the post-mortem examination is very real. There is circumstantial evidence that, from exposure during the necropsy in such a case, and within the space of seven months, at least five people developed active pulmonary tuberculosis, which was eventually fatal in one, and that four further cases occurred among their families, including two cases of tuberculous meningitis in children, one of whom died.[387] There

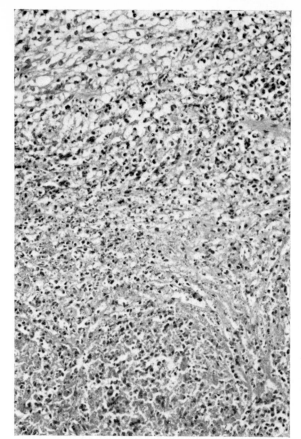

Fig. 9.76A. Lymph node involved in generalized non-reactive tuberculosis. The lower half of the field is necrotic and there is severe degeneration of the rest of the tissue, with much granular nuclear debris in both areas. Most of the few identifiable cells are lymphocytes and plasma cells, with a few larger cells that may be immunoblasts or small histiocytes. The illustration is typical of the whole of the biopsy specimen in showing no histologically specific evidence of the tuberculous nature of the disease. See Fig. 9.76B. *Haematoxylin–eosin.* × 160.

was no experimental evidence that the strain of tubercle bacillus was unusually virulent: the outbreak was attributed solely to the very great numbers of the organism that the patients were exposed to.

The nodes are often much enlarged. Usually they are soft, and when cut their substance may prove to be in part diffluent. Even before they are divided with the knife it may be possible to detect through their capsule the yellowish or greyish foci of necrosis. The finding of such changes in the lymph nodes at necropsy should make the pathologist alert to the possibility of this disease. In the majority of cases, and certainly in those that present the greatest danger of infection, immediate microscopical

examination of a film of aspirated debris from the nodes should disclose the presence of the bacilli and the imperative need to prevent their further dissemination. *The preparation of frozen sections of specimens that have not been sterilized by sufficiently prolonged storage in a suitable fixative solution is absolutely contraindicated* because of the great danger of contaminating the cryostat or other equipment used or of creating an airborne hazard by dispersing infective material through the laboratories by the propulsive effect of a carbon dioxide freezing jet.

Lymphadenitis Caused by Bacillus Calmette–Guérin (BCG)

Attempts to produce immunity to tuberculosis by the administration of tuberculin having failed,[388]

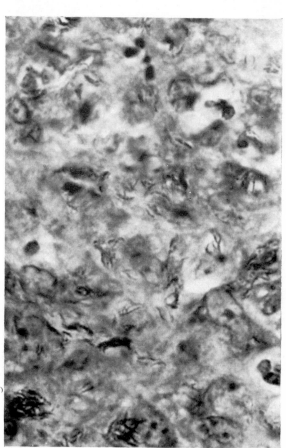

Fig. 9.76B. Same specimen as Fig. 9.76A. This field is from the margin of the necrotic zone and shows very large numbers of acid-fast bacilli. Some are obviously clustered in the cytoplasm of macrophages; elsewhere, similar clusters seem to mark the site of cells that have died. Single bacilli are scattered throughout the field. *Mycobacterium tuberculosis* was cultured from the node. *Ziehl–Neelsen.* × 1300.

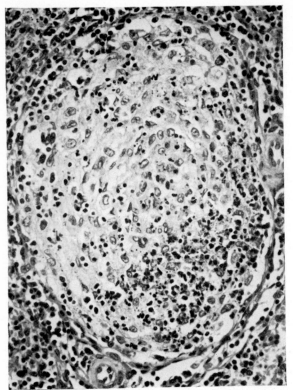

Fig. 9.77. Another case of non-reactive tuberculosis. A small tubercle-like aggregate of epithelioid histiocytes has formed in the lymph node. Necrosis has begun at one pole. A few neutrophils are present among the sparse lymphocytes throughout the focus, and there is extensive stippling with nuclear debris. Acid-fast bacilli were demonstrable in considerable numbers in Ziehl–Neelsen preparations. Changes elsewhere in the node were of the type illustrated in Fig. 9.76A. *Haematoxylin–eosin.* × 220.

vaccines composed of tubercle bacilli that had been grown on various media, killed in various ways, and extracted with various agents, were tried over the years. The outcome of these studies was the view that dead tubercle bacilli have little, if any, protective value. More recently, this conclusion has been questioned again, by various authorities,[389, 390] who would equate the effectiveness of killed organisms, under optimal conditions, with that of living bacillus Calmette–Guérin (BCG—see below). However, the general view is that living mycobacteria are the most effective agents for promoting acquired immunity to tuberculosis. The use of living virulent tubercle bacilli[391] was quickly abandoned as prohibitively dangerous. The choice is between living attenuated tubercle bacilli—specifically, BCG—and some other living mycobacteria, such as Wells's vole bacillus (*Mycobacterium microti*).[392]

The bacillus of Calmette and Guérin[393]—a strain of *Mycobacterium bovis* permanently stabilized in attenuated character as a result of subculture, at intervals of 3 weeks or so throughout a period of 13 years, on a glycerolated potato medium containing ox bile—proved to be effective in immunizing calves and guinea-pigs. It was first tried in man in 1921:[394] the recipient was the baby of a woman who had died of tuberculosis; the child remained well. Over the years, BCG has become the most widely used agent of immunization against tuberculosis: it has been given to many millions of people—its value is still the subject of controversy.[395]

The original French practice was to give BCG by mouth.[396] Later, subcutaneous inoculation was tried,[396] but this led to many instances of 'cold abscess' at the site, and the Scandinavian practice[397] of intradermal inoculation is that now generally adopted. Intradermal administration of about 0·1 mg of BCG to the previously uninfected individual is followed within 4 to 5 weeks by the formation of a local nodule that usually breaks down some 6 weeks later. The resulting ulcer heals in most cases in the course of a few weeks, sometimes with the development of a keloid scar.[398]

Lymphadenitis Following Injection of Bacillus Calmette–Guérin.—In most cases it is possible to recognize clinically that the lymph nodes draining the site of an intradermal inoculation of BCG are slightly or moderately enlarged. Predictably, this condition has been referred to by the deplorable terms 'BCG-itis' and 'becegitis'. The nodes break down in a proportion of cases, with extension of the infection into the surrounding tissues and the eventual formation of sinuses that discharge through the skin: this is particularly likely to happen following inoculation immediately after birth, is much less frequent when the inoculation is carried out from 1 to 24 months after birth and—in otherwise healthy and well nourished children—is an exceptionally rare complication if the BCG is given between the ages of 3 and 6 years (the frequency was 23·3 per cent, 2·3 per cent and nil among Chinese children in these three age groups[399]). The larger the dose, the greater the frequency of sinus formation: in a series in the Netherlands, the nodes broke down in 26·6 per cent of those infants who received two doses each of 0·1 ml, in 7·1 per cent of those who received two doses each of 0·05 ml and in 3·1 per cent of those who received two doses each of 0·03 ml.[400] In France, in contrast, the percentage of babies who developed this complication was 1·24.[401] Racial factors and variation in the pathogenicity of different strains of

BCG[402] may contribute to the liability to this complication, but the most important single factor is unquestionably the size of the inoculum. It has to be stressed that there is no good evidence that BCG can become converted back into a virulent tubercle bacillus: progressive, fatal infection following administration of BCG has been the outcome either of contamination of the vaccine by virulent mycobacteria, as in the Lübeck catastrophe (see footnote on page 606), or of a major deficiency in the immunological responsiveness of the patient.[403]

Subcutaneous inoculation with BCG is much likelier to lead to a severe regional lymphadenitis than intracutaneous or percutaneous administration. In a unique case, *intramuscular* inoculation (by an untrained person) of ten times the usual intracutaneous dose of BCG was followed by the formation of a large abscess at the site and an accompanying necrotizing regional lymphadenitis; the reconstituted BCG had become contaminated with a species of candida before the inoculation was made, and the fungus was isolated from the abscess in the muscle and from the lymph nodes, both of which also yielded BCG on culture: the child died of massive candida infection of the lungs, presumably haematogenous—BCG was not identified in the lungs.[404]

Histology.—In the very occasional case in which the regional lymph nodes draining the site of inoculation with BCG have been examined histologically when there has been no clinical evidence of breakdown of the nodes, the changes observed have been essentially of the nature of a simple histiocytosis, affecting the pulp as well as the sinuses, with great numbers of bacilli in the cells (Fig. 9.78).[405] Epithelioid cells and Langhans and other giant cells—and, indeed, all evidence of the formation of granulomas—being lacking, the usual designation of 'BCG granuloma' is quite inappropriate:* 'BCG histiocytosis' is a preferable term.[405]

Some fibroblastic activity is usual, particularly in the vicinity of the capsule and trabeculae, and extending to some extent between the bacillus-laden macrophages in the pulp. Necrosis may be absent, or there may be minute foci where groups of macrophages have begun to disintegrate. In those cases in which the lymph nodes break down and sinuses form, the necrotic material resembles that of rapidly developing caseation, with much particulate nuclear debris, large numbers of mycobacteria, and some-

---

* 'BCG lymphoma' is an even more ill-found term that has been applied to the lymphadenitis accompanying the development of the lesion at the inoculation site.

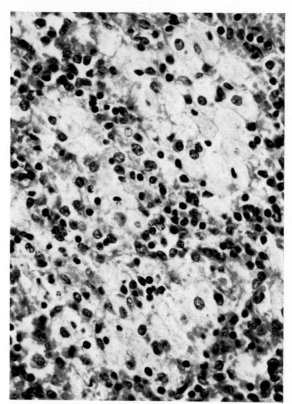

Fig. 9.78. Histiocytosis in a lymph node following intracutaneous inoculation of bacillus Calmette–Guérin (BCG). The patient was a medical student, aged 19 years, and otherwise in good health. There is an accumulation of large pale histiocytes with finely vacuolate or clear cytoplasm; large numbers of acid-fast bacilli were present in the cells. The picture is similar in many respects to that of lepromatous leprosy (see Fig. 9.81) and, except for the presence of the bacilli, to other forms of simple histiocytosis (see Figs 9.49 and 9.50, page 569). See also Fig. 9.278, page 860. *Haematoxylin–eosin.* × 350.

times a small number of neutrophils. When secondary infection develops, as it may once sinuses have formed, frank suppuration may develop.

When the lymphadenitis of BCG infection breaks down, and sinuses form, the enlargement of the nodes may persist for many months and has even been observed still to be present more than three and a half years after the inoculation.[400]

Differential Diagnosis.—In most cases the diagnosis will be evident from the history. In one case in which the clinician omitted to tell the pathologist that there was a history of inoculation with BCG, the latter interpreted the findings in the lymph node as those of lepromatous leprosy, an error that was facilitated by his observation of the great numbers of acid-fast bacilli in the macrophages.[387] The lymphadenitis of lepromatous leprosy[406] may closely resemble that of BCG infection (see page 608).

Lymphadenitis Following Administration of Bacillus Calmette–Guérin by Mouth.—Mesenteric lymphadenitis associated with the administration of BCG by mouth, as was practised formerly (see above), was an occasional cause of symptoms that—as in cases of acute non-specific mesenteric lymphadenitis (see page 574)—led to laparotomy because of the clinical suspicion that the patient was developing appendicitis. The clinical and surgical pictures in these two varieties of mesenteric lymphadenitis were identical. The histological findings were similar to those of the lymphadenitis following intracutaneous inoculation of BCG (see above), except that the infection was less heavy and the degree of histiocytosis correspondingly less marked.*

Lymphadenitis Caused by Killed Tubercle Bacilli

It is relevant to the continuing advocacy, by some authorities, of the use of killed tubercle bacilli in immunization against tuberculosis (see page 604)—and to the pathogenesis of the tubercle as the characteristic histological reaction to infection by tubercle bacilli—that typical tubercles, with caseation, may be seen after inoculation of killed tubercle bacilli into the tissues. This reaction to the dead organisms is believed to result from liberation of their constituents into the tissues as they are broken down by leucocytes. The lesion at the inoculation site, whether subcutaneous or deeper, is a 'cold abscess', with an initial accumulation of neutrophils, which are soon replaced by macrophages, with eventual liquefaction of the exudate and caseation or, occasionally, true suppuration. In the lymph nodes draining the site of inoculation the histological appearances are those typical of tuberculosis. Under experimental conditions, the inoculation of killed tubercle bacilli into the blood stream results in generalized tubercle formation

* Mesenteric lymphadenitis caused by BCG is quite distinct from the true tuberculous mesenteric lymphadenitis that was a characteristic finding in the children involved in the catastrophe that occurred in Lübeck, in northern Germany, in 1930, when 72 babies out of 251 who were given BCG by mouth died of tuberculosis, and all but 44 of the survivors developed clinical evidence of tuberculosis, as the result of contamination of the cultures of BCG by a virulent tubercle bacillus (Wilson, G. S., *The Hazards of Immunization*, chap. 6; London, 1967). The mesenteric lymphadenitis in these children was, of course, a manifestation of primary tuberculous infection and not due to BCG (see page 333).

throughout the tissues, an outcome that has been referred to as necrotuberculosis.[407]

Lymphadenitis Caused by Other Mycobacteria

In general, the commonest mycobacterial causes of lymphadenitis are *Mycobacterium tuberculosis* (see page 597), including the bacillus Calmette–Guérin (BCG—see page 604), and *Mycobacterium bovis* (see page 597). Other tubercle bacilli cause infection very rarely in man: the avian bacillus and the Battey bacillus are occasional causes of naturally occurring infection and may be isolated from infected lymph nodes (see pages 597 and 607); the murine bacillus (*Mycobacterium microti**) is probably not a cause of natural infection in man but, when used as an immunizing agent against tuberculosis, sets up a transient disease, with infection of the lymph nodes draining the inoculation site (see page 604); the organisms that cause tuberculosis in cold-blooded animals (*Mycobacterium chelonei* and related species) are rare causes of human infection (see below). The leprosy bacillus (*Mycobacterium leprae*) is commonly found in lymph nodes in cases of lepromatous leprosy and less often in cases of tuberculoid and 'intermediate' leprosy (see page 608).

In countries where tuberculosis, including infection by *Mycobacterium bovis*, has become significantly less prevalent, the incidence of clinically apparent lymphadenitis due to other mycobacteria has increased notably.[408] The organisms concerned are those that have variously been referred to as the anonymous, atypical, intermediate, opportunist, or tuberculoid mycobacteria;† representatives of each

* Formerly *Mycobacterium murium*, and renamed to avoid confusion with the saprophyte, *Mycobacterium muris*, which was isolated from the faeces of a mouse.

† The nomenclature of these mycobacteria is a problem. Many of them are no longer anonymous; they are no less typical of the genus *Mycobacterium* than the tubercle bacilli and the saprophytic mycobacteria; in pathogenicity they are intermediate between the tubercle bacilli, which are pathogenic, and the saprophytic acid-fast bacilli, which are not, and the designation 'intermediate' is perhaps less objectionable than the other names; to describe them as 'opportunist' recognizes their capacity to invade the tissues when conditions favour this occurrence, which, after all, is a capacity common to every organism that causes disease; and the designation 'tuberculoid', coined by analogy with the relation between diphtheria bacilli and diphtheroid bacilli, has the disadvantage that the same term is applied by histologists to a tissue reaction like that of tuberculosis but not caused by infection with tubercle bacilli (and not commonly caused by other mycobacteria). *See:* Wilson, G. S., Miles, A., *Topley and Wilson's Principles of Bacteriology, Virology and Immunity*, 6th edn, vol. 1, pages 565–566, 593–594; London, 1975.

of Runyon's four groups[409] (see page 328) have been responsible, at least presumptively, for lymphadenitis: most cases of lymphadenitis attributable to these organisms have been caused by members of Runyon's Groups II and III.

Lymphadenitis Caused by Mycobacteria of Runyon's Group I.—In Group I (the photochromogens, which produce yellow pigment on culture, but only if exposed to light), two species have been recognized as the cause of lymphadenitis, *Mycobacterium marinum* (*Mycobacterium balnei*) and *Mycobacterium kansasii*. *Mycobacterium marinum* causes 'swimming-pool granuloma' of the skin and may, in exceptional cases, spread to the lymph nodes that drain the affected region.[387] The rarity of lymphadenitis is probably related to the poor growth of this bacillus at body temperature (it grows best at 32–35°C). *Mycobacterium kansasii*, a cause of pulmonary infection (see page 328), has been isolated from the hilar lymph nodes in a fatal case of infection of the lungs;[410] ordinarily it does not cause serious, progressive disease and the opportunity to examine lymph nodes for its presence is rare.

Lymphadenitis Caused by Mycobacteria of Runyon's Group II.—In Group II (the scotochromogens, which produce a yellow-orange pigment on culture, whether in the dark or exposed to light), two species cause lymphadenitis, *Mycobacterium scrofulaceum* (see Fig. 9.79) and *Mycobacterium gordonae* (*Mycobacterium aquae*). These organisms, particularly the former, are now recognized so frequently among the causes of cervical lymphadenitis, especially in childhood,[411] that they are commonly known as the scrofulagenic bacilli, a name that once might have been coined for *Mycobacterium bovis* (see page 597), which they and *Mycobacterium tuberculosis* have superseded as causes of 'scrofula' (enlarged lymph nodes in the neck).*

Lymphadenitis Caused by Mycobacteria of Runyon's Group III.—In Group III (the 'non-chromogens'), there are again two species that cause lymphadenitis, *Mycobacterium intracellulare* (the Battey bacillus, named for the Battey State Hospital, Georgia,

* *Scrofula* is the diminutive of *scrofa*, the Latin word for a breeding sow, and is supposed to indicate the grossness of appearance that extensive lymphadenopathy may cause. It is one of two regionally distinct etymological sources of the pejorative 'scruffy' ('scroffy' in some dialects); the other source is scurfy, or scurvy, in the sense of dandruffy (implying unkempt).

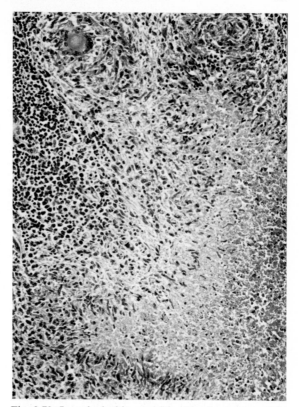

Fig. 9.79. Lymphadenitis caused by *Mycobacterium scrofulaceum*. The histological picture is not distinguishable from that caused by *Mycobacterium tuberculosis*. *Mycobacterium scrofulaceum* is now probably the commonest mycobacterial cause of cervical lymphadenitis in those parts of the world where infection by *Mycobacterium bovis* is no longer prevalent. Its presence in the case illustrated was recognized through its isolation in culture. *Haematoxylin–eosin.* × 140.

United States of America), which is closely related to *Mycobacterium avium*, and *Mycobacterium ulcerans*, which is often regarded as identical with *Mycobacterium burulii*, the cause of Buruli ulcer in Uganda. *Mycobacterium intracellulare* has been isolated occasionally from enlarged superficial lymph nodes, particularly cervical nodes (see page 597).[373] *Mycobacterium ulcerans* has not been isolated from lymph nodes, it seems, although the nodes draining the ulcerated region of the skin are commonly enlarged: this is usually explained by the fact that the organism grows poorly, if at all, at temperatures above 32°C, and therefore is unlikely to survive in the body except in the ulcerated skin. However, acid-fast bacilli have been found in histological preparations of the extensively necrotic tuberculoid tissue in the regional lymph nodes both in a case of rapidly progressive Buruli ulcer, in Uganda,[412] and in the caseating tuberculoid foci in the regional nodes in an Australian case of infection of the skin by *Mycobacterium ulcerans*:[413] the organisms were not cultured in either case, but their appearance in the sections was identical with that of the organisms in the cutaneous ulcers, from which 'Mycobacterium burulii' and 'Mycobacterium ulcerans' had been grown in the respective cases.

Lymphadenitis Caused by Mycobacteria of Runyon's Group IV.—In Group IV (the so-called 'rapid growers'—non-chromogenic mycobacteria that in subcultures produce colonies within about 3 days), there are only two species that have been recognized to cause disease of any sort in man. Some authorities doubt whether the differences justify separation of these species. They are *Mycobacterium fortuitum* (*Mycobacterium ranae*), which is usually regarded as identical with *Mycobacterium abscessus*, and *Mycobacterium chelonei* (*Mycobacterium friedmannii* —Friedmann's turtle bacillus). They are rarely seen as pathogens. They have been isolated from 'abscesses' at the site of injection of therapeutic drugs, antisera, vaccines and local anaesthetic solutions, and of drugs self-administered by addicts: the infection is presumably the result of contamination of the injectant or of the syringe or needle.[414]* *Mycobacterium fortuitum* has been isolated from soil. Lymphadenitis is an occasional accompaniment of these abscesses; rarely, it is the only clinical manifestation of the infection, and in a proportion of such cases a history of an injection— for example, of diphtheria, tetanus and pertussis vaccine ('triple vaccine'), or of a corticosteroid for relief of local 'rheumatism'—is elicitable, clinical examination then revealing a chronic 'injection abscess' or local induration consistent with its incomplete healing. Most of the strains of mycobacterium isolated from 'injection abscesses' have been identified as *Mycobacterium fortuitum* (*Mycobacterium abscessus*).[414] Only one instance of infection by *Mycobacterium chelonei* seems to be on record:[415] the infection, in a boy, aged 8 years, presented as cervical lymphadenitis four months after injection of a dental anaesthetic.

    Mycobacterium fortuitum infection, complicating a therapeutic injection, has been known to cause an ascending lymphangitis, with the development of

ulcerating nodules along the course of the affected vessels.[387] The picture resembled that of the corresponding form of sporotrichosis (see Chapter 39).

Histology.—There is nothing pathognomonic about the histological changes that result from infection by these 'atypical' mycobacteria (Fig. 9.79). The bacilli are often more readily demonstrated in the sections than the organisms of tuberculosis, mainly because they tend to be more numerous. However, it is noteworthy that some species, or at least some strains, are more easily decolorized by acid or alcohol than tubercle bacilli; some are strongly stained by unmodified Gram procedures.

    The lesions are tuberculoid granulomas, usually with caseous necrosis. The entire range of histological pictures associated with tuberculosis may be seen. The specific diagnosis requires identification of the organisms by microbiological means.

Leprosy

Tuberculoid Leprosy.—It is sometimes said that lymph nodes are not involved in cases of tuberculoid leprosy, or that no specific changes are to be found. In fact, the superficial nodes commonly show discrete epithelioid cell granulomas, with a variable number of multinucleate giant cells (Fig. 9.80); there is no necrosis.[406, 416] The granulomatous foci tend to undergo fibrosis and hyalinization. The picture may quite closely follow the pattern and evolution of the lesions of sarcoidosis (see page 747): the two diseases can be confused in biopsy material, particularly as the bacilli are very seldom demonstrable in the tuberculoid lesions of leprosy. The lepromin skin test shows a strongly positive late reaction (Mitsuda reaction) in tuberculoid leprosy; it is negative in sarcoidosis.

Lepromatous Leprosy.—In contrast to tuberculoid leprosy, lepromatous leprosy has long been recognized to give rise to a striking histiocytosis in lymph nodes (Fig. 9.81), at least in some cases, with a large number of leprosy bacilli in the cytoplasm of the macrophages. These cells are scattered singly or in clusters in the pulp of the nodes; they are large and rounded, and commonly appear to have a clear cytoplasm as a consequence of vacuole formation. These are the so-called lepra cells, or Virchow cells.[417, 417a] The vacuoles fuse and may reach a diameter of $30 \mu m$ and more; in haematoxylin–eosin preparations it is evident that some of them contain ill-defined amorphous or particulate material.

---

    * *Mycobacterium tuberculosis* is sometimes transmitted in this manner (see page 599). Other causes of such 'injection abscesses' include fungi (species of candida and of cladosporium, for instance) and, of course, pyogenic bacteria. Some 'injection abscesses' are sterile: these usually result from direct damage to the tissues by some constituent of the material injected.

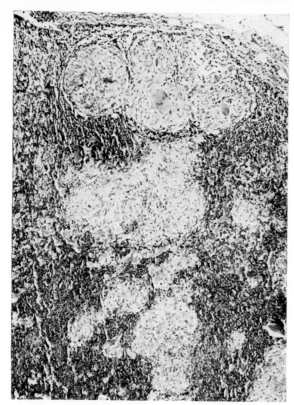

Fig. 9.80. Tuberculoid leprosy of a cervical lymph node. Discrete and confluent granulomatous foci are seen, some of them with multinucleate giant cells. There is no necrosis. The picture thus resembles that of sarcoidosis rather than tuberculosis. It is quite different from the picture of lepromatous leprosy (see Fig. 9.81). *Haematoxylin–eosin.* × 60.

When sections are stained by a Ziehl–Neelsen method this material proves to consist of aggregates of leprosy bacilli. The larger aggregates, which are known as globi,[418] are often rounded and may be so large that they are just distinguishable by the unaided eye (150 μm or so in diameter[419]). The contrast between these sharply outlined, rounded cells and the epithelioid cells of tuberculoid leprosy and other granulomas is distinct. Occasionally, multinucleate lepra cells are also seen:[420] they resemble the so-called Touton giant cells of xanthomatous lesions, their nuclei being dispersed throughout the foamy-looking cytoplasm, or centrally grouped, rather than at the periphery, as in the familiar Langhans giant cell of tuberculosis. Lepra cells are seldom found in the sinuses of the nodes, although some degree of simple sinus histiocytosis is usual. 'Hamazaki–Wesenberg bodies' (see page 562) may be present, both in the sinuses and among the lepra cells in the pulp: similar ceroid lipofuscin pigment may be seen, more finely dispersed or in the form of developing Hamazaki–Wesenberg bodies, in the nucleus or cytoplasm of the lepra cells.[421]

Necrosis is seldom a feature of the lepromatous histological reaction in the lymph nodes. The finding of necrosis is usually a manifestation of co-existent tuberculosis[422] or other incidental condition. This is of diagnostic importance in view of the liability of patients with lepromatous leprosy to develop fatal intercurrent infections, particularly tuberculosis.

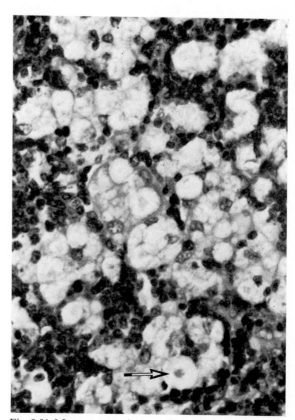

Fig. 9.81.§ Lepromatous leprosy of an axillary lymph node. Malaise and tender enlargement of superficial lymph nodes were the presenting symptoms of the patient's illness (Case 5 of Reference 424, page 871). The large pale histiocytes contain numerous leprosy bacilli; in some cells the bacilli form the rounded aggregates known as globi (one is arrowed). The picture in haematoxylin–eosin preparations is virtually indistinguishable from that of the silicone lymphadenopathy illustrated in Fig. 9.50 (page 569) and comparable to other forms of histiocytosis of similar pattern (see Figs 9.49 and 9.78, pages 569 and 605). The similarities indicate the need to consider the identity of the agent responsible for this type of cellular response. In the case of lepromatous leprosy the diagnosis is readily made by means of an acid-fast staining method appropriate for the histological demonstration of leprosy bacilli, which sometimes are significantly less acid-fast than tubercle bacilli. *Haematoxylin–eosin.* × 370.

The similarity of the picture of the lepromatous lymph node to that of silicone lymphadenopathy has already been noted (see page 569);[280] it may also be mentioned that confusion with certain types of lesion in cases of Hand–Schüller–Christian disease has been known (see Fig. 9.184, page 764).

'Borderline Leprosy'.—In cases of 'borderline' leprosy (dimorphous leprosy), which comprises those grades of the disease that are intermediate in their clinical and histological manifestations between the classic tuberculoid and lepromatous forms,[423] the changes in the lymph nodes approximate to those described above as characteristic of tuberculoid leprosy. The importance of recognizing the borderline cases lies in their instability: whereas the tuberculoid and lepromatous forms are practically stable, and thus unlikely to become transformed one into the other, the borderline cases tend to develop into the lepromatous form, which has a markedly worse prognosis, even with modern treatment, than the tuberculoid form. The finding of lepra cells, with their vacuolate cytoplasm and the readily demonstrable presence of leprosy bacilli, in lesions that are predominantly tuberculoid in histological pattern places a given case in the borderline-lepromatous category, with a particular liability to deterioration into the frankly lepromatous form.

Leprosy as a Diagnostic Problem Outside Endemic Regions.—In Britain, as in many other regions, there is no indigenous leprosy.* However, the disease is seen occasionally in patients who became infected while in parts of the world where it is endemic.[424] These patients may include returned expatriates.[424] The key to recognition of the disease is to think of its possible presence.

Lymphadenitis in Sarcoidosis

It is convenient to mention the lymphadenitis of sarcoidosis at this point, although there is no evidence that sarcoidosis is directly a manifestation of bacterial infection. Sarcoidosis has to be considered in the differential histological diagnosis of several of the conditions that have been discussed in this section of this chapter. The need to obtain confirmatory evidence before accepting a histological

diagnosis of sarcoidosis is considered later (see page 755), when the nature of sarcoidosis and the microscopical findings are discussed.

Lymphadenitis Caused by Corynebacterium ovis

The diphtheroid bacillus, *Corynebacterium ovis* (*Corynebacterium pseudotuberculosis ovis*, the Preisz–Nocard bacillus), is an invasive and potentially pyogenic organism, unlike *Corynebacterium diphtheriae* (see page 580); like the latter, it produces exotoxin, but the pathogenic significance of the toxin is uncertain. Its pyogenic capacity is seen mainly in horses and cattle,[425] which develop suppurative and ulcerative lymphangitis and suppurative or, sometimes, tuberculoid lymphadenitis; the disease in horses resembles glanders (see page 595). *Corynebacterium ovis* has sometimes been confused with *Corynebacterium pyogenes*, a commoner pathogenic diphtheroid, which causes suppurative lesions in animals, particularly cattle, sheep and goats.[426]* It has also been confused with *Corynebacterium ulcerans*, which is a rare cause of a diphtheria-like illness, with regional lymphadenitis (see page 581): it is said that the lymphadenitis in some of these cases may be due to infection of the nodes by *Corynebacterium ulcerans*, but in most it is attributable to absorbed exotoxin.

Infection of sheep by *Corynebacterium ovis* is of economic importance in many sheep-farming regions, especially in Australia,[427] where the disease is known to farmers as 'cheesy gland'. Only seven cases of human infection by this organism had been recorded up to 1974:[428] the condition presented as a granulomatous lymphadenitis in all these patients, as in two unpublished cases seen in Britain.[429] The histological picture in sheep and man is essentially the same,[429] and can be distinguished from that of chronic caseating tuberculosis only by the demonstration of the corynebacteria, which, in Gram preparations, are found without great difficulty at the periphery of the caseous matter (Figs 9.82A and 9.82B). Although ordinarily Gram-positive, many

---

* Since writing this, an 86-year-old woman, a lifelong resident in a home for mentally retarded patients, has been recognized to have developed lepromatous leprosy. She has never been out of the British Isles.

* *Corynebacterium pyogenes* occasionally causes infection in man, the patients usually being concerned with animals. It was isolated from an abscess in the calf of a veterinary surgeon's leg, following a penetrating wound by an infected knife that he had tried to catch with his legs as it fell from the necropsy table while he was dissecting a sheep that had died of pneumonia caused by the organism (Barson, G. J., Shrewsbury, J. F. D., Stammers, F. A. R., Symmers, W. St C., *unpublished observation, Birmingham*, 1949). The abscess was accompanied by the development in the groin of chronic necrotizing granulomatous lymphadenitis with suppuration ('suppurating granuloma'—see page 593).

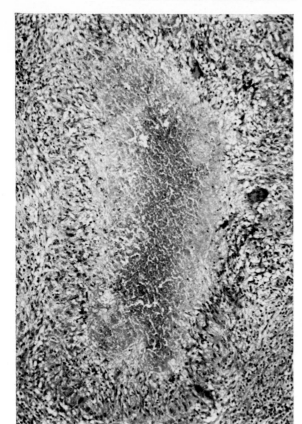

Fig. 9.82A. Lymphadenitis caused by *Corynebacterium ovis*. The patient was a sheep farmer in the north west of England. There was extensive caseation throughout the node, the picture exactly reproducing that of tuberculosis. The lesion illustrated was from a less heavily involved part of the node and shows an earlier stage in the reaction. The picture is identifiable from tuberculosis and other causes of such granulomas only by isolation of the causative organism, as in this case. See Fig. 9.82B. *Haematoxylin–eosin.* × 85.

of the organisms in sections are Gram-negative, probably because they were already dead when the specimen was obtained.* A confident diagnosis can be made only when the organisms have been identified by cultivation.

* I have mistaken *Mycobacterium avium* for *Corynebacterium ovis* through assuming that Gram-positive bacilli in a sheep shearer's tuberculoid lymph node were the latter, because the lymphadenitis followed a cutaneous infection complicating a wound by an electrical shearing tool. The flock of sheep was known to have enzootic corynebacterial infection; what was not known at the time was that some of the sheep were infected with *Mycobacterium avium*. Although Ziehl–Neelsen preparations of the lymph node had been examined, the mycobacteria were overlooked because they had been completely decolorized; they were stained well by the Gram method.

Syphilitic Lymphadenitis

There may be overt involvement of lymph nodes at any stage of acquired syphilis and in congenital syphilis. The occurrence of lymphadenitis is characteristic of the primary stage, in which the nodes draining the site of the chancre are affected, and of the florid secondary stage, in which there is generalized enlargement of the nodes throughout the body. Lymphadenopathy is a rarely observed manifestation of tertiary syphilis, usually occurring then in the form of gummatous lymphadenitis.

These varieties of syphilitic lymphadenitis may be considered in more detail below. It is a general experience that syphilis as the cause of lymphadenitis, as of other manifestations, is most frequently

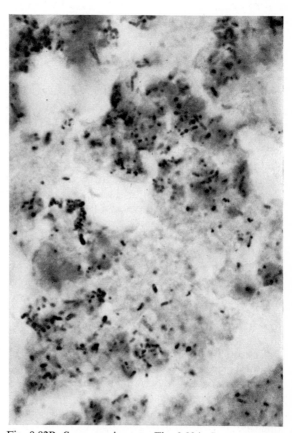

Fig. 9.82B. Same specimen as Fig. 9.82A. It may be very difficult to find the bacilli in sections. Ordinarily they are Gram-positive, but many of the bacilli in the tissues have died and become Gram-negative: this adds to the difficulty of detecting them, particularly when they are sparse. In the instance illustrated, although there are large numbers of the organisms in this field, it was exceptional to find more than one or two in the course of examining many other high-power fields, even at the margin of the necrotic areas, where they are likeliest to be present. *Gram.* × 1000.

overlooked because the possibility of its presence has not been thought of.[430] There are many reasons why the chancre responsible for a clinically recognized local lymphadenopathy should go unobserved by the doctor: the fault is not always his alone, although the clinician who remembers syphilis will not so often be taken in by the factors that tend to obscure its disclosure. A disinclination to cause embarrassment to a patient by requiring to examine the genitalia, a readiness to accept a patient's denial of having had symptoms of a sexual disease, the patient's reluctance to admit to such symptoms, which may seem to him irrelevant, and even a patient's wish not to embarrass a doctor, particularly a doctor of the opposite sex, or the nurse or students in attendance, by disclosing the presence of a sore or discharge, are all experiences that in the practice of a biopsy laboratory have been the background to cases of syphilitic lymphadenitis that had not been diagnosed prior to the histological recognition of the infection. Such diagnostic encumbrances most frequently relate to the lymphadenitis of early syphilis, particularly syphilis in the primary stage. In the case of an elderly doctor with gummatous lymphadenitis as the only sign of tertiary syphilis, which he expected his doctors to recognize without help from himself, the suggestion by the histologist that the biopsy findings indicated the need for serological tests to prove the tentative diagnosis of syphilis was turned down by the clinical specialists on the grounds that the medical father of a medical colleague would be affronted.*

Lymphadenitis of Primary Syphilis.—The regional lymphadenitis that develops in association with the primary lesion of syphilis is familiar as the painless, 'rubbery' induration and moderate enlargement of one or more nodes in the groups draining the site of the chancre. It is usually detectable a few days after the chancre itself becomes evident and it reaches its full development some 2 to 4 weeks later. It commonly persists for many weeks, even after the institution of effective treatment. When the chancre is on the external genitalia the lymphadenitis is usually bilateral, although often more marked on one side; in cases of extragenital chancre the lymph node involvement is usually unilateral, unless the lesion is near the midline—for instance, of the lower lip or tongue. The lymphadenitis accompanying a

chancre on the cervix of the uterus is usually internal, affecting only the iliac groups of nodes.

The enlarged superficial lymph nodes in the drainage region related to the primary lesions of syphilis have long been known as the 'satellite buboes', or 'sentinel buboes', or 'sentinel nodes',* of this stage of the disease.

Histologically,[431, 432] there is conspicuous hyperplasia of the follicles, with well developed germinal centres. Plasma cells are usually very numerous throughout the pulp of the node. Small clusters of epithelioid histiocytes may be sparsely or abundantly scattered through the lymphoid tissue, and are particularly concentrated in the paracortical region (see page 511); they may be accompanied by occasional, and sometimes quite numerous, multinucleate giant cells. There is some lymphocyte depletion in the paracortical region: it has been suggested that this is related to a deficiency of cell-mediated immunity and the consequent persistence of *Treponema pallidum* in the tissues.[432] The treponemes are readily found in sections treated by an appropriate silver impregnation method.

Fibrosing inflammatory changes are present in the wall of the blood vessels of the nodes (Fig. 9.83), both arteries and veins, and there is also fibroblastic proliferation and an infiltrate of plasma cells and lymphocytes in the capsule and trabeculae. Necrosis is not usually a feature, although it may occur in some of the larger epithelioid cell aggregates (Fig. 9.84). When it is of more than focal extent it is ordinarily a manifestation of coexistent infection by other organisms, such as *Neisseria gonorrhoeae*, *Haemophilus ducreyi* or the chlamydia of lymphogranuloma inguinale. In rare cases, massive necrosis is a result of initial overdosage with antitreponemal drugs: this is the Jarisch–Herxheimer reaction, in which extensive necrosis occurs, supposedly because of the liberation of toxic or allergenic products of the killed treponemes into the infected tissues. The Jarisch–Herxheimer reaction reaches its peak usually within 8 to 12 hours of injection of the drug responsible; it is accompanied by marked oedema in the region of the chancre and of the accompanying lymphadenitis. The other variety of massive necrosis of the lymph nodes draining the site of the primary chancre is that described on page 582), in the account of acute necrotizing non-suppurative and non-granulomatous lymphadenitis.

Very occasionally, the clusters of epithelioid

---

* The patient, when a student, had taken part in an unsuccessful trial of mercury ointment as a prophylactic against syphilis. The circumstances are believed to have been mentioned in: Gogarty, O. St. J., *Tumbling in the Hay*, chap. 20, pages 234–235; London, 1939.

* The term 'sentinel node' is also applied to a lymph node of the lower deep cervical group of the left side when it becomes enlarged as a result of involvement by the metastasis of a primary carcinoma of one of the viscera (see page 715).

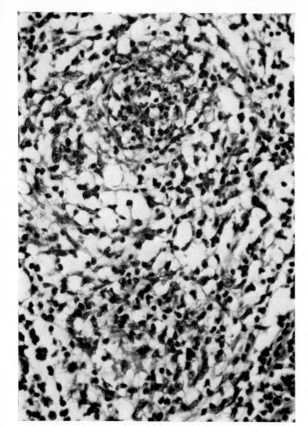

Fig. 9.83. Lymphadenitis of the primary stage of syphilis. Two small blood vessels are practically obliterated by infiltration of their wall and vicinity by lymphocytes and plasma cells and an occasional neutrophil. The eventual tendency for fibrosis to develop is not yet evident. The surrounding paracortical lymphoid tissue is depleted of cells and loose in texture. Treponemes were easily demonstrated in silvered preparations. *Haematoxylin–eosin.* × 250.

histiocytes in the lymph nodes in the primary stage of syphilis are large enough, and sufficiently sharply outlined, to resemble those of sarcoidosis.[431]

Lymphadenitis of Secondary Syphilis.—The appearances in sections of the lymph nodes in the secondary stage of syphilis are, in general, of the same type as those described above as characteristic of the primary stage. Follicular hyperplasia is more marked and the germinal centres are larger. Epithelioid cell clusters may be larger and more numerous (Fig. 9.85), but later tend to disappear, sometimes through fibrosis. Fibrosing endarteritis and periarteritis are more marked, and there may be considerable fibrosis of the trabeculae and capsule and of tissues round the nodes. Treponemes continue to be demonstrable in a few cases, particularly

among the epithelioid cells, but usually they cannot be found in histological sections at this stage.

The lymph nodes throughout the body are affected, including some that are comparatively seldom involved in other forms of 'generalized' infective lymphadenitis, such as the retroauricular (mastoid) and occipital nodes, the buccal (facial) and superficial parotid nodes, the prelaryngeal and pretracheal nodes, and the infraclavicular, pectoral, supratrochlear and popliteal nodes. The generalized involvement of the nodes, and their peculiarly firm but resilient consistency, was expressed in the term *polyscleradenitis* that was given to this manifestation of secondary syphilis, which, in the days before the introduction of the Wassermann reaction, in

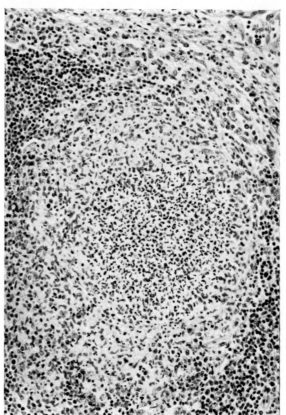

Fig. 9.84. Lymphadenitis of the primary stage of syphilis: another case. An unusually large aggregate of epithelioid cells has formed and undergone central necrosis. Most of the cells in the necrotic core are neutrophils, but there are also many plasma cells both there and elsewhere in the granuloma and adjoining lymphoid tissue. The lesion is basically similar to that in Fig. 9.59A (page 583), the latter being of massive extent. Necrosis is an infrequent feature of the lymphadenitis of the primary stage of the disease. *Haematoxylin–eosin.* × 170.

G

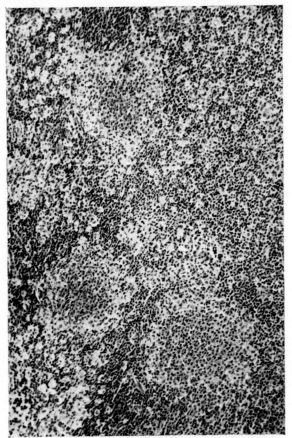

Fig. 9.85. Lymphadenitis of the secondary stage of syphilis. The field includes three clusters of epithelioid cells. Each has a core of smaller, darker histiocytes and a peripheral zone of larger, pale histiocytes; both zones are infiltrated by plasma cells and small lymphocytes. There is a well-marked scattering of large, rounded histiocytes through the rest of the field. *Haematoxylin–eosin.* × 100.

1906,[433] was considered to be of considerable diagnostic importance.

Lymphadenitis of Tertiary Syphilis.[434]—In most cases of syphilis in the tertiary stage there are no notable changes in the lymph nodes. Even in earlier times, when active tertiary syphilis was far from rare, changes in lymph nodes were seldom remarked either clinically or at necropsy. The occurrence of a massive form of gummatous lymphadenitis was recognized, and was familiar both macroscopically and in histological sections; a rarer form of lymphadenitis, characterized by the presence of miliary gummas throughout the affected nodes, was known only by its microscopical appearances and may therefore have tended to escape detection. Today, as

a result of earlier diagnosis and better treatment of syphilis, tertiary disease is less familiar, and massive gummatous lymphadenitis in particular is exceptionally rarely seen; the lymphadenitis characterized by miliary gummas is now relatively less rare than the massive gummatous form.

In the *massive form of gummatous lymphadenitis* (Figs 9.86A and 9.86B), which affects cervical and inguinal nodes rather than those elsewhere, much or all of the substance of the node is replaced by characteristic gummatous material, a 'ghost-like' pattern of the cells and stroma persisting, although staining only with eosin in haematoxylin–eosin preparations.[435] This pattern is particularly well seen in some cases when the sections are examined under the phase-contrast microscope (see also page 637). The nodes range from 2 to 6 cm in longest dimension, and may be even larger. There is usually a thin rim of tuberculoid granulomatous tissue at the margin of the necrotic mass, and an occasional multinucleate giant cell may be present. In a few cases none of the granulomatous tissue survives and the necrotic material abuts directly on the thick, hyalinized capsule of the node. There is marked fibrosis of the surrounding tissues, which may involve the skin. In some instances the necrotic nodes soften and sinuses lead to the surface, often then proceeding to the development of typical gummatous ulceration. Treponemes are demonstrable in only a very small proportion of these lymph nodes, and then only in small numbers (Fig. 9.86B), even when specific immunofluorescent techniques are used.[387] This variety of syphilitic lymphadenitis has to be distinguished from the gummatous forms of lymphogranuloma inguinale (see page 637) and of cat-scratch disease (see page 640).

In the *miliary form of gummatous lymphadenitis*, which also affects cervical and inguinal lymph nodes predominantly, but may be widespread, the affected nodes are little enlarged and there is little fibrosis round them. More or less numerous miliary gummas ('syphilomas'), indistinguishable from miliary tubercles, are scattered through the substance of the nodes; focal necrosis is common within them, and usually characterized by an abundance of particulate, haematoxyphile nuclear debris, although seldom lacking areas that more closely resemble caseous matter. Multinucleate giant cells are often, but by no means invariably, present: in the cases in which the multinucleate cells are lacking, the mononuclear epithelioid cells tend to be radially oriented round the necrotic core of the granulomatous foci.

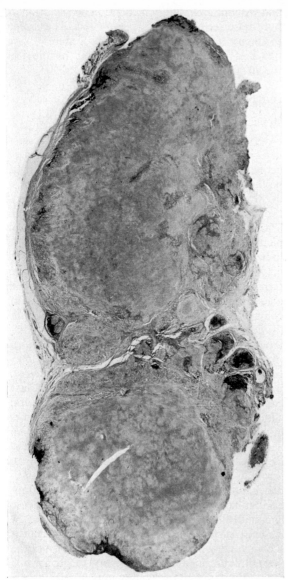

Fig. 9.86A. Massive form of gummatous lymphadenitis (tertiary stage of syphilis). Practically the entire substance of two adjoining nodes has been replaced by gummatous material in which the 'ghost' outlines of the earlier granulomatous foci and of the intervening lymphoid tissue can still be made out. The darkly stained areas at various points on the periphery of the nodes are surviving lymphoid foci, some of which are invaded by active granulomatous tissue. It is particularly in such areas of continuing activity that treponemes may be demonstrable by appropriate means (see Fig. 9.86B). It is probable that the foci of surviving lymphoid tissue develop as a compensatory phenomenon in the hilum and elsewhere in the vicinity of lymph nodes that have undergone slowly progressive destruction by such conditions as the gummatous stage of syphilis; the destructive process then involves them in their turn. *Haematoxylin–eosin.* × 5.

Lymphadenitis of Congenital Syphilis.[436]—Lymphadenitis as a manifestation of congenital syphilis may be observed in the stillborn infant or during the first months of life in those babies who survive. It corresponds in distribution and histology to the lymphadenitis of the secondary stage of acquired syphilis (see above), but the changes are less marked, and there is often atrophy rather than hyperplasia of the follicles. Minute foci of necrosis may be seen and are surrounded by a narrow zone of epithelioid cells, often with some infiltration by neutrophils. Treponemes are usually present in abundance and readily demonstrated in silvered preparations, particularly in the capsule and trabeculae and in the sinuses, where they may be free or within macrophages. Foci of haemopoietic cells are often scattered throughout the nodes.

Very rarely, massive gummatous lymphadenitis, confined usually to one group of nodes, and usually in the neck, is seen as a late manifestation of congenital syphilis, particularly during the second decade. It corresponds to the massive gummatous lymphadenitis of the tertiary stage of acquired syphilis. Sometimes, a condition corresponding to the miliary form of gummatous lymphadenitis of acquired syphilis is seen in the congenital disease. It should be remembered that these patients do not always show other clinical evidence of the infection: the diagnosis may then turn on the serological findings and the response to treatment.

Diagnosis of Syphilitic Lymphadenitis.—Tuberculosis, sarcoidosis and other varieties of tuberculoid lymphadenitis, infarction (see page 551), and necrotic tumours are the conditions that most frequently are diagnosed when the syphilitic nature of

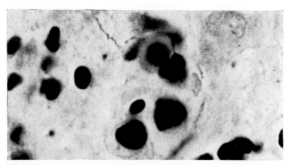

Fig. 9.86B. Same specimen as Fig. 9.86A. Treponemes were found in very small numbers, after a long search, in the still active granulomatous areas in the nodes illustrated in Fig. 9.86A. The field of this photograph was the only one to contain more than one treponeme, and one of the few in which the organisms were convincingly demonstrated. *Levaditi.* × 1500.

the changes in biopsy specimens of lymph nodes is not immediately recognized. Not to consider the possibility of syphilis when interpreting the significance of an epithelioid cell granuloma of uncertain causation is to run a risk that is no less dangerous than the assumption that every abnormality presented by a patient with syphilis is attributable to that infection.

Simple Histiocytic Lymphadenitis

Lymphadenitis may be described as simple histiocytic lymphadenitis when the essential response to the causative agent is proliferation of macrophages, predominantly within the pulp rather than within the sinuses, the cells retaining their identity as discrete, rounded units with pale cytoplasm that often is largely occupied by one or more coarse vacuoles. It must be understood that use of this term carries some risk of confusion with sinus histiocytosis (see page 559), which is a distinct and aetiologically different type of reaction.

Simple histiocytic lymphadenitis is seen in cases of lepromatous leprosy (see page 608), infection by bacillus Calmette–Guérin (BCG—see page 605) and scleroma (see page 589). It has also followed injection of silicone fluid into the tissues (see page 569).

Lymphadenitis Caused by Actinomycetes and True Fungi

Any actinomycete and any true fungus may set up a lymphadenitis. In the great majority of cases the lymphadenitis is subacute or chronic; an acute lymphadenitis caused by either of these types of organism is usually incidental to a rapidly progressive visceral infection, particularly in cases of acute nocardial pneumonia and of acute phycomycosis associated with a therapeutically-induced immunological deficiency. Lymphadenitis is very rarely the presenting manifestation of an actinomycetous or fungal infection: when it is, the diagnosis should be straightforward, as the causative organism can generally be isolated from the affected nodes or seen in histological sections of a biopsy specimen. Unfortunately, the diagnosis is overlooked in some cases because the organisms grown from the specimens are misinterpreted as saprophytes or contaminants, or because they escape detection in haematoxylin–eosin preparations. Any unexplained lymphadenitis, whatever the character of the histological picture, should prompt a search for actinomycetes and fungi,[437–439] among other organisms; the periodic-acid/Schiff reaction, with

and without preliminary incubation in a solution of pure diastase,[440] and the Grocott–Gomori hexamine (methenamine*) silver nitrate procedure[441] are particularly useful when examining histological preparations.

Lymphadenitis Caused by Actinomycetes

Actinomycosis

Lymphadenitis is a rare accompaniment of actinomycosis, but it may occur in the drainage area of actinomycotic lesions anywhere in the body. It is, perhaps, least rare in cases of thoracic actinomycosis, in which the bronchopulmonary and tracheobronchial nodes are sometimes extensively affected. The lesions in the nodes show the histological picture typical of the disease, and the diagnosis is indicated by the presence of the characteristic colonial 'grains' in small abscesses in their substance. Care must be taken not to mistake other microbial colonies and various inanimate structures for colonies of *Actinomyces israelii*.[442] *Actinobacillus actinomycetem-comitans*, a bacterium that is commonly present in association with colonies of *Actinomyces israelii* in cases of actinomycosis, may cause infection in the absence of the actinomyces: pure actinobacillary infections, which are not common, resemble actinomycosis in their general clinical and pathological characters, and the colonies of the two organisms are indistinguishable in haematoxylin–eosin preparations although readily identified in Gram preparations (the filaments of the actinomyces are Gram-positive whereas the actinobacilli are Gram-negative).[442] Species of actinobacillus have been described as a cause of mesenteric lymphadenitis,[443] and I have seen one case of bilateral actinobacillary axillary lymphadenitis accompanying multiple abrasions of the skin of the forearms sustained by a veterinary surgeon while engaged in research on 'woody tongue', the disease of cattle that is caused by *Actinobacillus lignieresii* (the organism isolated from the patient's lymph nodes was considered to be *Actinobacillus actinomycetem-comitans* on the equivocal grounds of its ready growth anaerobically as well as aerobically and its failure to produce indole[444]).

Nocardiosis

The nocardiae are fine, branching, Gram-positive, more or less acid-fast aerobic actinomycetes. Three

---

* Methenamine and hexamine are different names for the same compound. Methenamine is the name adopted in the *United States National Formulary* and hexamine is that adopted in the *British Pharmaceutical Codex*.

species are recognized to be pathogenic to man—
Nocardia asteroides, Nocardia brasiliensis and
*Nocardia caviae.** All three are causes of mycetoma;
Nocardia brasiliensis and *Nocardia caviae* are not
known to cause other types of disease; *Nocardia
asteroides*, in contrast, causes mycetoma only very
exceptionally and ordinarily is seen as the cause of a
rapidly progressive pneumonia developing in
patients whose resistance has been seriously lowered
by other diseases or by drugs that have an immunosuppressant effect (see page 348).

Lymphadenitis in Cases of Acute Infection by
Nocardia asteroides.—Acute suppurative lymphadenitis develops in the nodes draining the site of
acute infection caused by *Nocardia asteroides*,
particularly pneumonia (see page 348). The organism
is often very abundant in the purulent exudate, but
it may be difficult to see in haematoxylin–eosin
preparations. In infected tissue many of the nocardial
filaments lose their affinity for Gram's stain and the
presence of the organism can be overlooked in
Gram preparations. It is likelier to be seen by virtue
of its acid-fastness (Fig. 9.87), although this is less
marked than in the case of *Mycobacterium tuberculosis* and care is necessary to avoid overdecoloriza-
tion, particularly in paraffin wax sections.

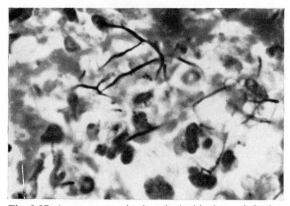

Fig. 9.87. Acute suppurative lymphadenitis due to infection
by *Nocardia asteroides*. The patient developed nocardial
infection of the elbow joint as a sequel of treatment of
'tennis elbow' by injection of hydrocortisone into the tissues
adjoining the lateral epicondyle of the humerus. The
arthritis was followed by regional lymphadenitis, septicaemia
and fatal nocardial meningoencephalitis. The section illustrated is from an axillary node. It shows the fine, branching,
acid-fast filaments of the nocardia. *Ziehl–Neelsen.* × 1200.

* The streptomycetes, *Streptomyces madurae, Streptomyces pelletieri* and *Streptomyces somaliensis*, which are
among the causes of mycetoma, were formerly considered to
belong to the genus *Nocardia* and some authorities still
hold this view.

Lymphadenitis in Cases of Nocardial Mycetoma.—
Slight enlargement of the regional lymph nodes is
often found in cases of longstanding mycetoma,
whether caused by actinomycetes or true fungi (see
page 628), and whether or not there is a significant
degree of secondary bacterial infection. Progressive
enlargement of the regional nodes, due to their
infection by the organism responsible for the
mycetoma, is observed only in exceptional cases; it
usually leads to early breakdown of the nodes, with
the formation of one or more sinuses. Of all the
causes of mycetoma, *Nocardia brasiliensis* is the one
likeliest to give rise to this complication; the
streptomycetes do so less frequently, but often
enough for this to be a development familiar to those
who see many patients with such mycetomas; true
fungi that cause mycetoma are seldom found to
involve the nodes. The lymphadenitis of nocardial
mycetoma is characterized by chronic suppuration,
with well-marked fibrosis round the abscesses in the
cases of long standing and the development of
sinuses that open through the skin. The colonial
grains of the nocardiae are comparatively seldom
large enough to be detected by the unaided eye, in
contrast to the so-called 'sulphur granule' colonies
of *Actinomyces israelii* and the sometimes massive
colonies of the madurellae. The nocardial colony
may even be so ill-defined and inconspicuous in
haematoxylin–eosin preparations that it escapes
notice: characteristically, it is a rounded or coil-like
structure, dull mauve, soft of outline and lying free
among the pus cells (Fig. 9.88).

Streptomycosis

The species of streptomycete that cause mycetomas
have been named in the footnote on this page. In the
rare instances in which they infect the regional nodes
draining the mycetoma the pathological changes
are comparable to those of the lymphadenitis of
nocardial mycetoma (see above), except for the
appearance of the colonies of the organisms, which
is peculiar to each species (Figs 9.89 to 9.91).[445]

Lymphadenitis Accompanying Infection Caused by True Fungi

Superficial Mycoses

The dermatomycoses, in which the infection is
ordinarily confined to the epidermis, hair and nails,
and the usual forms of candidosis, which involve the
superficial epithelium of mucous membranes, particularly those of the body's orifices, are seldom
accompanied by lymphadenitis. The rare occurrence

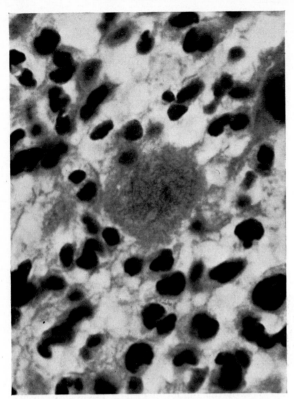

Fig. 9.88. A colony of *Nocardia brasiliensis* in an abscess in a cervical lymph node draining the site of a subcutaneous nocardial mycetoma. Mycetomas are very rarely accompanied by spread of the infection to lymph nodes. The patient was a Norwegian biology student who acquired the infection while trapping wild rodents in Mexico, presumably from contamination of one of the many skin wounds that he suffered from thorny scrubs. The colonies are often more extensive than this comparatively small, globular mass of nocardial filaments. The colonial growth of *Nocardia brasiliensis*, its more delicate filamentous structure and its lack of acid-fastness are among the microscopical features that distinguish it from *Nocardia asteroides*, which very rarely produces colonies in infected tissues. See Fig. 9.87. *Haematoxylin–eosin.* × 1500.

of enlargement of the regional lymph nodes in such cases is usually, if not always, a manifestation of non-specific lymphadenitis, in consequence of the inflammatory reaction in the skin or mucosae to the presence of the fungus or to scratching or the application of irritant drugs. In such instances, histological examination shows a non-specific lymphadenitis or the picture of dermatopathic lymphadenitis (see page 686). Among the fungi that cause dermatomycoses, species of trichophyton have been demonstrated in lymph nodes, but only when lymphadenitis complicates a chronic persistent granulomatous form of trichophytosis of the skin,

which is essentially a deep mycosis, although usually beginning as a simple superficial infection (see below).

Exceptionally, progressive enlargement of lymph nodes in association with a superficial mycosis is the initial manifestation of invasion of the deeper tissues by the fungus. *Trichophyton* species and *Candida* species may penetrate surface epithelia and set up progressive infection of the underlying tissues—and, eventually, of distant tissues—if the natural resistance of the body is lowered by disease or treatment that interferes with immunity. Trichophytic lymph-

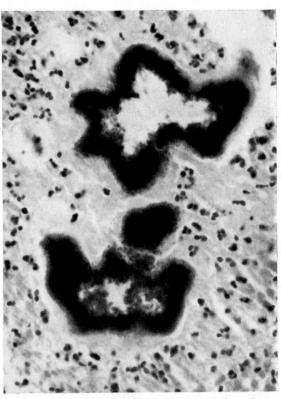

Fig. 9.89. Two colonies of *Streptomyces madurae* in an abscess in an inguinal lymph node draining a mycetoma of a foot caused by this organism. The irregular, ring-like growth, with dissolution of the core of the colony as it enlarges peripherally, and the intense haematoxyphilia are features that enable this species to be identified in histological sections (see Figs 9.88, 9.90 and 9.91). Sometimes the colonies of *Streptomyces madurae* have a well-developed surface zone of club-like projections, the result of precipitation of immunoglobulins and fibrin on the protruding filaments. Like all mycetomas, the streptomycotic infections rarely spread to lymph nodes. The patient was an Indian businessman, living in England when his infection began to be troublesome; it had been acquired in India some years earlier. On his first admission to hospital in England the condition was mistaken for actinomycosis. Compare with Fig. 9.70, page 596. *Haematoxylin–eosin.* × 480.

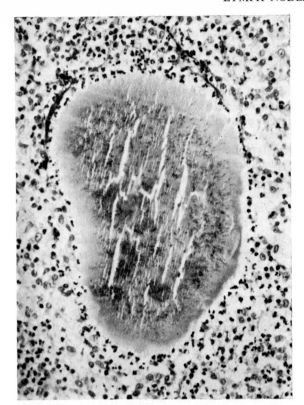

Fig. 9.90. A colony of *Streptomyces somaliensis* in an abscess in an inguinal lymph node draining a mycetoma of a foot caused by this organism. The colony is solid but shows characteristic parallel and crosswise fissuring, a peculiar artefact that is of help in identifying the organism. Another characteristic is the relatively narrow and pale peripheral zone and the faint radial striation immediately deep to it that results from the haematoxyphilia of the surviving filaments. Compare with the other streptomycetes in Figs 9.89 and 9.91. The patient was an Irish missionary who was able to date the infection of the foot to a deep prick by an acacia thorn in his garden in Ethiopia. *Haematoxylin–eosin.* × 215.

adenitis has been an early feature of a few of the very small number of observed cases of 'opportunistic' trichophytosis, preceding the onset of haematogenous dissemination of the infection (see page 621).[446] In cases of 'opportunistic' candidosis, which is appreciably less rare, the infection of the blood stream usually arises directly through the invasion of the mucosal vessels by the fungus as it grows through the tissues underlying the superficial foci of infection;[447] lymphadenitis is a feature in only a small proportion of cases.

Deep Mycoses

Any deep-seated mycosis—that is, a mycosis with ulcerative, visceral or haematogenous lesions—may

be accompanied by lymphadenitis. Some of the deep mycoses are caused by fungi that seldom, if ever, establish an infection unless the patient's resistance has been lowered by pathological or therapeutic conditions that interfere with the body's defences: these are the so-called '*opportunistic*' *mycoses*, which, by definition, are secondary to depression of immunity. Other fungal infections occur without predisposition and may conveniently be referred to as the *primary mycoses*: it is important to note that the conditions that predispose to the occurrence of the 'opportunistic' infections also predispose to the

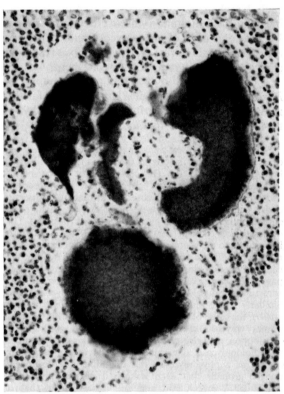

Fig. 9.91. Several portions of an irregularly shaped colony of *Streptomyces pelletieri* in an abscess in an axillary lymph node draining a mycetoma of a hand caused by this organism. The colony is solid, intensely haematoxyphile, with a somewhat denser peripheral zone and in places a fine, sharp linear outline. The intense staining is in part due to the presence of calcium salts, which commonly impregnate the colonies of this organism in tissues, accounting both for the peculiar density of the lesions when seen in radiographs and for the notable grittiness of the exudate. These features enable the organism to be recognized specifically in histological sections. Compare with Figs 9.89 and 9.90. The patient was a European expatriate working in Morocco. He came to hospital for diagnosis and treatment while at home on leave. The condition was mistaken for actinomycosis. *Haematoxylin–eosin.* × 235.

conspicuous histiocytosis characterized by the inclusion of more or less numerous cryptococci in the cytoplasm of mononuclear or multinucleate macrophages, to a tuberculoid reaction, with or without suppuration or caseation. Necrotic tissue may occupy most of the extent of the lesion; there may be heavy calcification. The appearance of the fungal cells is unmistakable when their diameter is within the average range (5 to 15 μm) and they have the characteristic, thick, halo-like, mucicarminophile, mucinous capsule. When the fungal cells are smaller and their mucinous capsule is thin, or apparently lacking, they may be mistaken for other organisms, particularly *Histoplasma capsulatum* and leishmaniae.

Sporotrichosis.—Enlargement of the regional lymph nodes is evident clinically in only a small proportion of cases of sporotrichosis of the skin,[456] which is by far the commonest site of the disease (see Chapter 39). It is an open question whether the clinically enlarged nodes are infected by the sporothrix or are merely a manifestation of non-specific lymphadenitis accompanying the necrotic, ulcerative lesions.[457] Enlargement of nodes is less infrequent in cases of solitary lesions than in the ascending lymphangitic form of cutaneous sporotrichosis. Although the latter is characterized by the slowly progressive proximal extension of the lesions from the site of inoculation along subcutaneous lymphatics, with the development of multiple ulcerating nodules along their course, involvement of lymph nodes is unusual. In cases of lymphangitic sporotrichosis involving a hand and forearm—the commonest distribution—any lymphadenitis is often confined to the supratrochlear node.[458]

The closer the initial lesion in the skin is to the regional nodes, the earlier and likelier is the development of lymphadenitis. The two manifestations may attract clinical attention almost simultaneously in cases of facial sporotrichosis.

The lymph nodes break down and discharge through the skin only in very exceptional cases. In some such instances the sporothrix has been cultured from the nodes.

In those cases in which the sporothrix infection can be proved to have involved the regional lymph nodes, the histological picture is that of a chronic suppurative lymphadenitis, with epithelioid histiocytes and scattered multinucleate giant cells around the foci of suppuration, which often are confluent. 'Asteroids' form about occasional cells of the causative organism, *Sporothrix schenckii*, in some cases, particularly when the infection was acquired

in southern Africa (see Chapter 39, Figs 39.179A and 39.179B). In most cases the organism cannot be seen in conventional histological preparations, even when special stains for fungi are used, including the periodic-acid/Schiff method following digestion by diastase,[440] and the hexamine silver (methenamine silver) method (Fig. 9.93). Isolation of the sporothrix in culture is usually needed for its demonstration.

Chromomycosis.—Cutaneous chromomycosis and subcutaneous chromomycosis (chromomycotic cold abscess) result from direct inoculation of the fungus (*Phialophora* species*) into or through the skin (see

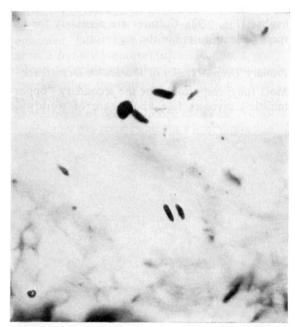

Fig. 9.93. Lymphadenitis in sporotrichosis. Biopsy of the moderately enlarged axillary lymph nodes in a case of localized sporotrichosis of the skin and subcutaneous tissue of the forearm showed an extensive tuberculoid granulomatous reaction with central suppuration in some foci and caseation in others. No asteroids were seen (see text), but—contrary to the usual experience—it was possible to demonstrate the fungal cells in sections stained by the periodic-acid/Schiff method and other 'fungal stains'. The field illustrated includes a large yeast-like form of the fungus, so-called cigar-shaped bodies (that is, cylindrical with pointed ends) and some bacilliform bodies. It is most unusual to be able to demonstrate the sporothrix in these characteristic forms in naturally occurring infections. The fungus was isolated in cultures from this specimen. *Grocott–Gomori hexamine (methenamine) silver.* × 1200.

* Although the genus name *Phialophora* is now widely accepted, some authorities still use such synonyms as *Hormodendrum* and *Fonsecaea*.

Chapter 39). They are most frequent under sub-tropical and tropical conditions, but may be seen as indigenous infections anywhere in the world. Lymphadenitis is a rare accompaniment of chromo-mycosis involving the skin. It has been seen in association with generalized haematogenous dis-semination of the infection in the absence of any evident involvement of the skin.[459] The brown, yeast-like fungal cells are seen in multinucleate giant cells or free in the pus in 'suppurating pseudo-tubercles' (see Chapter 39, Figs 39.180A and 39.180B).

Visceral forms of chromomycosis are rare. The association of lymphadenitis with the visceral lesions has not usually been a feature of published accounts, although there have been exceptions.[459] There was microscopical evidence of involvement of a bronchopulmonary lymph node excised during pulmonary lobectomy in a case of lung abscess caused by *Cladosporium trichoides* or *Cladosporium bantianum*.[387*]

Primary Deep Mycoses of Geographically Restricted Occurrence

The primary deep mycoses that have a more or less restricted distribution are the two types of histo-plasmosis (infection by *Histoplasma capsulatum* and infection by *Histoplasma duboisii*, the African histoplasma), coccidioidomycosis, 'North American' blastomycosis, paracoccidioidomycosis ('South American blastomycosis'), Lôbo's disease, mycet-omas caused by true fungi, subcutaneous phyco-mycosis and entomophthorosis, and a few rarer infections and infections by organisms that have not yet been identified. Lymphadenitis may develop in any of these conditions, either incidentally or as a clinically important manifestation.

Histoplasmosis.†—Infection by *Histoplasma cap-sulatum* is widely distributed throughout the

---

* *Cladosporium bantianum*, having been regarded in the 3rd edition of the *Medical Research Council Memorandum No. 23 (Nomenclature of Fungi Pathogenic to Man and Animals;* London, 1967) as a synonym of *Cladosporium trichoides*, is now again considered to be probably a distinct species (*Medical Research Council Memorandum No. 23*, 4th edn; London, 1977 [in press]).

† Generally, when the name histoplasmosis is used without qualification it is understood to mean histoplasmosis due to infection by *Histoplasma capsulatum;* infection by *Histo-plasma duboisii* is then usually described as African histo-plasmosis. However, in those parts of Africa where the latter is the more familiar in practice it is often referred to simply as histoplasmosis: doctors elsewhere may find this misleading until they learn the local usage.

Americas and in Africa, and in parts of southern Asia. It is rare, or does not occur at all under natural conditions, in the rest of the world. Its prevalence depends essentially on whether the environment can support the saprophytic phase of the fungus, which alone is the source of the infective conidia. Differences in environmental conditions, still only partly understood, account for the remark-able fact that an infection that is endemic throughout so much of North America, and that has been estimated to have affected at least 20 per cent of the population of the United States,[460] is not indigenous in, for instance, north-western Europe, including Britain and Ireland.

Lymphadenitis is probably the rule in cases of histoplasmosis in the initial stage. The primary focus of infection is ordinarily in the lungs and may be solitary or multiple and bilateral (see page 335): correspondingly, the associated bronchopulmonary lymphadenitis may be unilateral or bilateral. Just as in the course of the primary complex of tuberculosis (see page 332), the caseous nodes of the primary complex of histoplasmosis may compress bronchi or pulmonary blood vessels, or erode into their lumen, causing dissemination of the infection through the bronchial tree or by the blood stream throughout the body.[461] Sometimes the infected nodes form solid or pseudocystic masses up to 10 cm or so in greatest dimension.[462] Eventually, the caseous material becomes heavily calcified. When the foci of caseation have been discrete, confined to the centre of tuberculoid granulomas that have not become confluent, the resulting calcification has a similarly discrete and scattered character that gives a stippled appearance to both the naked eye and the radiological appear-ances of the nodes.[461] Comparable lymphadenitis develops in the regional nodes draining the site of a primary focus of histoplasmic infection of the skin,[463] which in exceptional cases may be the portal, particularly by accidental inoculation in the course of laboratory work.

Histoplasmic infection of lymph nodes may also be seen as an accompaniment of chronic ulcerative and visceral lesions that may follow the primary stage of the disease. It is inconstant in such cases, and there is often little to see macroscopically except for some enlargement of the nodes. Similarly, lymph nodes may be involved in the course of generalized haematogenous histoplasmosis, which occurs often-est as a consequence of a breakdown in immunity in the presence of diseases that interfere with the body's defences (for example, Hodgkin's disease and leukaemia) and as a complication of treatment of these or other diseases with cytotoxic drugs and other resistance-lowering agents.

Histologically, the reaction in the nodes ranges from histiocytosis (Fig. 9.94), with or without multinucleate cells, to a sclerosing tuberculoid granuloma closely resembling that of sarcoidosis but for the presence of the parasites in the cytoplasm of some proportion of the cells. Caseation, which is usually present in the nodes of the primary complex, may be confined to the centre of the discrete tuberculoid lesions or may become confluent and extend through most of the substance of the enlarged nodes. The histoplasmas, which in most cases are very abundant, are for the most part intracellular (Figs 9.94, 9.95A and 9.95B); they are readily seen in haematoxylin–eosin preparations in the majority of cases of active, progressive infection, but organisms that have been dead for some time—for instance, in caseous lesions—may be overlooked unless special methods for their demonstration, particularly the hexamine silver procedure (see page 616), are used (Figs 9.96A and 9.96B).

Care is needed to distinguish between *Histoplasma capsulatum*, the small forms of *Paracoccidioides brasiliensis* and of *Cryptococcus neoformans* (see page 622), leishmaniae,[464] and even small vacuoles and small birefringent ovoid inclusions that are

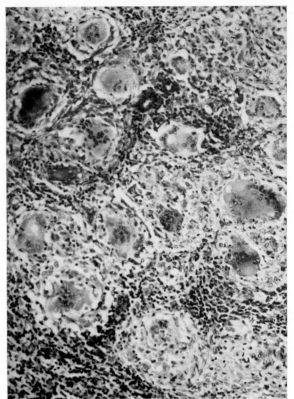

Fig. 9.95A. Another instance of histoplasmic lymphadenitis. Tuberculoid granulomatous reaction, with numerous large multinucleate giant cells. See Fig. 9.95B. *Haematoxylin–eosin.* × 140.

sometimes to be found in macrophages, particularly multinucleate giant cells, in any tuberculoid granuloma.

*African Histoplasmosis.**—Histoplasmosis caused by *Histoplasma duboisii* has been recognized only in the tropical belt of Africa, and particularly in its central and western parts. The source and mode of infection are still unknown. The fact that in some cases there has been good circumstantial evidence that the disease originated from inoculation of the skin does not exclude the possibility that, as in histoplasmosis caused by *Histoplasma capsulatum* (see above) and other primary systemic mycoses, the initial lesion is ordinarily in the lungs.

Lymphadenitis accompanies the cutaneous lesions in some cases, and particularly those in which the history suggests the possibility of infection by inoculation. The regional nodes are moderately or considerably enlarged and they may break down,

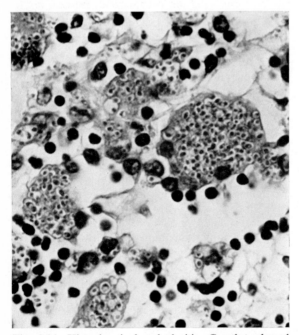

Fig. 9.94. Histoplasmic lymphadenitis. Greatly enlarged endothelial macrophages in a sinus. Their cytoplasm contains large numbers of rounded and ovoid, encapsulate organisms (*Histoplasma capsulatum*). See Figs 9.95A, 9.95B and 9.96B. *Periodic-acid/Schiff; Mayer's haemalum.* × 670.

* See footnote on page 623.

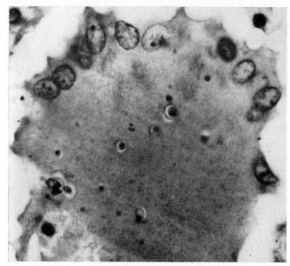

Fig. 9.95B. Same specimen as Fig. 9.95A, showing sparse histoplasmas in the cytoplasm of a multinucleate giant cell. The organisms could be seen in the haematoxylin–eosin preparations but were more easily demonstrated by 'fungal stains'. The patient acquired his infection in Britain; there was strong presumptive evidence that the infection was carried from North America through fomites (see: Symmers, W. St C., *Brit. med. J.*, 1956, **2**, 786). *Periodic-acid/Schiff; Mayer's haemalum.* × 860.

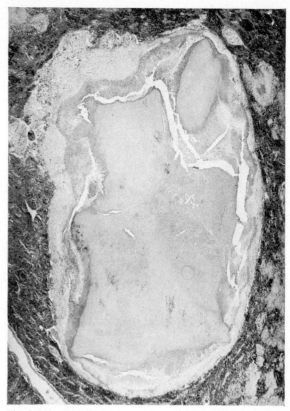

Fig. 9.96A. Encapsulate, caseous mass in a pulmonary hilar lymph node. The lesion was indistinguishable from the corresponding tuberculous lesion in this situation, until examination with the help of the hexamine silver stain showed it to be a manifestation of histoplasmosis. See Fig. 9.96B. *Haematoxylin–eosin.* × 9.

with the formation of sinuses and large ulcerated granulomas. In many instances there is no evident lymphadenitis, whether the presenting manifestations are cutaneous, skeletal or—least common—visceral. In cases of fatal disseminated disease it is usual to find widespread involvement of the nodes throughout the body,[465] probably as a result of haematogenous extension. Exceptionally, African histoplasmosis presents with lymph node enlargement and no other manifestations.[466]

The most characteristic feature of the histological reaction in most cases is the presence of large numbers of quite closely packed multinucleate giant cells of the so-called foreign body type, all of them containing several histoplasmas (Fig. 9.97). There are some mononuclear macrophages between the giant cells and there is a variable tendency to fibrosis. Necrosis is commonly seen and may be accompanied by suppuration or spreading caseation. The fungal cells are much larger than cells of *Histoplasma capsulatum*. They are round or, oftener, ovoid and they measure about 7 to 12 μm in their larger dimension. They have a well-formed cell wall and this encloses the cytoplasm, which often appears shrunken because of the effects of histological processing; sometimes a distinct nucleus is seen.

Histoplasma duboisii has been mistaken for

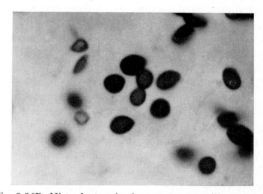

Fig. 9.96B. Histoplasmas in the caseous mass illustrated in Fig. 9.96A. The appearances are typical of *Histoplasma capsulatum*. The hexamine silver procedure can demonstrate histoplasmas that other methods fail to indicate, even fungal cells that are long dead taking the stain. *Grocott–Gomori hexamine (methenamine) silver.* × 1500.

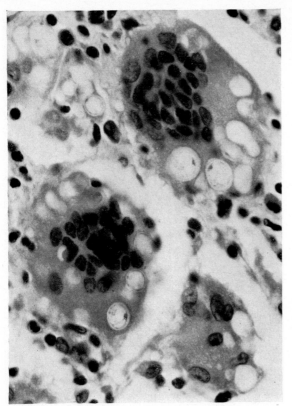

Fig. 9.97. African histoplasmosis. Three multinucleate giant cells, of 'foreign body' type, are seen in the sinus of a lymph node. The large, ovoid structures in the cytoplasm are cells of *Histoplasma duboisii*, an organism substantially larger than *Histoplasma capsulatum* (see Fig. 9.94). They have a distinct but fine double contour. *Haematoxylin–eosin.* × 650.

Blastomyces dermatitidis, Paracoccidioides brasiliensis, Loboa loboi and *Cryptococcus neoformans* in histological preparations. Apart from the patient's geographical history, which may help conclusively in eliminating some of these possibilities, all four organisms that have been confused with the African histoplasma can usually be seen in budding forms in the tissues, while the cryptococcus, when large enough to be of the same range of size as the African histoplasma, always has a well-formed, halo-like capsule of mucicarminophile material. Of all these conditions, infection by *Blastomyces dermatitidis* is likeliest to be confused with infection by *Histoplasma duboisii* because both diseases occur in the same geographical region.

Coccidioidomycosis.—A primary complex, with bronchopulmonary lymphadenitis, is less frequent in cases of primary pulmonary coccidioidomycosis (see page 358) than in those of primary pulmonary

histoplasmosis (see above).[467] In contrast, there is almost always a well-marked regional lymphadenitis in those comparatively rare cases in which the initial lesion of coccidioidomycosis is in the skin, in consequence of direct inoculation.[468] In cases of disseminated haematogenous coccidioidomycosis, lymph node involvement is the rule, but is merely one manifestation among many of the generalization of the infection.

The histological changes in the infected nodes range from occasional tuberculoid foci, often with central suppuration, to extensive caseating and fibrosing lesions, maybe with heavy calcification. The spherules are easily seen in haematoxylin–eosin preparations: their diameter varies widely, and there are always some that are filled with endospores (Fig. 9.98), although these may have to be searched for.

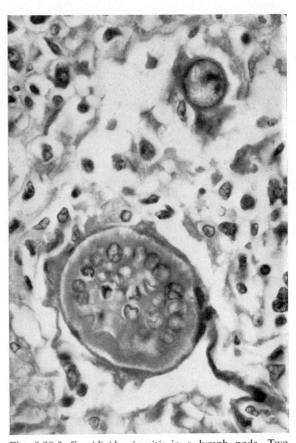

Fig. 9.98.§ *Coccidioides immitis* in a lymph node. Two spherules are seen, the larger containing endospores. From a case of coccidioidomycosis diagnosed in Britain and presenting atypically with bilateral axillary lymphadenitis as the only clinical manifestation (Case 2 in: Symmers, W. St C., in *Coccidioidomycosis*, edited by L. Ajello, page 301; Tucson, Arizona, 1967). *Haemaioxylin–eosin.* × 750.

The only fungal structures that are occasionally confused with the endosporulating form of the coccidioides are the sporangium of *Rhinosporidium seeberi* (see Fig. 4.13, page 211), which in exceptional cases may infect lymph nodes, and the sporangium of such 'opportunistic' phycomycetes as *Rhizopus* species (see Fig. 4.11, page 209). The sporangia of the rhizopus can form only when the mould is growing in a superficial lesion, exposed to air: from the practical point of view confusion with the coccidioides should not arise.

'North American' Blastomycosis.*—It seems that lymphadenitis is a comparatively rare accompaniment of the primary focus of blastomycotic infection in the lungs,[469] although it occurs more regularly in those infrequent cases in which the disease starts with inoculation of the organism into the skin.[470] The latter pathway is now recognized to be rare, although for many years it was believed to be the usual one. The lesions in lymph nodes may be of only microscopical dimensions.

Blastomyces dermatitidis multiplies in infected tissue by budding. The bud is solitary (see Fig. 7.51, page 359), a point that distinguishes this organism from *Paracoccidioides brasiliensis*, which forms buds over much of the surface of the parent cell. The need to differentiate between *Blastomyces dermatitidis* and *Histoplasma duboisii* has been mentioned above.

The tissue reaction is characteristically a tuberculoid granuloma with central suppuration ('suppurating pseudotubercle'). The lesions are of miliary size, but they tend to become confluent. Some are predominantly suppurative, the fungal cells lying free in the exudate. Elsewhere the fungi are within the

---

* The disease that is caused by *Blastomyces dermatitidis* has long been known as North American blastomycosis, this name serving both to distinguish it from 'European blastomycosis' (an occasional synonym of cryptococcosis—see footnote on page 621) and from 'South American blastomycosis' (paracoccidioidomycosis—see this page) and to intimate that it was recognized in, and believed to be confined to, North America. The geographical designation has proved to be inappropriate, for the disease is now known to be prevalent throughout much of Africa, from the Mediterranean coast to South Africa and from the Atlantic coast to the Red Sea and the Indian Ocean. Although mycologists are now arguing about the validity of the name *Blastomyces dermatitidis*, it seems reasonable to continue, at least for the present, to refer to the disease as blastomycosis (if this is felt to be ambiguous, in view of the continuing currency of 'South American blastomycosis' as a synonym of paracoccidioidomycosis and in view of the occasional use of 'chromoblastomycosis' as a synonym of chromomycosis, perhaps 'North American' blastomycosis is the preferable name).

cytoplasm of macrophages, including multinucleate giant cells. Caseation necrosis is less characteristic than suppuration, and tends to be seen particularly in the nodes draining the primary focus: often the caseous matter, when sections are stained appropriately, proves to consist in large part of the remains of dead fungal cells, which fail to show well in haematoxylin–eosin preparations but continue to be readily demonstrable by the hexamine silver (methenamine silver) method.

Paracoccidioidomycosis ('South American Blastomycosis').—Infection by *Paracoccidioides brasiliensis* may be found in almost all parts of South and Central America and in Mexico; it has not been recognized as an indigenous disease in any other part of the world. Its portal of entry into the body was long considered to be the mucous membrane of the mouth, throat and nose, and occasionally the skin, but evidence is collecting that the initial lesion is usually pulmonary.[471] Lymphadenitis is a common but not a constant accompaniment of the primary pulmonary disease:[472] when present, it is usually of no more than microscopical extent. In contrast, there may be conspicuous lymphadenitis in cases of primary infection by inoculation of the skin or mucous membranes, and in association with the mucocutaneous lesions—for instance, round the mouth and anus—that are now supposed to result from haematogenous dissemination of the fungi from a pulmonary focus.

Paracoccidioidomycosis may present with ulcerating mucosal or cutaneous granulomas accompanied by lymphadenitis, as in the original case described by Lutz in São Paulo, in Brazil, in 1905;[473] rarely, it presents with enlargement of lymph nodes and no other apparent manifestations.[474] There is also an unusual syndrome of intestinal malabsorption associated with marked enlargement of the abdominal lymph nodes, due to their infection by the paracoccidioides in the absence of other evidence of paracoccidioidomycosis.[475]

The fungus appears in tissues in two main forms. The more characteristic is a large yeast-like cell, 8 to 15 μm in diameter, with multiple small buds protruding outward from its surface (Fig. 9.99). When there are no buds, this type of cell may be mistaken for *Blastomyces dermatitidis* or for *Cryptococcus neoformans*, although the absence of the mucinous 'halo' should distinguish it from the latter. The other form is a small cell, often quite indistinguishable from *Histoplasma capsulatum*, except by the presence elsewhere of the larger cells with their multiple buds. The small cell, like the histoplasma, is found

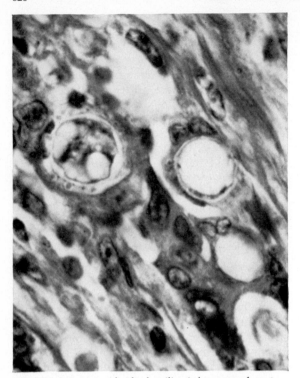

Fig. 9.99.§ *Paracoccidioides brasiliensis* in a granulomatous focus in the spleen. The multiplicity of buds at the periphery of the fungal cell above and to the left of the centre of the field is characteristic of this organism. The same phenomenon is seen, but not so strikingly, in the cell to the right of the centre. The cells at the bottom left and right lack buds. Same specimen as Fig. 9.131, page 679. *Haematoxylin–eosin.* × 1200.

within the cytoplasm of macrophages, which may be heavily parasitized.

Lôbo's Disease ('Keloidal Blastomycosis').—Lôbo's disease,[476] which is commonly referred to also as 'lobomycosis', has been recognized hitherto only in the tropical forest regions of the northern parts of South America and in parts of Central America.[477] The fungus that causes it has not yet been acceptably classified and is still known by various names, among them *Loboa loboi*, *Paracoccidioides loboi*, *Blastomyces loboi* and *Glenosporella loboi*. In infected tissue the organism resembles *Blastomyces dermatitidis* in size and general appearance, and in reproducing by the formation of a solitary bud; its tendency to grow in chain-like rows of cells is an occasional peculiarity that may help to identify it.

The infection is confined to the skin, forming firm, flat, tumour-like lesions ('keloid' lesions) that later may become verrucose, resembling the verrucose lesions of cutaneous chromomycosis. The lesions have little tendency to become ulcerated. They may be solitary or multiple, and they are thought to result from direct inoculation of the fungus. In some cases the infection spreads to the regional lymph nodes,[478] with or without clinically evident nodules along the course of the subcutaneous lymphatics. Visceral lesions have not been recognized, and the condition seems to have little, if any, effect on the patient's general health.

A condition quite comparable to Lôbo's disease has been recognized in dolphins from the Atlantic Ocean off the coast of Florida and from the Gulf of Mexico.[479] The fungus responsible is *Loboa loboi*. A dolphin is thought to have been the source of infection in the case of what is probably the first instance of Lôbo's disease to originate outside the endemic area of Central and South America.[480] The patient was an attendant at an aquarium in Europe who, about 3 months before the first sign of his infection, had helped to look after a dolphin that had recently been caught in the nets of a fishing boat in the Bay of Biscay. There were ulcerated and verrucose lesions on several areas of the animal's skin. The patient's lesion was a well-defined, indurated thickening of the skin of the dorsum of one hand, without ulceration. The supratrochlear lymph node was enlarged, tender and firm. There was no history of injury. Fungi with appearances consistent with those of *Loboa loboi* were present in the tuberculoid granuloma in histological specimens of the dolphin's lesions and of the patient's skin lesion and supratrochlear node (Fig. 9.100). Cultures were not obtained.

Mycetoma.*—Any mycetoma may be accompanied by a non-specific regional lymphadenitis. Very occasionally the organism responsible for the mycetoma is carried to the nodes and sets up a specific infection. Specific lymphadenitis accompanying mycetoma may be seen in any variety of mycetoma, whether caused by an actinomycete (see page 617) or by a true fungus. The true fungi are notably less likely to spread by way of the lymphatics, perhaps because of the larger size of their elements and of their greater tendency to grow cohesively, in the form of colonies that show little evidence of the

---

* The term mycetoma continues to be misapplied to fungal 'ball colonies' that form in cavities in the lungs—for instance, the familiar colony of an aspergillus in an old tuberculous cavity (see page 350). Such colonies should be referred to as aspergillomas, penicilliomas, and so forth, and the word mycetoma should be used only of the chronic granulomas with sinus formation that are considered here and in Chapter 39 (see footnote on page 347).

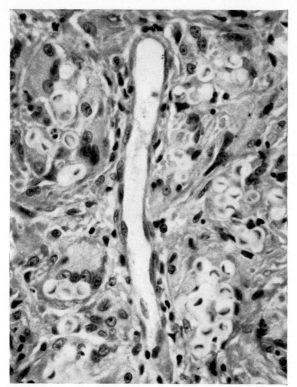

Fig. 9.100. Lymphadenitis associated with Lôbo's disease. The field is from a granulomatous focus that replaced part of the affected node. The cells of the granuloma are mostly multinucleate giant cells; there are a few mononuclear macrophages, plasma cells and lymphocytes among them. The yeast-like fungal cells are loosely clustered in the cytoplasm of the giant cells, and the picture is similar to that characteristic of the African form of histoplasmosis (*Histoplasma duboisii* infection—see Fig. 9.97). *Haematoxylin–eosin*. × 370.

type of superficial outgrowth that, in the case of actinomycetous colonies, leads to separation of bacilliform fragments, encouraging dispersal of the infection.

Of the true fungi that cause mycetomas, the madurellae (*Madurella mycetomi* and *Madurella grisea*) and *Allescheria boydii* (*Monosporium apiospermum*, *Petriellidium boydii*) are those least rarely found in the regional lymph nodes. It may be noted that *Allescheria boydii*, unlike the various other true fungi that are responsible for these lesions, is probably of worldwide distribution; it has been recognized as the cause of an indigenous mycetoma in Britain (see Chapter 39, Fig. 39.183).[481]

The histological picture in infected lymph nodes is essentially the same as that in the initial lesion. Chronic suppuration, with multiple sinuses and extensive fibrosis, and often the formation of tuberculoid granulomatous foci, is characteristic. In many instances the fungus can be identified generically, even specifically, from the appearance of its colonies.

Nothing is gained clinically by biopsy of lymph nodes that are thought to be possibly infected in cases of unequivocal mycetoma. If there is doubt about the nature of a primary mycetoma-like lesion, it should be itself the subject of further investigation. Excision of a lymph node that proves to be infected by the actinomycete or fungus concerned has been followed by the development of persistent sinuses and typical mycetomatous lesions in the biopsy wound in more than half the cases in which I have known this procedure to be adopted. A biopsy operation, as far as lymph nodes are concerned, is contraindicated. Moreover, enlargement of regional lymph nodes in association with a mycetoma is oftener due to non-specific lymphadenitis than to spread of the fungal (or actinomycetous) infection to the nodes.

Primary Subcutaneous Phycomycosis (Basidiobolomycosis).—Primary subcutaneous phycomycosis, which is caused by *Basidiobolus meristosporus*,* probably results from inoculation of the fungus into the tissues, an aetiological factor that it has in common with the mycetomas, sporotrichosis, and cutaneous and subcutaneous chromomycosis. It is generally to be regarded as a tropical disease; it was originally described in Indonesia[482] and is widely prevalent in other tropical regions of Asia, but it is recognized most frequently in Africa. Two cases have been recorded in which the infection was acquired in temperate regions (England[483] and Germany[484]).

The infection is ordinarily confined to the subcutaneous tissue, in which it spreads slowly, widely and in continuity. The regional lymph nodes are seldom enlarged; when they are, there is usually no evidence as to the cause of the enlargement. In two cases in which I have seen invasion of lymph nodes by the fungus, the nodes themselves were in regions into which the subcutaneous disease had spread directly, involving and incorporating them as it did

* The name *Basidiobolus meristosporus* (Greer, D. L., Friedman, L., *Sabouraudia*, 1965–66, **4**, 231) has been miscopied, through my own editorial unmindfulness, as *Basidiobolus meristophorus* (Symmers, W. St C., *Ann. Soc. belge Méd. trop.*, 1972, **52**, 365; this book, 2nd edn, vol. 1, pages 208 and 352, 1976). An outcome of this error exemplifies the difficulty of maintaining consistency of nomenclature: the erroneous rendering of the species name has already been perpetuated, in good faith, by others who were misled by its publication. '*On ne peut que s'excuser sans se disculper*'.

so. Some of the nodes remained unaffected within their capsule; the fungus had breached the capsule of others, invading their substance and converting it to the sclerosing inflammatory mass characteristic of the reaction of the tissues in this disease. The appearance of the fungus in sections of infected tissue is distinctive, its hyphae typically enclosed in a sleeve of eosinophile precipitate (see Chapter 39, Fig. 39.181). The tissue reaction comprises accumulation of macrophages, eosinophils and neutrophils, in varying proportions; there are quite extensive areas of necrosis in some cases, and there is an overall tendency to fibrosis.

Entomophthorosis (Rhinoentomophthoromycosis; 'Rhinophycomycosis'*).—Lymph node involvement has not been observed in the published cases of this uncommon disease of the nasal region, caused by the phycomycete *Entomophthora coronata*. In an exceptional case in which the infection had spread from the nose and nasal sinuses to the lungs[485] there was involvement of the bronchopulmonary and tracheobronchial lymph nodes: the appearances in the affected nodes were similar to those in the cases of basidiobolus infection of nodes involved in subcutaneous phycomycosis (see above).

Rhinosporidiosis.—Lymphadenitis seldom accompanies rhinosporidiosis. When it is present it is usually a manifestation of non-specific inflammation in association with ulceration and possibly secondary bacterial infection of the rhinosporidial lesions in the nose or nasal sinuses (see page 210) or, occasionally, in other parts of the body, particularly the conjunctiva or the external genitalia. The only instance of specific rhinosporidial lymphadenitis that I know of was in a case in which the infection had spread from the nose to the larynx, trachea and bronchi, with the eventual development of fatal staphylococcal pneumonia. There were extensive rhinosporidial lesions in both lungs, mainly in the vicinity of the bronchi, and typical rhinosporidial sporangia (see Fig. 4.13, page 211) were found in bronchopulmonary lymph nodes on both sides.

Multiple Infections in Cases of Primary Deep Mycoses.—The 'opportunistic', or secondary, mycoses tend to occur together because the factors that predispose to the occurrence of any 'opportunistic' infection tend to predispose to others

equally, with the result that in quite a considerable proportion of cases there is generalized infection by more than one species of fungus.[486]

It is unusual to see cases in which more than one primary deep mycosis is present. The associations that may be found reflect the range of pathogenic fungal flora that is present in a given geographical area. Difficult diagnostic problems may thus arise, both in clinical practice and in the laboratory. Among the combinations that have been observed are *Histoplasma capsulatum* infection and 'North American' blastomycosis,[487] *Histoplasma capsulatum* infection and *Histoplasma duboisii* infection,[488] *Histoplasma capsulatum* infection and paracoccidioidomycosis,[472] paracoccidioidomycosis and Lôbo's disease,[489] paracoccidioidomycosis and cryptococcosis,[490] coccidioidomycosis and cryptococcosis,[491] and others.

Sometimes, when resistance is lowered by other diseases and their treatment, an 'opportunistic' mycosis may be associated with dissemination of a previously dormant primary mycosis. In a recent case, in Ireland, generalized haematogenous aspergillosis and candidosis were associated with generalized haematogenous infection by *Histoplasma capsulatum* and by *Coccidioides immitis*, the two latter infections having presumably been acquired during residence in the United States of America some years earlier.[488] The patient was under treatment for chronic lymphocytic leukaemia.

Involvement of lymph nodes in the course of multiple infections is unlikely to be of practical importance, in clinical terms, for usually it will not be recognized prior to post-mortem examination. In any case, the examination of single nodes is unlikely to disclose the range of infections present. Nevertheless, it is important to remember that multiple infections may occur, and that the therapeutic requirements may then be correspondingly more complex.

The association of a mycosis with tuberculosis or other mycobacteriosis has also been observed repeatedly.

Lymphadenitis Caused by *Pneumocystis carinii*

Pneumocystis carinii, which some authorities believe may be a fungus while others consider it to be a protozoon, is very rarely seen outside the lungs (see page 360). In the exceptional cases, the extrapulmonary sites of the infection have been predominantly tissues of the lymphoreticular system, particularly lymph nodes, spleen and bone marrow.[492] Hypogammaglobulinaemia has been

---

* The name rhinophycomycosis should not be used as a synonym of entomophthorosis as it has been applied also to 'opportunistic' phycomycosis of the nasal sinuses caused by species of *Rhizopus*, *Absidia* and *Mucor*, particularly as a complication of severe diabetes mellitus (see page 208).

present in most cases, and in the others treatment with cytotoxic or immunosuppressant drugs, or corticosteroids, appears to have been a predisposing factor. Other 'opportunistic' infections have been present in several of the cases, particularly cytomegalovirus infection (see pages 324 and 646), which is so often associated with pneumocystis pneumonia, both in infancy and in later life.

The infection is readily recognized in haematoxylin–eosin preparations of lymph nodes, in which it presents as irregularly rounded, pale foci in the superficial cortex, abutting on the subcapsular sinus (Fig. 9.101). These foci range up to 3 mm or so

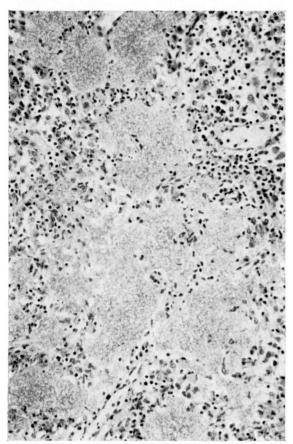

Fig. 9.101.§ Lymphadenitis caused by *Pneumocystis carinii*. The collections of the parasite have a characteristic, finely foamy appearance. They form mainly in the cortex adjacent to the subcapsular sinus, which may be involved, and the lymphoid tissue is displaced by their growth. They elicit remarkably little reaction; in particular, it is very unusual to see any host cells within the colonies. Some of the collections are outlined by a layer of epithelioid histiocytes. Elsewhere, immunoblasts and plasma cells are found in small numbers in their vicinity. Compare with the picture of pneumocystis infection of the lungs (Fig. 7.53, page 361). See also Fig. 9.102. *Haematoxylin–eosin.* × 160.

across. When seen under the higher powers of the microscope they have a characteristically foamy appearance, exactly reproducing the appearance that is seen within the infected pulmonary alveoli in cases of pneumocystis pneumonia (see Fig. 7.53, page 361). The foci give a positive periodic-acid/Schiff reaction. The organisms are demonstrated most easily in hexamine silver (methenamine silver) preparations (Fig. 9.102).

Lymphadenitis Caused by Algae

Infection by algae is very rare. The only genus known to cause disease in man is *Prototheca*.[493, 494] The lesions have been cutaneous in the published cases, with the exception of one in which the infection eventually spread from the skin to the regional lymph nodes.[494a] In one of the two cases that I have seen, biopsy of the lesion of the skin[494b] was followed within a few weeks by progressive painful enlargement of the regional nodes; biopsy of the latter showed the characteristic organisms within tuberculoid granulomas (Fig. 9.103). The algal cells are round or ovoid and range from 8 to 30 μm in their longest dimension. They reproduce by internal sporulation, and may contain from two to several daughter cells, which have flattened surfaces where they abut one on another (see also Chapter 39, Fig. 39.191).

The absence of external budding distinguishes the algal cells from *Blastomyces dermatitidis* and *Paracoccidioides brasiliensis*. The large size, relatively small number and flattened surfaces of the daughter cells make it unlikely that the alga could be mistaken for the endosporulating spherules of *Coccidioides immitis*.

Lymphadenitis Caused by Rickettsiae

There may be a moderate enlargement of the lymph nodes throughout the body in any form of rickettsial infection, and this is commonly accompanied by some degree, usually slight, of splenomegaly. In some forms of rickettsial disease, in which there is a local lesion at the site of inoculation of the organism into the skin, regional lymphadenitis is a conspicuous feature of the clinical picture.

In epidemic typhus fever (exanthematic or classic typhus; louse-borne typhus), which is caused by *Rickettsia prowazekii*, the severity of the illness is such that the accompanying lymphadenopathy is an insignificant detail in its course. In the mild, chronic, endemic form of typhus that is known as Brill's disease,[495] Brill–Zinsser disease[496] or 'larval

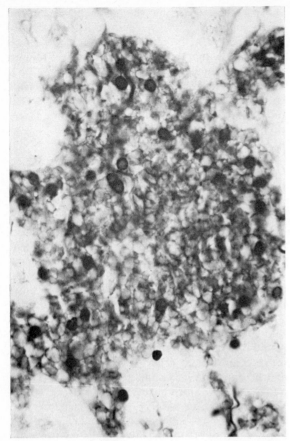

Fig. 9.102. Lymphadenitis caused by *Pneumocystis carinii*. Another case. It often is difficult to demonstrate the individual organisms clearly. The material in the fine interstices between them contains mucopolysaccharides and gives a moderately intense periodic-acid/Schiff reaction. It also blackens diffusely in hexamine silver preparations. Its presence tends to obscure the minority of the organisms that may have an affinity for these reagents, but with care these can be seen as darker, well-defined, round or ovoid bodies, sometimes lying in pairs: several organisms are visible in the field illustrated. The organisms that do not show well may be dead. *Grocott–Gomori hexamine (methenamine) silver.* × 700.

typhus', first recognized among the immigrant Jewish population of New York City in 1898, and also caused by *Rickettsia prowazekii*, slight enlargement of the lymph nodes may be the clue to the diagnosis; even in patients without symptoms the rickettsia has sometimes been recoverable from such nodes.

In endemic murine typhus (flea-borne typhus), caused by *Rickettsia mooseri* and of worldwide distribution, the much milder clinical illness may mean that the moderate generalized lymph node enlargement, when present, is likelier to be observed. Comparable lymph node enlargement was occasion-

ally noted in cases of trench fever ('five-day fever'), caused by *Rickettsia quintana* and epidemic in the battle zones of Europe in both world wars.

Generalized enlargement of lymph nodes is often a notable clinical feature in cases of American tick-borne typhus (Rocky Mountains spotted fever), which is caused by *Rickettsia rickettsii*. In the North American form of this disease there is no lesion in the skin at the site of the bite by which the infection

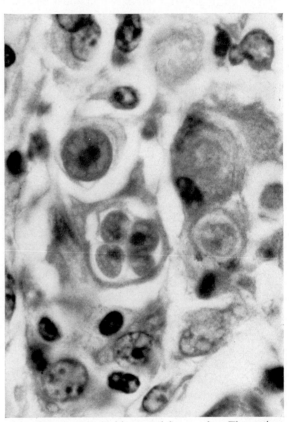

Fig. 9.103. Lymphadenitis caused by an alga. The patient was a German technician working in Britain who had had a verrucose thickening in the skin of the dorsum of one foot for 5 years. Biopsy of the skin lesion showed the presence of an organism that was identified morphologically as a prototheca. Within a few weeks the lymph nodes of the lateral axillary group had become enlarged and tender. Lymph node biopsy showed the picture illustrated. In this field there are several algae within macrophages and one free in the tissue space. One of the parasites has undergone internal division with the formation of four daughter cells ('autospores'). The tissue reaction throughout the infected tissue was characterized by a simple accumulation of macrophages, including multinucleate cells, with occasionally some semblance of tuberculoid granuloma formation. Cultures were not obtained. The disease was treated by surgical excision; there has been no recurrence during 6 years following the operations. *Haematoxylin–eosin.* × 1200.

was initiated; in the South American form, particularly in the State of Minas Gerais, in Brazil, a small ulcer develops at the inoculation site and this is accompanied by regional lymphadenitis, as in European and African tick-borne typhus (see below).

In contrast to the rickettsial infections mentioned already, in which lymphadenitis is usually relatively inconspicuous, enlargement of lymph nodes is a characteristic feature of the European form of tick-borne typhus (*fièvre boutonneuse*—'spotty fever') and of the tick-borne typhus of Africa. These European and African infections are caused by *Rickettsia conorii*. The lymphadenitis is most marked in the regional nodes draining the site of inoculation, which is regularly marked by the development of a small nodule that rapidly undergoes necrosis and ulcerates. Similar tick-borne infections occur in the Far East, where they are caused by *Rickettsia siberica*, and in Queensland, where the cause is *Rickettsia australis*.

The development of a necrotic focus in the skin, at the site of inoculation, and local lymphadenitis are characteristic also of mite-borne typhus (scrub typhus, tsutsugamushi disease,* Japanese river fever) which is caused by *Rickettsia tsutsugamushi* (*Rickettsia orientalis*).[497] The local lymph nodes may become massively enlarged: the mites tend to bite particularly in the region of the head and neck, and it is usually therefore the cervical nodes that are most affected. Later, nodes elsewhere become involved, but their enlargement is never so great.

Another mite-borne rickettsial infection is the so-called rickettsial pox, caused by *Rickettsia akari*. It is endemic in parts of New York and of Boston and some other North American cities, and in parts of the Soviet Union and of Africa. Ulceration at the inoculation site, regional lymphadenitis and a more or less generalized skin eruption are the usual features.[498]

Diagnosis.—Serological studies, particularly the complement fixation and Weil–Felix tests, and, when

* *Tsutsuga-mushi*, in Japanese, means 'misfortune (-bringing) mite', or, at a more popular level, 'evil bug', approximately. *Mushi*, now used to mean a mite, in the sense of a minute living creature, and, more technically, a mite in the sense of an acarine mite, formerly had the same meaning as miasma, an evil (vaporous) emanation that, before microbes were discovered, might be the source of certain diseases. I am obliged to Professor C. J. Dunn, Professor P. G. O'Neill and Mrs Goodliffe, of the School of Oriental and African Studies, University of London, for their interest and help in interpreting the Japanese name of this form of rickettsial infection.

facilities allow, isolation of the causative organism are the means of specific diagnosis. Biopsy is not a generally useful procedure, but in exceptional circumstances examination of sections of an infected lymph node has suggested the possibility of a rickettsial disease when such a diagnosis has not previously been considered.

Histology.[499]—The changes in the lymph nodes are essentially the same in all rickettsial infections, including Q fever (see below). There is an accumulation of inflammatory cells in the sinuses and cortex, particularly of cells that resemble the 'immunoblasts' that are seen characteristically in the lymph nodes in infectious mononucleosis (see page 650), with rather basiphile cytoplasm and a relatively large, pale nucleus. Some of the cells are binucleate or have several nuclei and may be reminiscent of the Sternberg–Reed cells of Hodgkin's disease. Similar, usually mononuclear, cells may be present in considerable numbers in the peripheral blood, which characteristically shows a 'monocytosis' in many cases of these infections. Neutrophils and plasma cells are also present in the sinuses of the lymph nodes, but are less numerous than the large mononuclear cells.

Vascular changes are more characteristic. However, they are a feature of the severer infections and may be little developed in other cases (Fig. 9.104). The changes comprise thickening of the vessel wall by oedema and an infiltrate of large mononuclear cells, plasma cells, lymphocytes and neutrophils, in varying proportions. Similar infiltration is seen in the tissue immediately surrounding the vessels. The endothelium is swollen, the nucleus of the cells often enlarged and the cytoplasm remarkably conspicuous. The endothelial cells are heavily parasitized by the rickettsiae, but these are not often to be recognized in conventional histological preparations: when the tissue has been suitably fixed immediately after excision it may be possible to demonstrate the organisms, particularly in Giemsa-stained sections. Thrombus may be present, evidently forming through platelet aggregation on the surface of the enlarged endothelial cells and partially or completely obliterating the lumen. The more or less extensive areas of necrosis in the substance of the nodes, often with local haemorrhage, are attributable to these occlusive vascular lesions.

Q Fever

Lymphadenitis is a major clinical feature in a comparatively small proportion of cases of Q

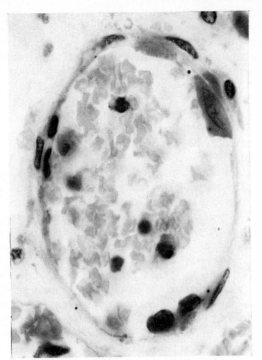

Fig. 9.104. This small blood vessel is in the hilum of an axillary lymph node. It shows a range of changes in the endothelial cells, including swelling and faint stippling of the cytoplasm and a variable degree of enlargement and hyperchromasia of the nucleus. In Giemsa preparations it was possible to make out the presence of rickettsiae in the cytoplasm of similar cells in adjoining vessels. The specimen was obtained at biopsy in a case of unexplained fever accompanied by monocytosis in the peripheral blood. Serological tests for infectious mononucleosis were negative although the changes in the substance of the lymph node were thought to be consistent with that diagnosis. The chance finding of a positive Weil–Felix reaction led to questioning the patient about his 'geographical history': it was only then learnt that he had been bitten by a tick while on a picnic near Pretoria, South Africa, 5 weeks earlier. The significance of the initial lesion at the site of the bite, which was over the sacrum, and of the resulting regional lymphadenitis had been overlooked. Complement-fixing antibodies against *Rickettsia conorii* were present in high titre. It may be noted that hypertrophy and hyperplasia of the endothelium of blood vessels in lymph nodes are commonly found in a wide variety of inflammatory states (see, for instance, Fig. 9.64, page 589). *Haematoxylin–eosin.* × 750.

fever,* which is due to infection by *Coxiella burnetii* (*Rickettsia burnetii*), an organism that is

* Q fever was recognized first in Queensland, among workers in a slaughter-house in Brisbane (Derrick, E. H., *Med. J. Aust.*, 1937, **2**, 281). The common statement that the 'Q' stands for Queensland is wrong: it indicated the questionable nature of the disease—'query fever', hence 'Q fever'—before its rickettsial nature was discovered (Burnet, F. M., Freeman, M., *Med. J. Aust.*, 1937, **2**, 299).

believed in most cases to enter the body through the lungs, in dust contaminated by infected cattle, sheep or goats, or through the alimentary tract, in infected milk. The disease is transmitted among animals by ticks, a means of infection that is rarely responsible for its occurrence in man. In man, Q fever presents oftenest as a simple, acute fever; pneumonia develops in a small proportion of cases (see page 327) and very occasionally infective endocarditis (see page 33). A syndrome of fever, pharyngitis, lymphocytosis, enlargement of cervical lymph nodes and splenomegaly is sometimes seen.[500] This syndrome was common in some of the outbreaks of a disease that occurred among troops in the Eastern Mediterranean during the latter part of the second world war (*Balkan-Grippe*, Balkan fever) and that is now considered to have been Q fever. It is reminiscent of infectious mononucleosis; in this context it may be noted that a rickettsia (*Rickettsia sennetsui*) has been recognized as a cause of a comparable syndrome in Japan (see page 649).

The histological changes in the lymph nodes in cases of Q fever are similar to those in other rickettsial infections (see above).[501]

Chlamydial Lymphadenitis and Similar Infections

The organisms that cause ornithosis (see page 325) and lymphogranuloma inguinale, and the TRIC agents, which cause trachoma and inclusion conjunctivitis (see Chapter 40), have until recently been referred to as the psittacosis-lymphogranuloma-trachoma group (PLT group). At first they were thought to be large viruses, but it was recognized that they are more closely related to rickettsiae than to viruses and their bacterial status is now presumed. Their taxonomical position remains debatable: they are usually gathered into a single genus, *Chlamydia*,[502] this name having precedence[503] over the still occasionally used *Bedsonia*.[504] Some authorities use the generic name *Miyagawanella* for the agents that cause ornithosis and lymphogranuloma inguinale and restrict *Chlamydia* to the TRIC agents. In this book *Chlamydia* is applied in the wider sense indicated above.

The chlamydiae multiply only within host cells. They may be seen in a variety of forms, ranging from 'elementary bodies' (200 to 400 nm in diameter) to the larger and less frequent structures known as initial bodies (0·5 to 1·0 μm in diameter). They are basiphile, and when stained appropriately, as with Giemsa's stain, they can be seen with the light microscope. However, their demonstration in conventional histological sections is unconvincing to most microscopists: film preparations, by contrast, are often invaluable.

Lymphadenitis in Ornithosis

Lymphadenitis is found at necropsy in a proportion of cases of psittacosis and other forms of ornithosis (see page 325). The pulmonary infection being usually the major manifestation, it is typically the bronchopulmonary nodes that are affected. Histologically, the nodes may show only non-specific inflammatory changes, sometimes with small foci of simple necrosis. Less frequently, there are appearances that are reminiscent of the early changes of lymphogranuloma inguinale (see below), with foci of amorphous, haematoxyphile, necrotic material surrounded by a zone of more or less radially oriented histiocytes; neutrophils are generally present, but in comparatively small numbers. The lesions are less extensive than those of lymphogranuloma, and the star-shaped foci of necrosis characteristic of the fully developed stages of the latter are not seen.

Lymphogranuloma Inguinale*

Lymphogranuloma inguinale has several synonyms —lymphogranuloma venereum,† lymphopathia venerea, poradenitis inguinalis (see below), climatic bubo, the 'sixth venereal disease'‡ and Nicolas–

* Few medical terms can have so much difference in meaning in different countries as *lymphogranuloma*. When used without qualification in English-speaking countries it usually refers to *lymphogranuloma inguinale* (lymphogranuloma venereum, or Nicolas–Favre disease); in most European countries other than Britain and Ireland it implies Hodgkin's disease ('*lymphogranuloma malignum*'), but in Scandinavia it is commonly used as a synonym of sarcoidosis ('*lymphogranuloma benignum*'). The confusion is not always avoided even when care is taken to limit the ambiguity by using the name appropriate for the disease in English when appending an English summary to a paper written in, say, German (see footnote on page 703).

† Lymphogranuloma inguinale (lymphogranuloma venereum) must not be confused with granuloma inguinale (granuloma venereum), which is caused by *Donovania granulomatis*, an intracellular parasite that is possibly related to *Klebsiella pneumoniae* (Rake, G., *J. Bact.*, 1948, **55**, 865). Granuloma inguinale (see page 593 and Chapters 26, 27 and 39) is sometimes known as donovaniosis. The intracellular organisms are known as Donovan bodies, a further source of confusion as the name is so similar to Leishman–Donovan bodies (*Leishmania donovani*) (see page 659).

‡ The 'numerical' classification of sexually transmitted (erstwhile venereal) diseases has long been out of fashion but still figures in lists of synonyms. The enumeration varied somewhat between regions, but a widely used sequence was: first venereal disease, syphilis; second, gonorrhoea; third, chancroid; fourth, fusospirochaetosis; fifth, granuloma inguinale; sixth, lymphogranuloma inguinale.

Favre disease (Durand–Nicolas–Favre disease[505]). It is a chlamydial infection that is usually transmitted by sexual intercourse (see also Chapters 26, 27 and 39). It occurs throughout the world, but its prevalence is greatest in warm climates, and particularly among socially and economically backward communities. In countries with cooler climates the disease is rarely seen except among seafaring men and travellers, and those with whom they associate sexually. A small papule or vesicle, which may ulcerate, develops within 1 to 3 weeks at the site of inoculation, which is usually on the genitalia: it is usually painless, and generally heals spontaneously within a few days, being therefore easily overlooked by the patient. In women, the primary lesion is rarely on the vulva: it may be in the vagina or, much oftener, on the cervix, and in these situations must even more frequently escape detection. The cervical distribution of the primary lesion has important consequences in terms of the differential distribution of the resulting lymphadenitis in the two sexes: this involves the inguinal nodes in men but the iliac nodes in women. Iliac lymphadenitis may cause peritoneal irritation and therefore hypogastric discomfort or pain; in many cases it may go unremarked. Iliac lymphadenitis also occurs, in both sexes, when the infection has resulted from anal intercourse, the inoculation lesion presumably being in the rectum.

In men, after an interval that ranges from 2 to 10 weeks, the inguinal nodes on one or, less often, both sides become painful, enlarged, matted together and fluctuant; the overlying skin becomes stretched and cyanotic, and sinuses form when the nodes break down. The resulting cavitation of the lymph nodes accounts for one of the now rare synonyms of the disease, '*poradenitis*'. The lymphadenitis may subside spontaneously at any stage, even before sinuses develop, and it seldom persists for more than 3 to 4 months at most.

In those cases in which the site of inoculation is extragenital the affected lymph nodes are in the group that drains the site of inoculation, which may be anywhere on the body surface, including the conjunctiva and mouth. In some cases the disease becomes chronic, or it may be reactivated after a long latent period following apparent cure. Chronic forms are met with oftener in women: elephantiasis of the vulva ('esthiomene'—see below), due to lymphatic obstruction, and vaginal or rectal strictures may be among these. There is a specific skin test, the Frei test,[506] which becomes positive early in the course of the infection and generally remains positive for many years after the disease has completely subsided clinically; the test is carried out by injecting the specific antigen intradermally. The Frei antigen was formerly prepared from pus aspirated from the buboes in known cases of infection; the chlamydia can be cultivated now, in the chick embryo and in cultures of some strains of human cells, and this provides more convenient sources of antigen. A complement-fixation test is also available.

Histology[507, 508]

Discrete and confluent foci of histiocytic proliferation replace much of the normal structure of the infected lymph nodes. In the earliest stages, and in as yet relatively little affected nodes in the vicinity of those in which the disease is more advanced, the histiocytes may be epithelioid and grouped in small clusters, the picture resembling that of toxoplasmic lymphadenitis (see page 654). Soon, the foci fuse and enlarge rapidly. Neutrophils accumulate in the central part of these foci, which become necrotic and present a core formed of pus cells and abundant, granular, haematoxyphile debris (Figs 9.105 and 9.106). The histiocytes abutting on the areas of necrosis tend to become radially arranged, in palisade formation, and there may be occasional multinucleate cells among them and at the periphery of the lesion. Plasma cells are a regular feature of the reaction and sometimes are very numerous. They are present from the initial stages and persist throughout the course of the disease. Eosinophils may also be found. The neutrophils gradually disappear after the earlier stages and the necrotic material loses its purulent character and becomes an amorphous, granular mass containing much haematoxyphile nuclear debris. Where it borders on the histiocytic zone the necrotic material may be patterned with sharply outlined, rounded spaces that contain recognizable remnants of a mononuclear cell. Histological processing usually causes the necrotic mass to shrink away from the tissue that encloses it (see Fig. 9.108). These lesions, which for convenience may be referred to as abscesses, although their contents are purulent only in the earlier part of the course of the disease, commonly extend and fuse in such a manner that they form a characteristically rambling or star-shaped cavity ('stellate abscess') .They may erupt through the capsule of the node, to track across the soft tissues and point through the skin. The resulting sinuses may continue to discharge for long periods, sometimes even for years, although they may dry and close spontaneously.

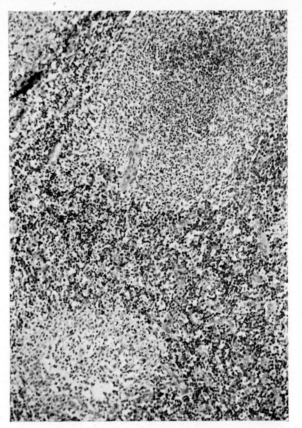

Fig. 9.105. Early stage of the lymphadenitis of lymphogranuloma inguinale. Two focal aggregates of epithelioid histiocytes are seen; central suppuration is more advanced in the larger. There are single histiocytes and small clusters of these cells among the lymphoid cells throughout the rest of the field. This picture is not pathognomonic. It may be seen in the early stages of cat-scratch disease, listeria infection and other conditions noted in the text (page 638). See also Fig. 9.106. *Haematoxylin–eosin.* × 140.

Eventually, the necrotic matter in the lymph nodes becomes less haematoxyphile, more eosinophile and at the same time more homogeneous. It may be in part absorbed, the cavity closing as the apposed histiocytic zones come in contact and fuse. Fibrosis proceeds, forming a capsule-like zone round the granulomatous mass. The fibrous tissue involves the tissues round the nodes themselves, obstructing the lymphatics in the vicinity and leading to lymphoedema in the drainage area (vulvar 'esthiomene', for instance, although some authorities deny the association of this condition with lymphogranuloma inguinale[509]).

In some cases the necrotic material forming the core of the granulomatous foci is recognizably composed of the shadowy remains of mononuclear cells,

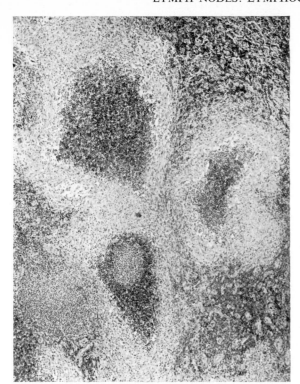

Fig. 9.106. Lymphadenitis of lymphogranuloma inguinale at a stage rather later than that in Fig. 9.105. The histiocytic granulomas are larger and confluent and there is much haematoxyphile nuclear debris among the pus cells at their centre. The next stage is identical with that illustrated in Fig. 9.108, although the latter shows the lesion of cat-scratch disease. *Haematoxylin–eosin.* × 55.

well stained with eosin in haematoxylin–eosin preparations. Sometimes when this feature is not immediately evident on examination under the conventional microscope it may be demonstrated by phase-contrast microscopy,[510] as in some instances of syphilitic gummatous lymphadenitis (see page 614). In the cases in which this picture predominates,[511] the condition is sometimes referred to as '*gummatous lymphogranuloma inguinale*'. The gumma-like appearance may be recognizable, within a dense fibrous scar in the nodes, even many years after the initial infection:[510] the interval was 33 years in one substantiated case (Fig. 9.107)—the patient had been seen first in 1940 with a primary infection of the uterine cervix and a positive Frei test; she eventually developed symptoms from a rectal stricture, in 1973, and the gumma-like condition was recognizable in a biopsy specimen from enlarged, fibrotic iliac lymph nodes obtained during laparotomy (she did not have syphilis).[512]

Occasional Features

In exceptional cases there are conspicuously numerous binucleate or multinucleate cells that appear to be atypical plasma cells, and there may also be many uncommonly large mononuclear plasma cells. These are usually in the surviving lymphoid tissue immediately adjoining the granulomas. In early cases, or when the granulomas are relatively small, this picture has been known to suggest the possibility of Hodgkin's disease, but this interpretation misjudges the significance of the large

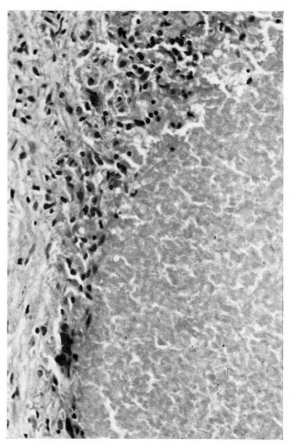

Fig. 9.107. The rare 'gummatous' form of lymphadenitis as a late manifestation of lymphogranuloma inguinale. The 'ghost' outlines of the cells of the necrotic tissue are discernible. There is a narrow zone of persistent granulomatous tissue between the dead matter and the surrounding fibrotic zone. From the patient whose case is noted in the text. Such lesions can be distinguished from the gummatous lymphadenitis of tertiary syphilis (see Fig. 9.86A, page 615) only by the history and by the result of serological investigations. The Frei test for skin sensitivity to lymphogranuloma inguinale antigen is not always positive when the gummatous lesion is found, which may be many years after the infection occurred. *Haematoxylin–eosin.* × 250.

cells, which in fact do not have the characteristics of Sternberg–Reed cells.

Several authors have described what they have interpreted as the infective agent in the cytoplasm of large mononuclear cells, particularly in the vicinity of fresh abscesses in the early stages of infection of the lymph nodes. These include the so-called Miyagawa 'granulocorpuscles'[513] ('Miyagawa bodies'), which at their largest are about 0·5 μm in diameter, and the Gamna–Favre bodies,[514, 515*] which range from 1·0 to 5·0 μm in diameter. The nature and significance of these bodies are debatable: it is usually considered that the Miyagawa bodies are the elementary bodies of the chlamydial parasite, and that the Gamna–Favre bodies may be 'initial bodies' (page 634) and, in part, nuclear debris.

Differential Diagnosis

Histological appearances that are indistinguishable from those of lymphogranuloma inguinale may be found in a variety of other diseases of lymph nodes. These include cat-scratch disease (see below), and some cases of listeria infection (see page 577), glanders (see page 595), melioidosis (see page 595), yersinial mesenteric lymphadenitis (see page 584) and tularaemia (see page 586).

While, exceptionally, the chlamydia of lymphogranuloma inguinale may cause an initial infection in the facial region or in the mouth, with therefore the development of the characteristic lymphadenitis in nodes of the cervical region, it may be noted that in most cases of what has sometimes been rather quaintly called 'lymphogranuloma inguinale of the neck' there has been another cause of the histological findings. Listeria infection certainly accounts for some of these (see page 577); cat-scratch disease has been responsible for others (see below).

A positive Frei test and complement fixation reaction indicate the diagnosis of lymphogranuloma inguinale, provided the results are considered in relation to the clinical picture (cross reactions occur in patients infected by other chlamydiae: for instance, both tests may be strongly positive in cases of ornithosis—see page 325). Isolation of the responsible chlamydia is specific evidence of the diagnosis. The other conditions that may be confused histologically with lymphogranuloma inguinale can be recognized by appropriate immunological and microbiological studies.

* Gamna–Favre bodies, oddly, are sometimes confused with Gandy–Gamna nodules, which are the siderofibrotic foci that are found in the spleen in cases of congestive splenomegaly (see page 731).

Cat-Scratch Disease

Although the agent responsible for cat-scratch disease has not been discovered, the clinical and pathological pictures and the diagnostic significance of a delayed sensitivity reaction to the intradermal inoculation of antigen prepared from the necrotic exudate in affected lymph nodes of other cases—a procedure comparable to the Frei test, differing only in the source of the antigen—are so closely similar to the corresponding characteristics of lymphogranuloma inguinale that this seems the appropriate place to consider the condition.[516]

Synonyms.—Cat-scratch disease has many synonyms.[517] They include cat fever, cat-scratch fever, felinosis,[518] benign inoculation lymphoreticulosis,[519] benign infectious lymphoreticulosis, benign virus lymphadenitis,[520] non-bacterial regional lymphadenitis,[521] Petzetakis's disease[522] and others. As the disease is occasionally acquired from sources other than cats, has very occasionally been blamed for a patient's death, and is not known for certain to be caused by a virus, a proportion of these names may be thought unsuitable. Those names that designate the disease as a 'lymphoreticulosis' are objectionable on the grounds that this term, related to 'reticulosis', has connotations that are better not perpetuated (see page 537). Cat-scratch disease,[523] the name that is most widely familiar, may serve until the cause is known, when a more specific term may become applicable.

The earliest recorded cases for which a retrospective diagnosis of cat-scratch disease may be correct were seen in the United States of America in 1932 by Foshay, who originally took them to be cases of tularaemia.[524, 525] The disease is sometimes known as Foshay's disease.

Aetiology

Occurrence.—The disease is probably of worldwide occurrence. It was seldom seen before the 1950s, its greatest prevalence was in the first half or so of that decade, and since then it has become infrequent. The reason for this rise and fall in its incidence is unknown, and may well prove to be of aetiological importance if eventually it is recognized. The peculiar concentration of cases in that short period is reflected in the chronology of the published cases and in the personal series of some authorities.[526] In a series of 46 cases that I saw during the period from 1946 to 1975 inclusive, in the United Kingdom and the Republic of Ireland, 36 presented during the years 1952–56.[527]

The disease may be commoner in autumn and winter than at other times.

Source.—About a third of the patients are under 10 years old. Among adults, women are appreciably oftener affected, perhaps because they have more to do with looking after cats as household pets. Sometimes, a number of members of a household may develop the disease at about the same time. There is usually a definite history of being scratched by a cat; occasionally, a cat bite may be responsible. The cat is usually free from signs of disease, but in some instances has been ill, although not seriously. It has been suggested that cats are vectors, carrying an infection from birds or small rodents to man, but the disease has been acquired in some instances from hand-reared kittens that have not begun to hunt.[527] In a few instances the source of the disease seems to have been a scratch by a rabbit or a mole,[527] insect bites, contamination of superficial wounds while working in a slaughter-house, and scratches or pricks by vegetation. Some patients cannot recall any incident that might have been the origin of their illness. It has been suggested that the infection may sometimes enter through mucous membranes.[528]

Nature.—The nature of the infecting agent remains unknown. Most attempts to transmit the disease to animals have been unsuccessful. Intracutaneous and subcutaneous inoculation of material freshly aspirated from the infected lymph nodes of two patients failed to produce any disease in cats, birds, mice, rats, rabbits, guinea-pigs, ferrets and monkeys;[529] an assistant in the animal house, who, during this study, accidentally pricked her hand with an infected needle, developed a local lesion, enlargement of the supratrochlear and axillary lymph nodes, and a positive skin reaction to cat-scratch disease antigen. Successful intracutaneous inoculation of monkeys has been reported.[530] The mainly negative results of such investigations make it doubtful whether the source of the so-called Greek virus, isolated from the lymph nodes of patients whose clinical illness (described in the 1930s[531]) has in retrospect been considered typical of cat-scratch disease,[522] was indeed the latter and not a further addition to the range of infections that are known to reproduce its clinical and pathological features (see opposite). Various minute granules and larger 'inclusions' that have been described by different observers in the cytoplasm or nuclei of cells in the lymph nodes[530, 532] are of doubtful significance. Attempts to isolate organisms by inoculation of chick embryos or of tissue cultures have been unsuccessful. In particular, the search for a chlamydia, encouraged by the similarities between cat-scratch disease and lymphogranuloma inguinale, has failed to support this hypothesis of the nature of the infection.

The isolation of photochromogenic mycobacteria from 7 out of 8 cases of cat-scratch disease[533] has not been followed by similar findings in other series and again may merely underline the difficulties of distinguishing clinically and pathologically between infections caused by different organisms.

Course

An inflammatory reaction at the site of the initial injury to the skin is often remarked by the patient, but may be no more than would ordinarily accompany such a wound. It may subside completely and then, after a few days to several weeks, the site may again become red, swollen and painful. A small area of ulceration may appear and discharge a little seropurulent exudate. In many cases there is no longer any trace of active inflammation at the site of inoculation when the regional lymph nodes begin to enlarge, which usually occurs some 3 weeks after the scratch or other injury. Less often, the lymphadenitis does not begin to appear until after an interval of 2 to 3 months. The nodes may remain enlarged for many weeks, and in rare cases even for as long as 2 years.[525] They do not necessarily persist for the longest time in those cases in which sinuses form.

The patient with cat-scratch disease shows a positive delayed hypersensitivity reaction to an intradermal inoculation with specific antigen (a heat-sterilized preparation of exudate aspirated from the affected nodes in known cases of the disease). The test is comparable to the Frei test in lymphogranuloma inguinale. The development of the positive reaction at the test site may be accompanied by accentuation of the lymphadenopathy and recurrence or aggravation of the inflammatory signs at the site of the scratch or other injury. There is no reaction to Frei-test antigen, and the complement fixation test with lymphogranuloma inguinale antigen gives a low titre result or is negative.

Serious complications of cat-scratch disease have been described, including encephalitis, myelitis and meningitis.[525, 528] Other manifestations are said to have included infection of pharyngeal lymphoid tissue, conjunctivitis, acute mesenteric lymphadenitis (see page 574) and pulmonary involvement of the type described sometimes as 'primary atypical pneumonia' (see page 326). Death has been attributed to the disease[518] but this is exceptionally rare, and the diagnosis may not have been unequivocal.

Histopathology

Microscopical examination of the affected lymph nodes (Figs 9.108 and 9.109) shows a picture that cannot be distinguished from lymphogranuloma inguinale (see page 636). The changes reproduce any of the range of appearances that may be seen in that disease, including the gumma-like variant. Although various attempts have been made to define features that distinguish the lymphadenitis of cat-scratch disease from that of lymphogranuloma inguinale, the range of histological pictures is such that any appearance seen in the one disease may be seen in some cases of the other. The distinction between them depends on the clinical history and the results of other laboratory and clinical investigations.

Viral Lymphadenitis and Infectious Mononucleosis

Lymphadenitis is frequently an accompaniment of infection caused by viruses. In this context it must

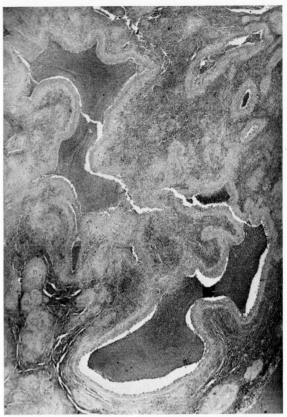

Fig. 9.109. Fully developed lymphadenitis of cat-scratch disease. Confluence of the abscesses has produced an excavation of somewhat stellate outline ('stellate abscess'). The contents have shrunk away from the lining in places. The lining is a well-defined, relatively pale zone, formed of epithelioid histiocytes. This histological picture cannot be distinguished from that of comparably advanced cases of lymphogranuloma inguinale and of the other conditions that may be the cause of this type of lesion (see page 638 of text). Compare with Figs 9.55 and 9.60, pages 577 and 584. *Haematoxylin–eosin.* × 10.

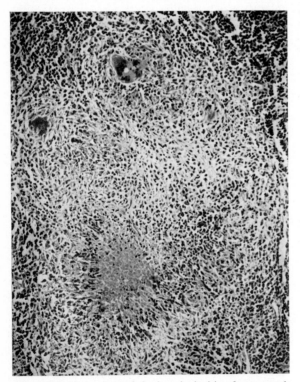

Fig. 9.108. Early stage of the lymphadenitis of cat-scratch disease. There is palisading of histiocytes round the necrotic core of the epithelioid cell granuloma. A few multinucleate giant cells are seen. Compare with the tuberculous granuloma illustrated in Fig. 9.73, page 600. *Haematoxylin–eosin.* × 95.

be noted that some diseases that formerly were classed among the viral infections are now considered apart from the latter, the organisms that cause them being no longer regarded as viruses: chlamydial infection—specifically, lymphogranuloma inguinale (see page 635)—is a case in point. Again, the discovery of the Epstein–Barr virus and its relation to the tumour that is now generally known as Burkitt's lymphoma (see page 824),[534] and, later, the demonstration of an association between this virus and infectious mononucleosis (see page 648),[535] necessitated reconsideration of the role of viruses in the aetiology and pathogenesis of diseases of the lymphoreticular system. It is no longer appropriate to equate viral infection of the lymphoreticular system simply with 'inflammatory' changes in the constituent organs and tissues of the system—lymphadenitis, for instance. The changes that characterize 'inflammation' ordinarily involve a variety of cells, contributing within a useful quantitative range to the body's reaction to the inflammatory stimulus: most viruses that affect the lymphoreticular tissues produce changes that, while often distinctive, fall within the bounds of what most pathologists could accept as an 'inflammatory' response. Some regard infectious mononucleosis as an exception, considering it to be characterized by a proliferation of lymphoreticular cells that, while benign and self-terminating, is quantitatively determined by the pathogenic agent rather than by the body's own response to the latter. Burkitt's tumour is usually regarded as frankly neoplastic.

The viral infections that cause lymphadenitis in the conventional sense of a reaction that is simply related to the neutralization and elimination or containment of the pathogenic agent will be considered here. Infectious mononucleosis will also be considered in this section. Burkitt's lymphoma, because of its quite different pathological nature and clinical course, will be dealt with later in the chapter, among the other lymphomas (see page 824).

Lymphadenitis Accompanying Diseases Caused by Ribonucleic Acid Viruses (RNA Viruses)

Measles (Morbilli)

The most characteristic finding in the lymph nodes in measles, which is caused by a paramyxovirus, is the presence of the peculiar multinucleate giant cells that ordinarily are known only in relation to infection by the measles virus.* These cells are usually referred to as Warthin–Finkeldey cells,[536, 536a] although they were noted more than 20 years earlier by Ciaccio[537] and Alagna.[538] They are found only during the prodromal stage of the infection and, at most, the first 3 to 5 days following the appearance of the skin eruption (information about their occurrence after the prodromal stage is based on small numbers of post-mortem studies[538a]). They are to be seen in the germinal centres of the lymphoid follicles, in which they may be numerous, and—often—in the lymphoid tissue immediately abutting on the follicles. They are of irregular shape, sharply outlined, and notably haematoxyphile because of the multiplicity of their nuclei, which contain abundant chromatin: there may be from three nuclei to many

hundreds of nuclei in a cell, and the cells range from 20 to 400 μm in their longest dimension, although they exceed 150 μm only exceptionally (Figs 9.110A and 9.110B). Warthin–Finkeldey cells are distinct from the very large, sometimes multinucleate, macrophages that in some cases of measles are conspicuously numerous in the germinal centres, their cytoplasm heavily laden with the hyperchromatic, rounded remnants of dead nuclei that they have ingested (Fig. 9.111). These macrophages, which may also be found in the sinuses in the affected nodes, are immediately reminiscent of the similar, but smaller, cells that, with their content of Flemming's 'stainable bodies' (see page 512), are so familiar a feature of the follicles in cases of simple follicular hyperplasia (see page 553).

It should be noted that Warthin–Finkeldey cells are quite different in appearance from the multinucleate giant cells that are a feature of the lungs in cases of measles pneumonia (see page 323 and Fig. 7.35). The cells of giant cell pneumonia have pale cytoplasm and relatively small, often palely stained nuclei that are scattered through the cytoplasm rather than seeming to crowd the latter into a comparatively very small volume. The crowding and overlapping of the nuclei of the Warthin–Finkeldey cells earned them the name 'mulberry cell'.

Warthin–Finkeldey cells, found on examination of sections of tonsils, including the pharyngeal tonsil ('adenoids'), when these have been excised, by chance, during the prodromal stage of measles, may enable the histologist to foretell the clinical development of the exanthematous stage.* Similarly, the changes in the mesenteric lymph nodes during the prodromal stage, or obstruction of the appendix by hyperplasia of the lymphoid tissue in the mucosa and submucosa, may cause abdominal symptoms that lead to laparotomy because of the possibility of appendicitis: Warthin–Finkeldey cells in the lymphoid tissue of the appendix itself, or in mesenteric lymph nodes, the swelling and hyperaemia of which may sufficiently attract the surgeon's concern to lead to biopsy, again enable the microscopist to diagnose measles.[539] This may be an unimportant achievement when the community in which he practises is one among which measles is a disease of low mortality; but it has occasionally been life-saving in regions where measles is more dangerous,

---

* The occurrence of similar cells in some cases of the so-called 'Mediterranean lymphoma' is noted on page 847.

* Usually, by the time the report on the sections reaches the clinician who is looking after the child—this happens most frequently in childhood—the rash has already developed, the diagnosis of measles has been made at the bedside, and the pathologist's achievement is appreciated only by himself.

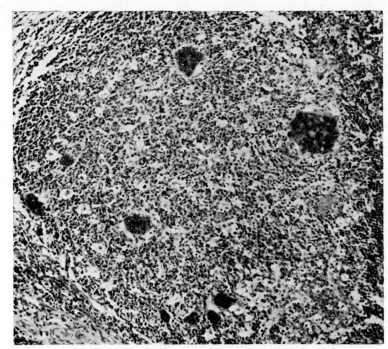

Fig. 9.110A. Cervical lymph node in a case of measles. This large germinal centre in a follicle contains nine multinucleate giant cells of the Warthin–Finkeldey type, characteristic of measles. The largest of these is shown at higher magnification in Fig. 9.110B. The patient was the 9 years old daughter of a doctor who, noticing the rapid enlargement of the child's cervical nodes and fearing that they might indicate the development of acute leukaemia, arranged for a biopsy. The measles rash appeared 5 days after the operation. There was no other abnormality. *Haematoxylin–eosin.* × 120.

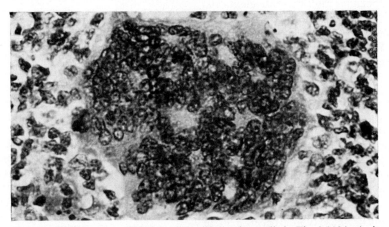

Fig. 9.110B. Higher magnification of one of the giant cells in Fig. 9.110A. As is characteristic of this variety of measles giant cell, which occurs only in the lymphoreticular tissues, the nuclei are distributed throughout the cytoplasm and vary considerably in intensity of staining and in size. These cells are quite different from the multinucleate giant cells that are found in the lungs in cases of measles pneumonia (see Fig. 7.35, page 323, Volume 1). *Haematoxylin–eosin.* × 500.

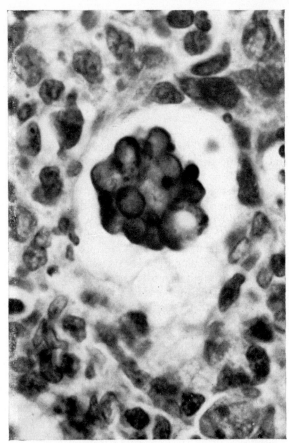

Fig. 9.111. Nuclear remnants, probably derived from Warthin–Finkeldey giant cells, in the vacuolate cytoplasm of a multinucleate macrophage in a cervical lymph node removed 2 days before the appearance of the skin rash of measles. Typical, intact giant cells were still present elsewhere in the node. These rounded, haematoxyphile remnants are akin to Flemming's 'stainable bodies' (see Fig. 9.4, page 513), although larger, and usually fused, as in the cluster illustrated. *Haematoxylin–eosin.* × 1200.

where its rash may be overlooked because of cutaneous pigmentation, and where delay in recognition may increase the risks accompanying its complications.

The other changes in the lymph nodes in measles are non-specific. They include simple follicular hyperplasia (see page 553) and sometimes a degree of sinus histiocytosis (see page 559).

Lymphadenitis Accompanying Immunization against Measles.—Inoculation of live attenuated measles virus subcutaneously or into muscle is followed in some cases by considerable enlargement of the regional lymph nodes, which develops within a period of a few days to 2 weeks or so after the injec-tion.[539a] The cause of the lymphadenopathy is easily overlooked clinically if the history of inoculation is not known, as has been the case repeatedly when the mother of a young child has not understood what has been done at a clinic, and when the family doctor has not been informed of the inoculation. Incarcerated hernia has been suspected in cases of gluteal inoculation with subsequent inguinal adenitis,[480, 539a] leading to surgical exploration, the discovery of enlarged lymph nodes, and biopsy excision of one of these.

The infected nodes show a proliferation of immunoblasts in the pulp, often with accumulations of plasma cells, shrinkage or, occasionally, hyperplasia of the follicles, and a variable number of typical Warthin–Finkeldey cells (see page 641). The last are not always present, but when they are found in their fully developed form they are pathognomonic.

Rubella (German Measles)

Rubella virus is an unclassified RNA virus. Enlargement of lymph nodes, characteristically including the retroauricular and occipital nodes, is the earliest sign of the disease and the sign that is last to disappear. It may be detected from 4 to 2 days before the skin eruption, and it may still be present 6 weeks and more after the eruption has faded. Not surprisingly, in relation to a disease that has a very low mortality and in which there is no indication for biopsy, little is known about the changes in the lymph nodes. In the only fatal case that I have seen, in which the child died of encephalitis on the eighth day of the illness, the findings in the nodes—allowing for post-mortem autolysis—seemed to be no more than hyperaemia and some hyperplasia of plasma cell precursors, as in a published instance.[540]

Rubella lymphadenitis is an occasional cause of the syndrome of acute mesenteric lymphadenitis (see page 574).

Poliomyelitis

Poliovirus is a picornavirus, specifically an enterovirus, and, like the viruses that cause measles and rubella, is one of the RNA viruses. The changes in the lymph nodes in cases of poliomyelitis in the acute stages are not specific, comprising some degree of hyperaemia, follicular hyperplasia and sinus catarrh. These changes in the abdominal nodes may be sufficiently marked to cause symptoms from peritoneal irritation, and this may lead to laparotomy, particularly when the symptoms develop during the preparalytic stage of the disease. As laparotomy during the preparalytic stage of poliomyelitis may predispose to more extensive paralysis than otherwise might have developed, clinical judgement of the need for surgical exploration becomes uncommonly important. There is no question but that some cases of 'acute non-specific mesenteric lymphadenitis' (see page 574) occurring in the course of outbreaks of poliomyelitis are instances of poliovirus infection, even when neurological manifestations are, fortunately, lacking.

Occasionally, compact multinucleate cells of about 15 to 20 μm in diameter are seen in the lymph nodes in cases of infection by poliovirus.[541] They are probably derived from reticulum cells or from plasma cells or their precursors.

Lymphadenitis Accompanying Diseases Caused by Deoxyribonucleic Acid Viruses (DNA Viruses)

Smallpox

The superficial lymph nodes may be appreciably enlarged in cases of classic smallpox (variola major) and of alastrim (variola minor), which are caused respectively by highly virulent and less virulent strains of the variola virus (*Poxvirus variolae*). It is generally said that the enlargement of the nodes is secondary to the destruction of tissue at the sites of the skin lesions, and to pustulation of the latter and, in some instances, superimposed bacterial infection. However, in some cases, microscopical foci of necrosis are found in the nodes: these foci are distinct from any foci of suppuration that may have resulted, perhaps from infection by pyogenic bacteria. Sometimes, and this seems to be exceptional, spherical or ovoid, palely eosinophile inclusions, from 3 to 10 μm in longest dimension, homogeneous or rather granular, and sharply or hazily outlined, are found in the cytoplasm of large mononuclear cells in the sinuses of the nodes and, more rarely, in the vicinity of the necrotic foci in the pulp: these inclusions correspond in appearance to the characteristic Guarnieri bodies in the infected epidermal cells in the skin lesions of smallpox and of vaccinia (see Chapter 39, and Fig. 39.163), which are aggregates of viral particles in a gelatinous matrix.[542]

Vaccinia

Two forms of lymphadenitis have been recognized to occur in the regional nodes draining the site of a vaccinial lesion resulting from prophylactic immunization against smallpox with vaccinia virus (*Poxvirus officinale*). One is a lymphadenitis that accompanies the development of the cutaneous lesion at the site of the inoculation. The other is usually regarded as a sequel of vaccinia and is particularly important because, if its association with the infection is for any reason overlooked, it is sometimes misinterpreted histologically as a lymphoma.

Lymphadenitis Accompanying Vaccinia.—The nodes draining the site of a successful vaccination against smallpox become moderately enlarged and painful. In instances of primary vaccination—that is, vaccination of the individual who has not been vaccinated before—the reaction in the lymph nodes begins to attract the patient's attention at about the time when the lesion at the site of inoculation is becoming vesicular (about the fifth day). The lymphadenitis is at its most marked when the pustule that develops from the vesicle is at its most florid (about the 10th to the 12th day). If the vaccinial lesion in the skin becomes infected by pyogenic bacteria, suppuration may develop in the lymph nodes. In the typical case, however, the lymphadenitis subsides quite quickly once the pustule dries and the scab forms, although the affected nodes tend to remain rather enlarged and tender for 2 to 4 weeks after healing of the skin.

In instances of revaccination, in which partial immunity leads to an accelerated reaction to vaccinia virus, the regional lymphadenitis is less marked, in keeping with the less severe cutaneous reaction. Indeed, in some cases no involvement of lymph nodes is evident: this is most frequently so when the patient's immunity is such that the cutaneous reaction does not reach the stage of vesiculation.

The pathological changes in the lymph nodes draining the site of vaccination have seldom been studied during the course of the vaccinial infection. In two cases, the patients having died of unrelated causes while the vaccinial infection was at its height,[543] the nodes draining the site of the cutaneous lesion showed a marked follicular hyperplasia, with large germinal centres. There was also a notable proliferation of large, pale cells among the lymphocytes of the superficial cortex and paracortical region: these cells ranged from 10 to about 25 μm in longest dimension and contained a relatively large, round, vesicular nucleus with a small but conspicuous eosinophile nucleolus. These cells are now commonly regarded as transformed lymphocytes (immunoblasts).[544] In one of the two cases, eosinophile inclusions, identical with the inclusions in the cutaneous lesion (see Chapter 39, Fig. 39.163), and presumably the vaccinial equivalent of the Guarnieri body of smallpox (see opposite), were present in some of these cells.

Persistent Lymphadenitis Following Vaccination ('Postvaccinial Lymphadenitis').—Occasionally, the lymphadenitis that results from vaccination, particularly successful primary vaccination in adults, persists for many weeks instead of subsiding once the cutaneous lesion has dried and the scab has formed under which scarring takes place. In some cases, lymph nodes that had more or less completely returned to their normal inconspicuous state begin to enlarge again and may form a mass big enough to cause considerable concern to the clinician. Such nodes may be painless, and this serves both to mask the possibility that their enlargement is inflammatory and to support the impression that the condition may be neoplastic. Biopsy is then likely to be undertaken. Unless the pathologist who examines the sections is told of the recent vaccination his findings may seem to indicate the presence of a lymphoma (see below). The clinician himself may not have elicited the history of vaccination, or he may not recognize the possibility of a relation between the vaccination and the lymphadenopathy —for instance, if the affected nodes are not those topographically nearest to the vaccination site (as an example, vaccination over the region of the deltoid muscle may cause cervical, not axillary, lymphadenitis).

The histological picture in the lymph nodes affected by persistent lymphadenitis following vaccination (Figs 9.112A and 9.112B) is essentially the same as that described above as accompanying vaccinia, although inclusions seem not to have been described in published series[545] and were not present in any of the five cases that I have seen.[546] It is misinterpretation of the nature of the large, pale cells in the pulp (Fig. 9.112B), referred to above as transformed lymphocytes (immunoblasts),[544] and described also as 'reticular lymphoblasts',[545] that tends to direct the microscopist toward the possibility of a lymphoma, particularly Hodgkin's disease. In fact, a diagnosis of malignant lymphoma was mistakenly made in nine of a series of 20 cases of 'postvaccinial lymphadenitis'[545] and in three of the five cases that colleagues have shown to me.[546] Nonetheless, the similarity to Hodgkin's disease is slight, and Sternberg–Reed cells are not a feature. The condition is benign, and eventually subsides completely.

H

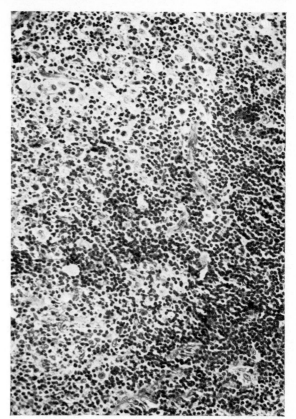

Fig. 9.112A. Persistent lymphadenitis following vaccination against smallpox ('postvaccinial lymphadenitis'). Large pale cells are scattered through the interfollicular tissue (see Fig. 9.112B). There is a follicle with germinal centre in the bottom left corner of the field. *Haematoxylin–eosin.* × 160.

Cowpox

The cowpox virus (*Poxvirus bovis*) was long considered to be identical with vaccinia virus (*Poxvirus officinale*), but the two are now recognized to be distinct. Cowpox is an occupational disease of those who work with cattle, particularly in dairy farming.* The initial lesions are usually on the hands, and if the individual has been vaccinated against smallpox previously they may be so trivial that their significance is overlooked. The unvaccinated person who becomes infected with cowpox develops lesions in the inoculated area of skin that closely resemble those of vaccinia, although they have a greater tendency to be haemorrhagic; lymphangitis and, oftener, lymphadenitis may accompany the cutaneous eruption. In a classic instance, in which the patient was a final year medical student who had

* Conversely, vaccinia has been known to be transmitted from the recently vaccinated person to cows (Downie, A. W., Dumbell, K. R., *Ann. Rev. Microbiol.*, 1956, **10**, 237).

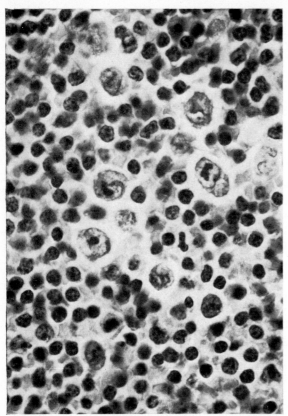

Fig. 9.112B. Same specimen as Fig. 9.112A. The large pale cells in the interfollicular tissue have a large, vesicular nucleus with one or more distinct nucleoli. Some nuclei are more heavily stained. The cytoplasm is relatively sparse in most instances, but tends to stain well. The cells are probably immunoblasts. Immature and mature plasma cells are present among the lymphocytes. A few cells in mitosis are seen. There is nothing in this instance that should cause confusion with Hodgkin's disease, but in some cases a larger proportion of hyperchromatic cells and more numerous mitotic figures may be misleading, especially when the history of recent vaccination is overlooked. See also Fig. 9.6C, page 515. *Haematoxylin–eosin.* × 600.

never been vaccinated against smallpox, and who spent a holiday working on a dairy farm, the changes in the axillary lymph nodes, at biopsy, were virtually identical with those described above as typical of the lymphadenitis accompanying primary vaccination, except that no inclusions were found.[547] Meningo-encephalitis has been recorded as a fatal complication of cowpox.[548]

Other Poxvirus Infections

Orf (contagious pustular dermatitis), which is a worldwide disease among sheep and goats that occasionally infects man (see Chapter 39), *camelpox*, and *pseudo-cowpox* and '*milkers' nodules*' are caused by related viruses that have been referred to as the paravaccinia viruses.[549] Lymphadenitis is an occasional clinical accompaniment of any of these conditions but, with rare exceptions, histological examination has not been undertaken. In a case of orf, in which necropsy was performed because the patient was killed in a road accident, the appearances in the regional lymph nodes, allowing for post-morten change, were those of a non-specific lymphadenitis with follicular hyperplasia, marked sinus dilatation and considerable numbers of neutrophils throughout the node.[550]

Varicella and Zoster

Current opinion favours the view that varicella (chickenpox) and zoster (herpes zoster, zona) are caused by the same virus, *Herpesvirus varicellae*. Varicella is regarded as the primary manifestation of infection by the virus, zoster being a manifestation of reactivation of a dormant infection. Inflammatory enlargement of superficial lymph nodes may accompany both diseases, being generalized in its distribution in cases of varicella and confined to the regional nodes in cases of zoster. In zoster, in fact, there may be no clinical evidence of lymph node involvement at all: in those cases in which the nodes are enlarged it is likely that this reflects merely the reaction to the local destructive lesions in the skin. In those rare instances in which there is overt secondary bacterial infection of the zoster lesions in the skin, as when they become the site of impetiginous involvement, the lymphadenitis is probably the manifestation of a streptococcal or staphylococcal infection. Similarly, the lymphadenitis of varicella may be essentially due to the extensive vesiculation and pustulation of the cutaneous lesions. However, in some cases there is the added feature of widespread formation of multinucleate giant cells in the lymphoid tissues, including the tonsils as well as lymph nodes. These giant cells have been likened to those of measles (see page 641),[551] an observation that begs the question whether there has been a double infection in such instances. Very occasionally, both in zoster[552] and in varicella, intranuclear inclusions, identical to those in epidermal cells in the skin lesions (see Chapter 39), may be seen in endothelial macrophages in the sinuses of lymph nodes and in mononuclear cells—possibly immunoblasts—in the pulp.

Cytomegalovirus Infection

Like the virus of varicella and zoster, cytomegalovirus is a herpesvirus. In cases of congenital infection the presence of cells in lymph nodes that show the characteristic changes is no more than incidental to the generalized disease. It is usually the endothelial macrophages of the sinuses and, less frequently, reticulum cells in the pulp that are affected.[553] The changes in the infected cells are characteristic— in the nucleus the development of a large, initially somewhat haematoxyphile and later eosinophile inclusion body, on average about 8 to 10 μm in diameter, and in the cytoplasm a compact collection of moderately haematoxyphile inclusions, each within the range 0·5 to 3·0 μm in diameter. A clear, halo-like zone surrounds the intranuclear inclusion body, giving it a characteristic 'owl eye' appearance.

The peculiar tendency for cytomegalovirus infection to be associated with infection by *Pneumocystis carinii*—an association seen in many cases of pneumocystis pneumonia, both in the neonatal period and in adults (see pages 324 and 361) —is evident in some cases of lymph node involvement: collections of the pneumocystis (see page 630) may be present as well as the changes characteristic of cytomegalovirus infection.

'*Cytomegalic Mononucleosis*'.—Cytomegalovirus is an occasional cause of the syndrome of glandular fever (see *Infectious Mononucleosis*, below),[554] which more frequently is associated with the Epstein–Barr virus (page 648); other causes include *Listeria monocytogenes* (page 578) and *Toxoplasma gondii* (page 653). The heterophile-antibody test (Paul–Bunnell test) is negative in typical cases of mononucleosis accompanying infection by cytomegalovirus, listeria and toxoplasma, and antibodies to Epstein–Barr virus do not appear in the course of uncomplicated infection by these organisms. The distinction between the three may be made by isolation of the organism and by serological studies.[555] It is sometimes said that absence of enlargement of lymph nodes favours the diagnosis of cytomegalovirus infection as a cause of 'infectious mononucleosis': this is an unreliable criterion, as there may be definite, if moderate, enlargement of superficial nodes, particularly in the neck, in such cases. The histological changes in the nodes are of the same character as in classic cases of infectious mononucleosis, except that the typical inclusions may be present in a proportion of the cells. It should be noted that the finding in the peripheral blood of cells that show the changes characteristic of infection by cytomegalovirus is exceptionally rare.

Cytomegalovirus infection as a cause of mononucleosis may be accompanied by manifestations of visceral involvement, including myocarditis, hepa-titis and pneumonia, and peripheral neuropathy, but these are not invariably present.[554, 555] In some cases the infection is a manifestation of depression of resistance, as is usually the case when adults develop disease due to cytomegalovirus (see page 324). However, it has been observed repeatedly following transfusion of fresh blood or the use of fresh blood for perfusion during operations on the heart, and in these cases is clearly the straightforward consequence of direct inoculation of the virus into the blood stream of a patient who has not previously been infected by it.[556] Blood that has been stored for not less than 48 hours is said to be free of this hazard.

Mononucleosis associated with cytomegalovirus infection is generally self-limiting, with return of the blood to normal within about 6 weeks, and disappearance of any associated manifestations. The greatest danger to the patient is that the failure of resistance that is responsible for most cases will enable other 'opportunistic' infections to set in, and any of these may be quickly fatal (see page 362).

Infectious Mononucleosis—Glandular Fever

Infectious mononucleosis and glandular fever are terms that have been used synonymously by some authorities and with different meanings by others. In general, they relate to a syndrome comprising fever, enlargement of lymph nodes and the presence in the blood of atypical mononuclear cells. The condition is regularly named *infectious mononucleosis* when, in addition to its three basic components, the syndrome includes particular serological findings—the presence of antibodies that agglutinate sheep erythrocytes (heterophile antibodies) and that are distinguishable from Forssman antibodies (for instance, by the Paul–Bunnell–Davidsohn test), and the presence of antibodies to the Epstein–Barr virus. When neither heterophile antibodies nor antibodies to the Epstein–Barr virus are present, the disease is now commonly regarded as distinct from classic infectious mononucleosis and referred to instead by the older term, *glandular fever* (see *Nomenclature*, below).

The name glandular fever was introduced by Pfeiffer, in 1889.[557] He described the disease as an acute infectious fever among children, characterized by soreness of the throat, fever and transient swelling of the lymph nodes of the neck. The condition had been referred to as idiopathic adenitis by N. F. Filatov, 4 years earlier.[558] The association with peculiar changes in the circulating white blood cells was recognized by Türk, in 1907.[559] The name infectious mononucleosis was used first by Sprunt and Evans, in 1920.[559a] The introduction of the Paul–Bunnell test for heterophile antibodies, in 1932,[560] and of the Davidsohn differential test[561] which excludes the diagnostically non-specific heterophile antibodies of Forssman type, and the recognition in 1968 of the association between the Epstein–Barr virus and the syndrome,[535, 562] made it possible to distinguish between cases that present specific serological features and those that lack them.

Until lately, infectious mononucleosis—or glandular fever—was regarded as an acute or, oftener, chronic and tedious illness, almost always benign and self-limiting and seldom demanding more than the symptomatic treatment that, in fact, remains the limit of therapeutic capability except in the small minority of cases caused by organisms that are sensitive to treatment with antibiotics. In the rarest of cases a patient may die of meningoencephalitis,[563] acute polyneuritis (Guillain–Barré syndrome),[564] rupture of the spleen,[565] hepatitis,[566] hypoplastic anaemia[567] or other complications:[565] for such reasons the disease has never been a condition to consider lightly. Now, advances in knowledge of the aetiology of the syndrome have brought much additional interest to the pathologist, as to the clinician. First, from the immediately practical point of view, is the need to investigate the cause in every case, particularly as this may be the means to counter the very rare, but potentially mortal, complications that require effective, and particular, treatment. Second, and more theoretically, infectious mononucleosis represents a remarkable meeting of influences that span the division between benign and cancerous diseases of the haemopoietic and lymphoreticular systems: recognition of the role of the Epstein–Barr virus in the causation of infectious mononucleosis, which is essentially a benign disease, and of Burkitt's lymphoma (see page 827) and nasopharyngeal carcinoma (see page 243), which are unequivocally malignant neoplasms, has introduced a new concept into our knowledge of the aetiology and pathogenesis of these diseases, and this is a concept that perhaps may have much wider implications.

There has always been speculation about the nature of 'infectious mononucleosis', whatever name we may give to it. One unusual view that may be noted is the thoughtful, and provocative, supposition that the disease might be regarded as a self-limiting (benign) form of leukaemia.[568] Certainly, infectious mononucleosis is in no way to be likened to leukaemia in prognostic terms, but it

would be rash to deny its unique characteristics and their great interest in relation to the role of viruses in the development of certain forms of malignant disease in man.

Nomenclature.—While *infectious mononucleosis* is the term most widely used for the conditions under discussion, and, interpreted literally, might be accepted as appropriate, whatever the nature of the infecting organism and whatever the identity of the cells involved, there is currently a trend to confine its use to cases associated with the presence both of heterophile antibodies that are not absorbed by guinea-pig kidney and of antibodies against the Epstein–Barr virus. All other cases of the syndrome would then be designated *glandular fever*. This seems to be a regrettably arbitrary restriction on the use of the term infectious mononucleosis, which literally specifies neither a particular cause of the disease nor a particular identity of the reacting cells and therefore is ill-suited to be used in an aetiologically specific way. It would be preferable to specify the cause of the infection, accepting for the time being the ambiguous 'mononucleosis', a term that is as applicable to proliferation of any other variety of mononuclear cell as to that of monocytes or lymphocytes, and that must stand until the identity of the circulating cells—not necessarily the same in cases of different causation—has been defined, as will surely be achieved in the foreseeable future. As most authorities seem to accept now that the cells usually are atypical lymphocytes, although whether T cells or B cells, or both, remains debatable,[569] maybe the time is coming when we may look forward to a more rational terminology.

Other synonyms that have been used to designate the *syndrome* include Pfeiffer's disease,[557] Filatov's disease (which should have precedence over the more commonly used eponym),[558] monocytic angina (see footnote on page 991), acute lymphadenosis and acute benign lymphoblastosis.*

Causation

The syndrome may be divided into three groups: those cases in which there are both heterophile antibodies and antibodies to the Epstein–Barr virus, those cases in which there are no heterophile anti-

---

* Infectious mononucleosis has also acquired unusually many inadmissible names, originating in mistranslation or misunderstanding. These include Piper's disease, pipers' disease, Druses' fever and Drusenfieber's disease (the last two may be traced to the title of Pfeiffer's original paper, *Drüsenfieber*, of which 'glandular fever' is the translation).

bodies although antibodies to the Epstein–Barr virus are present, and those cases in which there are neither heterophile antibodies nor antibodies to the Epstein–Barr virus. In the first two of these groups it is assumed that the cause of the syndrome is the Epstein–Barr virus. In the third group the recognized causes include *Listeria monocytogenes* (see page 577), *Toxoplasma gondii* (see page 653) and cytomegalovirus (see page 647). In Kyushu, in Japan, an essentially similar syndrome, presenting as an illness known locally as Kagami fever, is caused by a rickettsia, *Rickettsia sennetsui*.[570] It should be possible to distinguish by name each of these aetiologically distinct varieties of the syndrome; in practice, unfortunately, the organism responsible is not always demonstrable, and the non-specific terminology is likely to remain current (see above).

The known infective causes of the syndrome have been mentioned in the preceding paragraph. It is relevant to add that certain drugs may cause a similar syndrome (see page 696). These include the hydantoin group of anticonvulsant drugs, phenylbutazone, aminosalicylic acid and its salts (for instance, sodium aminosalicylate—'sodium PAS')[571] and sulphones.[572] In many cases in which drugs are responsible there are other side effects that should indicate the cause (for instance, haemolytic anaemia, conspicuous rashes, synovial reactions, peripheral neuropathy, renal disturbances, and jaundice resulting from damage to the liver): however, the various infective causes of mononucleosis may also cause such manifestations (see below)—the most important guide to the recognition of a drug-induced mononucleosis is awareness of the possibility.

Pfeiffer showed remarkable comprehension when, in his original account of 'glandular fever',[557] he made the point that he anticipated that its clinical picture would prove to be the manifestation of various disease processes that would be differentiated by bacteriological and morbid anatomical investigation.

Manifestations[565, 573]

Infectious mononucleosis of the usual type—that is, associated with Epstein–Barr virus—may occur at any age from infancy to extreme old age, but most of the patients are between 15 and 30 years, with no particular preponderance of either sex. It is difficult to define an incubation period, but circumstantial evidence from small outbreaks among groups of students suggests that it ranges between 4 and 8 weeks. Apart from some prodromal malaise, the most consistent initial manifestation is soreness of the throat: it is usually at this stage that lymphadenopathy becomes evident, the nodes in the neck, including particularly those below the angles of the jaw, being most markedly affected, although the involvement is commonly generalized. A rash, often morbilliform, is present in some cases but seldom lasts more than 2 to 3 days. Fever is usual: it seldom rises above 39°C. The spleen, although soft, is palpable in about half the cases; it rarely reaches 5 cm below the costal margin. About 10 per cent of the patients develop jaundice. In another 10 per cent the symptoms are much severer and resemble those of typhoid fever. The illness occasionally presents with abdominal pain that may lead to laparotomy.

Blood Picture.—The changes in the peripheral blood (see page 476) are characteristic. The white cell count usually reaches its highest levels in the third week of the clinical illness and rarely exceeds $20 \times 10^9/1$, although in exceptional cases, mainly in children, there may be a leukaemoid reaction, with counts up to $75 \times 10^9/1$. It is not the absolute cell count that is diagnostic, but the presence of a substantial proportion of atypical cells: if the proportion of these cells is from 13 to 19 per cent of the white cell count the condition is regarded by some authorities as probably infectious mononucleosis and if it is 20 per cent or above the diagnosis is considered to be definite.[574] In most cases the atypical cells account for 60 per cent or more of the white cell count. The atypical cells (see Fig. 8.26C, page 477) are now generally believed to be lymphocytes, although it is not yet determined whether they are T cells or B cells (the tumour cells of Burkitt's lymphoma, which is also associated with the Epstein–Barr virus, are usually identified as derived from B lymphocytes —see page 833).[569]

Complications.—Haemolytic anaemia is a rare complication and appears to be related to the development of a substantial titre of anti-i antibody (see page 465), which is a feature of many cases of infection by the Epstein–Barr virus. Not fewer than 50 per cent of patients with infectious mononucleosis show anti-i antibody in their serum, and it is assumed that the patients who develop frank haemolysis are those whose antibody titre reaches a sufficient level.[567]

Acute hypoplastic anaemia (aplastic anaemia)[567] and agranulocytosis[575] may occur but are very rare. Either may be fatal. Thrombocytopenia of a moderate degree is very frequently found; rarely, excessive bleeding results.[576]

It is said that a quarter of the patients have abnormalities of the cerebrospinal fluid and that a third have an abnormal electroencephalogram.[565] It is not surprising, then, that various neurological complications occur, with occasional fatality. Some degree of functional disturbance of the liver is to be found in a large proportion of cases,[577] in keeping with the frequency of hepatitis and of collections of atypical lymphocytes in biopsy specimens of the liver (see page 1226);[578] jaundice occurs in 5 to 10 per cent of cases and sometimes is the presenting sign.[579] Evidence of renal disturbance is sometimes found;[566] the nature of the lesions in the kidneys is uncertain. There is a predisposition to rupture of the enlarged spleen.

Cell-mediated immunity may be deficient, possibly because the infection interferes with the function of T lymphocytes. This may be demonstrated in some cases by a temporary failure of the normal cutaneous reaction to tuberculin. From the practical, clinical point of view it may predispose to certain types of 'opportunistic' infection, including systemic mycoses and generalized non-reactive tuberculosis: however, this occurs much more rarely than in, say, Hodgkin's disease, perhaps because patients who are recognized to have infectious mononucleosis are not treated by irradiation or with drugs that also lower resistance.

Pathology of the Lymph Nodes[580, 580a]

Lymph node biopsy is comparatively seldom the first indication of the correct diagnosis in cases of infectious mononucleosis. Ordinarily, the clinical picture leads to examination of the peripheral blood: the finding then of a substantial proportion of atypical lymphocytes is followed by investigation for the presence of circulating heterophile antibodies. When the clinical and haematological findings indicate the possibility of infectious mononucleosis but the Paul–Bunnell test for heterophile antibodies is negative and antibodies against the Epstein–Barr virus are not present the search for evidence of infection by any of the other types of organism that are known to cause the syndrome (for instance, *Listeria monocytogenes* and *Toxoplasma gondii*— see pages 577 and 653 respectively) is likely to be undertaken before deciding to recommend biopsy.

The nodes are usually only moderately enlarged, seldom exceeding 2 cm in any dimension. At present it does not seem possible to define a histological picture that is diagnostic of infectious mononucleo-sis, even if the attempt to find such a picture is made exclusively on the basis of examination of biopsy specimens from patients whose blood shows the classic qualitative and quantitative cytological changes and contains heterophile antibodies (not of Forssman type) and antibodies against the Epstein–Barr virus. In retrospect, earlier attempts to identify pathognomonic histological changes[581] may be considered to have indicated no more than the findings that should put the microscopist in mind of the disease, although they may prove to have some other cause.

The most striking changes in many cases are a marked hyperplasia of the pulp of the nodes, follicles often then being few and small, widely spaced, and almost—or totally—lacking germinal centres. Similarly, the sinuses are generally inconspicuous, although some degree of the condition known as 'immature sinus histiocytosis' (see page 561), is commonly found, mainly in the subcapsular sinus, and may be very marked. The cells in the sinuses, some of which are in mitosis, encroach somewhat on the adjoining pulp (Fig. 9.113). In the pulp itself there is a very varied proliferation of cells, their proportions and the extent to which they are intermingled differing widely from case to case and sometimes in different parts of a single node: reticulum cells, plasma cells and lymphocytes, and the precursors of these cells, and the large pale cells that are now considered to be transformed lymphocytes ('immunoblasts'—see page 522) make up a pleomorphic picture. The number of mitotic figures and the presence of binucleate and sometimes multinucleate cells may add to an overall ominous impression, particularly as the degree of cellular proliferation is such that the normal structure of the node may seem to have been destroyed, unless the reticulin pattern is carefully studied in silvered preparations. It is a feature of the binucleate and multinucleate cells that their nucleoli are relatively small and more haematoxyphile than those of Sternberg–Reed cells, with which they tend to be confused, sometimes leading to a misdiagnosis of Hodgkin's disease (Fig. 9.114).

In a small proportion of cases, small epithelioid cell clusters form and the picture may be difficult or impossible to distinguish from that of toxoplasmosis and other conditions that present this pattern (see page 656). Some of these are, in fact, cases of toxoplasmosis, which is one of the known causes of the syndrome of 'infectious mononucleosis', but without an accompanying development of heterophile antibodies (see page 648). Some are in other respects classic cases of infectious mononucleosis with

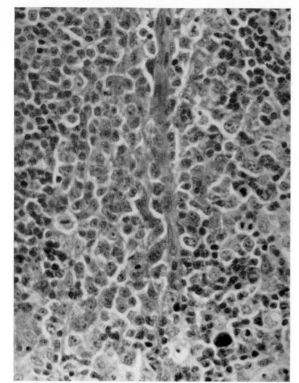

'A confident diagnosis of infectious mononucleosis cannot be made by histological means alone, although in some cases the histological findings suggest the possibility of this diagnosis; it is always necessary to obtain confirmation by haematological and serological means'.

Infectious Lymphocytosis[585]

There is doubt whether the condition that was described in 1941 as infectious lymphocytosis[586] is a variant of infectious mononucleosis (see above) or an entity. It is probably the latter. It occurs mainly in young children and, in typical cases, is characterized by fever, enlargement of lymph nodes and splenomegaly, and a large increase in the number of small lymphocytes in the circulation. The lymphocytes are of normal appearance. The total white cell count is usually within the range $30–50 \times 10^9/1$ but has been known to exceed $100 \times 10^9/1$. There may be an accompanying eosinophilia. No serological

Fig. 9.113. Lymph node in a case of infectious mononucleosis. The sinus on each side of the trabecula shows sinus histiocytosis of the 'immature' type, characterized by the accumulation of large, pale mononuclear cells. There is some extension of these cells into the adjoining pulp. Several mitotic figures are present and there is one large, hyperchromatic cell. Compare with the picture of 'sinus catarrh' (Fig. 9.38B, page 559) and simple sinus histiocytosis (Fig. 9.40, page 560). The more uniform appearance of the cells, their smaller size and compact association, and the conspicuous nucleoli are points of distinction from simple sinus histiocytosis. Infectious mononucleosis is one of the conditions that is most frequently accompanied by 'immature' sinus histiocytosis, the others including toxoplasmosis and brucella infection (see page 591). It can, sometimes, be very difficult to distinguish between this picture and the accumulation of leukaemic cells in the sinuses of lymph nodes, particularly in cases of acute monocytic leukaemia. The diagnosis of infectious mononucleosis may be suggested by the histologist, but it always requires confirmation by haematological and serological studies. See also Fig. 9.114. *Haematoxylin–eosin.* $\times 320$.

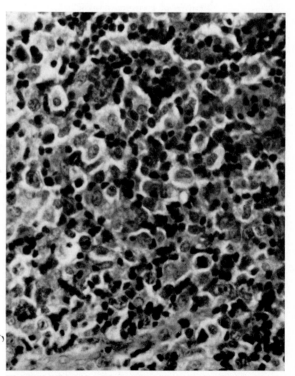

Fig. 9.114. Lymph node in another case of infectious mononucleosis, showing an unusually pleomorphic cellular picture such as is liable to be taken for that of Hodgkin's disease. Elsewhere, the node included changes in the sinuses such as are illustrated in Fig. 9.113: but for this, it is unlikely that the correct diagnosis would have been suggested on histological grounds. *Haematoxylin–eosin.* $\times 360$.

heterophile antibody formation[582] and antibodies against the Epstein–Barr virus.[583]

In the first edition of this book, 10 years ago, I wrote, '. . . although with experience a confident histological diagnosis of infectious mononucleosis can sometimes be made it is always necessary to obtain confirmation by haematological means'.[584] With more experience, now, I would modify this to,

abnormalities have been found. The lymphocytosis ordinarily subsides within 3 to 6 weeks. Respiratory symptoms are present in some cases, and the differential diagnosis from pertussis requires consideration. Meningeal symptoms, rashes and diarrhoea are occasionally present.[587] Both rubella and measles are liable to be simulated. The most serious diagnostic problem is related to the distinction from lymphocytic leukaemia, particularly as there may be a very marked proliferation of small lymphocytes in the bone marrow, even exceeding 90 per cent of the nucleated cells.[588] Lymph node biopsy may similarly suggest a leukaemic state, for the normal structure may seem to be largely or totally replaced by a great proliferation of small lymphocytes. Yet all these changes may revert to normal within a few weeks.

Adenovirus type 12 has been isolated in a number of cases[589] and enteroviruses have been isolated in some others.

Protozoal Lymphadenitis

While almost any protozoal infection may be accompanied by lymphadenitis, it is comparatively unusual for this to be a conspicuous feature of the clinical picture. For instance, lymphadenitis is not frequently observed in the course of malaria or amoebiasis, nor is it a recognized accompaniment of such frequent conditions as giardia infection of the intestine (see page 1079) and trichomonas infection of the genital tract. In the case of the two last-named conditions it may be that the organism does not pass to the lymph nodes; alternatively, lymph node involvement may be overlooked because it is clinically inapparent—for instance, *Balantidium coli*, a protozoon appreciably larger ($30–150 \times 25–120\,\mu$m) than either *Giardia lamblia* ($12–16 \times 6–8\ \mu$m) or *Trichomonas* species ($8–30 \times 3–16\ \mu$m), has been found in mesenteric nodes (Fig. 9.115) in some cases of severe ulcerative balantidial colitis (see page 1115):[590] it may be that specific protozoal lymphadenitis, caused by such organisms, is likely to be detected only in such rare circumstances.

In other protozoal infections, lymphadenitis may be an important diagnostic feature (for instance, in the course of the reaction to the initial infection in cases of trypanosomiasis), or a familiar clinical manifestation (for instance, in visceral leishmaniasis), or the presenting and most frequent clinical feature (for instance, in acquired toxoplasmosis).

Some of these conditions may be considered in more detail.

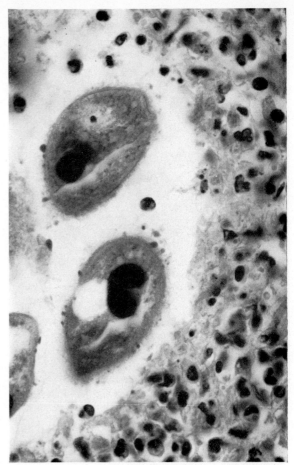

Fig. 9.115. Infection of a paracolic lymph node by *Balantidium coli*. The patient, an alcoholic with severe nutritional deficiencies, developed perforation of the sigmoid colon. The perforated bowel was resected successfully. Its mucosa was extensively ulcerated, and it was one of the ulcers that had perforated. Histological examination showed a heavy infection of the ulcerated area by balantidia. The organisms were present in several of the lymph nodes in the mesocolon. They had caused focal suppuration, mainly in the region of the subcapsular sinus. The photograph shows two trophozoites. The cilia covering the delicate cuticle of the organism, the reniform macronucleus, and various inclusions in the cytoplasm are seen. It is exceptionally rare for the balantidium to be found apart from the immediate vicinity of the intestinal lesions. *Haematoxylin–eosin.* × 630.

Toxoplasmosis[591, 592]

It is probable that toxoplasmosis is one of the most prevalent, and geographically the most widespread, protozoal infection of man. *Toxoplasma gondii*, a coccidian parasite of worldwide distribution, was discovered independently, in 1908, by Nicolle and Manceaux,[593] in the Pasteur Institute in Tunis, where they recognized it as the cause of a disease in

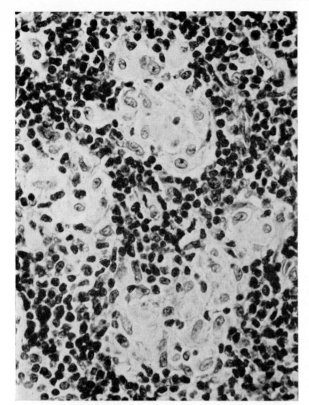

Fig. 9.116B. Same specimen as Fig. 9.116A. Higher magnification of the epithelioid cell clusters. *Haematoxylin–eosin.* ×375.

gates; necrosis elsewhere in the affected nodes is mentioned below. There is no tendency to fibrosis. In general, the architecture of the nodes is well maintained.

Some degree of sinus histiocytosis is always present. It is of the type described as 'immature' (see page 561) (Figs 9.116C and 9.117). There may be necrosis in the accumulations of histiocytes in the sinuses; phagocytosis of nuclear debris by larger macrophages is then a feature, and occasionally a local infiltration of neutrophils, and sometimes of eosinophils, may be seen. In a small proportion of cases there is a diffuse scattering of solitary, large, pale cells in the pulp (Fig. 9.118): this may mimic the picture of 'immunoblastic lymphadenopathy' (see page 703), except that the vascular proliferation characteristic of the latter is lacking and some of the cells have a hyperchromatic nucleus or may be binucleate. The finding of hyperchromatic and binucleate cells may cause the microscopist to suspect the presence of Hodgkin's disease (Fig. 9.119), a problem in differential diagnosis that is the more difficult to resolve because some cases of

Hodgkin's disease in its early stages are characterized by the formation of epithelioid cell clusters (see page 797).

Follicular hyperplasia is a frequent finding and there may be uncommonly large germinal centres. Foci of necrosis may appear in the pulp, without relation to the epithelioid cell aggregates: such foci are marked by local oedema and a scattering of nuclear debris, some of it engulfed by macrophages.

The Parasites in Histological Preparations.—Toxoplasmas are demonstrable in the sections of the nodes only in the most exceptional cases of toxoplasmic lymphadenitis.[627] They may be found in the form of the typical parasitic cysts, which vary

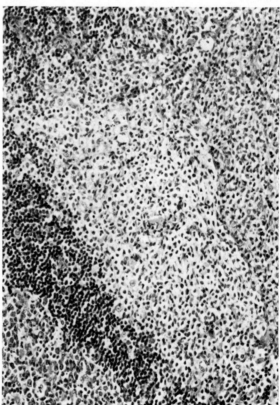

Fig. 9.116C. Same specimen as Figs 9.116A and 9.116B. Sinus histiocytosis of the 'immature' type. The line of the capsule of the node is seen toward the right of the picture. The subcapsular sinus is filled uniformly by relatively small, pale histiocytes. These cells encroach on the adjoining lymphoid tissue, including the follicle (below, left), and, as an unusual feature, in this instance have infiltrated the capsule also. See also Fig. 9.43 (page 562), which is an enlargement of part of this field, and compare with other examples of immature sinus histiocytosis illustrated in Figs 9.113 (page 651) and 9.117 (the latter from another case of toxoplasmosis). *Haematoxylin–eosin.* ×150.

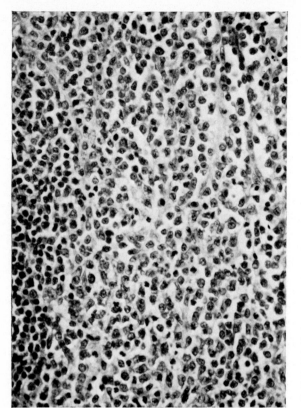

Fig. 9.117. Toxoplasmic lymphadenitis. Sinus histiocytosis of the 'immature' type. The cells appear to have less cytoplasm than those in Fig. 9.116C and the general appearance of the lesion is consequently different. To some extent such a difference between specimens may be due to differences in fixation and other technical effects. It may be noted that the demarcation between the cellular accumulation in the sinus and the adjoining lymphoid tissue is blurred by the encroachment of the histiocytes on the latter. *Haematoxylin–eosin.* × 275.

considerably in size but are commonly of the order of 60 μm in diameter; the cysts are filled with merozoites. When cysts are found they usually appear to lie free in the tissues, without any reaction to their presence; sometimes it is possible to make out that a cyst is in fact within the cytoplasm of a macrophage. Occasionally, in the vicinity of a recently ruptured cyst, the released merozoites—which at this stage come to be known as trophozoites—may be seen free in the tissues, or within macrophages, in the bow-shaped (crescentic) form to which the toxoplasma owes its name. The trophozoites measure within the range of 4–7 × 2–4 μm. They vary in shape, those that are extracellular being more typically crescentic, with pointed ends, while those that are within cells tend to be shorter, with rounded ends, and may be almost spherical. Their recognition

in sections can be very difficult (Fig. 9.120), particularly as they tend to degenerate; moreover, various particles of nuclear or cytoplasmic debris that may be present in any lymph node, normal or pathological, may take on a particularly confusing aspect when the histologist is looking for parasites as elusive as the toxoplasma.

Differential Diagnosis.—There are important diagnostic considerations in relation to every case in which multiple, small, discrete, epithelioid cell aggregates are found in lymph node biopsy specimens. These aggregates are not pathognomonic of toxoplasmosis. They are seen in identical form in

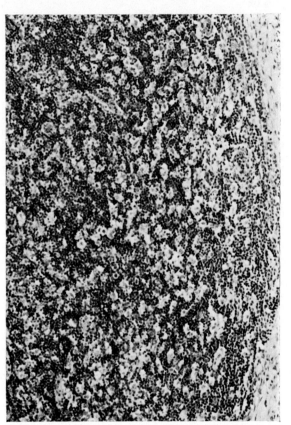

Fig. 9.118. Toxoplasmic lymphadenitis. In this field there is a quite uniform pattern of pale cells scattered among the lymphocytes of the cortex. Some of the pale cells are grouped in clusters, but these are appreciably smaller than the epithelioid cell clusters that are the most characteristic feature of the lymphadenitis of toxoplasmosis; other cells lie singly, are round, and have a large nucleus and abundant cytoplasm. The picture in general, at this order of magnification, resembles the appearances associated with proliferation of immunoblasts in the lymphoid tissues (see Fig. 9.153, page 704). The node illustrated also contained areas of the character shown in Figs 9.116A and 9.116B. *Haematoxylin–eosin.* × 100.

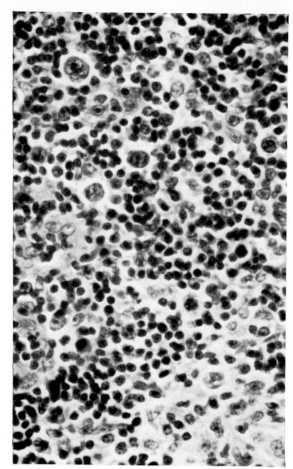

Fig. 9.119. Toxoplasmic lymphadenitis. Appearances such as are shown in this field led to an initial diagnosis of Hodgkin's disease in this case, but with the comment that toxoplasmosis was the alternative possibility in view of the presence of epithelioid cell clusters such as those in Figs 9.116A and 9.116B (which illustrate another case). Part of one such cluster is seen at the bottom of the picture. The serological tests for toxoplasmosis proved to be strongly positive. The binucleate and hyperchromatic cells included in this field, whatever their nature—atypical reticulum cells or atypical immunoblasts—remain a perplexing feature of some cases of toxoplasmosis, as of brucella infection (see Fig. 9.67, page 592); their presence demands consideration of the possibility that the patient may have Hodgkin's disease. *Haematoxylin–eosin.* ×400.

and cat-scratch disease (page 640), immunoblastic lymphadenopathy (page 704), some instances of the granulomatous lymphadenitis that may affect nodes draining the site of a carcinoma (page 682), some instances of the lymphadenitis accompanying fatal granulomatous disease of childhood due to deficiency of the bactericidal activity of the neutrophils (page 710), and a variant of Hodgkin's disease (page 806).

In individual cases there may be particular features that exclude certain diagnostic possibilities —for instance, the absence of sinus histiocytosis of the so-called 'immature' type (see page 561) in nodes affected with tuberculosis or sarcoidosis may help to

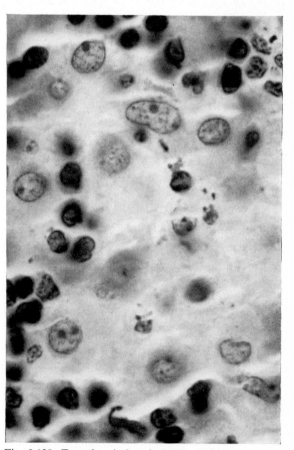

Fig. 9.120. Toxoplasmic lymphadenitis. This field, at the margin of an epithelioid cell cluster adjoining a trabecular sinus, contains several free trophozoites of *Toxoplasma gondii*, some rounded and some elongated and bowed. The parasites were more easily demonstrated under the microscope, with the advantage of being able to focus throughout the thickness of the section. It must be noted that some of the particles in this field are probably fragments of tissue debris. Unless toxoplasma cysts are seen, the parasites can rarely be identified with certainty from other particulate structures. *Haematoxylin–eosin.* ×1200.

specimens that represent a remarkable range of different diseases. These include early stages in the development of sarcoidosis (see page 747) and of mycobacterial lymphadenitis (page 600), primary and secondary syphilis (pages 612 and 613), infectious mononucleosis (page 650), certain forms of listeria infection (page 578), yersinia infection (page 585), tularaemia (page 588), brucella infection (page 591), lymphogranuloma inguinale (page 636)

distinguish between early stages of these conditions and toxoplasmosis, in which this type of sinus reaction is almost the rule (Figs 9.116C and 9.117). In leishmanial lymphadenitis, the only difference from toxoplasmic lymphadenitis is the readily discernible presence of the leishmaniae in the cytoplasm of the epithelioid cells (Figs 9.121A and 9.121B, page 662).

Although toxoplasmosis is the condition that most frequently shows this picture of multiple, small foci of epithelioid histiocytes in lymph nodes, the biopsy problem is less straightforward than the striking appearances might suggest. The difficulties reflect the range of diseases that may present the same, or essentially the same, picture, and the variety of special investigations that must be undertaken in order to identify the cause. In most cases the histologist can do no more than indicate the possibilities, and the eventual solution depends on the findings of his colleagues in other laboratories. In a small but not insignificant proportion of cases the diagnosis remains elusive until the clinical course of the disease discloses other features that provide the key. Sometimes the lymphadenitis subsides undiagnosed.

Diagnosis of Toxoplasmosis.[591, 593]—The histological picture is not itself diagnostic unless unmistakable toxoplasmas are seen in the sections, and this is a finding of quite exceptional rarity: even then, other investigations are essential in order to confirm the identity of the parasite. Isolation of the organism provides the most conclusive evidence, but care still needs to be taken because of the possibility that the toxoplasma has been dormant, coincidentally, in tissue affected by another disease.* Inoculation of possibly infected material into the peritoneal cavity of mice remains the most frequently used means of isolating the toxoplasma, and ordinarily is very much more sensitive than attempts to grow it in chick embryos or in tissue cultures. Great care is necessary to ensure that the animals are free from enzootic toxoplasmosis. Positive results are likeliest in the early weeks of the disease.

The dye test of Sabin and Feldman[628] ('cytoplasm-modifying test') becomes positive within 8 to 14 days of the clinical onset, the haemagglutination test rather later and the complement fixation test within a month.

---

* I have blundered at least once in such a situation: in this case the subsequent course indicated that the lymphadenopathy had been, in fact, an early manifestation of infection by *Mycobacterium scrofulaceum* (see page 607). The patient was the fiancé of a colleague.

Source of Infection.—Toxoplasmosis, which appears to be caused by the same species, *Toxoplasma gondii*, in all the varieties of animals and birds in which it has been recognized, is so widespread that it cannot be surprising that subclinical and clinical infections are as frequent as they are. There are several sources and means of infection. The two most important are ingestion of infected animal tissue and faecal contamination. Infection in man may result from eating raw or undercooked meat[629, 630] (pork, and lamb or mutton, rather than veal or beef[631]): the infection is then due to the presence of toxoplasma cysts in the muscle fibres.[632] Faecal contamination is commonly to be blamed on cats,[633] which contaminate the environment with oocysts of the parasite that are infective to other carnivores, to herbivores and to man.[634] Occasional sources of infection, other than the transplacental route (which is a special case—see page 653),[635] include accidental inoculation in laboratories[636] and during necropsy,[637] organ transplantation[614] and—particularly rarely—blood transfusion.[638] Saliva of patients with lymphadenitis has been found to contain toxoplasmas;[639] the significance of this observation as a means of transmission of the infection is unclear. The parasites have also been demonstrated in the milk of infected animals, including cattle, goats and sheep,[640] but there is no evidence that this is a source of infection of man; it may be noted that the toxoplasma is destroyed by pasteurization.

Leishmaniasis

The leishmaniae and the trypanosomes are the only members of the family Trypanosomatidae, the haemoflagellates, that are pathogenic to man. The leishmaniae are predominantly intracellular parasites, infecting the cells of the reticuloendothelial system (see page 525). The two main varieties of leishmanial disease, visceral leishmaniasis (kala azar) and cutaneous leishmaniasis, are caused by different species of leishmania. Visceral leishmaniasis is characterized by infection of the reticuloendothelial cells throughout the body, great enlargement of the spleen and liver being among its typical manifestations. In cutaneous leishmaniasis the infection is usually confined to the skin or, in American leishmaniasis, to the skin and the mucocutaneous junctional regions. Involvement of lymph nodes is regularly present in visceral leishmaniasis as part of the generalized infection of the reticuloendothelial system. In contrast, lymphadenopathy is seldom evident in cases of cutaneous leishmaniasis.

All forms of leishmaniasis are transmitted by phlebotomine sandflies.[641] The female sandfly is a blood-sucking insect and becomes infected while feeding, taking up with her blood meal some of the leishmaniae that are present in the macrophages in the dermis—for instance, in dogs, which are often a reservoir of the infection—or, particularly when man is the reservoir, acquiring the parasite in the blood itself, where it may occasionally be demonstrated in the cytoplasm of monocytes and, more rarely, of polymorphonuclear leucocytes, in cases of visceral leishmaniasis. The sandfly ingests the parasite in the so-called amastigote (flagellum-less) or 'leishmanial' form in which it is found in the mammalian hosts. In the midgut of the sandfly the ingested amastigote develops into the promastigote (flagellate) or 'leptomonad' form, which is not seen in infected vertebrates. The elongated, motile promastigotes migrate to the fore part of the midgut and eventually are expelled into the bite when the insect starts to feed. Once in the new host, the promastigotes are taken up by macrophages, undergo binary fission and multiply rapidly, now in the amastigote form, to fill the cytoplasm of the parasitized cells. The latter rupture, liberating the organisms, which are ingested by further phagocytes and establish the disease.

Morphology of the Leishmania.—The various species of leishmania that cause diseases in man and other mammals cannot be distinguished by their appearances, either in films or sections of infected material or in cultures. The only means of differentiating them is Adler's test:[642] in this test the organism under investigation is grown in culture in the presence of specific antisera, which inhibit the formation of the flagellum, the serum having no effect on the normal development of the promastigotes of the species other than the one against which it has been prepared.

The amastigote—the familiar intracellular Leishman–Donovan body—is a rounded or ovoid structure of about 3–4 μm in its main dimension. It is seen readily enough in haematoxylin–eosin preparations of biopsy specimens, but may be difficult to distinguish from small intracellular fungal cells, particularly *Histoplasma capsulatum* (see page 624) and also small forms of *Paracoccidioides brasiliensis* (see page 627) and of *Cryptococcus neoformans* (see page 622). The leishmaniae do not give a positive periodic-acid/Schiff reaction and are not blackened in Grocott–Gomori hexamine (methenamine) silver preparations (see page 616). Unlike most strains of cryptococci they are not mucicarminophile. In contrast to the fungal cells, leishmaniae stain distinctively with Romanowsky stains, particularly Giemsa's stain, but these are really helpful only when the tissue has been freshly fixed in Zenker's solution or a similar fixative in place of formalin. In good Giemsa-stained histological preparations the nucleus of the leishmania is well defined, purplish, and 1–2 μm in diameter; nearby is the kinetoplast, a rod-shaped or ovoid structure, dark purple or dark blue, and about 0·5–1·0 μm in length. The kinetoplast comprises the blepharoplast, from which—in the flagellate (promastigote) form of the parasite—the flagellum originates, and the parabasal body, which is a clump of mitochondrial deoxyribonucleic acid. These cytological details are much more readily seen in Romanowsky-stained films, and, where possible, a histological diagnosis of leishmaniasis should always be subjected to confirmation by study of films—for instance, of bone marrow or of aspirates from enlarged lymph nodes, or other viscera, in cases of visceral leishmaniasis, or from the ulcerated lesions in cases of cutaneous and mucocutaneous leishmaniasis.

When examining histological sections, it is sometimes helpful that silver methods for impregnating reticulin fibres blacken the complex formed by the nucleus and kinetoplast of the leishmaniae: provided the cytoplasm of the macrophages that contain the parasites is not itself too heavily silvered, this characteristic may be a guide to the diagnosis.

The need to distinguish leishmaniae from fungal cells has been mentioned above. They must also be distinguished from other protozoa. There should be no serious difficulty in telling them from toxoplasmas, including the rounded merozoites liberated from the cysts, which are likelier than the crescent form to be confused with leishmanial amastigotes. In contrast, it is very difficult to see any difference between leishmaniae and the amastigote form of *Trypanosoma cruzi*, the cause of American trypanosomiasis (Chagas's disease) (see also page 666, and Fig. 1.40, page 47), although experts may find it possible to recognize one from the other by the larger size of the kinetoplast of the latter.

Visceral Leishmaniasis (Kala Azar*)

Visceral leishmaniasis, wherever it occurs, is caused by *Leishmania donovani*. Some authorities recognize

---

* *Kala azar* is the Assamese vernacular name for the disease, *kala* meaning 'black' and *azar* meaning 'sickness'. Dr Sharat C. Desai, of King Edward Memorial Hospital and Seth G. S. Medical College, Bombay, and Canon Kenyon

subspecies, including *Leishmania donovani infantum* (*Leishmania infantum*) as the cause of Mediterranean visceral leishmaniasis, which affects young children particularly, *Leishmania donovani nilotica* as the cause of visceral leishmaniasis in the Sudan, and *Leishmania donovani chagasi* as the cause of visceral leishmaniasis in Brazil. It seems that the main reason for distinguishing these subspecies is geographical, for there is no agreed criterion for differentiating any of them on microbiological grounds.

Epidemiology.—Epidemiologically, visceral leishmaniasis may be considered in three groups, distinguished by different reservoirs of infection

that are the source from which the sandflies acquire the parasites and so maintain the endemic, epidemic or sporadic incidence of the disease in man. Throughout the Mediterranean basin and across the Middle East and the southern parts of the Soviet Union to Central Asia and China the reservoir is canine (the dog in towns, and the dog, fox, wolf, or jackal in rural areas). The infected animal is sick and emaciated, and its skin is thickened and often extensively ulcerated. Dogs and foxes are also the reservoir in Brazil, where the disease occurs mainly in the north east.[643] In all these regions the disease affects infants or children in the first decade, with the greatest frequency within the first 5 years of life.

In Africa,[644] visceral leishmaniasis occurs mainly in the Sudan, northern Kenya, Ethiopia and Somalia. The reservoir animals are species of rodents. The disease is seen oftenest in the second decade.

In north-eastern India[645] and in Bangladesh man is himself the reservoir of infection. Most of the patients are adolescents and young adults.

The frequency of the disease, its distribution, and its clinical and epidemiological pattern vary appreciably.[646] In has become less prevalent in Assam and West Bengal, the regions of India in which it has long been most frequent, and the same is true of Bangladesh, but natural catastrophes, such as floods, drought and famine—and, possibly, other epidemic diseases, particularly cholera—can be followed by its recrudescence. Its recognition has become commoner and more widespread in China,[647] in East Africa,[644] and in the north-eastern states of Brazil,[643] which are the main centres of its prevalence in South America (visceral leishmaniasis is not known to occur in Central America or North America).

In some regions where leishmaniasis has been prevalent, control of malaria by attacking the mosquito vector also reduced the number of sandflies and so lowered the incidence of leishmanial infection: when the local eradication of malaria had been achieved, the insecticidal measures ended and the sandflies eventually returned, to resume the transmission of leishmaniasis from the reservoirs of infection to fresh hosts.

Clinical Manifestations.—Fever, weakness, emaciation, anaemia, and enlargement of the liver and spleen are the main clinical features in classic cases. The characteristic, but inconstant, darkening of the skin is mentioned in the footnote on page 659:[648] the pigmentation is not usually accompanied by the demonstrable presence of the parasites in the skin,

E. Wright, of the International Development Centre, Coventry Cathedral, have kindly helped in interpreting the range of other meanings of the term. The words are common to the Hindi and Bengali languages as well as belonging to Assamese, all three languages being of Sanskrit origin, and the meaning is the same in all and may be taken either literally or metaphorically. It has become usual, in western writings, to interpret *kala azar* as the 'black disease' in terms of the increased pigmentation of the skin of the patient, which may be noticeable, especially over the abdomen and at the extremities, even in normally dark-skinned people. In fact, it is likelier that the words were originally used with the sense of 'black' as 'deadly'—the 'deadly illness' (the great epidemic in Assam in the last decades of the nineteenth century had a mortality, at its height, of close on 100 per cent, and before the introduction of antimonial therapy the disease was fatal in 70 to 90 per cent of cases, wherever it occurred). The mortality is so high, in the absence of chemotherapy, that some etymologists have suggested that the name *kala azar* was derived originally not from *kala* but from *kal*, meaning 'death'—the 'death sickness', which, figuratively translated, became *kala azar*, the 'black sickness' (those inclined to see an analogy with 'Black Death', the vulgar synonym of bubonic plague, should read the history of this name: Shrewsbury, J. F. D., *A History of Bubonic Plague in the British Isles*, page 37; Cambridge, 1970).

The name *Dum Dum fever*, also a synonym of visceral leishmaniasis (and possibly the source of the misnomer *Stummfieber*—'dumb fever'—listed among its names in a publication in German), is, with the dumdum bullet, a memento of the military cantonment at Dum Dum, the region of the outskirts of Calcutta where the city's international airport is now situated. Visceral leishmaniasis was prevalent among British and Indian troops stationed there. Leishman discovered the parasite of the disease when, while on leave in 1900, he made a post-mortem examination in the case of a British soldier who had been invalided from Dum Dum to England (Leishman, W. B., *Brit. med. J.*, 1903, **1**, 1252); Donovan's independent discovery of the parasite, while serving in Madras, was published shortly afterwards (Donovan, C., *Brit. med. J.*, 1903, **2**, 79).

Leishman's account of the disease, published before the 1914–18 war, is still read with advantage (Leishman, W. B., in *A System of Medicine by Many Writers*, edited by C. Allbutt and H. D. Rolleston, vol. 2, part 2, page 226; London, 1912).

and it is quite unrelated to the so-called 'post-kala-azar dermal leishmanoid': the latter is a widespread nodular lesion, containing the organisms, that develops in a variable proportion of cases after treatment of visceral leishmaniasis and that may persist for many years.[649]

Moderate enlargement of lymph nodes is often evident: in some instances enlarged nodes are the most conspicuous clinical finding.[650] In cases of visceral leishmaniasis occurring on the Mediterranean littoral, where the disease is seen mainly in young children ('infantile kala azar'), generalized lymphadenopathy is commonly a feature; there may be no evident enlargement of the liver and spleen. There are regional differences in the findings. In Malta, for instance, although the disease is becoming less common it is still among the more frequent causes of lymph node enlargement in children.[651] Among the Maltese it is almost exclusively children in the first 4 years of life who acquire the disease:[652] the clinical picture is that of visceral leishmaniasis as it occurs elsewhere, and the notable involvement of the spleen is recognized in the former local name, marda tal-biċċa ('splenic disease'), although the first sign of the infection may be enlargement of superficial nodes, particularly in the neck. Adults who acquire the disease in Malta are usually immigrants and other foreign residents from parts of the world where leishmaniasis does not occur:[653, 654] again, lymphadenopathy is often obtrusive in these cases, and it may be the only clinical finding, as was not infrequently found when the disease affected British service personnel stationed in the Maltese Islands.[655] The occasional misdiagnosis of leishmanial lymphadenitis as acute leukaemia in children who became infected in the Mediterranean region is referred to on page 663.

Lymph node enlargement is often conspicuous in cases of visceral leishmaniasis in East Africa. In many of these cases it is the inguinal nodes that are most markedly involved.[656] A doctor, working in East Africa, had had a benign pigmented naevus removed from one leg some months before the appearance of enlarged nodes in the groin of the same side: a clinical biologist in Europe misinterpreted the leishmania-laden macrophages as melanoma cells, and the patient took his own life; necropsy disclosed the presence of visceral leishmaniasis.

In India, lymphadenopathy is rarely remarked as a manifestation of visceral leishmaniasis.[649] In Brazil, a slight degree of lymph node enlargement is said to be usual but clinically unobtrusive. However, massive enlargement of cervical and axillary lymph nodes, in the absence of enlargement of the liver and spleen, was the presenting sign in the case of a student from Ceará, in north-eastern Brazil, who became ill while working in Britain.[657]

Diagnosis.—Demonstration of the leishmania is the simplest and most effective means of diagnosis, and is better undertaken on film preparations than in histological sections, although the latter are sufficient provided care in interpretation avoids confusion with other organisms (see page 659). Most clinicians prefer aspiration to open biopsy. Aspirated bone marrow is suitable, but the operation, although safer than needling the spleen or liver, is viewed with such apprehension by many patients that it is more usual for the sample to be obtained from the latter organs. Unless they are markedly enlarged, superficial lymph nodes seem less likely to give positive results than the spleen, liver or bone marrow.

Occasionally, the diagnosis requires inoculation of hamsters, and evidence of infection may not develop in these animals for many months. Cultures and serological investigations (complement fixation, fluorescent antibody and haemagglutination tests) are occasionally helpful. The leishmanin skin test (Montenegro test[658]) indicates delayed hypersensitivity and is of very limited value: it becomes positive some weeks after completion of successful treatment, but only in cases of visceral leishmaniasis of East African origin;[659] it also becomes positive during the course of cutaneous leishmaniasis, and as it remains positive for life its significance in individual cases has to be interpreted circumspectly.

Pathology.—Infection of the cells of the reticulo-endothelial system (see page 525) by the leishmania, their enlargement and their great proliferation are the essential histopathological feature of visceral leishmaniasis. This accounts, directly or indirectly, for all the manifestations. In addition to the enlargement of the affected organs, the proliferation of the parsitized macrophages in bone marrow may, rarely, be so extensive that anaemia, leucopenia and thrombocytopenia result: a picture may thus develop that has been likened to a leucoerythroblastic anaemia (see page 462). Anaemia and pancytopenia in cases of visceral leishmaniasis have been attributed also to hypersplenism as an effect of the gross splenomegaly (see page 724).[660]

In general, the pathological picture in the various organs reflects the distribution of their reticulo-endothelial components. Its general features are exemplified in the lymph nodes. The pathognomonic feature of the lymphadenitis of leishmaniasis is the presence of the leishmaniae in large numbers in the cytoplasm of macrophages.[661] These are seen both in the sinuses and in the pulp. In the former they may remain attached to the stroma or lie free. In the pulp they may be sparse or quite numerous, and disposed singly or, less often, in clusters of two to four cells; exceptionally, multinucleate forms appear. In other cases, the macrophages in the pulp undergo epithelioid metamorphosis:[655, 662] the picture may then come to resemble non-caseating tuberculosis or sarcoidosis;[655] or much smaller aggregates of epithelioid cells form that, except for the readily identifiable presence of the leishmaniae (Figs 9.121A and 9.121B), exactly reproduce the picture described on page 654 as typical of toxoplasmosis.[662] There is also a very marked proliferation of plasma cells and their precursors throughout the pulp;[663] they are commonly accompanied by many Russell bodies and by eosinophile protein crystals.

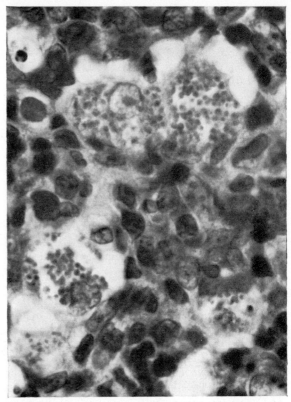

Fig. 9.121B. Same specimen as Fig. 9.121A. The leishmaniae (Leishman–Donovan bodies) have to be distinguished from other parasites that may be ingested by macrophages, including the amastigote form of trypanosomes (particularly in cases of American trypanosomiasis—see Fig. 9.123, page 666) and *Histoplasma capsulatum* (see Fig. 9.94, page 624). *Haematoxylin–eosin.* × 1000.

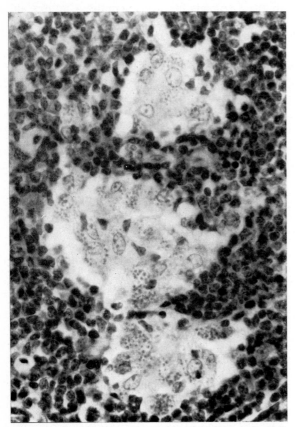

Fig. 9.121A. Lymphadenitis of visceral leishmaniasis (kala azar). The three clusters of epithelioid histiocytes differ from those in toxoplasmosis only in the presence of the leishmaniae in the cytoplasm of the cells (see Fig. 9.116B). See also Fig. 9.121B. *Haematoxylin–eosin.* × 430.

Histological Differential Diagnosis.—The possibility of confusing leishmaniae in histological sections with other protozoa and with fungi has been mentioned (see page 659). By coincidence, after drafting that paragraph I was asked to act as a referee of a paper submitted for publication in a West European journal by a group of doctors of whom one occasionally works in Malta while the others seem to have no serious professional knowledge of the islands. The paper purported to be about the first cases of histoplasmosis to be recognized in Malta: there were no cultures, and there had been 'no opportunity' for serological or histoplasmin tests, but the appearance of the intracellular parasites in sections of lymph node biopsy specimens was described as characteristic of *Histoplasma capsulatum* on the grounds of the authors' experience of histoplasmosis as an endemic disease in their own country. An opportunity to review the histological preparations showed the parasites to be leishmaniae; the authors were informed. They revised the paper and (in 1976) resubmitted it for publication as an account of the first cases of leishmaniasis to be recognized in Malta. It has been turned down again.

In the period 1968–76 I saw, in western Europe, five children, all under the age of 7 years, in whose case a diagnosis of acute leukaemia had been made and who had in common wealthy parents with holiday homes in the Mediterranean region (Malta, Sicily and Corfu). The illness presented with fever, progressive anaemia, splenomegaly and enlargement of superficial lymph nodes in the neck or elsewhere. The blood contained abnormal cells that were taken to be leukaemic 'blast' cells; similar cells were found in the bone marrow. Acute leukaemia was diagnosed. Three of the children were put on treatment accordingly. Further investigation showed that all five had visceral leishmaniasis; four were treated successfully for leishmaniasis, including a pair of twins whose family doctor had advised the parents to have a second paediatric opinion before agreeing to the treatment for leukaemia (the consultant who gave the second opinion saw the children with his registrar, a Maltese doctor who suggested the correct diagnosis). The fifth child died of an 'opportunistic' fungal infection as a complication of the treatment given for leukaemia. None of these five children had leukaemia. A sixth child, with a comparable geographical history, whose illness presented with similar manifestations during this period, proved to have acute leukaemia; leishmaniasis was not present.

Cutaneous Leishmaniasis ('Oriental Sore')

In contrast to visceral leishmaniasis (see above), cutaneous leishmaniasis is very seldom accompanied by the development of lymphadenitis. In many of the cases in which the regional lymph nodes become enlarged it is likely that this is no more than a non-specific reaction associated with ulceration of the leishmanial lesion of the skin, possibly with secondary bacterial infection in a few cases. Rarely, corynebacterial infection is superimposed on a leishmanial ulcer (see page 580).

Ulceration and secondary infection occur more frequently in cases of rural cutaneous leishmaniasis. This is caused by *Leishmania tropica* of particular virulence (*Leishmania tropica major*) and is seen particularly in Central Asia and parts of Iran. It is in this type of cutaneous leishmaniasis that satellite foci may be seen along the line of the regional lymphatics, and leishmanial infection of the regional nodes has sometimes been demonstrated. The urban variety of cutaneous leishmaniasis, caused by *Leishmania tropica minor*, is a less rapidly developing, longer lasting infection, with less tendency to ulcerate and correspondingly less scarring. It is seen in many cities in the Middle East and throughout much of the Mediterranean littoral and also in Pakistan and north-western India.

Cutaneous and visceral leishmaniasis may co-exist. Neither appears to provide immunity against the other. In general, however, there is notably little geographical overlap of the two forms of leishmaniasis.

American Cutaneous and Mucocutaneous Leishmaniasis

Cutaneous leishmaniasis is more widespread in the Americas than visceral leishmaniasis, which is practically confined to parts of Brazil (see page 660). The cutaneous infection is caused by *Leishmania brasiliensis* and transmitted by phlebotomine sandflies of the genus *Lutzomyia*. The disease has many exotic vernacular names and some exotic scientific ones. In Mexico, particularly in Yucatán, and in parts of Guatemala and of Belize, it is familiar as the chicleros' ulcer (chicle ulcer),* which is a destructive lesion that most frequently affects the auricle (pinna): the organism that causes it is sometimes considered to be a distinct species, *Leishmania mexicana*, but usually is regarded as a subspecies of *Leishmania brasiliensis*.[664] A form of the infection that occurs particularly frequently in Venezuela is sometimes known as leishmaniasis tegumentaria diffusa (diffuse cutaneous leishmaniasis):[665] this is a spreading, usually non-ulcerative, nodular infiltration that, in the course of many years, may come to cover much of the body, and that may exactly reproduce the clinical picture of lepromatous leprosy.[666, 667] A condition very similar to the diffuse cutaneous leishmaniasis of South America is seen sometimes in East Africa in cases of infection by *Leishmania tropica*:[668] in some cases there is an accompanying leishmanial infection of the superficial lymph nodes, as in the case of an Ethiopian student recently seen in London.[657]

Cutaneous leishmaniasis goes by the name *uta* in

* *Pace* those who imply that the disease was described by Chiclero, it is in fact an occupational disease of *chicleros*, the labourers who collect the coagulated milky juice (latex) obtained by tapping the sapodilla, a wild-growing tree in tropical and subtropical America. The coagulum is *chicle*, or chicle gum, once imported into North America as a substitute for rubber and later to become the basic ingredient of chewing gum, until synthetic substances took its place.

Peru and Chile; it has become rare in these countries. In Brazil the disease is known as *espundia*.

With the exception of the chicleros' ulcer, any manifestation of American cutaneous leishmaniasis may spread ('metastasize') to involve muco-cutaneous junctional regions, particularly the mouth and nostrils and sometimes the eyelids and the anal, vulvar and penile areas. This occurs most frequently in the Brazilian cases. The route of such extension of the infection is uncertain; it is thought to be the blood stream. Some enlargement of the regional lymph nodes is not uncommon in these cases; aspiration may show them to contain leishmaniae.

Trypanosomiasis

Lymphadenitis is an accompaniment of trypanosomiasis at some stage in the disease in every case, and most frequently in the initial period of the infection, when enlargement of the nodes draining the site of entry of the parasites into the body is of diagnostic importance.

African Trypanosomiasis[669]

Conventionally, two forms of trypanosomiasis are recognized in man in Africa, Gambian trypanosomiasis (mid-African sleeping sickness), which is caused by *Trypanosoma gambiense*, and Rhodesian trypanosomiasis (East African sleeping sickness), which is caused by *Trypanosoma rhodesiense*. These trypanosomes are generally considered to be morphologically indistinguishable from each other and from *Trypanosoma brucei*, which does not cause disease in man but is the cause of the disease of cattle and other domestic animals known as nagana, and also of enzootic infection in animals in the wild. Some authorities regard all these organisms as subspecies of *Trypanosoma brucei* (*Trypanosoma brucei gambiense*, *Trypanosoma brucei rhodesiense* and *Trypanosoma brucei brucei*).[670] They can be differentiated in various other ways, including their species pathogenicity, their sensitivity to certain drugs, particularly tryparsamide, and by the inhibitory action of normal human serum (which destroys *Trypanosoma brucei brucei*). All are transmitted by the bite of species of the tsetse fly, *Glossina*,[671] in which they pass through a series of morphological changes. When they enter the vertebrate host, already in the trypanosomal form, they spread rapidly through the tissues and gain the blood stream. In man, an inflammatory reaction (the so-called *trypanosomal chancre*) develops at the site of the bite, with accumulation of neutrophils and macrophages. This lesion may be evanescent in cases of infection by *Trypanosoma brucei gambiense* but tends to be larger and longer lasting, and to become ulcerated, in cases of infection by *Trypanosoma brucei rhodesiense*, which, in general, causes the more rapidly progressive illness. The parasites make their way from the inoculation site through the tissue spaces and in the lymph: as a consequence, the regional lymph nodes become infected.

Lymphadenitis.—The characteristic lymph node enlargement in the initial stages of African trypanosomiasis may involve any group of superficial nodes but most frequently those in the neck, including the retroauricular and occipital nodes. Enlargement of the nuchal and posterior cervical nodes is the classic Winterbottom's sign.[672] The distribution of the lymphadenitis depends on the situation of the 'chancre', and this in turn reflects the habit of the tsetse vector. *Glossina fuscipes* (*Glossina palpalis*), which transmits *Trypanosoma brucei gambiense*, *Glossina tachinoides*, which transmits *Trypanosoma brucei gambiense* and *Trypanosome brucei rhodesiense*, and *Glossina morsitans*, which transmits *Trypanosoma brucei rhodesiense*, tend to fly high and to bite on the head, particularly the face: the eventual lymphadenitis is, accordingly, cervical. *Glossina pallidipes*, a vector of *Trypanosoma brucei rhodesiense*, tends to fly low and to bite on the legs: the lymphadenitis accompanying the resulting 'chancre' affects the corresponding inguinal nodes.

Aspiration of material from the enlarged lymph nodes and its immediate microscopical examination allow of recognition of the actively motile trypanosomes, which cannot be mistaken for other parasites. The wet preparation can then be fixed and the organisms readily demonstrated by use of any Romanowsky stain, Giemsa's solution being among the most satisfactory. A positive result is said to be obtained from the enlarged nodes in 80 to 90 per cent of early cases and from peripheral blood in only 40 to 50 per cent[673] (see also *Diagnosis*, below).

Histological examination of the lymph nodes in the early stages shows sinus catarrh, follicular hyperplasia with the development of large germinal centres, an increase in the number of lymphocytes, plasma cells and large pale cells (possibly immunoblasts) in the pulp, and sometimes marked hyperaemia.[674] Trypanosomes may be very abundant, especially within the sinuses, but they are not so readily seen in sections as in film preparations. At a comparatively early stage they seem mostly to become ingested by proliferating macrophages, which destroy them; for a time it may still be possible to recognize intact parasites in the lumen of the blood vessels in the sections. Later, considerable fibrosis develops: I know of a case in which this led to a mistaken histological diagnosis of Hodgkin's disease, although the resemblance in fact was not at all close and the pathognomonic features of the latter were lacking (Fig. 9.122); a similar observation is on record,[675] and this may be another instance of the need to consider a patient's geographical history with special care. In the sclerotic stage it is evidently exceptional to be able to demonstrate trypanosomes in the sections.

Diagnosis.—The diagnosis of trypanosomiasis depends on demonstration of the trypanosomes. The most sensitive method depends on separation of the parasites from the blood by passing a sample through an anion-exchange column, which removes the blood cells, leaving the organisms in the eluate, in which they may be identified by examining the deposit after centrifugation.[676] In a comparative study of a series of 62 patients known or suspected to have Gambian trypanosomiasis, trypanosomes were shown to be present in 47 per cent by the column-separation method, in 34 per cent by examination of fluid aspirated from a cervical lymph node and in only 10 per cent by examination of thick films of peripheral blood.[676a] It was noted that each of the three methods missed infections that where shown by one of the others to be present.

Trypanosomiasis among Travellers from Africa.— Cases of African trypanosomiasis have been diagnosed in North America[676b] and in Europe: the patients are tourists or other visitors who have returned from Africa, or Africans travelling abroad. It is almost the rule in such cases that there is some delay before the correct diagnosis is considered. In some cases the presenting symptom has been enlargement of lymph nodes, and in some of these instances the diagnosis has been made at biopsy.[676c]

American Trypanosomiasis (Chagas's Disease)[677]

Lymphadenitis is a common finding in the initial stages of American trypanosomiasis (Chagas's disease[678]), which is caused by *Trypanosoma cruzi*. The infection is carried by reduviid bugs, particularly species of *Triatoma* and *Rhodnius*. These vectors are blood-suckers: they contaminate the skin by depositing infected cloacal contents while feeding, and they do not inoculate the bite directly,

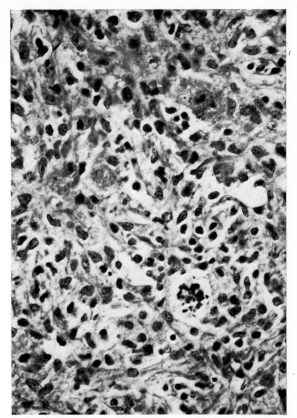

Fig. 9.122. Part of an extensive area of subcapsular fibrosis in a retroauricular lymph node. The original biopsy report was that the patient had Hodgkin's disease. This interpretation was accepted, if with some reservations, by the pathologists at the therapeutic centre to which the patient was transferred. A course of chemotherapy was given. This was followed by the rapid development of personality changes that were thought to be schizophrenic. It was then learnt that the patient had been found to have trypanosomiasis 11 months earlier while working in central Africa; he had been treated with suramin, but received only two injections before he was transferred to work in England. He had not been told the nature of his disease. He died of cerebral involvement, in spite of further treatment. There was no evidence of any lymphoma. The fibrotic changes in the biopsy specimen are believed to have been an outcome of the trypanosomal lymphadenitis of the initial stage of his infection. No trypanosomes could be found in the node. There were a few large cells, probably macrophages, in the fibrotic tissue, and occasional unequivocal macrophages that had ingested nuclear debris, but the picture lacks the diagnostic criteria of Hodgkin's disease. Compare with Fig. 9.220, page 809. *Haematoxylin–eosin.* × 400.

in contrast to the tsetse fly vector of African trypanosomiasis (see opposite). *Trypanosoma cruzi*, once placed on the skin, may enter the tissues by way of the bite or of abrasions caused by scratching; oftener, it penetrates an intact mucous membrane, particularly the conjunctiva. The conjunctival sac, usually on one side only, is said to be the portal of the infection in about 50 per cent of cases: an initial infection by this route presents a characteristic 'oculonodal complex' (*Romaña's sign*[679]), which comprises acute unilateral conjunctivitis, with very marked oedema of the soft tissue of the upper and lower eyelids, and an accompanying enlargement of the superficial parotid lymph nodes on the same side. In about 25 per cent of cases of American trypanosomiasis the skin is the evident portal of infection, as indicated by the development of an inflammatory nodule or ulcer at the site of the contaminated bite or abrasion, and of infection of the regional lymph nodes, which become enlarged. The initial cutaneous lesion has come to be known by the inelegant jargon names 'chagasoma' and 'chagoma'. In the remaining 25 per cent of cases there are no local signs of the initial stage of the infection, which presents merely with fever or other general manifestations that go undiagnosed unless the trypanosomes are looked for in the blood.

The great importance of American trypanosomiasis lies in its very high prevalence in areas where it is endemic, and the morbidity and mortality that it causes. About 5 per cent of those infected die during the acute phase, usually from encephalomyelitis or myocarditis; the rest recover from the acute stage of the infection, usually within 3 months, although there may be residual splenomegaly and enlargement of the liver for some time longer.[680] The initial conjunctivitis or cutaneous lesion and the accompanying lymphadenitis subside within a month of the onset. Most of the patients are children. It is often many years—perhaps 10 to 40—before the chronic infection kills the patient, most frequently through myocardial damage (see volume 1, page 46) and occasionally as a result of chronic dilatation of hollow viscera (megoesophagus and megacolon, for instance—see pages 1004 and 1103), chronic encephalomyelitis or indurative pulmonary haemosiderosis. It has been said that Chagas's disease causes the death of more than 30 per cent of all adults in some highly populous parts of Brazil,[681] and that there are at least 7 million people with this infection in Latin America.[682]

Lymphadenitis.—The lymph node enlargement that is a feature of the majority of cases of this disease in its initial phase is confined at first to the nodes draining the site at which the parasite entered the body. Later it may be generalized, subsiding eventually as the other manifestations of this phase subside. Its occurrence is of practical importance, both as an index of the presence of the infection and

as a source of material in which to demonstrate the parasite. During the first days of the development of the initial lymphadenopathy it may still be possible to identify occasional trypanosomes that have made their way to the sinuses of the nodes. Most of the invading trypanosomes are taken up immediately by macrophages, in which they proliferate and at the same time undergo metamorphosis to the amastigote (leishmanial) form: the histological picture now reproduces that of leishmaniasis (see page 659, and compare Figs 9.123 and 9.121B). The parasitized cells break down, liberating their content of parasites: some of the latter have by this time developed

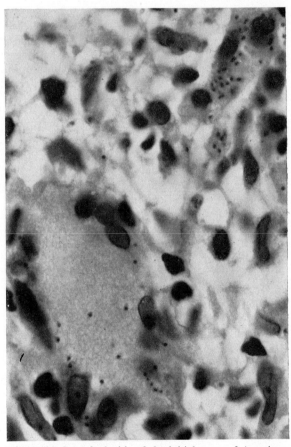

Fig. 9.123. Lymphadenitis of the initial stage of American trypanosomiasis (Chagas's disease). A multinucleate giant cell and several smaller macrophages contain the leishmanial form of *Trypanosoma cruzi*. The similarity to *Leishmania* species is obvious (see Figs 9.121A and 9.121B). The lymph node was involved as part of the primary 'oculonodal complex' (see text). The patient had returned to Europe from a tour in Brazil 3 days before unilateral conjunctivitis developed. He had spent some weeks living in Brazilian villages where he slept in bug-infested adobe huts. The field illustrated is from the subcapsular sinus. *Haematoxylin–eosin.* × 1000.

into trypanosomal forms (trypomastigotes) and these alone are found in the blood, in which they circulate, setting up intracellular infection in other organs and tissues. The reticuloendothelial system is notably involved in the earlier stages of the disease. Later, it is more and more the cells of the parenchyma of other organs that are colonized, and this eventually leads to the characteristic myocardial involvement and to the destruction of ganglion cells in the wall of hollow viscera and of cells of the central nervous system: these are the effects that underlie the serious visceral disease that makes American trypanosomiasis so grave a condition.

Malaria

Little seems to have been written about the changes in the lymph nodes in malaria. Enlargement of the superficial nodes is rarely a feature of the clinical findings, although it is occasionally observed in children from non-endemic areas when they acquire infection by *Plasmodium falciparum* (malignant tertian malaria), which is usually very severe in these unprotected patients. Enlarged nodes may also be found in some patients with any form of chronic malaria that has produced the clinical state of cachexia.

At necropsy, in cases of *Plasmodium falciparum* infection, the lymph nodes are often unusually conspicuous, although little if at all enlarged: this results from the purplish grey pigmentation that they share with other organs with a substantial reticulo-endothelial component, particularly the spleen (see page 730) and liver. The peculiar colour is attributed to the presence in the reticuloendothelial cells of malaria pigment, which is a relatively insoluble particulate deposit of brownish-black pigment derived from the haemoglobin of parasitized erythrocytes and consisting of haem and denatured protein.[683] Malaria pigment ('haemozoin') cannot be distinguished histochemically or otherwise from formalin pigment: it can, however, be seen in suitable microscopical preparations of unfixed material and in sections of material that has been fixed in solutions other than those that contain formalin. Like formalin pigment, it is often birefringent. It is seen, in blood films, both in the trophozoites and schizonts of the parasite and, after release from the red cells, in the cytoplasm of monocytes, and, in sections, of other reticuloendothelial cells.

Lymphadenitis.[684]—The sinuses of the lymph nodes are often widened and contain many macrophages and lymphocytes and some erythrocytes. The macrophages contain malarial pigment and ingested erythrocytes. The follicles are usually small and their germinal centres are relatively small or, sometimes, absent. The only distinctive feature is the presence of parasitized erythrocytes in the blood vessels, and these are likely to be conspicuously numerous only in the most serious cases (Fig. 9.124).*

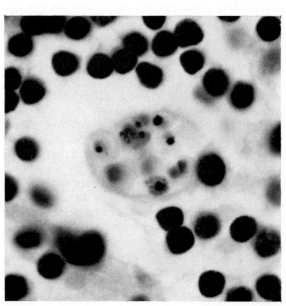

Fig. 9.124. Erythrocytes parasitized by *Plasmodium falciparum* in a capillary blood vessel in an abdominal lymph node. The patient died of cerebral malaria, clinically unsuspected, a few days after returning to Europe from a visit to West Africa. The small, very dark structures are particles of malaria pigment in the red cells; the related parasites are not so readily seen, appearing as grey areas in the photograph. Two of the red cells contain a schizont (seen particularly well in the cell at the centre of the lower margin of the capillary). Schizonts are comparatively rarely found in the peripheral blood; they are readily seen in the capillaries of the internal organs. *Haematoxylin–eosin.* ×1500.

* In an unusual case, a young doctor, trained in a country where infection by *Plasmodium falciparum* is still endemic, could not find a cause for the coma of a patient, a flyer recently returned from equatorial Africa to Europe and there found unconscious in his bed. The doctor noticed that there was a slightly enlarged lymph node in one axilla: he excised this and sent it for an urgent histological examination as he thought it might indicate that the patient had cancer of the lungs with metastasis to the brain and to the lymph node. The sections, not examined until a few hours later, showed that there were large numbers of malarial parasites in the blood in the node. When the doctor was informed, he replied that the report was no longer required as the patient had died. Death had been certified as due to uraemia. There was neither a *post mortem* nor an inquest, but it may reasonably be presumed that the patient died of cerebral malaria.

Babesia Infection (Babesiosis; Piroplasmosis)[685, 686]

Many species of *Babesia* cause disease in domestic and wild animals and are of veterinary importance. They are worldwide in distribution. Like the malarial parasites, they infect the circulating red blood cells, and they also are classed as members of the order Sporozoa. The malarial parasites belong to the suborder Haemosporidea and the babesiae to the suborder Piroplasmidea; the babesiae (and the theileriae, which are comparable blood parasites in animals) are therefore also known as piroplasmas.

Human infection by a piroplasm was first observed in 1956, by Škrabalo, in Zagreb, in Yugoslavia.[687] The patient died of renal failure, after a short illness. A few further cases have been reported, from Ireland,[688] California[689] and Nantucket Island, Massachusetts.[690] The three patients infected in Europe[685, 688] died, and it is significant that all three had previously had a splenectomy for some other illness. One of the American patients had also had a splenectomy,[689] but his infection, although severe, was not fatal. None of the other American patients died, and it is thought possible that their organism was of a species distinct from that found in Europe, which probably is *Babesia bovis* or *Babesia divergens*.

Although lymphadenopathy has not been a feature of the published cases, the infection is noted here because of a personal recollection of a tantalizingly undocumented case that may have been an instance of this condition. At a laboratory meeting in the Institute of Pathology of the Queen's University of Belfast, in 1939, blood films and sections of a lymph node biopsy specimen were demonstrated by a physician from a county hospital in Northern Ireland as an instance of indigenous malaria, a disease that had long since disappeared from Ireland.* The patient had presented with anaemia, and had been found to have enlargement of cervical lymph nodes and of the spleen. There was a history of a tick bite, and the physician suggested the possibility of transmission of 'malaria' by this means. The minute parasites in the red cells in the blood film and in red cells in the sections of the lymph node, including cells that had been engulfed by macrophages in the sinuses, had been interpreted as trophozoites of a malarial plasmodium: in retro-

* Probably the last major outbreaks in Ireland of an intermittent fever that may well have been malaria were those in the region of Cork in the middle decades of the nineteenth century, and particularly after the return of the soldiery from the malarial battlefields of the Crimean War (1854–56) to barracks in the swampy Ballincollig district (Cummins, N. M., *Some Chapters of Cork Medical History*, chap. 18; Cork, 1957).

spect, it seems possible that this was an example of babesia infection, as was suggested during discussion of the demonstration by Dr N. C. Graham and Sir Thomas Houston.

Bartonella Infection

Although *Bartonella bacilliformis*, the cause of Oroya fever and of the infection of the skin known as *verruga peruana*, is generally agreed to be a bacterium,[691] these diseases may be considered here because, in common with the malarial plasmodia (see page 667) and the babesiae (see above), the bartonella parasitizes red blood cells primarily. The cells of the reticuloendothelial system also become infected, and lymphadenopathy is commonly evident.

Oroya Fever (Carrión's Disease*)

This acute febrile illness, which is characterized by rapidly progressive haemolytic anaemia and enlargement of the liver, lymph nodes and, sometimes, spleen, has a mortality ranging from 10 to 50 per cent. It occurs in the steep Andean valleys between the equator and the 15th parallel of latitude to the south, with its greatest frequency in Peru and Colombia, and endemic foci and occasional epidemics in Ecuador and in northern Chile and western Bolivia. An epidemic in the Guaitara valley in the south of Colombia in 1936 killed over 4000 of the population of about 100 000;[692] much larger outbreaks have been recorded, and the name Oroya fever originally referred to those that resulted in the death of at least 7000 construction labourers in the Mantaro Valley in Peru when the railway from Callao and Lima to La Oroya and thence north and south along the valley was being built in the early 1870s. The infection occurs almost exclusively within the altitude range of 700 to 3000 m. It is conveyed by species of *Lutzomyia* sandflies, which bite

* Daniel Alcides Carrión, a medical student in Lima, in Peru, suspected that there might be a causal relation between Oroya fever, an acute and very dangerous disease, and the chronic and disfiguring, but harmless, skin disease known as *verruga peruana*. Disregarding the advice of colleagues, he persuaded a doctor to inoculate him with material from a *verruga*: Oroya fever developed and Carrión died 39 days later. Ernesto Odriozola, a Peruvian physician, introduced the name 'Carrión's disease' in recognition of his former colleague's experiment and the proof that it provided of the relation between the two diseases (Odriozola, E., *Monit. méd.* [*Lima*], 1895, **10**, 309). The causative organism was discovered in a case of Oroya fever ('fiebre verrucosa') in Callao, near Lima, in 1905 (Barton, A. L., *Crón. méd.* [*Lima*], 1909, **26**, 7).

only after dark and are apparently restricted to quite small areas—for instance, particular ravines—with the practical consequence that, when these areas are known, the infection can be avoided by restricting work in them to the hours between sunrise and sundown.

Pathology.—Bacillary forms of the pleomorphic bartonella are seen on the surface of infected erythrocytes and within their substance. They can be recognized easily in good Romanowsky preparations of blood films, Giemsa's stain being particularly suitable. A very high proportion of the circulating red cells may be affected. The disease is essentially a form of septicaemia. The infected erythrocytes are taken up by reticuloendothelial cells, particularly Kupffer cells and the endothelial macrophages of the sinuses of lymph nodes; the macrophages of the spleen are often notably less involved. A marked proliferation of the reticuloendothelial cells of the liver and lymph nodes results. Their cytoplasm is laden with haemosiderin, in consequence of the very severe haemolysis, and also contains many bartonellae.[693]

When the disease is fatal, as it is in up to 50 per cent of cases, death usually occurs after about 2 to 3 weeks of illness. Severe salmonella infection, septicaemic in nature (see page 1070), is a frequent accompaniment of severe Oroya fever,[694] possibly because of the frequency of subclinical infection by salmonellae among the population. The usual organism is *Salmonella typhimurium*. It is possible that Oroya fever, whether because of its intrinsic severity or through interference with the defensive functions of the reticuloendothelial system, specifically lowers resistance to such infections.

Cutaneous Infection by Bartonella

The cutaneous lesions of bartonella infection are generally known by the Spanish name, *verruga peruana* (Peruvian wart). They may develop independently of Oroya fever, in which case the incubation period is about 2 months, or, oftener, they appear in the course of the latter. Oroya fever itself has an incubation period of about 3 weeks: those patients who survive become gradually less feverish and less anaemic over a period of about 3 to 4 months. The skin eruption begins to appear 4 to 6 weeks after the onset of the fever. It occurs in two forms—one relatively common, characterized by multiple small lesions, and a rarer form in which the lesions are few and comparatively large. In the commoner form (sometimes described as 'miliary',

although in most cases the lesions are too large to be so described—see page 335), granulomatous nodules, up to about 0.5 cm in diameter, appear, mainly on the face and the extensor surface of the limbs. Mucous membranes are sometimes affected also, and dysphagia from oesophageal involvement may be troublesome. In the rarer form (sometimes described simply as 'nodular'), there is a small number of sessile or, sometimes, pedunculate, lesions that range up to as much as 10 cm in diameter: these are usually in the region of the elbows or knees, but may occur anywhere, including the face, and they tend to develop in crops. Mucosal involvement is exceptional in cases of the nodular form, but has been observed in a recent instance, seen in London (the patient had worked as a member of a film unit in the Andean valleys).

The cutaneous forms of bartonella infection are disfiguring, and leave a visible stigma in the form of a scar or an area of excessive pigmentation or depigmentation, but they seldom endanger the patient's life. Death has been known to occur from the effects of starvation or dehydration accompanying oesophageal lesions, from haemorrhage from these or other mucosal lesions, and from relapse into the septicaemic form of the disease (Oroya fever).

Amoebiasis

While *Entamoeba histolytica* may infect lymph nodes, being carried to them in lymph draining regions that are the site of an amoebic infection, this is seldom apparent clinically, and is a very rare histological finding (Fig. 9.125). I have seen amoebic lymphadenitis only twice, and in both instances it accompanied a so-called 'amoeboma' of the rectum (see page 1113) that had been mistaken for a carcinoma and treated by abdominoperineal excision; the affected nodes were in the pararectal group in each case. The amoebae were confined to small foci of necrosis involving the sinuses and immediately adjacent pulp. The nodes showed the changes of chronic non-specific lymphadenitis with some fibrosis; there was some hyperplasia of the endothelial macrophages in the sinuses, and a few of these cells had ingested lymphocytes and erythrocytes but could readily be distinguished from the parasites, some of which also contained erythrocytes.

Metazoal Lymphadenitis

Lymphadenitis demonstrably due to the presence of metazoal parasites or their ova in the nodes is a rare observation. Most histopathologists from time to

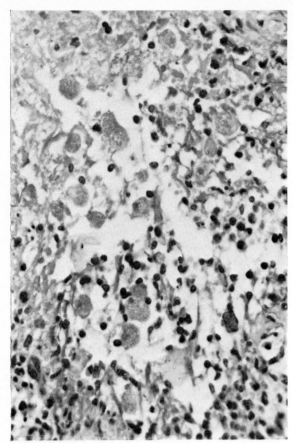

Fig. 9.125. Lymphadenitis caused by *Entamoeba histolytica*. The tissue is necrotic and there is at least a score of amoebae in the field. The parasites are ill-defined, larger than any of the host's cells and contain a relatively small, round, poorly stained nucleus. Some have ingested red blood cells, but these cannot be distinguished from the nucleus of the amoeba in the photograph at this magnification. The patient had an amoebic granuloma ('amoeboma') of the rectum, which was mistaken for a carcinoma and treated by radical excision. The amoebae had infected some of the pararectal lymph nodes, one of which is illustrated. *Haematoxylin–eosin*. × 400.

time see lesions in lymph nodes—as in other organs and tissues—that give the impression that they may be associated with a late stage in the disintegration of a metazoal parasite: the evidence may be no more than an irregular fragment of intensely eosinophile, refractile or hyaline, material that looks as if it might be a remnant of cuticular membrane or body wall of a parasite; sometimes such structures are heavily calcified. Exceptionally, in similar instances, it is possible to demonstrate structures that are identifiably of parasitic origin, such as echinococcal hooklets (see Fig. 21.40) or the denticulate cuticle of the larva of a linguatula. Such fragments,

recognizable or not, are so much more frequently seen in histological practice in areas where there is a high incidence and wide variety of metazoal parasites in the population that it seems reasonable to believe that some of them may be of this nature, not only in such regions but also in those where parasites are, in general, less frequently seen.

With few exceptions, lymph node involvement in cases of metazoal infestation is unusual and incidental. However, it is a common, if not commonly recognized, event in the course of some infestations: for example, in schistosomiasis a stage of the developing parasite may migrate by the lymphatic pathways, and in the forms of filariasis in which the adult parasites have their station in the lymphatics the microfilariae may be seen with some frequency in the lymph nodes of the vicinity.

For convenience, the infestations will be considered in sequence under the headings of nematodes (round worms), cestodes (tape worms), trematodes (flukes) and pentastomids.

Nematode Infestation

The occasional finding of larval nematodes in histological sections, whether of lymph nodes or of any other organ or tissue, invariably poses a problem of identification. The recognition of the larvae of different species of ascarid, for instance, or the differentiation of ascarid larvae from those of strongyloides, depends on minute study of morphological details: these details are often distorted by histological processing or deficient because only part of the larva is present in the planes of the available sections. Painstaking three-dimensional reconstruction from studies of serial sections that include parts of many individual larvae may be helpful, but they commonly fail to provide even the experienced specialist in human parasitology with sufficient information for confident diagnosis. In many cases the identity of the parasite remains unknown; in some others it is possible to deduce the identification with reasonable certainty from associated pathological findings, such as the known presence of adult parasites.

Ascariasis

It is said that, at the middle of this century, there were more than 600 million people in the world infested by *Ascaris lumbricoides*,[695] the common round worm: there is no doubt about the very great frequency of ascariasis throughout the world. It may therefore be surprising how seldom its larvae present in histological specimens (see pages 365, 1081 and 1235). A proportion of the newly hatched larvae that penetrate the mucosa of the bowel may enter lymphatics rather than venules, and these are carried to the regional lymph nodes (Fig. 9.126): some continue on their way to the lungs through successive lymphatic channels and the systemic venous return; others are trapped in the nodes, die, and become the centre of an inflammatory reaction. Initially, the inflammatory cells are eosinophils with a proportion of neutrophils; soon, histiocytes collect round the larva, a zone of eosinophils often forming the periphery of the lesion, while the larva itself, now showing more or less advanced lytic changes, becomes covered by a variably thick layer of intensely eosinophile precipitate that contains both globulins and fibrin (an example of the so-called Splendore–Hoeppli phenomenon—see page 750). The histiocytes in some cases undergo epithelioid metamorphosis and at the same time the eosinophils disappear and the peripheral zone of the lesion comes to be formed of varying proportions of lymphocytes and plasma cells; often, by the time this tuberculoid stage is well developed, the larva has completely disappeared or is represented only

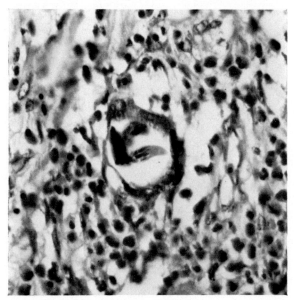

Fig. 9.126. Larva of *Ascaris lumbricoides* in a sinus in a mesenteric lymph node. The identification is presumptive only, and based on the presence of a heavy infestation of the bowel by mature ascarids and the likelihood of repeated reinfestation through swallowing ova. Neutrophils, eosinophils and plasma cells are present in the vicinity of the larva. The specimen was obtained at laparotomy, necessitated by acute obstruction of the ileocaecal valve by a tangle of more than 40 mature ascarids. *Haematoxylin–eosin.* ×480.

by a remnant of its body wall at the centre of what persists of the globulin-fibrin precipitate, sometimes with the formation of multinucleate giant cells that abut on the latter.

The sequence described in the preceding paragraph is a manifestation of the condition that is often referred to by the term 'visceral larva migrans'. This term is applicable also to the comparable lesions of toxocariasis, strongyloidiasis, ancylostomiasis and a number of other nematode infestations (see below).

When there is a heavy infestation of the bowel by the adult worms it is said that there may be some atrophy of the lymphoid tissue of the abdominal lymph nodes and an accompanying increase in the numbers of plasma cells and, particularly, of eosinophils in their pulp.[696] My own limited experience has been that there are no constant changes in the mesenteric lymph nodes; the presence of eosinophils, usually in moderate numbers only, has been the most frequent finding.

Toxocariasis

When man, or—more precisely—the child, ingests the ova of *Toxocara canis* (the dog ascarid) or of *Toxocara catti* (the cat ascarid), granuloma formation follows death of the larvae that have migrated through the tissues (see page 1242). As in cases of infestation by *Ascaris lumbricoides* (the ascarid of man—see above), the 'larva migrans' may reach and die in a mesenteric lymph node. The resulting lymphadenitis takes the form of a focal lesion corresponding to that described above in similarly exceptional cases of ascariasis. However, it seems that the toxocara larvae are more active in their capacity to bore their way through tissues: whereas the larva of *Ascaris lumbricoides*, when it leaves the lumen of a blood or lymph vessel, including the lymph sinuses in lymph nodes, tends to die in the immediate vicinity, that of a toxocara is able to cover considerable distances, its track being marked by necrosis of the tissue traversed, with deposition of fibrin and local infiltration by neutrophils and, characteristically, eosinophils. Many histological sections may have to be searched before a larva is found to account for such a track, and very often it totally eludes the search.

Strongyloidiasis

Infestation by *Strongyloides stercoralis* is acquired when the filariform larvae penetrate the skin. The larvae migrate in the blood to the lungs, where they mature, the adult worms then migrating by way of the bronchi and trachea to the oesophagus and so to their definitive habitat in the upper reaches of the small bowel (see page 1082). It is possible that during its migration the filariform larva—one variety of 'larva migrans' (see above)—may reach and lodge in tissues other than those on its normal pathway. It has been suggested that it may occasionally enter lymphatics and so pass to lymph nodes draining the site of cutaneous penetration (ordinarily on the feet or lower part of the legs).

The female adult burrows into the intestinal mucosa to lay her eggs but otherwise lives in the lumen of the intestinal glands. The rhabditiform larva that hatches from the egg ordinarily makes its way directly through the overlying tissue of the mucosa to enter the lumen of the bowel; some larvae take the opposite direction and enter the submucosa and may even reach the serosa, where it seems they perish.

In recent years many instances have been recognized in which lowering of the host's immunity by the administration of drugs with an immunosuppressant action has led to widespread dissemination of strongyloides larvae (see page 1083). The drugs include corticosteroids and their analogues, cytotoxic compounds used in the treatment of cancer, and drugs, such as azathioprine, that are specifically used for their immunosuppressant action in cases of organ transplantation. Heavy infestation of the mesenteric lymph nodes and often of the pre-aortic nodes has been a feature of all five cases of this condition that I have seen and has been illustrated by others.[697] There are many larvae in the sinuses of the infested nodes, often with little or no reaction to their presence, but in some instances with the development of reactions indistinguishable from those occurring in relation to ascaris larvae (see page 671), in spite of the depression of immune responses (Figs 9.127A and 9.127B).

Ancylostomiasis (Uncinariasis)

Like the strongyloides (see above), the hookworms— *Ancylostoma duodenale* and *Necator americanus*— establish infestation when their filariform larvae (third stage larvae) penetrate the skin of the new host, usually on the feet (see page 1082). The larvae enter capillary blood vessels or lymphatics and so eventually reach the lungs in the systemic venous blood and thence migrate by way of the airways and gullet to the intestine. Those larvae that travel initially by the lymphatics have to traverse the regional lymph nodes, usually those in the groins, and it is believed that many are held up there and

die. In cases of heavy initial infestation (such as affected those participants in a recent medical symposium who went barefoot on the grass between their residence and its swimming pool, against the advice of their hosts), there may be painful enlargement of the inguinal nodes as a transitory symptom following the pruritus at the sites of entry of the larvae through the skin of the feet. In the only instance of which I have seen sections the histological appearances in the node were similar to those associated with the presence of ascaris larvae (see page 671), except that eosinophils were all but lacking from the tissues; tuberculoid foci were not present, but the period between exposure to the risk of infestation and the biopsy was 13 days, and probably too short for this type of response to be evoked, assuming that it occurs at all in cases of infestation by the ancylostome larvae.

There are conflicting accounts of the findings in the lymph nodes of the mesentery in the presence of

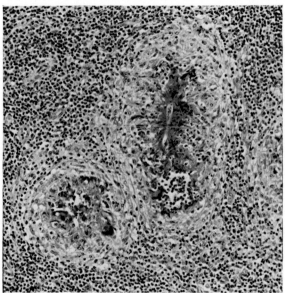

Fig. 9.127A. Tuberculoid granulomas associated with infestation of a mesenteric lymph node by larvae of *Strongyloides stercoralis*. The granulomas consist of a zone of epithelioid histiocytes round a core of intensely eosinophile material enclosing the larva. The eosinophile deposit consists of immunoglobulins, often admixed with fibrin (Splendore–Hoeppli reaction—see page 750). Multinucleate giant cells have formed in relation to the eosinophile material. Eosinophils are numerous and in the larger granuloma form a microabscess. The patient had acquired asymptomatic strongyloides infestation of the small intestine while working in South America. Later, back in Europe, she developed fatal disseminated larval strongyloidiasis while under intensive treatment with corticosteroids for rheumatoid arthritis. See Fig. 9.127B. *Haematoxylin–eosin.* × 120.

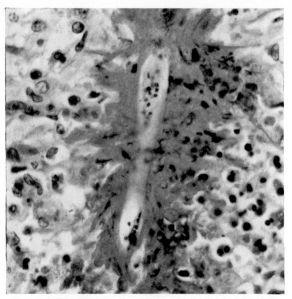

Fig. 9.127B. Higher magnification of the larger granuloma in Fig. 9.127A, to show the larva more clearly within the deposit of immunoglobulins. *Haematoxylin–eosin.* × 560.

Lymph nodes become infested both during the initial phase of larval migration from the bowel and, rather later, by way of their arterial blood supply. The histological appearances at the latter stage are essentially those already described in cases of ascariasis (see page 671).[701] They are very rarely seen. In the case of a child who developed abdominal symptoms necessitating laparotomy 7 days after eating about 200 g of raw pork that was known to be suspect and had been set aside—insufficiently carefully—for veterinary inspection, one of the enlarged and hyperaemic superior mesenteric lymph nodes was excised and proved to contain free larvae in its sinuses; there was no other particular histological feature. The slide flocculation test and other serological tests for trichinelliasis became positive and trichinellae were eventually demonstrated in a muscle biopsy specimen after peptic digestion and centrifugation.[702]

infestation of the bowel by adult hookworms. One report noted considerable atrophy of the lymphoid tissue, sparsity of eosinophils and absence of plasma cells.[696] Another described the opposite condition—follicular hyperplasia and well-marked focal infiltration by eosinophils, with numerous plasma cells and plasma cell precursors.[698]

Trichinelliasis (Trichiniasis)[699, 700]

Larvae of *Trichinella spiralis*, encysted in the muscle fibres of undercooked or raw meat, particularly pork (in Europe and in North America), become free in the stomach, pass at once to the duodenum and upper part of the jejunum, and there mature. The adult female ejects from 1000 to 2000 larvae in the course of about 5 weeks. The larvae at once penetrate the mucous membrane of the bowel, enter lymph spaces and migrate along lymphatics and through the lymph nodes to reach the systemic venous return and so the lungs, traversing the pulmonary capillary bed and eventually gaining their destination, which is the skeletal musculature, in the arterial blood supply. Larvae that are unable to lodge in striated muscle cells die and ordinarily are disposed of without trace; those that encyst in muscle reach their full development within a month and may remain alive and capable of repeating the cycle in a fresh host for periods of 20 years and more.

Oxyuriasis (Enterobiasis)

Unlike the helminths considered already, *Oxyuris vermicularis (Enterobius vermicularis*—the threadworm, pinworm or seatworm) does not ordinarily enter the tissues of its host: its entire life cycle is passed within the lumen of the bowel. Intrusion of the adult worm into the tissues is a misadventure of rare occurrence: as it commonly results in death of the parasite, and as the intrusive parasite is usually an egg-carrying female, ova may be shed into the tissues and their presence leads to the development of an abscess and, later, of a tuberculoid granuloma. Ordinarily, the gravid female leaves the rectum to deposit ova on the circumanal skin: she then dies, or returns to the bowel, or—rarely—loses her way. As an errant oxyuris may stray through the vagina to the uterus, the uterine tubes and the peritoneal cavity, or into the urethra or other natural or pathological orifice, the eventual abscess or granuloma is in such sites as the uterus, a uterine tube, one of the pelvic peritoneal pouches, the prostate gland, or—when it is a pathological sinus that is entered—the subcutaneous tissue or some deeper inflammatory lesion.

It is exceptionally rare to find an oxyuris in the bowel wall with a local inflammatory reaction as evidence that the penetration occurred while the tissues were living. In contrast, threadworms that are trapped in the lumen of an appendix that has been removed surgically may penetrate deeply into the dead tissue of the appendix wall before they also die, even when there has been no abnormality of the organ other than the presence of the parasites in its lumen: in such instances there is no evidence of an inflammatory reaction to the passage of the parasites through the tissues. When an oxyuris is seen to have entered living bowel tissue, as may be shown by the presence of a granulomatous or other inflammatory reaction that clearly is related to the parasite, there is always some ulcerative condition that may have facilitated the invasion, such as acute appendicitis or some form of ulceration of the colon.

It must be even rarer for an oxyuris to make its way to a lymph node. The circumstances in which this might occur are speculative. Even assuming the rare event of penetration of the mucosa of the bowel by the worm, it is difficult to believe that it could enter and pass along lymphatic vessels. Certainly, the mature female oxyuris (6–13 × 0·3–0·5 mm) would seem to be too large to do so. The smaller dimensions of the mature male (2–5 × 0·1–0·2 mm) may be such that it could move within lymphatics, and in the only published instance of an indisputable oxyuris indisputably in a lymph node,[703] the photomicrographs show the parasite to be a male (Fig. 9.128). In other cases that purport to be examples of invasion of a lymph node by an oxyuris,[704, 705] there seems to be little doubt, on reviewing the published accounts,[706] that the lesion was not in a lymph node and that it was in fact an abscess or granuloma that had formed when the parasite died after reaching the abdominal cavity, probably by way of the genital tract (both the patients were women).

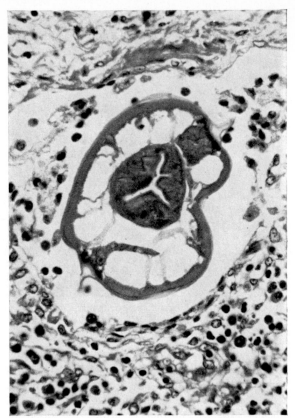

Fig. 9.128.§ Cross-section of an adult threadworm, *Oxyuris vermicularis* (*Enterobius vermicularis*), in the subcapsular sinus of a mesenteric lymph node. The internal structure indicates that the parasite is a male. The lateral cuticular crests appear as pointed, clear projections; they are not peculiar to the oxyurids but their presence is supporting evidence for this identification. *Haematoxylin–eosin.* × 400.

Trichuriasis

Like *Oxyuris vermicularis* (see above), *Trichuris trichiura* (*Trichocephalus dispar*, the whip worm) passes its life cycle wholly within the lumen of its host's bowel. However, the adult parasites attach themselves to the mucosa, particularly in the caecum and ascending colon: the attenuate, whip-like anterior three-fifths of the parasite terminates in a 'mouth spear' by which it becomes anchored to the tissues, sometimes penetrating to the muscularis mucosae and even deeper. The female is from 30 to 50 mm long when fully grown and the male from 25 to 45 mm long: the thicker part of the body is about 1·8 mm in diameter in the female and about 1·3 mm in the male. It is difficult to conceive of the adults making their way to the lymph nodes. However, there were large numbers of larval nematodes in a lymph node that was included in the intussusceptum in a case of ileocaecal intussusception complicating an exceptionally heavy infestation of

the large bowel by the trichuris: whether the larvae were trichuris larvae is debatable, but no other nematodes were recognized to be present.[707] The patient was a technician in a parasitological laboratory in a west European country and was assisting in research relating to trichuriasis; she was in the habit of eating her midday sandwiches while sampling faecal specimens by what had been designed as a no-touch technique.

The Filarial Diseases

Various filarial worms may be the cause of lesions in lymph nodes. The most notable are *Wuchereria bancrofti* and *Brugia malayi*, which are essentially parasites of the lymphatic system and therefore regularly set up a lymphadenitis. Other filariae involve lymph nodes occasionally.

Infestation by Wuchereria bancrofti.—*Wuchereria bancrofti* (*Filaria bancrofti*,* *Filaria sanguinis hominis*) is very widely distributed throughout tropical and subtropical regions of the world. Infestation is very much more frequent than resulting morbidity. The latter most characteristically is the outcome of infestation of lymphatics by the adult parasites, and results particularly when these die, for it is then that lymphangitis and consequent obstructive fibrosis occur, leading to lymphoedema, of which elephantiasis is a manifestation (see page 160). Obstructive lymphangitis leads to progressive distension of the sinuses of the lymph nodes distal to the obstruction, as is manifest, for instance, in the condition known clinically as 'varicose groin glands'. In some cases the adult parasites are within lymph nodes, and they may be readily identifiable in sections, if they were alive at the time when the specimen was obtained; if they had died before then, their remnants, more or less recognizable, are the centre of a tuberculoid granulomatous reaction, often with numerous eosinophils in the vicinity.

Microfilariae may also be found in lymph nodes.[708] This may be an accompaniment of microfilariaemia, in which case any node may be infested by the microfilariae. There is generally no reaction to their presence, which is ordinarily a chance finding when a node is examined for some unrelated reason. In other cases the nodes are enlarged and show follicular hyperplasia and a general increase in the number of cells in the pulp, with many plasma cells and many eosinophils: in addition, and most striking, there are focal collections of eosinophils, sometimes forming abscess-like collections and sometimes enclosing a microfilaria (Fig. 9.129) or a small tuberculoid granuloma that has formed round an amorphous eosinophile structure.[709] The latter may contain recognizable remnants of a microfilaria, although these may be no more than fragments of cylindrical appearance. Sometimes the parasitic remnant is the centre of a stellate, hyaline, intensely eosinophile precipitate that is probably an immunoglobulin complex. Lymphadenitis associated with the presence of microfilariae is found oftenest in cases of what is referred to as *occult filariasis* (the Meyers–Kouwenaar syndrome[710]):[711] this condition is

* It is generally accepted that *Filaria bancrofti* is a synonym of *Wuchereria bancrofti*. However, some authorities use the name as a synonym of *Dirofilaria magalhaesi*, which probably is identical with *Dirofilaria immitis* (see page 677). It is said that *Dirofilaria magalhaesi*, when first described, was taken for the parasite that we now know as *Wuchereria bancrofti* (Brumpt, E., *Précis de parasitologie*, 6th edn, vol. 1, page 927; Paris, 1949).

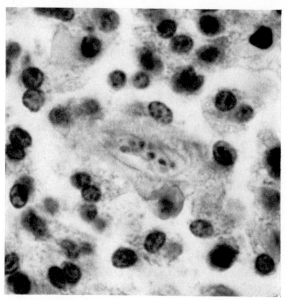

Fig. 9.129.§ Microfilaria of *Wuchereria bancrofti* in an eosinophil 'abscess' in an axillary lymph node. There is incipient development of the hyaline deposit of eosinophile material characteristic of the Splendore–Hoeppli phenomenon (see Figs 9.127A and 9.127B). *Haematoxylin–eosin.* × 1500.

characterized by marked eosinophilia in the blood, pulmonary symptoms (see page 366), enlargement of lymph nodes and the absence of microfilariae from the blood although they are present and usually readily demonstrable in the nodes.[709] The condition is probably a manifestation of hypersensitivity, specifically to microfilariae.

In longstanding cases of infestation by wuchereria no trace of the parasites may be found in lymph nodes. At this stage even nodes from the vicinity of the obstructed lymphatics show only non-specific changes, often mainly in the nature of obliterative fibrosis.

Infestation by Brugia malayi.—The pathological changes in cases of infestation by *Brugia malayi* are essentially the same as in filariasis due to *Wuchereria bancrofti* (see above). The lymphadenitis of brugia infestation is usually inguinal, and accompanies the episodic febrile illness that is often characteristic of the disease.[712] It is due in some cases to the presence of the adult parasites in the nodes and in others to the inflammatory reaction round the worms that have died in the regional lymphatics.

Lymphadenitis associated with the presence of microfilariae in the nodes occurs as in cases of wuchereria infestation (see above). The syndrome of *occult filariasis* was originally described in cases of what in retrospect may be identified as infestation by *Brugia malayi* (see above).

Like the wuchereria, brugia causes symptomless, subclinical infestation much oftener than clinically apparent disease.

Onchocerciasis.—Onchocerca volvulus (Onchocerca caecutiens) is best known as the cause of onchocerca nodules, the fibrotic masses that form round the adult parasites in the subcutaneous tissue, and of blindness (see Chapter 40). It is widespread and rife in parts of tropical Africa, and known, but less frequent, in Central America and in the Yemen. It is believed to have been introduced to America and Arabia by slaves brought from Africa (and it may have been introduced to Mexico in the nineteenth century by French soldiers from the Sudan). The microfilariae that are produced by the mature female worms in the onchocerca nodules may spread widely in the skin and subcutaneous tissue. They do not circulate in the blood, but they are not infrequently to be found in superficial lymph nodes, both those draining the regions in which the nodules are situated and those at a distance. In the earlier stages of the lymphadenitis, collections of histiocytes are found in the sinuses and in the pulp, and there are often many eosinophils and plasma cells; the microfilariae are usually to be found without difficulty in the nodes, particularly in the sinuses and in the capsule and trabeculae. It is characteristic of the later stage of the lymphadenitis in African cases of onchocerciasis that extensive fibrosis develops as a consequence of the infestation;[713] obstruction to the lymph flow may lead to lymphoedema and elephantiasis.[714]

The adult onchocerca is only very rarely found apart from the classic nodule but has been said occasionally to lie free in the subcutaneous tissue. The female ranges from 200 to 500 mm in length and 0·25 to 0·4 mm in diameter and the male from 15 to 45 mm in length and 0·1 to 0·2 mm in diameter. Each nodule includes one or more female worms and twice as many males, embedded in dense, cellular fibrous tissue within which many free microfilariae are seen. The nodules are usually from 5 to 25 mm in diameter and only seldom exceed 50 mm. They are situated in subcutaneous tissue, adherent to the skin and, very occasionally, to underlying structures, such as periosteum. In a case recently observed in Britain, the nodule, 30 mm in diameter, overlay and was adherent to an enlarged pectoral lymph node; the capsule of the node had been destroyed where it was in contact with the nodule, and the substance of the two structures merged imperceptibly (Fig. 9.130).

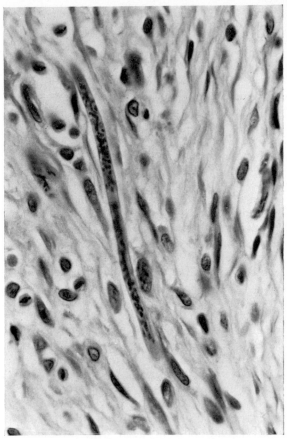

Fig. 9.130. Microfilaria of *Onchocerca volvulus* in fibrosing tissue in a lymph node abutting on an onchocerca nodule. The lack of reaction to the larva as it makes its way through the tissues is characteristic. The fibrosis is part of the reaction to the presence of the mature parasites in the nearby nodule. *Haematoxylin–eosin.* × 630.

The patient was one of two European medical students who acquired the infestation while on vacation work in West Africa.[657]

Loiasis.[715]—*Loa loa*, the so-called eye worm, is found only in the equatorial rain forest and swamp forest areas of Africa, from the west coast to about longitude 30° East. Its intermediate hosts are species of mangrove flies (*Chrysops*). Little is known of the development of the parasites in human tissues following inoculation by the bite of the fly. It is believed that the period required for maturation is at least 6 months. The microfilariae produced by the mature female are released into the adjoining tissues and make their way to the blood stream: they may, therefore, be found in many organs and tissues, including lymph nodes, but ordinarily without producing any reaction. In other cases, perhaps in association with the development of hypersensitivity, an inflammatory reaction develops round the microfilariae, particularly those that have died. The histological picture is then of the same general type as in cases of lymphadenitis, or of inflammation in other organs and tissues, associated with sensitivity to other metazoal parasites (see page 671).

Dirofilariasis.—It has been recognized only comparatively recently that the common and worldwide dirofilariae, which are intracardiac or subcutaneous parasites of domestic animals, particularly dogs and cats, and of some wild carnivores, are capable of setting up infestation in man.[716] Two species are recognized. *Dirofilaria immitis*, which may be identical with *Dirofilaria magalhaesi* (see footnote on page 675), is the familiar canine heart worm: it may cause pulmonary infarcts in man and has been described on several occasions as an incidental finding in the cavities of the human heart at necropsy.[717] *Dirofilaria conjunctivae* is a name currently given to any dirofilaria identified as the cause of conjunctival or subcutaneous infestation in man: it is probably identical with *Dirofilaria tenuis*,[718] a subcutaneous parasite of the racoon in various parts of North America, and possibly with similar parasites of various other animals. The infestation is believed to be mosquito-borne. The larvae, when inoculated into a fresh host, moult and then migrate through the tissues, usually only developing to maturity once they reach their most favoured site (chambers of the right side of the heart, or conjunctiva, or subcutaneous tissue, according to the species of parasite). In the course of its migration an occasional larva must pass through lymph nodes. It is possible that dirofilarial lymphadenitis might then result. A published case that could be so interpreted concerned a filarial infestation of an inguinal lymph node in a resident of New York City:[719] however, the possibility of an indigenous infestation by *Wuchereria* species or *Brugia* species seems to have been regarded as likelier, although no less remarkable.

Dracontiasis (Dracunculiasis)

Lymphadenitis is a common accompaniment of infestation by *Dracunculus medinensis*, the Guinea worm.[720] In most cases it is secondary to bacterial infection of the infested tissue, and this usually is a complication of maladroit attempts to extract the adult parasite. In rare instances, a lymph node has formed part of the tissues occupied by the mature female worm.[721] Guinea worm infestation is occasionally seen in practice in parts of the world where it is not endemic: most of the patients are newly arrived from endemic areas, but an English engineer first developed symptoms more than 5 years after visiting a West African country, his only excursion to a known source of the disease. It occurs in parts of Africa (the Nile Valley and southward into Uganda, the region of Lake Chad, and on the west from Mauritania to the Republic of the Congo, but not including the basin of the Congo River), it is very widespread in Asia, and in the past it was known in limited areas of the northern parts of South America and near Salvador (Bahia) in Brazil.

Cestode Infestation

Cestodiasis—infestation by a tapeworm or by tapeworm larvae—involves lymph nodes only when man acts as the intermediate host; even then it is exceptionally rare to find that a larva has developed in a node. When ova of a tapeworm are swallowed, they hatch in the small intestine and the hexacanth embryo—the onchosphere—escapes and passes through the epithelial lining to enter venules or, sometimes, lymphatics and so make its way to the eventual site of its encystment, where it develops into the fully formed larva.

Cysticercosis

The larva of *Taenia solium*, the pork tapeworm, is still known, in its final form, as *Cysticercus cellulosae*, the name that it was given before its identity as a stage in the life cycle of the taenia was recognized. Cysticercosis in man seems to have been recorded only once as indisputably caused by *Cysticercus bovis*, the mature larva of *Taenia saginata*, the beef tapeworm;[722] in all other cases of cysticercosis, and it is not a particularly rare condition, the larvae have been those of *Taenia solium*. The cysticerci of the two species are readily distinguishable, the most notable characteristic of that of *Taenia solium* being the rows of unmistakable hooklets, usually numbering from 20 to 50, on the invaginated scolex; the cysticercus of *Taenia saginata* is without hooklets. Cysticerci develop quite quickly, reaching their full size (about $10 \times 5 \times 5$ mm) within some 10 weeks. The wall of the bladder-like body cavity of the larva has three layers—an eosinophile, corrugated cuticle, an intermediate nucleate layer, and an inner 'parenchymatous' layer formed of a fine meshwork of fibrils among which further nuclei are rather sparsely scattered; these

I

features and the invaginated scolex enable the parasite to be identified in histological sections.

In two cases of cysticercosis involving abdominal lymph nodes,[723] the cysts were taken for secondary deposits of mucinous carcinoma by the surgeon during laparotomy and were correctly identified under the low power of the microscope without histological sectioning being immediately necessary.

In another case,[723] lymph node involvement was part of a widespread and very heavy cysticercosis that had developed as an endogenous larval infestation, the result of treatment of taeniasis with niclosamide. The patient was believed to have had three adult tapeworms in the intestine. Through an oversight, no purgative was given after the treatment. Regurgitation of viable ova is a recognized hazard of treatment with niclosamide, predisposing to cysticercosis and contraindicating the use of this drug in cases of infestation by *Taenia solium*: purgation following the treatment diminishes the risk but does not eliminate it.

Echinococcosis (Hydatid Disease)

Abdominal lymph nodes may be involved in the progressive extension of the rare alveolar type of hydatid cyst, which is the larval form of *Echinococcus multilocularis* (*Echinococcus alveolaris*), a parasite of limited geographical distribution (see page 1240) that has its adult existence in various canine species.[723a]

The commoner echinococcus, *Echinococcus granulosus* (*Taenia echinococcus*), another of the dog tapeworms, is much more widespread; its typical larval form is the classic hydatid cyst (see page 1237). I have seen a hydatid cyst, 2 cm in diameter, in a lateral aortic lymph node in the abdomen, a chance post-mortem finding; the substance of the node was somewhat atrophic through being stretched over the enlarging cyst. Presumably, the growth of such a cyst in a lymph node could eventually obliterate all traces of the latter, the hydatid then appearing as a retroperitoneal structure of otherwise indeterminate situation.

Sparganosis[724]

The term sparganum is applied to the plerocercoid larval stage of the pseudophyllidean tapeworms (it is the stage that develops in the second intermediate host). For example, the sparganum of *Diphyllobothrium latum*, the so-called fish tapeworm that is a cause of vitamin B_{12} deficiency and consequent anaemia (see page 456), develops in fresh-water fish and is ingested by man. In many instances the adult worm of which a sparganum is the plerocercoid stage is unknown, and the name sparganosis is given to cases of infestation by such unidentified solid larval tapeworms. Cases of sparganosis, in this sense, have been reported from many parts of the world, and such infestation is probably worldwide. The spargana range from 2 to about 50 cm in length and are up to 1 cm in width and 0·2 cm thick. They may be found in many situations in man, including subcutaneous tissue and the eyes (see Chapter 40). Lymphatic sparganosis may lead to elephantiasis. The presence of an encysted sparganum in an inguinal lymph node and of three identical larvae in the lymphatics in the femoral triangle of the same side had caused severe lymphoedema of the leg in a young woman who, 14 months earlier, had taken a camping holiday in Norway that had included several meals of freshly caught fresh-water fish that had been eaten after inadequate cooking on a pointed stick over an open fire.[725]

Trematode Infestation

Schistosomiasis

Lymph nodes may be involved at various stages in the course of development of schistosomiasis (see page 1236). During the initial migration of the schistosomules from the skin, where they are formed from the cercariae as these lose their tail during penetration of the epidermis, it is probable that the pathway is the lymphatic plexus of the skin and subcutaneous tissue rather than the blood. Schistosomules have been found in the regional nodes draining the invaded area of skin and in more centrally situated nodes; they may be demonstrated both in histological sections and in films of aspirated material.[726, 727] Depending on the species of schistosome, a period of from 4 to 9 weeks passes between the initial cercarial invasion of the skin and the deposition of the first ova by the mature flukes at their site of election within the venous system. The end of this period is sometimes marked by a so-called 'toxaemic' or hypersensitivity phase of the infestation, with abdominal pain, diarrhoea, malaise, and fever up to 40°C; there may be generalized enlargement of lymph nodes during this phase, probably as a manifestation of the hypersensitivity reaction.

In the later stages of schistosomiasis, ova may be an incidental finding on examination of any lymph node, as of any other tissue (Fig. 9.131), during investigation of specimens removed in the course of diagnosis or treatment of other diseases or, occa-

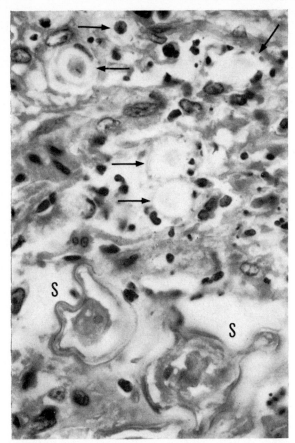

Fig. 9.131.§ Part of an extensive granulomatosis of the spleen of a South American patient who died in Britain of chronic myocarditis due to American trypanosomiasis. Splenomegaly was associated with fibrosis of the liver due to infestation by *Schistosoma mansoni*. This field includes schistosomal ova (S, S) and several cells of *Paracoccidioides brasiliensis* (centre and upper part of picture, arrowed). There had been recent haematogenous generalization of the fungal infection; its point of origin was not found at the necropsy. The same specimen is illustrated in Fig. 9.99, page 628. *Haematoxylin–eosin.* × 800.

sionally, of complications of the infestation itself. The ova may be few or numerous; even when plentiful they are usually spaced apart. They may be well preserved, and with care the presence, position and size of the spine that projects from their surface can be made out and the species of schistosome thereby identified. Alternatively, they may be so heavily calcified that little detail can be seen. The recently deposited ovum is surrounded by a compact accumulation of inflammatory cells, histiocytes predominating, with varying proportions of neutrophils, eosinophils, lymphocytes and plasma cells. There may be an eosinophile precipitate of immuno-

globulin on the ovum,* particularly when the cellular reaction is becoming more overtly histiocytic; at this histiocytic stage the lesion may be outlined by a narrow zone of eosinophils. Later, the reaction is frankly tuberculoid, the histiocytes undergoing epithelioid metamorphosis; the ovum may then become enclosed by multinucleate giant cells. Eventually, concentric fibrosis reduces the extent of the cellular component of the granuloma until all traces of the earlier reaction are obliterated and the ovum lies enclosed in dense, hyaline, collagenous tissue. As the granulomatous reaction runs its course to fibrosis, the ovum becomes increasingly distorted and fragmented, but identifiable traces can generally be found.

Paragonimiasis[728]

Paragonimus westermani, the lung fluke, is widespread in the Far East; related or identical species are known in parts of West Africa and of the Pacific coastal belt of South America. It causes 'endemic haemoptysis', which is the outcome of the predilection of the adult flukes for the lungs, in which they form cyst-like lesions that tend to suppurate and open into the bronchial tree (see page 364). The infestation is sometimes known as pulmonary distomiasis, or distomatosis, after an obsolete name of the parasite (*Distoma westermani*), The fully grown fluke is ovoid and measures from 8 to 20 mm in length by 4 to 8 mm in diameter.

The infestation results from ingestion of raw or under-cooked fresh-water crabs, or from contamination of other food by the encysted metacercariae from the crabs. Once swallowed, the larvae follow a complicated path from the small bowel to the lungs, the penultimate stage of which is access to the pleural cavities by traversing the diaphragm. They may go astray at any time during their transit, and correspondingly the mature flukes may develop in extrapulmonary situations, which include lymph nodes in the abdomen and mediastinum, and sometimes farther afield, as in the groins or axillae. The flukes themselves tend to move about within the infested tissues, leaving a trail of necrosis littered with their ova, which are often sterile and collapsed. The most serious complication is involvement of the central nervous system, which is disabling, has a high

---

* This phenomenon, the so-called Splendore–Hoeppli phenomenon, was originally described by Splendore in relation to sporotrichosis and by Hoeppli in relation to experimental infestation with *Schistosoma japonicum* (see page 750).

mortality in spite of appropriate treatment, and occurs in about 1 per cent of patients with active pulmonary infestation.[729]

Infestation by Liver Flukes

Fasciola hepatica, the common liver fluke of sheep, goats and various other domestic and wild animals, is of worldwide distribution. In man (see page 1235), as in other hosts of the mature parasites, the pathway by which the metacercariae that have excysted in the duodenum pass to the biliary ducts is controversial: generally it is believed that they penetrate the wall of the bowel to reach the peritoneal cavity, in which they then move to the liver, penetrating its capsule and passing through its substance to reach the biliary ducts, where they develop into mature flukes. This is a transit from which the immature parasites may deviate, with the consequent development of 'ectopic' fascioliasis in other organs or tissues, including lymph nodes. Such ectopic infestation occurs very rarely.

Clonorchis sinensis, the Chinese liver fluke (see page 1236), and *Opisthorchis* species, liver flukes that occur in limited areas of Asia and Europe (see page 1236), seem not to give rise to 'ectopic' infestation in man. Their metacercariae enter the biliary passages directly through the orifice of the hepatopancreatic ampulla, following excystment in the duodenum: this pathway does not offer the same possibilities for the larvae to stray.

Pentastomiasis

Infestation by Larvae of Linguatula serrata

The lymph nodes in the mesentery and alongside the abdominal part of the aorta are on the path followed by the first stage larva of *Linguatula serrata*, the so-called tongue worm (see page 1242), a parasite that is found mainly in temperate regions. The characteristic larval cyst is occasionally an incidental finding at laparotomy or necropsy. The larva dies within a year or two, the cyst collapses, and a firm nodule, later calcified, takes its place. Its nature will continue to be recognizable in histological sections if identifiable remnants of the larva are present, such as its denticulate cuticle and annulate structure.

Like cysticerci (see page 678), fresh linguatulid larvae in abdominal lymph nodes are liable to be mistaken at laparotomy for secondary deposits of a mucinous carcinoma. The degenerate, calcified cysts are often assumed to be old tuberculous foci.

Infestation by Larvae of Armillifer Species

Lesions comparable to those of larval linguatuliasis may be seen in abdominal lymph nodes in cases of infestation by larvae of *Armillifer* (*Porocephalus*) species (see page 1243), which are found in some tropical parts of Asia and Africa (Fig. 9.132).

Lymphadenitis without Animate Cause
Sarcoidosis

Sarcoidosis is considered on page 745.

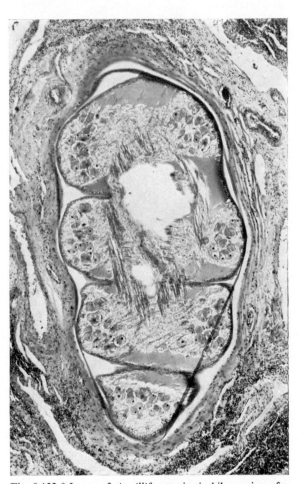

Fig. 9.132.§ Larva of *Armillifer* species in hilar region of a mesenteric lymph node. The segmental appearance represents the annulation of the vermiform body of the larva, only part of which is included in the plane of the section. It lies in a well-defined cyst-like structure, walled by a delicate membrane of parasitic origin and surrounded by a fibrotic capsule formed by the host tissue. The lining membrane has contracted tautly across part of the larva, an effect of histological processing. The specimen is one of the series studied in Malaysian aborigines by: Prathap, K., Lau, K. S., Bolton, J. M., *Amer. J. trop. Med. Hyg.*, 1969, **18**, 20. *Haematoxylin–eosin.* × 45.

Berylliosis[730]

Lymph nodes may be involved as an accompaniment of both the acute pneumonic form and the chronic granulomatous form of pulmonary berylliosis (see page 386)[731] and in the course of generalized berylliosis as beryllium salts become carried through the body from the site initially involved.[732] In some cases in which the disease has not otherwise extended beyond the lungs and mediastinal lymph nodes there may be involvement of cervical nodes.[733] The cutaneous lesion that may result from direct inoculation of beryllium[734] may be accompanied by the development of the typical lesions in the regional lymph nodes; like the granuloma in the skin itself, the regional lymphadenitis may become manifest only years after the inoculation, a delay that is reminiscent of the comparable period of latency between implantation of siliceous foreign material into the skin and the development of the sarcoid type of granuloma that may eventually follow (see page 757 and Chapter 39).

In the lymphadenitis accompanying the acute pulmonary disease there is a striking degree of proliferation of the endothelial macrophages in the sinuses, with phagocytosis of nuclear debris and of erythrocytes and lymphocytes. There is no evident tendency to form discrete cell aggregates such as are characteristic of the chronic disease. In the latter, tuberculoid foci range from loosely constructed, rather ill-defined collections of epithelioid histiocytes, with an occasional multinucleate giant cell, to well-developed, compact, discrete and confluent foci that are virtually indistinguishable from the lesion that typifies sarcoidosis. Necrosis may occur in some of the granulomatous foci: it may be fibrinoid in character; very rarely it resembles early caseation (Fig. 9.133). Concentrically layered, rounded structures, 10 to 150 μm in diameter, are sometimes present in the granulomatous tissue; they are sometimes haematoxyphile and sometimes eosinophile, sometimes calcified and sometimes impregnated with iron. They are often referred to as 'conchoids' or 'conchoidal bodies'. They closely resemble the Schaumann bodies of sarcoidosis (see page 748): some pathologists have noted them to lack an affinity for stains for elastic tissue,[735] which are said to react strongly with Schaumann bodies, but my own experience does not confirm that the latter can regularly be stained in this manner or that such stains distinguish reliably between them and the concentric bodies of berylliosis.

The diagnosis of berylliosis from sarcoidosis can be exceptionally difficult.[732, 736] A history of exposure to beryllium or its salts, the spectrographic

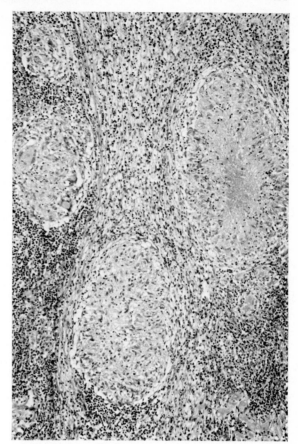

Fig. 9.133. Involvement of one of the inferior deep cervical lymph nodes ('scalene node') in berylliosis. Four epithelioid cell granulomas are seen. The two smaller lesions include a number of multinucleate giant cells; the two larger lesions show central necrosis; the necrosis is frankly caseous in the largest. There is some lymphocyte depletion in the lymphoid tissue in parts of the field: this, like the caseation, is not typical of berylliosis. Cultures for mycobacteria and other organisms were sterile. The Kveim test was negative. Beryllium was demonstrated in the specimen by spectrography. There was a history of industrial exposure to beryllium salts. The biopsy was performed in the course of investigating the nature of generalized mottled shadowing in both lungs, with enlargement of the hilar lymph nodes. *Haematoxylin–eosin.* × 70.

demonstration of beryllium in urine,[737] and a positive skin reaction to patch tests with beryllium salts[732] support, but do not confirm, a diagnosis of berylliosis. Spectrographic demonstration of beryllium in tissue—for instance, in a lymph node that shows the characteristic histological picture—is conclusive but requires particular facilities and skills. The Kveim test on patients with berylliosis is usually negative or equivocal; on occasion it has been reported as positive by experienced specialists.

In fact, the distinction between berylliosis and sarcoidosis is generally best made on the basis of clinical judgement by an experienced physician.

Lymphadenitis of Crohn's Disease (Regional Enteritis)

It is commonly said that in most cases of Crohn's disease the changes in the regional lymph nodes are non-specific, and comprise only follicular hyperplasia and sinus catarrh, the latter often associated with dilatation of the sinuses.[738] However, the more thorough the histological examination of the nodes that are included in resection specimens the larger the proportion in which other, and diagnostically important, changes are to be found, and if time and resources permit the preparation of sections at several levels in each lymph node very few cases will be found without epithelioid cell clusters or frankly tuberculoid foci (Fig. 9.134A).[738] It is notable that these foci may be absent from the larger nodes yet numerous in small ones in the same case (see page 1075). In some cases there is fibrosis of many of the foci (Fig. 9.134B). Necrosis is not infrequently seen at the centre of the foci (Fig. 9.135); it is said never to be caseous, but I have seen typical caseation, though of restricted extent, in a few confluent granulomatous foci in four cases of Crohn's disease in which microbiological examination of the same nodes showed no mycobacteria in films and cultures or by guinea-pig inoculation.

In two otherwise typical cases of Crohn's disease of the terminal ileum that I have seen, the lymph nodes in the mesentery were without aggregates of epithelioid cells and tuberculoid foci but showed many solitary multinucleate giant cells throughout the pulp (Fig. 9.136). A similar observation is on record.[739] The same picture may be seen without known causation, in the absence of other disease; in such cases the observed changes have been in superficial nodes (see page 684).

Cholegranulomatous Lymphadenitis

This condition has been considered on page 588.

Lymphadenitis Accompanying Neoplasia in the Drainage Area

The occurrence of simple sinus histiocytosis in lymph nodes draining the site of a primary malignant tumour, particularly a mammary or gastric car-

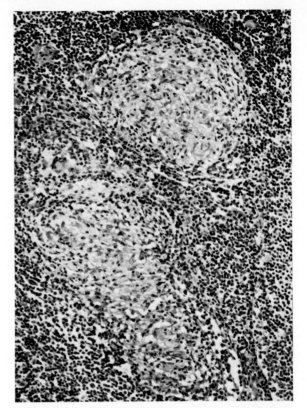

Fig. 9.134A. Lymphadenitis of Crohn's disease (regional enteritis). Early stage in the development of epithelioid cell granulomas. The lesions in the lymph nodes may range, in any case, from clusters of a few histiocytes through well-formed tuberculoid granulomas to sclerosing foci: different stages may be seen in a single node, or the lesions in different nodes may be at different stages. See Figs 9.134B, 9.135 and 9.136. *Haematoxylin–eosin.* × 140.

cinoma, has been mentioned on page 561. Such histiocytosis has no obvious relation to the tuberculoid granulomatous reaction that similarly may be seen in nodes draining these or other primary tumours. The tuberculoid reaction is infrequent: in a series of 500 surgical specimens of malignant tumours it was found in 29 cases (6 per cent);[740] in a series of 2000 cases of visceral cancer in which lymph nodes were sectioned histologically at the time of examination of the resected primary growth it was found in 79 instances (4 per cent).[741] The changes range from a more or less widespread clustering of epithelioid cells that reproduces the picture seen in, for example, toxoplasmosis (see page 654) to a characteristic tuberculoid granulomatosis with discrete or confluent epithelioid cell and giant cell foci (Figs 9.137A and 9.137B). The granulomatous foci are often more 'angular' in

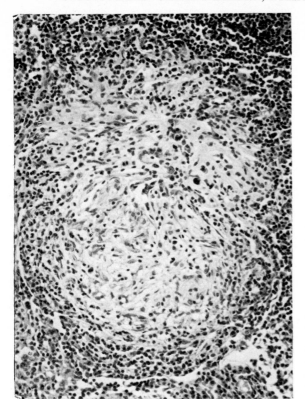

Fig. 9.134B. Same specimen as Fig. 9.134A. Epithelioid cell granuloma with well-marked hyaline fibrosis at one pole. *Haematoxylin–eosin.* ×165.

also accompanied carcinoma of the liver, kidneys and adrenals, seminoma, dysgerminoma, thyroid and prostatic carcinoma, malignant melanoma, squamous carcinoma, and transitional cell carcinoma of the urinary tract.

The pathogenesis of this type of lymphadenitis is uncertain. It is presumed to be the result of carriage to the nodes of breakdown products of the related tumour or of the tissues invaded by it. The tuberculoid reaction has no prognostic implications.

It must not be forgotten that any condition that causes a tuberculoid lymphadenitis, not least tuberculosis itself, may be present in the lymph nodes of a region of the body in which a cancer coincidentally develops. It can be prognostically important not to overlook this possibility and the need to treat the condition responsible for the granuloma as well as the cancer.

outline than those of sarcoidosis and tuberculosis. They may show minimal necrosis, sometimes with the accumulation locally of a small number of neutrophils; oftener, the necrosis is fibrinoid, although of such restricted extent—sometimes in the form of eosinophile 'threads' among the centrally placed epithelioid cells—that it is scarcely noticeable. Concentrically laminate structures like the Schaumann bodies of sarcoidosis are not infrequent, and 'asteroids' may be present (see page 748). It is most unusual for the nodes that show these changes to be demonstrably invaded by secondary deposits of the related cancer.

Similar tuberculoid changes may be seen in the stroma of the primary tumour in these cases, but this is relatively rare. Very occasionally, other organs are similarly affected, the liver perhaps least rarely.[742] The primary tumours may be in any organ or tissue; usually they are carcinomas. As noted above, carcinomas of the breast and stomach have predominated (respectively 30 and 20 cases in a review of 96 examples[743]), but such a lymphadenitis has

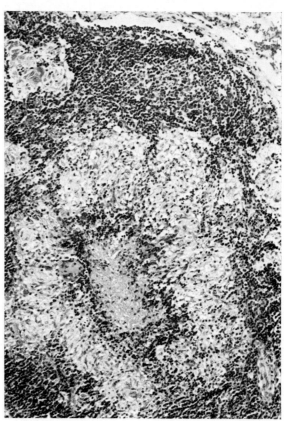

Fig. 9.135. Lymphadenitis of Crohn's disease. Another case, showing what appears to be a large group of confluent epithelioid cell granulomas, with necrosis at the centre of the group. The necrotic core is outlined by a zone in which neutrophils, lymphocytes and particulate nuclear debris are collected. *Haematoxylin–eosin.* ×100.

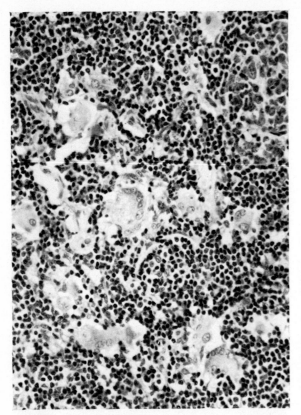

Fig. 9.136. Lymphadenitis of Crohn's disease. Another case. There were no epithelioid cell granulomas in this instance. Instead, there was widespread proliferation of small multinucleate macrophages, sometimes solitary and sometimes in small groups, scattered throughout the lymphoid tissue, particularly in the cortex of the node. See Figs 9.134A, 9.134B and 9.135. Compare with the 'pure giant-celled lymphadenitis of unknown causation' illustrated in Fig. 9.138. *Haematoxylin–eosin.* × 230.

Histologically Distinctive Forms of Lymphadenitis of Unknown Causation

Pure Giant-Celled Lymphadenitis of Unknown Causation

There is a very rare form of lymphadenopathy that is characterized by the widespread formation throughout the pulp of the nodes of large rounded giant cells, 20 to 75 μm in diameter, with opaque eosinophile cytoplasm and a small number—3 to 10 in the plane of a section—of round or, oftener, ovoid pale nuclei, most of them situated at the margin of the cytoplasm (Fig. 9.138). A variable proportion of the cells may contain an asteroid body (see page 749). When the giant cells are numerous they may seem to form clusters, but these give the impression of an

association resulting simply from their formation in propinquity rather than as a manifestation of any focal cellular proliferation such as occurs, for example, in the development of the epithelioid cell granulomatous foci of sarcoidosis (see page 747). Mononuclear histiocytes are infrequent among the giant cells; when present they are in the form of simple rounded macrophages without evidence of epithelioid metamorphosis. There is no necrosis.

There may be some proliferation of endothelial macrophages in the sinuses, but this is inconstant, and giant cell formation within sinuses is unusual.

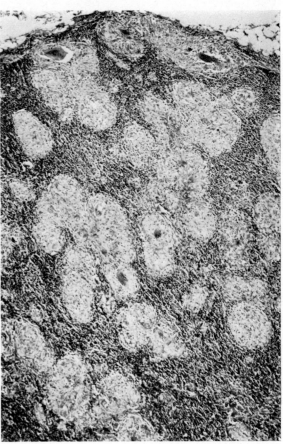

Fig. 9.137A. Tuberculoid granulomatous lymphadenitis in a lymph node draining a primary mammary carcinoma. The primary growth was a scirrhous infiltrating carcinoma without unusual features; there was no associated retention of secretion or necrosis, products of which might have been the cause of the changes in the regional nodes. Multinucleate giant cells are conspicuous in several of the granulomatous foci. Some of the foci appear to be centred on the subcapsular sinus but most are within the pulp. There is no sinus histiocytosis (see Fig. 9.42, page 562). The picture suggested the possibility of sarcoidosis, but there was no evidence of granulomatosis elsewhere in the body. *Haematoxylin–eosin.* × 50.

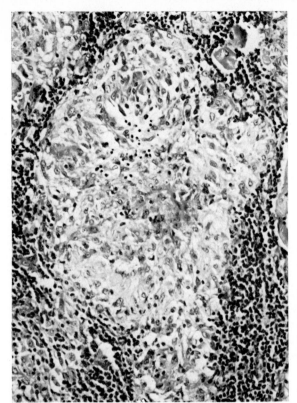

Fig. 9.137B. Same specimen as Fig. 9.137A. There has been some necrobiosis within this granuloma, as shown by the loss of cells and the particulate nuclear debris in one area. Below that area there is some 'fibrinoid' change. *Haematoxylin–eosin.* ×165.

There is no particular disturbance of the general structure of the nodes and the follicles are normal and usually contain a well-formed germinal centre.

In the only case of this condition in which I have seen sections of the spleen, this organ showed the presence of occasional giant cells of the same appearance as those in the nodes. They were confined to the lymphoid tissue.

The cause and nature of this peculiar form of lymphadenopathy are unknown. An identical picture is seen in mesenteric lymph nodes in a small minority of cases of Crohn's disease in place of the more usual tuberculoid reaction (see page 682). Similarly, the lymphadenopathy associated with the presence of prosthetic joints made of silicone rubber is histologically comparable, only the foreign material that is visible in some of the cells distinguishing the two pictures (see page 570).

The clinical picture is that of a moderate degree of generalized enlargement of superficial lymph nodes. There have been no other obtrusive manifestations

in the few cases that I know of. The patients have been young adults, of either sex, and in good general health. The disease appears to be self-limiting and to have no sequelae.

'Stengel–Wolbach Sclerosis'

The condition that is sometimes known as Stengel–Wolbach sclerosis[743a, 743b] is a generalized tuberculoid granulomatosis that affects the lymphoid tissues, often with predominant involvement of the spleen. The lesions in lymph nodes are mainly in the sinuses and their vicinity.[743c] The granulomatous foci are of about the size of miliary tubercles; they

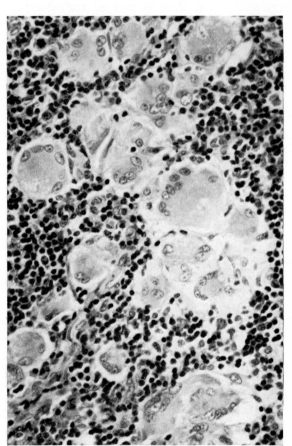

Fig. 9.138. Pure giant-celled lymphadenitis of unknown causation. The lymphoid tissue throughout the node was studded with giant cells of the type illustrated here: the cells are rounded, solitary or juxtaposed one to another; they have several vesicular nuclei, mainly placed at the periphery of the cell, which has opaque cytoplasm. An occasional cell is partly vacuolate, and, as in the cell to the right above the centre of the field, may contain an 'asteroid' body (see Fig. 9.180, page 751). See also Figs 9.51A and 9.51B (page 570) and Fig. 9.136. *Haematoxylin–eosin.* ×300.

1*

are discrete or, when the disease is particularly extensive, confluent. They consist of comparatively sparse epithelioid histiocytes among which large multinucleate giant cells are numerous and conspicuous (Fig. 9.139). It is a characteristic feature that the giant cells contain one or more well-formed asteroid bodies (see page 749 and Fig. 9.180). There is no necrosis, or, exceptionally, a few dead cells are seen in an occasional granuloma, maybe with a few neutrophils in their vicinity. Fibrosis within and round the granulomas is always a notable feature, and in the spleen may lead to considerable loss of both white and red pulp.

This is a rare form of granulomatosis and its cause is not known. It is sometimes regarded as a variant of sarcoidosis, but there is nothing that seems to justify this. The Kveim test was negative in the two cases in which I know it to have been carried out.

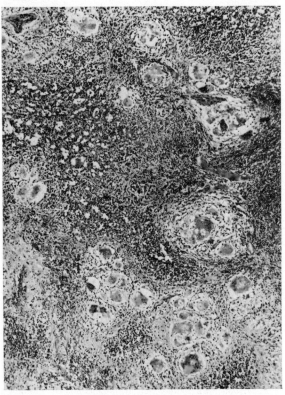

Fig. 9.139. Giant-celled tuberculoid granulomatosis of the spleen in 'Stengel–Wolbach sclerosis'. Even at this low magnification it is clear that epithelioid cells account for only a small part of the size of the granulomatous foci, which consist mainly of very large, discrete, multinucleate giant cells. Many of the giant cells contain one or more 'asteroids' (see Fig. 9.180, page 751). The appearances in the lymph nodes are essentially the same as those illustrated here in the spleen. *Haematoxylin–eosin.* × 55.

Splenomegaly and anaemia are the striking clinical features in most cases, the latter perhaps being a manifestation of 'hypersplenism' (see page 724).

Focal Epithelioid Cell Folliculitis of Lymph Nodes

Another unusual and rare form of granulomatous lymphadenitis is of interest because the histological changes are confined to the deep aspect of the germinal centre of the lymphoid follicles, usually within the mantle (see page 512) and occupying up to half or two thirds of the germinal centre. The foci comprise numerous small, discrete or partly confluent, clusters of closely packed epithelioid cells (Fig. 9.140). Some of the cells are binucleate; multinucleate giant cells are not found. The nuclei are pale and rather small and the cytoplasm is opaque and faintly eosinophile. There is no necrosis and, in my limited experience (five cases), no fibrosis. The clusters are generally smaller and more compact than those of, for example, toxoplasmosis (see page 654), and their situation is quite different from that of toxoplasmic foci. The lymph nodes otherwise show no noteworthy features, and there is neither formation of immunoblasts nor accumulation of plasma cells or any other feature that might be a clue to functional changes.

Clinically, the condition presents as a moderate enlargement of superficial lymph nodes, particularly in the neck but also to some extent in the axillae and groins. The patient, usually an adult, of either sex, seldom has any other symptoms, but may give a history of a recent, mild, influenza-like illness.

The cause and nature of this peculiarly localized epithelioid cell folliculitis are quite unknown. The location of the lesions indicates the likelihood of a particular disturbance in the cellular responses of a restricted part of the germinal centres, and perhaps specifically the part deep to the 'cap' that includes the 'dendritic reticular cells' (see page 514). Microbiological and serological investigations provided no clues to the nature of the condition in any of the three cases in my series in which it was possible to try to find evidence of the nature of the disease.

Dermatopathic Lymphadenitis

The changes in the lymph nodes that are characteristic of dermatopathic lymphadenitis (dermatopathic lymphadenopathy) may be associated with various skin diseases (see below). It is a mistake to believe that this form of lymphadenitis is anything other than a reaction of the lymph nodes to an

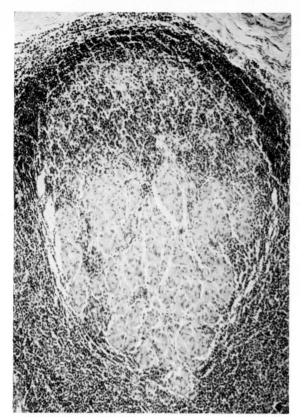

Fig. 9.140. Focal epithelioid cell folliculitis of lymph nodes. Multiple, discrete, pale clusters of epithelioid cells occupy most of the deeper half of the lymphoid follicle. Shrinkage of the tissues during histological processing has accentuated the general tendency of the cellular foci to remain separate. A few similar, smaller foci are present in the more superficial part of the follicle also. *Haematoxylin–eosin.* × 90.

inflammatory stimulus reaching them through the lymph stream: there are no good grounds for perpetuating the former view that such changes were a primary manifestation of a specific disease involving the lymph nodes and the skin—in all cases the skin changes, whatever their nature, precede and are the cause of the lymphadenopathy. The histological picture of dermatopathic lymphadenitis was first described by Pautrier and Woringer in 1932,[744] and they later suggested the name lipomelanic reticulosis:[745] this name is still in use, but it would be as well if it could be replaced by a term free from the connotation of malignancy that the word reticulosis has for so many clinicians (see page 537). The most florid form of dermatopathic lymphadenitis occurs in association with generalized exfoliative dermatitis (Fig. 9.141A).[746] A mild degree of the same changes, showing all the diagnostic features, may be seen in cases of many localized skin diseases, particularly

those that cause pruritus or that are accompanied by hyperaemia or desquamation of the affected area of skin. These less severe skin conditions include psoriasis and various psoriasiform dermatoses, lichen planus and other lichenified eruptions, pityriasis rosea, sunburn, and even drug rashes and insect bites.

Histology[747]

The essential microscopical feature is the formation of a pale, peripheral zone in the affected nodes, due to histiocytic proliferation in the subcapsular sinus and to a less extent in the trabecular sinuses: the histiocytes are rather loosely packed and have an unusually pale, vacuolate cytoplasm. This proliferation is not confined to the lumen of the sinuses but extends into the pulp. The cytoplasm of the histiocytes usually, but not always,[748] contains neutral fat and sometimes a small amount of other lipids. Often, melanin is present in a considerable proportion of the cells, either in the form of a fine powdering of the cytoplasm or, in contrast, as abundant, dark

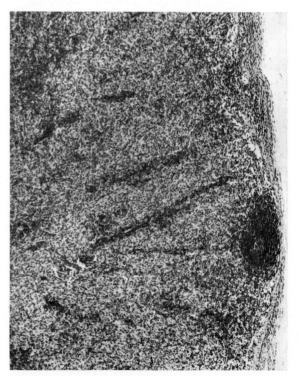

Fig. 9.141A. Dermatopathic lymphadenitis in a case of generalized exfoliative dermatitis. Widespread proliferation of macrophages accounts for the paler areas. The proliferation starts in the sinuses and spreads into the adjoining pulp. See also Fig. 9.141B. *Haematoxylin–eosin.* × 55.

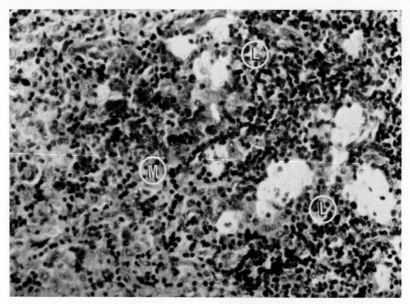

Fig. 9.141B. Same specimen as Fig. 9.141A. L, L: Clusters of large macrophages with clear cytoplasm (lipophages from which the lipid contents have been dissolved during preparation of the section). M: Although not readily seen in the black-and-white reproduction, many macrophages in the area above the letter are laden with melanin. Elsewhere in the field are macrophages with pale, opaque cytoplasm: they account for the greatest part of the increased cellularity of the lymph nodes affected by this condition (see Fig. 9.141A). *Haematoxylin–eosin.* × 275.

brown or blackish clumps (Fig. 9.141B); sometimes it is altogether lacking.[749] Haemosiderin is also found in many examples. Eosinophils are often conspicuous among the histiocytes, but may be absent. This histological picture is so characteristic that from its presence the microscopist can suggest the likelihood of a disease of the skin as the cause of enlargement of the lymph nodes—often in such cases the causal significance of some chronic dermatosis or dermatitis is overlooked until the clue is provided by the finding of these changes in an excised lymph node.

Prognosis

As dermatopathic lymphadenitis is sometimes mistakenly looked upon as an entity, and one that may have a bad prognosis, it is important to stress that it itself has no prognostic significance. The prognosis in a case of dermatopathic lymphadenitis is, in fact, the prognosis of the skin condition that is its cause. It should be remembered, however, that generalized exfoliative dermatitis, which is one of the most impressive causes of dermatopathic lymphadenitis, may itself be symptomatic of Hodgkin's disease; more rarely, exfoliative dermatitis is an accompaniment of other types of malignant lymphomatosis. In such cases the histological picture of the underlying lymphoma and that of dermatopathic lymphadenitis may be associated in a single biopsy specimen, or dermatopathic lymphadenitis and the lymphoma may be found respectively in successive specimens. The lymphoma predisposes to the dermatitis and is not a consequence of it.[747] The pathogenesis of the skin changes is obscure. Involvement of the skin by the malignant process is rarely observed in these cases: when it occurs it affects a small proportion of the skin, whereas the dermatitis is widespread and may affect even the whole surface of the body. An autoimmune mechanism may be involved.

Lymphadenitis with Eosinophil Infiltrate

Eosinophils may be found in any lymph node: their presence in small numbers in an inflamed node is therefore commonly without special significance. In certain conditions, particularly when the pathological process has an allergic basis, and notably in some forms of metazoal infestation, eosinophils may be very numerous in the nodes.

Lymph Nodes in Allergic Diseases

In allergic diseases the lymph nodes themselves are seldom directly involved in the allergic reaction but often contain many more eosinophils than is normally the case. For instance, eosinophils may be very numerous in bronchopulmonary and tracheo-bronchial nodes in cases of severe bronchial asthma, at least as judged by post-mortem findings in cases of status asthmaticus. In other conditions in which an allergic type of sensitivity reaction may be involved—for example, some cases of polyarteritis—there may be specific lesions in the nodes (see page 693).

Lymph Nodes in Metazoal Diseases

The types of metazoal parasites that may infest lymph nodes have been considered already (see pages 669 to 680). Not all of these infestations are characterized by an increase in the number of eosinophils in the nodes. Equally, the presence of eosinophils in lymph nodes in cases of metazoal infestation of other organs—for example, the bowel—seldom indicates extension of the infestation to the nodes themselves: it is commonly found that there are many eosinophils in the nodes of the mesentery and elsewhere in the abdomen when there is heavy infestation of the bowel by worms, as is particularly frequently the case in the tropics.

Rare Forms of 'Eosinophil Lymphadenitis'

There are several rare conditions in which eosinophils are a main participant in inflammatory changes in lymph nodes. They constitute the small group of diseases that are sometimes classed together under the name 'essential eosinophilic lymphadenitis'.

'Allergic Granulomatosis'.—'Allergic granulomatosis' is the term applied to a very rare, fatal condition in which a histiocytic or tuberculoid granulomatosis of periarterial and other connective tissues, with infiltration of the tissues by eosinophils and eosinophilia in the blood, is associated with severe asthma and fever.[750] There may be focal fibrinoid necrosis, mainly at the core of the granulomas; however, necrosis may be absent from particular lesions and it is not seen in all lymph node biopsy specimens, even when frequent in other tissues.

It remains uncertain whether this disease is an entity and whether the histological picture is a manifestation of an allergic state. No allergen has been identified. In one of two cases that I have seen that may have been instances of 'allergic granulomatosis' of this type, there was an unequivocal history of sensitization to sulphonamides and the fatal illness developed soon after a course of treatment with a proprietary suspension of sulphamethoxazole and trimethroprim: the doctor knew that the patient had a history of dangerous sensitivity to sulphonamides but was unaware that the suspension prescribed contained a sulphonamide (sulphamethoxazole).

Necrotizing Eosinophil Granulomatosis.[751]—This condition, which is also fatal, is even rarer than 'allergic granulomatosis', of which it may be a variant. It is possibly related to polyarteritis and to Wegener's disease (see page 693). Multiple miliary or confluent foci of necrosis in the lymph nodes throughout the body and in the spleen are the essential histological feature: in addition to fibrinoid necrosis there are collections of eosinophils that merit description as 'eosinophil abscesses' as well as a considerable infiltration of the nodes as a whole by eosinophils. There is eosinophilia in the blood. There may be a necrotizing angitis.

The condition has been mistaken for Hodgkin's disease. The presence of eosinophils and occasionally of hyperchromatic and enlarged reticulum cells, and the destruction of the normal architecture of the nodes, may explain this error. The resemblance to Hodgkin's disease is very tenuous: in particular there are no Sternberg–Reed cells and the abnormal reticulum cells do not have the uncommonly large nucleolus characteristic of the atypical reticulum cells of Hodgkin's disease.

Eosinophil Suppurative Lymphadenitis.—In contrast to the rare fatal conditions just described, there is an apparently self-limiting form of localized lymphadenitis that is also characterized by particularly heavy infiltration by eosinophils.[752, 753] It is usually confined to the nodes in one groin but sometimes affects other superficial groups as well, or alone. The affected nodes are enlarged up to 4 cm in their largest dimension. Histologically, they are heavily and widely infiltrated by eosinophils, often in such numbers that the picture is aptly enough designated an eosinophil abscess. There are also more or less numerous aggregates of large pale cells, usually described as reticulum cells or histiocytes: the centre of the aggregates may be necrotic, and there is then a heavy local accumulation of eosinophils. Confluence of adjoining lesions may lead to massive destruction of the nodes, but without evident tendency to extend beyond their capsule.

The cause of this benign condition is unknown. In two cases in which it was confined to the inguinal nodes on one side the patients were women who previously had suffered from oxyuriasis, but there is little reason to believe that there was any causal relation between this history and the lymphadenitis.[752] An identical lymphadenitis developed in the inguinal nodes of a patient who was being treated for rheumatoid arthritis by 'apiotherapy', prescribed and applied by her vicar:[753] the lymphadenopathy followed stings by four bees that, at a single session, were offered an area of skin on the thigh of the same side. The patient had no manifestations otherwise of an untoward response to the stings, and the local lesions in the skin were in no way remarkable. In another case, the affected lymph nodes were in the axilla of the side on which a child had been bitten on the forearm by an adder (*Vipera berus*) in an English garden some 5 weeks earlier;[753] an hour after the bite polyvalent snake venom antiserum was injected into the bitten area and also intravenously—during the intravenous injection the patient collapsed with dyspnoea and acute arterial hypotension, evidently anaphylactic in nature, and he subsequently developed severe urticaria.* Swelling of the lymph nodes in the axilla was apparent within 3 days of the injections and reached its peak a week later. The relation between such events and the the development of eosinophil lymphadenitis is equivocal.

Lymph Nodes in Hand–Schüller–Christian Disease and Letterer–Siwe Disease

Eosinophils are commonly associated with the histiocytosis of these two conditions (see pages 763 and 858), which therefore may need to be considered in the differential diagnosis of lymphadenopathies of which an eosinophil infiltrate is a feature.

Lymphadenitis Associated with Connective Tissue Diseases

Lymph nodes are very commonly, if not invariably, affected in the course of diseases that primarily involve the connective tissues,[754] in the sense of the latter as a system of cells and their derivatives that are distributed throughout the body as a metabolically active, ennourishing, mediatory and

---

* But for the fact that the child's mother was a doctor, who considered it an obligation, although she was not in practice, to maintain a comprehensive kit for use in medical emergencies, he would not have received the antivenom so promptly (and possibly needlessly: Editorial, *Lancet*, 1976, **2**, 185); nor would the means of treating the anaphylactic reaction have been so ready to hand.

supportive stromal complex. The connective tissues in this sense are comparable to the cells and cell derivatives of the analogous, but functionally distinct, lymphoreticular system; indeed the two systems—the connective tissue system and the lymphoreticular system—are in certain respects inseparable (for instance, the relation between the reticuloendothelial cells and the reticulin fibres). The diseases of the connective tissues, in the broadest context, are the diseases of all other tissues and organs. In a narrower sense, of diseases primarily affecting the connective tissues, there is the group of conditions that are still generally known, at least among general physicians, by the unsatisfactory term 'collagen diseases' (or, worse, 'collagenoses'). The lymphadenopathies that are to be referred to in this section are those that accompany this group. In particular, there are notable changes in lymph nodes in rheumatoid arthritis, systemic lupus erythematosus and polyarteritis. Lymph node involvement in cases of anaphylactoid purpura (Schönlein–Henoch purpura), dermatomyositis, polymyalgia rheumatica and systemic sclerosis must also be noted. So must that in thrombotic thrombocytopenic purpura and in Wegener's disease, although these conditions are less clearly in the same general nosological category as the others and, at practical level, are more usefully considered among haematological diseases (see page 493) and diseases of the upper respiratory passages and lungs (see pages 213 and 371) respectively. 'Allergic granulomatosis' probably belongs to this category also (see page 689).

Rheumatoid Arthritis

Rheumatoid arthritis (see Chapter 38) is very commonly accompanied by generalized enlargement of lymph nodes.[755] This is particularly marked in cases of the so-called Felty syndrome (rheumatoid arthritis, splenomegaly and leucopenia)[756] and its childhood equivalent (Chauffard–Ramon–Still syndrome[757, 758]). In some cases of rheumatoid arthritis, particularly in younger women, the enlargement of the axillary and inguinal nodes results in considerable masses that may lead the clinician to suspect the presence of a lymphoma. In some cases the clinical impression then influences the histologist to interpret the changes in the nodes as malignant when in fact they are benign (see below).

Histology

Follicular hyperplasia, often with considerable enlargement of follicles as well as an appreciable increase in their number, and with correspondingly large germinal centres, is associated with some degree of sinus catarrh. Neutrophils are often numerous in the sinuses. Some of the hyperplastic endothelial macrophages are multinucleate, but compact and hyperchromatic: they have sometimes been mistaken for Sternberg–Reed cells, but should be readily distinguishable from them by the presence of ingested cells or other material in their cytoplasm and by the small size of their nucleoli. A misdiagnosis commoner than that of Hodgkin's disease is follicular lymphoma: the latter may be quite closely simulated in those comparatively rare cases in which the germinal centres are either not conspicuous or are composed largely of lymphocytes of intermediate size that occupy almost the whole of the follicles. Usually, however, macrophages containing ingested nuclear debris (Flemming's 'stainable bodies'—see page 512) are very numerous in the germinal centres of the hyperplastic follicles.[759]

Plasma cells are sometimes abundant in the pulp. There may be an inverse relation between the degree of follicular hyperplasia and the intensity of the plasma cell accumulation.

Amyloidosis.—Amyloid is demonstrable in the lymph nodes in about 10 per cent of cases, in conformity with the frequency of amyloidosis as an accompaniment of rheumatoid arthritis.[760, 761]

Systemic Lupus Erythematosus

There is said to be involvement of lymph nodes in about 50 per cent of all cases of systemic lupus erythematosus.[762] Sometimes the histological picture in a lymph node biopsy specimen is the first evidence of the nature of an illness: enlargement of cervical nodes was the first clinical manifestation in nine (1·7 per cent) of a series of 520 cases and generalized lymph node enlargement was the first clinical manifestation in five (1 per cent) of this series.[762] Clinically, cervical nodes are involved most frequently, followed by axillary nodes; at necropsy the abdominal and mediastinal nodes are commonly found to be affected also.

Histology

In most cases of systemic lupus erythematosus in which there are changes in the lymph nodes these are non-specific. In the earlier stages there may be follicular hyperplasia. It is often said that there is no phagocytosis of nuclear debris by macrophages in the germinal centres of the hyperplastic follicles,[763]

and this has been thought to have some significance as a point in favour of the diagnosis of systemic lupus erythematosus when other evidence indicates the possibility; my own experience is that this must be an inconstant finding, for I have seen Flemming's 'stainable bodies' in macrophages in the germinal centres in several cases.

The features that have diagnostic value are necrosis and the peculiar structures known as haematoxyphile bodies (see below). Necrosis takes the form initially of necrobiotic foci, starting with pyknosis or karyorrhexis of the nucleus of individual cells and developing into more extensive areas of colliquative necrosis, with dissolution of cells, oedema and maybe some accumulation of neutrophils (Fig. 9.142). Elsewhere, foci of fibrinoid necrosis may appear, perhaps oftener in the centre of the follicles than elsewhere, but in the later stages, when the follicles are often no longer clearly discernible, in any part of the pulp (Fig. 9.143). Sometimes, necrosis seems to be associated with changes in the vasculature of the node: these changes are of

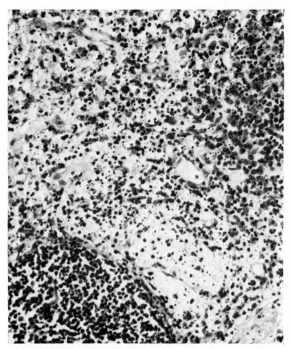

Fig. 9.142. Lymph node in acute systemic lupus erythematosus. Extensive colliquative necrosis with nuclear debris and oedema. There is marked depletion of lymphocytes although plasma cells persist and in places form aggregates (above, right). Inexplicably, adjoining areas of lymphoid tissue, separated from the areas of destruction only by an intact trabecula, appear to be unaffected (below, left). See also Figs 9.143 and 9.144. *Haematoxylin–eosin.* × 190.

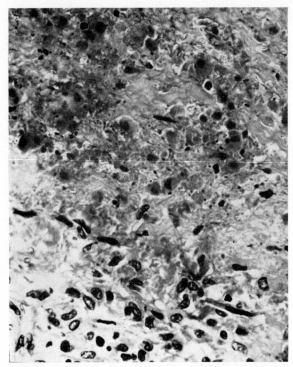

Fig. 9.143. Lymph node in acute systemic lupus erythematosus. This biopsy specimen is characterized by extensive fibrinoid necrosis, with karyolysis of the cells of a follicle. Occasional haematoxyphile bodies ('H-bodies') are seen—for instance, upper left corner of field. See also Figs 9.142 and 9.144. *Haematoxylin–eosin.* × 450.

the types familiar elsewhere in this disease and include necrotizing arteriolitis and the formation of concentric rings of fibrosis round small arteries (see page 733); they are not pathognomonic.

In some cases there is a striking accumulation of plasma cells in the pulp of the nodes, often with many Russell bodies or similar hyaline, eosinophile structures.

Haematoxyphile Bodies.—In some case the haematoxyphile bodies ('haematoxylin bodies', or 'H-bodies') that are a characteristic feature of the histological picture of the lesions of systemic lupus erythematosus in other parts of the body are found in the lymph nodes (Fig. 9.143), maybe in considerable numbers.[764] Their appearance is usually a late phenomenon, and they are observed in post-mortem material much oftener than at biopsy. They consist of deoxyribonucleic acid, gammaglobulin and polysaccharide.[764, 765] They are structureless and their outline is rather indistinct; their haematoxyphilia varies greatly, so that in haematoxylin–eosin preparations they range in colour from lilac red to

darkest blue. Their diameter is usually from 5 to 12 μm, the smaller bodies within this range being spherical and the larger ovoid. Much larger, and then usually much more intensely haematoxyphile, examples may be found (Fig. 9.144), especially *post mortem*; they probably form through coalescence of smaller bodies. Most of these haematoxyphile bodies, at least in lymphoid tissue, are thought to be formed from the nuclei of lymphocytes; some are derived from the nuclei of granular leucocytes and other local cells.

It is a characteristic of the haematoxyphile bodies that they lie free in the tissues. In lymph nodes they may be seen in the vicinity of necrotic foci (Fig. 9.143) or in the sinuses. Eventually, they probably dissolve and disappear. Very occasionally, a haematoxyphile body is clearly seen to have been ingested by a phagocyte, which is usually a macrophage but sometimes a neutrophil: this is the

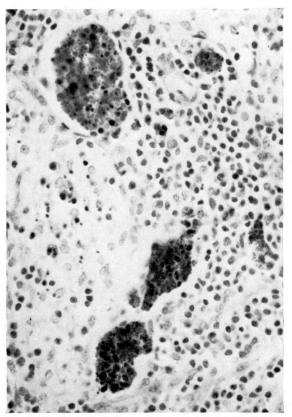

Fig. 9.144. Systemic lupus erythematosus. Several agglomerates of haematoxyphile bodies are seen in the sinuses and nearby pulp of a lymph node from the mediastinum. Postmortem specimen. As may be the case when these bodies coalesce in this way, the intensity of their haematoxyphilia is seen to vary considerably. *Haematoxylin–eosin.* × 400.

in-vivo counterpart of the 'lupus erythematosus cell' as demonstrated *in vitro*.[766] The haematoxyphile bodies themselves, in sections, are considered to be the histological manifestation of the altered nuclear material that is ingested by a neutrophil (or, occasionally, by a monocyte) in the blood to form the so-called lupus erythematosus cell (LE cell—see Fig. 8.4D, page 435). Like LE cells, haematoxyphile bodies are occasionally seen in other conditions, including a small proportion of cases of rheumatoid arthritis.[767] By analogy with the genesis of the LE cell, it is presumed that they are a manifestation of the presence of antinuclear antibody (the LE cell factor, which is an immunoglobulin of class G).

Polyarteritis

Characteristic polyarteritic lesions may be found in small arteries in the vicinity of a lymph node, including the hilum, and sometimes in arterioles within its substance. Their presence in a lymph node biopsy specimen has, rarely, led to recognition of the disease when it had escaped diagnosis previously. Polyarteritis is a rare cause of infarction of lymph nodes (see page 551) (Fig. 9.145).

In some cases of polyarteritis there is a peculiar granuloma-like change in the germinal centre of the follicles,[768] which are often hyperplastic in this disease. A similar 'granulomatoid folliculitis' may be seen in the spleen (see page 732). This lesion is characterized by necrobiotic changes in a proportion of the cells, with the accompanying formation of a small number of epithelioid histiocytes; a frank tuberculoid aggregation does not develop. The reticulin fibres within the follicle may be thickened and have a fibrinoid appearance.

The changes in the lymph nodes in Wegener's disease, which is often considered to be a variant of polyarteritis, are described on page 694.

Lymphadenopathy in Other Connective Tissue Diseases

Anaphylactoid Purpura.—'Granulomatoid folliculitis', identical with that occasionally seen in polyarteritis (see above), is sometimes found in the lymph nodes and spleen in cases of anaphylactoid purpura (Schönlein–Henoch purpura—see page 495 and Chapter 39).

Dermatomyositis.—Only non-specific changes have been described in lymph nodes in cases of dermatomyositis.[769]

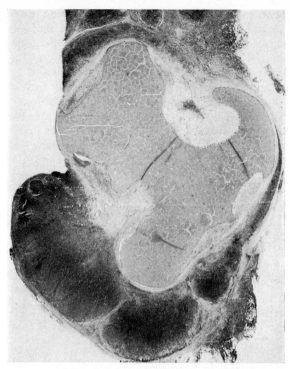

Fig. 9.145. Infarction of an axillary lymph node due to obliteration of an artery in its hilum by polyarteritis. Sudden local pain and progressive enlargement of the node, leading to diagnostic biopsy, were the first manifestations of the arterial disease. The inflammatory cellular infiltrate round the artery forms a dark crescent within the pale area of fibrous tissue that has developed in the hilum (above, right of centre). The specimen was obtained 25 days after the acute onset of the symptoms. *Haematoxylin–eosin.* × 7.

'Polymyalgia Rheumatica' and Giant Cell Arteritis. —The condition that is known as 'polymyalgia rheumatica' is often said to be a manifestation of giant cell arteritis (see Chapter 36). A patient with polymyalgia developed manifest giant cell arteritis, confined clinically to one temporal artery: this development was accompanied by painful swelling of a superficial parotid lymph node on the same side. The histological picture in the node was that of partial infarction, caused by obliteration of a small artery in the hilum that showed the classic changes of giant cell arteritis.[770]

Systemic Sclerosis.—The lymph nodes seem not to have had much consideration in published reports of systemic sclerosis ('generalized scleroderma'). In an unpublished case, necropsy showed no unusual changes in superficial lymph nodes (two were examined, one from the neck and one from a groin); in contrast, the four visceral lymph nodes sectioned (a tracheobronchial node, two bronchopulmonary nodes and a node from the mesentery in the ileocaecal angle) showed marked fibrosis of the capsule and trabeculae, with partial obliteration and obstruction of the sinuses, concentric fibrosis of the intima and adventitia of arterioles, and foci of fibrosis extending through the pulp (Fig. 9.146).[770] The disease had involved the lungs severely, causing 'honeycomb lung' (see page 369); there was severe oesophageal fibrosis (see page 1003); and the cause of death was peritonitis from perforation of an area of the caecum that had become gangrenous as a result of ischaemia complicating fibrosis of the intima of the arterial branches in its wall.

Thrombotic Thrombocytopenic Purpura

In an exceptional case of thrombotic thrombocytopenic purpura (see page 493), the illness presented

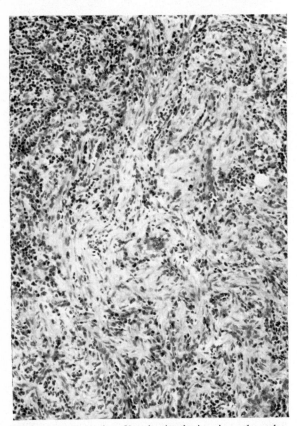

Fig. 9.146. Extensive fibrosis developing in a bronchopulmonary lymph node in a fatal case of untreated systemic sclerosis (the patient refused treatment). The sinuses are obliterated and the fibrosis extends into the pulp. The fibroblasts traverse the field in a somewhat whorled pattern and are separated by small collections of lymphocytes and plasma cells. *Haematoxylin–eosin.* × 140.

with generalized enlargement of lymph nodes. Biopsy showed many small arterioles and capillaries in an axillary node to be the seat of the thrombotic microangiopathy that is characteristic of the disease (see page 493); the only other notable finding was follicular hyperplasia.[771] Enlargement of lymph nodes is a rare observation in this condition. The involvement of their vasculature (Fig. 9.147) is a manifestation of the generalization of these lesions throughout the body.

Wegener's Disease

Lymph node involvement is almost always found at necropsy in cases of Wegener's disease (Wegener's granulomatosis, rhinogenic polyarteritis)[772, 773] but is seldom clinically obtrusive. The clinical manifestations of the disease are pre-eminently those affecting the nose (see page 213) and lungs (see page 371), and, terminally, the kidneys (see Chapter 24). The nature of Wegener's disease is uncertain, but it is usually regarded as an immunological disorder associated with an unidentified antigen reacting primarily in the upper and lower parts of the respiratory system.

Enlargement of the upper deep cervical nodes and, less often, of the submandibular nodes may be found when the disease is well established in the nose or nasal sinuses, but is rarely marked. Involvement of nodes in the mediastinum is often demonstrable radiologically in cases of extensive disease in the lungs but is always incidental to the latter.

Exceptionally, biopsy of an enlarged cervical lymph node has provided the first evidence of Wegener's disease. In one such case the only other manifestation at the time of diagnosis was opacity of the maxillary sinus of the same side;[774] in another case, in which a seemingly healthy patient was found to have 'coin' shadows on radiological examination of the lungs, biopsy of the so-called scalene lymph nodes (lower deep cervical or paratracheal nodes in the vicinity of the lower attachment of the anterior and middle scalene muscles) showed the classic picture associated with Wegener's disease.[774]

Histology

The most striking feature of the lesions of Wegener's disease, as seen in lymph nodes, is extensive necrosis. The foci of necrosis range from the size of small tubercles to vast confluent masses associated with enlargement of the nodes up to 5 cm in diameter. The necrotic material may have the look of caseation, but is often more stippled with haematoxyphile particles than tuberculous caseating matter. The

and tracts of fibrinoid necrosis in the capsule or trabeculae of the nodes and sometimes within the parts of the pulp that are not destroyed in the 'caseating' process. The angitis is not always demonstrable in lymph nodes. When present, it may be accompanied by thrombosis and focal infarction, but such ischaemic lesions do not appear to be the cause of the more extensive foci of necrosis. Sometimes, inflammation and thrombosis of blood vessels in the nodes is clearly secondary to their involvement in the spreading granulomatous lesion; elsewhere,

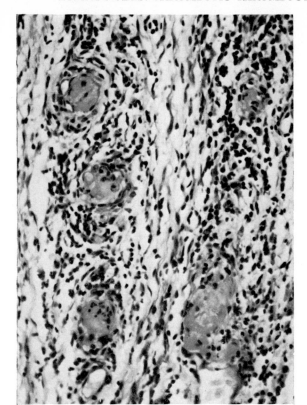

Fig. 9.147. Lymph node in an unpublished case of thrombotic thrombocytopenic purpura. Small blood vessels in the capsule (left) and abutting on the subcapsular sinus (right) are distended by eosinophile thrombus consisting mainly of blood platelets. The thrombus is partly hyaline and in some vessels has begun to shrink, with partial reopening of the lumen. There is a characteristic microaneurysm with contained thrombus (below, right). Similar appearances, but accompanied by local accumulation of neutrophils, may be seen in some instances of acute systemic lupus erythematosus and, rarely, in drug-induced angiopathies (Schönlein–Henoch purpura and the like). The cells in the vicinity of the vessels in the specimen illustrated are lymphocytes and an occasional plasma cell and appeared to be merely part of the associated chronic non-specific lymphadenitis. The node was from the cervical region. *Haematoxylin–eosin.* × 235.

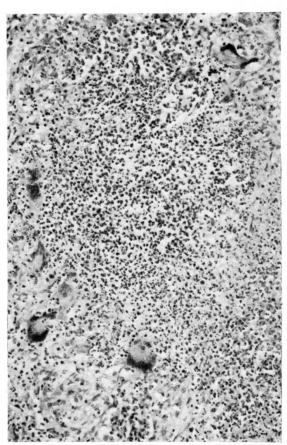

Fig. 9.148. Lymphadenitis in Wegener's disease. In this instance there are so many neutrophils in the necrotic core of the lesion that it may be described as suppurating. The giant cells among the epithelioid cells of the granuloma show characteristic hyperchromasia of the majority of their nuclei. In this case the initial interpretation of the biopsy was that an infective cause should be looked for: the diagnosis of Wegener's disease was not made until the presence of pulmonary and renal lesions was recognized and the true significance of maxillary sinusitis—previously thought to be incidental—was shown by biopsy. The patient's only serious complaint had been related to the painful swelling of lymph nodes in the neck and armpits. *Haematoxylin–eosin.* × 160.

foci are bounded by a relatively narrow zone of small, compactly disposed epithelioid cells among which there are almost always some of the multinucleate giant cells that are characteristic of the disease, although not pathognomonic: these cells have opaque and intensely eosinophile cytoplasm, and their nuclei are small, oval and often so hyperchromatic that they appear almost structureless, as if pyknotic.[775] Neutrophils may be numerous (Fig. 9.148); eosinophils are few or, usually, absent.

In addition to the granulomatous changes there are usually others, particularly necrotizing angitis however, angitis occurs apart from the latter, and especially in the small arteries in the hilum of the nodes and in arterioles in the capsule. Multinucleate giant cells, like those in the necrotic foci, may be present in the wall of the affected vessels or in the immediately surrounding tissue; the picture must not be mistaken for that of a giant cell arteritis (see page 214).

IATROGENIC LYMPHADENOPATHY

Drugs (including hormones and synthetic analogues of hormones), immunizing agents, antisera, radiotherapy and surgery are responsible for a considerable variety of pathological changes in lymph nodes. Some of these are considered in the section of this chapter that deals with factors that affect the lymphoreticular system (see page 533)—radiotherapy, cytotoxic drugs, antilymphocyte serum and corticosteroid hormones all cause significant atrophy of the nodes. Surgery may result in infarction of parts or the whole of a node through interference with its arterial blood supply.

Some drugs have the effect of stimulating a highly atypical proliferation of the lymphoreticular tissues, particularly of lymph nodes. These are considered below (this page). Some other effects of drugs and immunizing agents may be summarized first.

Iatrogenic Infection of Lymph Nodes

Infective lymphadenitis is a natural and expected consequence of the use of living micro-organisms as immunizing agents—for instance, bacillus Calmette–Guérin (see page 603) and vaccinia virus (see page 644). In contrast is the misadventure, potentially fatal, of infection resulting from bacterial contamination of material injected subcutaneously or into muscle.

Iatrogenic Siderosis of Lymph Nodes

Siderosis of the regional nodes follows intramuscular administration of iron dextran in the treatment of anaemia. The pharmacopoeial iron dextran injection is a sterile colloidal solution of a complex of ferric hydroxide with dextrans of low molecular weight; it contains 50 mg of iron in each millilitre, and a full course entails the injection of a considerable quantity (each gram of haemoglobin that needs to be made good requires about 6 ml of iron dextran injection). The injections are usually placed in the gluteal muscles. The inguinal nodes on both sides may become considerably enlarged in some cases,[776] through proliferation of macrophages, which become heavily laden with iron. This enlargement may lead to biopsy, and it has been known for melanoma to be diagnosed as a result of misinterpretation of the iron pigment when the history of iron injections has not been elicited. The iron in the nodes is in the ferric state and gives a positive Prussian blue reaction (Perls's test); it should not be mistakable for melanin. The converse diagnostic problem arose in a case in which the presence of iron that had been carried to the nodes from the site of iron dextran injections obscured the recognition of melanin in a case of melanoma: the tumour cells, which were sparse, were mistaken for macrophages.

Generalized enlargement of lymph nodes has occasionally been observed following intravenous administration of iron dextran.[777] The affected nodes show proliferation and siderosis of the endothelial macrophages in the sinuses and maybe small collections of siderotic macrophages in the pulp. Fever, urticaria and splenomegaly may accompany this reaction.

Miscellaneous Drug-Induced Lymphadenopathies

Enlargement of lymph nodes throughout the body is a common finding in cases of drug allergy of the type that resembles serum sickness, with fever, urticaria or other rashes, and sometimes arthralgia and oedema of soft tissues. It occurs in serum sickness itself,[778] and in cases of allergy to many different types of drugs, particularly sulphonamides[779] and thiouracils.[780] Little is on record about the histological changes.

A syndrome resembling that of glandular fever has been associated with taking aminosalicylic acid, sulphones, phenylbutazone and hydantoin drugs (see page 649). Phenylbutazone and, more frequently, the hydantoins also cause lymphoma-like changes: these are more important and are considered below.

The role of hypersensitivity to drugs in the causation of some instances of the condition known as immunoblastic lymphadenopathy is referred to on page 705.

Drug-Induced Lymphoma-Like Lymphadenopathies and Their Relation to Lymphomas

The most important drug-induced changes in lymph nodes are those that may be misinterpreted as lymphomatous, either clinically or histologically, and those that may be in fact lymphomatous. Both categories are seen oftenest as side effects of the hydantoin group of anticonvulsant drugs (hydantoin lymphadenopathy). More rarely, other drugs may be responsible (see below).* It is relevant that the histological picture of immunoblastic lymphadenopathy (see page 703) is liable to be misinterpreted as Hodgkin's disease, although in fact always distinguishable from the latter and from other lymphomas: in contrast, the most lymphoma-like examples of hydantoin-induced and similar lymphadenopathies are histologically close to the picture of Hodgkin's disease or, sometimes, of some other lymphoma, and they may become lymphomatous. The clinical syndrome of immunoblastic lymphadenopathy closely resembles that of hydantoin lymphadenopathy: fever, malaise and morbilliform or scarlatinaform rashes are common to both; anaemia, which may be haemolytic and associated with a direct positive Coombs test, lymphocytopenia, eosinophilia and sometimes neutrophil leucocytosis are also found in both. In immunoblastic lymphadenopathy it is a characteristic that there is hyperglobulinaemia involving any or all of the classes of immunoglobulin; in hydantoin lymphadenopathy it is possible that there is a deficiency of immunoglobulins rather than an increase.† The most striking differences between these two conditions are the high mortality of immunoblastic lymphadenopathy and its predominant occurrence in the 6th and 7th decades; hydantoin lymphadenopathy occurs most frequently in the 1st to the 3rd decade (as would be expected of a complication of the treatment of an illness that is most frequent among young people). Immunoblastic lymphadenopathy is essentially an immunological disorder: in a proportion of cases it is the manifestation of hypersensitivity to a drug, and it is notable that the drugs that may cause it include hydantoins. Hydantoin lymphadenopathy presents clinical and other features that indicate the possibility of hypersensitivity as the pathogenetic mechanism, and in some cases hypersensitivity to hydantoins has been demonstrated.

It is evident from such observations that there is an appreciable overlap between immunoblastic lymphadenopathy and the drug-induced lymphadenopathies that are typified by hydantoin lymphadenopathy. What distinguishes the latter is their remarkable affinity with the lymphomas, particularly Hodgkin's disease. Most cases of immunoblastic lymphadenopathy and most cases of hydantoin lymphadenopathy have features that are peculiar to their own group and that enable them to be identified. As the former condition becomes more familiar, a reconsideration of some cases in which reactions to other drugs were equated with hydantoin lymphadenopathy suggests that they belong rather to the category of immunoblastic lymphadenopathy.

Lymphadenopathy Accompanying Anticonvulsant Therapy (Hydantoin Lymphadenopathy)

Various anticonvulsant drugs may cause lymph node enlargement. In the cases that have been examined histologically, the range of appearances is the same whatever the drug: they are exemplified in the lymphadenopathy caused by the hydantoins, which are the drugs oftenest associated with this remarkable side effect. The hydantoins have been known to cause lymphadenopathy since the first compound of this group to be used clinically, 5-ethyl-5-phenylhydantoin (generally known by its proprietary name, Nirvanol*), was introduced as a sedative and hypnotic in the 1920s and was found to have some inhibitory effect on the involuntary movements of rheumatic chorea: enlargement of the lymph nodes was one of the signs that were considered to indicate that a course of treatment had been sufficiently prolonged. Nirvanol was abandoned because of its inevitable and potentially serious side effects: these constituted the so-called *Nirvanol disease*—a syndrome with many features in common with immunoblastic lymphadenopathy and hydantoin lymphadenopathy (see above).[781] Very little is known about the histological changes in the lymph nodes in Nirvanol disease: it was an era of comparatively rare recourse to biopsy,† and as the lymph-

* The occurrence of lymphomas in patients under treatment with immunosuppressive drugs is pathogenetically distinct from the drug-induced development of lymphomas under discussion here (see page 770).

† There is evidence that about a fifth of patients who are under treatment with phenytoin (diphenylhydantoin) show a fall in class A immunoglobulins (IgA) and other manifestations of immunodeficiency (Sorrell, T. C., Forbes, I. J., Burness, F. R., Rischbieth, R. H. C., *Lancet*, 1971, **2**, 1233).

* Nirvanol is no longer marketed. Valnoctamide, a minor tranquillizer that is marketed in France and some other countries under the proprietary name Nirvanil, is not related to the hydantoins.

† I know a patient personally who, while under treatment with Nirvanol for chorea, as a child in the 1920s, developed enlargement of lymph nodes that was diagnosed histologically as 'lymphadenoma' (Hodgkin's disease). As soon as she was convalescent from the chorea, it was decided to send her to London for treatment with X-rays: however, before going to England her parents took her on a pilgrimage to Lourdes, and the lymphadenopathy subsided. No treatment was given for the 'lymphadenoma'. The administration

adenopathy subsided when the drug was withdrawn there was no indication for microscopy.

Nirvanol was not used as an anticonvulsant and the occasional observation that patients with epilepsy had fewer attacks while receiving the drug as a sedative or hypnotic was attributed to sedation. The use of hydantoins as anticonvulsants dates from the introduction, in 1937–38, of phenytoin (diphenylhydantoin), which was developed for this purpose.[782] The proportion of patients who suffer side effects of treatment with a hydantoin anticonvulsant is very high, and enlargement of lymph nodes is one of the most frequent manifestations, some degree being recognizable clinically in almost every patient. Other side effects are noted above (see page 697) and are usually present as well as the lymphadenopathy. Another remarkable side effect that is very commonly present in some degree is hypertrophy of the gums, particularly of the upper jaw and particularly in relation to the incisor and canine teeth (hydantoin 'gingivitis' and hydantoin 'fibromatosis' are synonyms that give an incorrect impression of the pathology of this condition, which is neither inflammatory nor neoplastic but a hyperplastic state of the connective tissue).

The anticonvulsant with the greatest liability to cause troublesome side effects is methoin (mephenytoin), which is 5-ethyl-3-methyl-5-phenylhydantoin: it is metabolized in the body to the 5-ethyl-5-phenyl compound—that is, Nirvanol—by 3-demethylation.[783] Ethotoin (3-ethyl-5-phenylhydantoin) is the least toxic hydantoin, but also the least therapeutically effective. Phenytoin (5,5-diphenylhydantoin) is, at present, by far the most widely prescribed of all anticonvulsants; for this reason it accounts for the largest proportion of the observed complications, including lymphadenopathy. The undesirable effects of the hydantoins have encouraged the search for other anticonvulsants: some of these have proved also to cause lymphadenopathy (see below).

Hydantoin lymphadenopathy may be the only side effect of the drug; more usually it is accompanied by others. It may begin to develop within 2 to 3 weeks of the start of treatment, or the treatment may have been in progress for several months before the nodes are noticed to be enlarging. All the superficial groups of nodes may be affected at about the same time; oftener, the cervical nodes are affected first, and most, followed by the axillary and inguinal

of Nirvanol had been ended shortly before the pilgrimage. The patient, now a physician, regards this history, in retrospect, as typical of the usual non-progressive type of hydantoin lymphadenopathy (see text).

nodes. Involvement of thoracic and abdominal nodes has been observed in radiographs and at laparotomy respectively. Laparotomy may show the spleen to be moderately enlarged also, although the extent of the enlargement is very seldom such that the organ can be felt through the abdominal wall.

Histology of Hydantoin Lymphadenopathy.[784–786]— Four grades of hydantoin lymphadenopathy have been recognized.[787] In the *first grade*—much the commonest—there is a pleomorphic hyperplasia of the pulp of the nodes, but with maintenance of normal structural relations. The follicles persist, although they are often small and lack germinal centres. The cells predominantly involved in the hyperplasia are variously said to be immunoblasts, reticulum cells or histiocytes; in addition, untransformed lymphocytes, plasma cells and plasma cell precursors, eosinophils and neutrophils participate in varying proportions. Some of the large mononuclear cells are hyperchromatic and some contain two or more large nucleoli. Binucleate or multinucleate cells may be present (Figs 9.149 and 9.150). There may be many cells in mitosis. Usually there is no necrosis. The hyperplastic cells seldom encroach on the capsule or trabeculae. Complete reversion to normal follows withdrawal of the drug: resumption of treatment is likely to result in recurrence of the lymphadenopathy, which may present the same histological characteristics as before or those of a severer grade.

In the *second grade*, which in general corresponds to the picture seen in immunoblastic lymphadenopathy (see page 703),[788] the pleomorphic hyperplasia is more extensive, replacing the normal structure of the node more or less completely and infiltrating the substance of the trabeculae and capsule. In some cases there are conspicuous accumulations of eosinophils. The lymphoid tissue of the node may be virtually completely obliterated. There may be foci of necrosis: these may be small and few, or numerous, or—through their confluence—they may occupy much of the affected node. The smaller foci may be related to dilated blood capillaries that contain thrombus, but oftener there is no evident vascular lesion. More rarely, there is a thrombosing arteritis with consequent focal infarction of the nodes. Haemorrhage is seen in some of the necrotic foci. When the drug is withdrawn there is complete clinical regression of the lymphadenopathy. Lack of histological observations makes it impossible to confirm a return to normal structure; the only specimen that I have seen, apparently obtained 18 months after stopping hydantoin therapy, showed

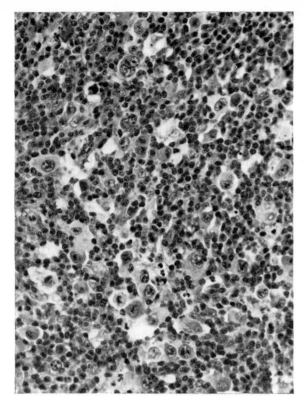

Fig. 9.149. Hydantoin lymphadenopathy. Striking proliferation of large mononuclear cells in a lymph node from a young adult under treatment with phenytoin sodium (sodium diphenylhydantoin) for epilepsy. The field includes cells with a hyperchromatic nucleus, with two nuclei, and with two or more large nucleoli. There are some in mitosis. The identity of the cells involved in this reaction to hydantoin drugs is controversial. Whatever their identity ('immunoblasts', reticulum cells or histiocytes), their atypicality makes it easy to take such a picture for that of Hodgkin's disease. In the case illustrated the condition subsided completely when the hydantoin was replaced by phenobarbitone, and there has been no further lymphadenopathy during the period of 12 years since then. It may be noted that barbiturates occasionally cause the same type of lymphadenopathy, and that prescribing a barbiturate in place of a hydantoin will not necessarily lead to regression of the changes in the nodes. See also Figs 9.150, 9.151, 9.152A and 9.152B. *Haematoxylin–eosin.* × 275.

no abnormality except considerable fibrous scarring of the node, probably consequent on necrosis.

The *third grade* comprises those cases that conform to the criteria of the second grade with the important exception that, having seemed to regress following permanent cessation of treatment with hydantoins, lymph node enlargement returns, but with the histological characteristics and clinical behaviour of a true malignant lymphoma.[787] These

cases are very rare. The tumour seems usually to be undifferentiated and rapidly progressive.

The *fourth grade,* intermediate in frequency between the second and third grades, comprises those cases in which the initial biopsy examination shows the lymphadenopathy to have the histological characteristics of an unequivocal malignant lymphoma. Most frequently the picture is that of the classic form of Hodgkin's disease (Hodgkin's disease of mixed cellularity);[789] sometimes the tumour is a lymphocytic lymphoma,[789] a 'histiocytic' ('immunoblastic') lymphoma[787] or a follicular lymphoma.[790] The clinical behaviour is that of a lymphoma.

Terminology.—The second of the two grades just described has been referred to as hydantoin pseudolymphoma and the third as hydantoin pseudo-pseudolymphoma. As these terms have been applied in different senses by different authors their further use can cause only confusion.

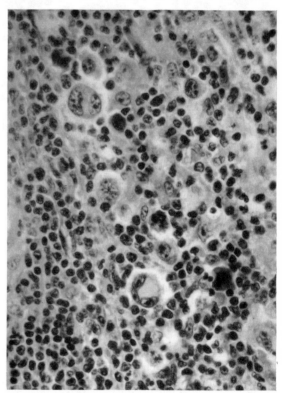

Fig. 9.150. Another example of hydantoin lymphadenopathy —in this case a complication of the treatment of epilepsy with phenytoin sodium and methoin (mephenytoin) simultaneously. As in the case illustrated in Fig. 9.149, the condition subsided when administration of the hydantoin drugs was stopped. The picture in the field shown could not be distinguished from that of Hodgkin's disease. *Haematoxylin–eosin.* × 400.

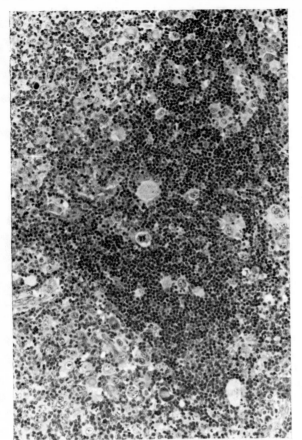

Fig. 9.152A. Simulation of Hodgkin's disease by lymphadenopathy induced by phenylbutazone. The patient was an ageing sportsman who dosed himself with phenylbutazone to minimize the pain of mild osteoarthritis. There is a striking proliferation of large pale cells, some of which are binucleate or multinucleate (see Fig. 9.152B). Multiple nucleoli are a feature of many of the cells. The condition subsided when the patient was persuaded to stop taking the drug. It did not recur during a follow-up period of 7 years. *Haematoxylin–eosin.* × 160.

Immunoblastic Lymphadenopathy

Although clinical and histological reconsideration of lymph node biopsy material seen during the last 30 years (1946–75) shows that the condition referred to here as immunoblastic lymphadenopathy has been represented among this material throughout the period under review, it is clear that it has been seen notably more frequently during the most recent decade. The condition seems to have been described first in 1972[796, 797] or 1973.[788] Since then several series of cases have been published, relating to altogether 111 patients.[788, 798–800] It is doubtful if all these cases are instances of the same disease, but there is a common clinical background to the sometimes confusingly different histological terminology, and it seems to be clear that the concept of a clinicopathological entity is well founded. Not surprisingly, several synonyms are current: they include angioimmunoblastic lymphadenopathy with dysproteinaemia,[798] chronic pluripotential immunoprolifera-

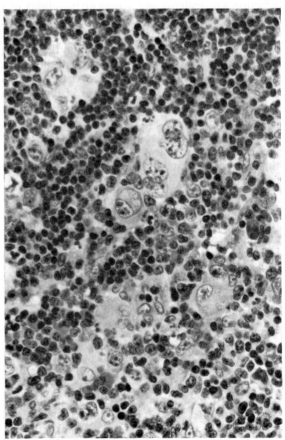

Fig. 9.152B. Higher magnification of part of field of Fig. 9.152A, to show detail of cells. *Haematoxylin–eosin.* × 400.

to which the failure of the body's defences predisposes; very occasionally it is the occurrence of lymphadenitis in such cases that attracts attention to the underlying deficiency.

Three disorders that have an immunological basis may be considered separately here, because of the obtrusive nature of the lymphadenopathy that is an essential accompaniment, or a consequence, of their presence. These are the so-called immunoblastic lymphadenopathy, primary macroglobulinaemia and the condition known variously as congenital dysphagocytosis, progressive septic granulomatosis and fatal granulomatous disease of childhood.

tive syndrome,[797] 'lymphogranulomatosis X'*[799] and immunoblastic lymphadenopathy. The last is simple and reasonably unambiguous and, provided the cytological concept of the immunoblast is accepted (see page 522), informative.

Clinical Picture

Most of the patients are in the 6th or 7th decade. There is no record of the condition under the age of 21 years. Neither race nor sex appears to be relevant. The illness usually presents as a rapidly developing, febrile lymphadenopathy, sometimes with enlargement of the spleen and liver, and often with various skin rashes. The cervical nodes are commonly those most markedly affected and they may be massively enlarged; in most cases there is involvement of the lymph nodes elsewhere as well. Some cases present with abdominal pain, the result of involvement of nodes in the mesentery, the initial picture thus resembling that in other types of acute mesenteric lymphadenitis (see page 574). Some degree of anaemia is frequent; the anaemia may be haemolytic, with a positive direct Coombs test. Leucocytosis or leucopenia, lymphopenia, eosinophilia and thrombocytopenia are often found. There is almost always an increase in the amount of immunoglobulins of any or all classes (polyclonal hyperglobulinaemia), most frequently involving class G (IgG) and class M (IgM).

Course and Prognosis.—The mortality in the reported series has ranged from 44 to 80 per cent. The relatively short period of follow-up in many cases before they were collated for publication suggests that the mortality is likely to be nearer the upper limit of this range, for death may occur within a period that has ranged from 1 month to several years. Remissions may occur, the disease then reappearing after a very variable interval: they are commonly a result of radiotherapy or treatment with cytotoxic drugs, prescribed in the belief that the

---

* The authors who originally used the term '*Lymphogranulomatosis X*' did not include it in the English summary that accompanied their German text but translated it by 'immunoblastic adenopathy'. Ignoring this, some English-speaking authorities, including clinicians, have already shown a tendency to prefer the trendy-seeming 'lymphogranulomatosis X', and then sometimes to misinterpret it as indicating that the condition is a form of 'histiocytosis X' (see page 858) or a manifestation of Hodgkin's disease (because they know that German-speaking colleagues may refer to the latter as 'lymphogranuloma'—see footnote [*] on page 635.

disease is lymphomatous; spontaneous remissions also occur.

Death is usually from infection, which is liable to progress rapidly because of the immunodeficiency that is a part of the syndrome. The hazard of infection is greatly increased by treatment with cytotoxic drugs and similar agents prescribed following histological misinterpretation of the lymphadenopathy as lymphomatous. There is some evidence that symptomatic treatment alone, including treatment for any infective complications, may be less dangerous than more active therapy, because of the risk of further lowering resistance by giving large doses of immunosuppressant or corticosteroid drugs.

In exceptional cases death has resulted from the development of some variety of lymphoma as a frankly sarcomatous transformation in lymph nodes involved in the immunoblastic lymphadenopathy.[788, 800a]

Histology

The most immediately striking feature of the histological picture is that the normal structure of the nodes is completely, or in large part, obliterated by pleomorphic cellular tissue in which immunoblasts preponderate (Fig. 9.153). The cellular tissue extends into the trabeculae and capsule, giving an impression of invasion, and encouraging interpretation of the condition as lymphomatous. Follicles are lacking. When the cells are examined critically it is evident that they lack features that support a diagnosis of malignancy. They include, in differing proportions, lymphocytes, plasma cells and plasma cell precursors, and immunoblasts (the last still being more familiar to many practising histopathologists as 'reticulum cells', although distinguishable from true reticulum cells by the pyroninophilia of the cytoplasm, which is characteristic of the immunoblast—see page 522). There are no hyperchromatic immunoblasts, and the nucleoli are small and amphiphile in haematoxylin–eosin preparations. Occasional binucleate immunoblasts, and even some with three, four or five nuclei, may be seen, but their nuclei are not abnormal and the appearances are quite distinct from those of Sternberg–Reed cells, with which they tend to be equated by the microscopist trying to find criteria to support his first impression that the condition is some form of Hodgkin's disease. Unusually large or multinucleate plasma cells may also be present, but are infrequent (Fig. 9.154); they tend to be more difficult to distinguish from Sternberg–Reed cells, largely because their nuclei are often hyperchromatic and have an irregular

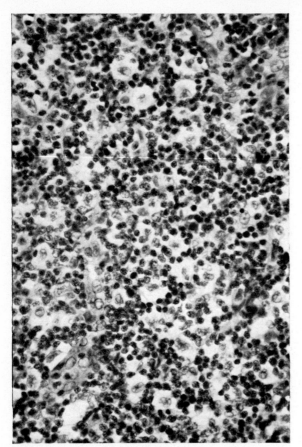

Fig. 9.153. Immunoblastic lymphadenopathy. Most of the node was replaced by tissue with the appearance shown here. The pale cells are immunoblasts and the others are small lymphocytes and plasma cells, with an occasional eosinophil and neutrophil. Numerous small blood vessels ramify among the cells (see Figs 9.155A and 9.155B), several being seen in this field; the endothelial cells of the vessels are large and conspicuous. Compare with Fig. 9.276, page 857. *Haematoxylin–eosin*. × 250.

histological picture. A further and diagnostically very important feature is the abundance of small blood vessels that ramify through the cellular tissue. These are often very difficult to make out in haematoxylin–eosin preparations but they may be seen well in preparations silvered to show reticulin (Figs 9.155A and 9.155B) and also in periodic-acid/Schiff preparations. Exceptionally, some vessels are particularly conspicuous because of hyperplasia of their endothelium (Fig. 9.155A).

In places there are deposits of amorphous eosinophile material between the cells and alongside the blood vessels; these deposits are occasionally quite extensive. The nature of the material has not been determined in detail, but it can be shown to contain polysaccharides and globulin. In one case it had a curiously spiky outline in places, giving an impression reminiscent of the homogeneous, coalescent, eosinophile, crystalline deposits that are occasionally seen in exudates that are rich in plasma cells.[793] Amyloid appears not to have been found in the lesions of immunoblastic lymphadenopathy. Foci of necrosis are sometimes present; they are usually small.

It has been said that the proliferation of immunoblasts, the arborization of many small blood vessels and the amorphous eosinophile deposits constitute a

distribution of chromatin, but their dusky and pyroninophile cytoplasm and their usually well defined cell margin are helpful pointers to the correct interpretation.

Scattered neutrophils and, usually more numerous, eosinophils are present among the immunoblasts and plasma cells. Clusters of histiocytes, usually showing epithelioid metamorphosis, are a feature of some cases; they may be difficult to see in areas of immunoblast predominance and are observed oftener in the surviving lymphoid tissue when such is still present. They do not differ essentially from the comparable epithelioid cell clusters that are a feature of so many other forms of lymphadenopathy (see page 656).

The cellular proliferation is only one aspect of the

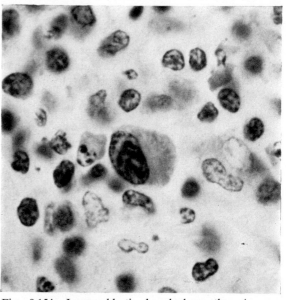

Fig. 9.154. Immunoblastic lymphadenopathy. An uncommonly large plasma cell is seen at the centre of the field. Its cytoplasm shows faint radial striation, the result of protein crystallization. The other cells include immunoblasts, plasma cells and lymphocytes. *Haematoxylin–eosin*. × 1200.

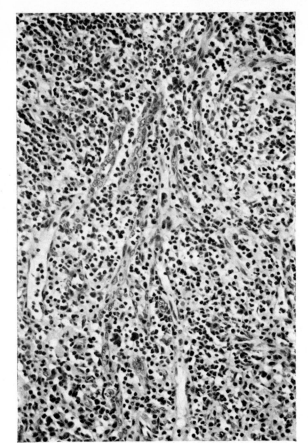

Fig. 9.155A. Immunoblastic lymphadenopathy. Many blood vessels ramify throughout the pulp of the node. The endothelial cells of some of the vessels are much increased in number and size; in other vessels they are flat and inconspicuous. Plasma cells predominate among the cellular component of this field and range considerably in size. See also Fig. 9.155B. *Haematoxylin–eosin.* × 175.

histological triad that is characteristic of this disease.[788]

Comparable changes are found at necropsy in the spleen, liver and bone marrow, and sometimes in the lymphoid tissue or interstitial tissue of other organs,[788] including the dermis.[799]

Aetiology

Immunoblastic lymphadenopathy is regarded as a non-neoplastic proliferation of B lymphocytes, with uncommonly marked transformation to immunoblasts. It is presumed to be determined by hypersensitivity. In most cases the precipitating factors are unknown. In perhaps a quarter of the recorded cases the quite abrupt onset of the illness has been related to medication and the circumstances have

been consistent with drug hypersensitivity in the allergic sense. The drugs that may have been responsible include various antibiotics (most frequently penicillin),[788, 799] oral antidiabetic agents,[799] chloroquine,[799] cyclophosphamide,[799] carbimazole,[793] dipyrone,[799] furazolidone,[793] hydantoins,* [788, 800] nitrofurantoin,[793] primidone,* [800] procaine,[799] sulphonamides[788, 800] a thiazide diuretic (buthiazide)[799] and trimethoprim.[793] Other drug-induced lymphadenopathies that may be related to immunoblastic lymphadenopathy include some of the changes that are caused by hydantoins

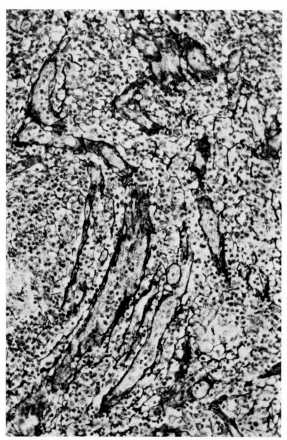

Fig. 9.155B. Immunoblastic lymphadenopathy. Field corresponding to that of Fig. 9.155A. The extent of the increased vascularity of the pulp of the lymph nodes in this condition is not always readily appreciated in haematoxylin–eosin preparations: silvering the reticulin framework shows the vessels unusually clearly. *Silver impregnation of reticulin; haematoxylin.* × 175.

* It seems probable that immunoblastic lymphadenopathy occurring in patients who are hypersensitive to hydantoins or other anticonvulsant drugs, including primidone, is not distinct from the second grade of histological reaction in cases of hydantoin lymphadenopathy (see page 698).

and other anticonvulsants (see page 697) and by the drugs noted on page 701: however, there are important distinctions, either in histological and biological character—the hydantoin-induced true lymphomas, for example—or in age incidence and prognosis.

In one instance the condition developed following a single intravenous dose of 5 mg of mustine (mechlorethamine) as treatment for Kaposi's sarcoma (see page 711): the patient had been treated successfully with this drug 2 years before, without untoward effects.[793]

Macroglobulinaemia

There is normally about a gram of macroglobulin in each litre of serum. A pathological increase may occur as a primary condition or, oftener, develops secondarily, in the course of some other disease.

Primary Macroglobulinaemia (Waldenström's Macroglobulinaemia[801]*)

The clinical and biochemical features of primary macroglobulinaemia are noted in Chapter 8 (page 498). There is a moderate degree of lymph node enlargement, which may be generalized or, occasionally, only evident in certain groups of nodes, particularly the cervical nodes. Biopsy is commonly undertaken, and often before the characteristic changes in the plasma proteins have been found: the histological picture may then be mistaken for that of a lymphocytic lymphoma. It has been said that the correct diagnosis is not to be expected of a histological examination, but a study of a large series of lymph nodes made it clear that there are appearances that justify a provisional diagnosis of this disease and indicate the need for the appropriate biochemical investigation.[801a]

Histology.[801a]—The nodes range from 0·7 to 2·0 cm in longest dimension. In haematoxylin–eosin preparations their normal structure is largely obliterated

* If the eponymous term is used it should be in the form Waldenström's macroglobulinaemia and not 'Waldenström's disease', for the reason that Waldenström was the eponym also of at least two other conditions—acute thyrotoxic encephalopathy (Waldenström, J., *Acta med. scand.*, 1945, **121**, 251) and a form of chronic active hepatitis (Sherlock, S., *Acta med. scand.*, 1966, suppl. 445, 426)—that are occasionally referred to as Waldenström's disease.

The form of macroglobulinaemia that Waldenström described is the primary disorder considered in this section. It is only to this form that the eponym is appropriate (Harrison, C. V., in *Recent Advances in Pathology*, 8th edn, edited by C. V. Harrison, page 216; London, 1966).

by a uniform accumulation of small, darkly stained cells. The identity of these cells is uncertain, but they are usually regarded as atypical lymphocytes: they are probably derived from B lymphocytes and related to plasma cells, and many pathologists describe them as plasma cells. They have more cytoplasm than is usual for lymphocytes of their size. Although the cytoplasm is not pyroninophile, the nucleus may contain aggregates of chromatin that are disposed in a manner recalling the pattern characteristic of the plasma cell. A variable, and usually very small, proportion of the cells contains an intranuclear inclusion in the form of a round or ovoid, homogeneous body, from 3 to 5 μm across, often with a halo-like clear zone about it. These bodies give a positive periodic-acid/Schiff reaction, the intensity varying from inclusion to inclusion. They are sometimes called Dutcher–Fahey inclusions[802] and they have been regarded by some pathologists as pathognomonic of primary macroglobulinaemia. However, they are occasionally to be seen in lymphocytes in other pathological conditions and in normal lymph nodes:[801a] even when numerous enough to be found readily—and this is unusual—their presence in a given lymph node biopsy specimen provides no more than an indicator of the possibility that the case is one of primary macroglobulinaemia.

Lymphoid follicles are usually lacking; when present they are very sparse, and often they can be recognized only when their site is made evident by demonstration of the reticulin pattern in sections impregnated with silver. The sinuses usually remain visible because of some degree of proliferation of the endothelial macrophages, the pallor of these cells in haematoxylin–eosin preparations contrasting with the dark background of the lymphocytic mass. In exceptional cases the sinuses may be distended with lymph that is deeply eosinophile or amphiphile in haematoxylin–eosin preparations. Plasma in blood vessels in the nodes and their vicinity stains with similar intensity.

The atypical lymphocytes that replace the normal substance of the nodes infiltrate in great numbers into the trabeculae and through the capsule to invade the tissue round the node, including its hilum. The infiltrate is so densely cellular that it may be difficult to identify the position of the original capsule except in reticulin preparations. However, the cells seldom extend far beyond the limits of the node, only exceptionally infiltrating the adjoining adipose tissue to a distance of a millimetre beyond the capsule. Such a picture is understandably liable to be misinterpreted as that of a lymphocytic lymphoma or leukaemia. Two points that weight interpretation against the usual forms of neoplastic disease are that mitotic figures are very infrequent and that there is usually a considerable proportion of mature plasma cells among the lymphocytes that make up the bulk of the infiltrate.

Another finding that has been regarded as potentially helpful in the differentiation of this disease from lymphomas and from leukaemia is the presence of mast cells, which are said to be significantly rarer in the two latter conditions than in primary macroglobulinaemia.[803] It has not been my impression that the relative numbers of mast cells in any of these diseases are sufficiently different to be diagnostically significant, but I have seen only four cases of primary macroglobulinaemia.

Necropsy.—Changes comparable to those in the lymph nodes are found *post mortem* in the spleen, liver and bone marrow, and occasionally in lymphoid tissue in other parts of the body, including the tonsils, bowel and lungs.

Course and Prognosis.—Primary macroglobulinaemia is eventually fatal. Its advance is very slow, and when the symptoms become incapacitating they may be relieved by treatment. Alkylating agents such as chlorambucil and cyclophosphamide must be given over many months in order to effect a significant reduction in the level of the macroglobulinaemia. Clinical emergencies resulting from the greatly increased viscosity of the blood include a rapidly progressive retinopathy, ischaemic encephalomyelopathy, and congestive cardiac failure: these may respond to treatment by plasmaphaeresis (removal of the patient's plasma and return of his blood cells in normal plasma). Eventually, such measures fail, and the patient may die of heart failure or neurological complications. In other cases death is due to infection, to which the frequent deficiency of immune response predisposes. Very rarely, after a course of many years, the condition becomes transformed into a rapidly progressive lymphocytic or undifferentiated lymphoma.

Generalized amyloidosis develops as a complication in some cases of primary macroglobulinaemia.[804] It may be noted in this context, therefore, that secondary macroglobulinaemia develops as a complication in some cases of amyloidosis (see below).

Nature of Primary Macroglobulinaemia.—Primary macroglobulinaemia is often considered to be a very slowly progressive lymphoma formed of functionally specialized, macroglobulin-elaborating cells. The alternative is to regard it as a non-neoplastic proliferation, or hyperplasia, of cells of the lymphocyte and plasma cell line that are rendered both morphologically atypical and functionally disordered: what the stimulus might be that would lead to this continuing response is speculative. For the present it seems as reasonable to include the disease under the general heading of immunological disorders as to classify it among the lymphomas, which are considered at the end of this chapter (see page 767).

Secondary Macroglobulinaemia

Secondary macroglobulinaemia is much less rare than primary macroglobulinaemia. It is most frequently an accompaniment of a malignant lymphoma, particularly a lymphocytic lymphoma;[805] occasionally it accompanies myelomatosis,[806] chronic lymphocytic leukaemia, and—rarely—carcinoma, bronchial carcinoma particularly. It may occur in association with amyloidosis, including amyloidosis as an accompaniment of ageing (see page 43),[807] and it was found in an unusual case of medullary thyroid carcinoma in which the presence of amyloid in the stroma (a frequent finding in this tumour—see Chapter 31) was accompanied by generalized secondary amyloidosis.[807] Other conditions that have been associated with macroglobulinaemia include rheumatoid arthritis (and other connective tissue diseases, notably systemic lupus erythematosus and polyarteritis),[808] chronic hepatitis and visceral leishmaniasis (kala azar).[808] It is notable that macroglobulinaemia may be found in a variety of conditions that predispose to amyloidosis as well as in association with established amyloidosis.

The manifestations of secondary macroglobulinaemia are those of the associated disease, with the addition of the effects of increased viscosity of the blood (see opposite and page 498). The increase in viscosity is sufficient to cause symptoms only when there is a substantial rise in the level of macroglobulins in the blood; such levels are comparatively rarely reached in the secondary form of macroglobulinaemia.

Histology.—The lymph nodes are only moderately enlarged. Their structure is maintained, although there is a considerable reduction in the number and size of the follicles. The atypical lymphocytes that are so characteristic of the histological picture of primary macroglobulinaemia are not a feature (see opposite). Occasionally it is possible to find an intranuclear inclusion of the type described in the account of the primary form of macroglobulinaemia; as such inclusions may be seen sometimes in normal nodes and in other pathological conditions their presence is of limited significance. There is no striking cellular infiltration of the trabeculae and capsule. Plasma cells are numerous throughout the pulp (Figs 9.156A and 9.156B).

'Heavy Chain' Diseases

Because of their relation to lymphomas, the so-called 'heavy chain' diseases—diseases in which immunoglobulins lacking light chains are present

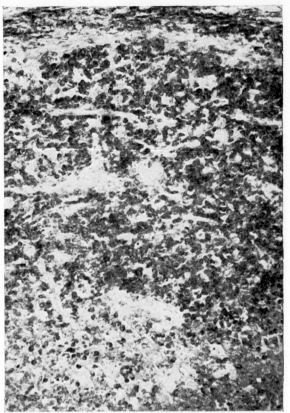

Fig. 9.156B. Same specimen as Fig. 9.156A, and corresponding field. The plasma cells in this preparation appear darker than the lymphocytes because of the pyroninophilia of the ribonucleic acid in their cytoplasm. *Unna–Pappenheim.* × 160.

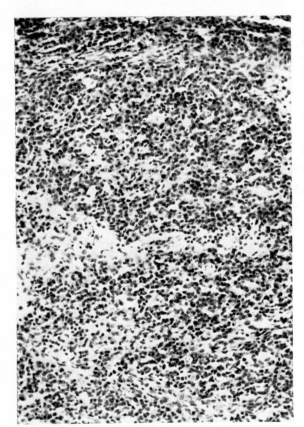

Fig. 9.156A. Lymph node in a case of secondary macroglobulinaemia. There is an exceptionally dense accumulation of plasma cells in the pulp just deep to the capsule of the node (above). The plasma cells appear to occupy the subcapsular sinus as well as the adjoining area of the cortex. This area merges, below, into a zone where lymphocytes predominate. The distinction between these zones is seen better in the Unna–Pappenheim preparation (Fig. 9.156B). The patient had longstanding rheumatoid arthritis. She died 3 years after this specimen was obtained, having subsequently developed amyloidosis (of which there was no evidence at the time of the lymph node biopsy). *Haematoxylin–eosin.* × 160.

in the serum—are considered in the section on lymphomas later in this chapter (see page 847).

Fatal Granulomatous Disease of Childhood Due to Deficiency of Bactericidal Activity of Neutrophils[809, 810]

This disease, which was described first in 1957,[811, 812] is characterized by a peculiar inborn functional deficiency of the neutrophile polymorphonuclear leucocytes. Although phagocytosis proceeds normally, the cells fail to destroy micro-organisms at a normal rate.[813] Predisposition to infection, from infancy onward, eventually proves fatal. The infections, which involve the skin, lymph nodes, lungs and other parts, are often caused by *Staphylococcus aureus* but also with notable frequency by organisms that ordinarily are of relatively low pathogenicity, such as klebsiellae, *Enterobacter* species, *Serratia marcescens*, enterococci, 'viridans' streptococci and species of salmonella and proteus. In the terminal stages, overwhelming pneumonic and septicaemic infections are frequent and may be caused by *Nocardia asteroides* or species of aspergillus and candida, as in other conditions that predispose to such 'opportunistic' infections (see page 362).

The large majority of the patients have been boys, and until the recognition of exceptional instances in girls[814] the condition was thought to be a sex-linked anomaly. In the affected child, failure to kill the ingested bacteria is a characteristic of all the neutrophils. In contrast, the child's mother possesses different clones of neutrophils, some with normal activity and some with the defect; the former suffice to compensate fully for the incapacity of the latter.[815-817]

There is no evident deficiency of the activities of reticuloendothelial cells. In-vitro studies show that bacteria that thrive and proliferate in the cytoplasm of neutrophils from affected children do not multiply in macrophages from the same children but quickly shrink and begin to undergo lysis;[817] similarly, they are digested normally after phagocytosis by neutrophils from normal people.[818] The disease is very frequently accompanied by hyperglobulinaemia, the gammaglobulins in particular being raised: the explanation is unknown. There is no impairment of antibody formation and both humoral and cell-mediated immunity remain normal.[819]

Nomenclature

Many names are in use and none of them describes the disease unambiguously, succinctly or accurately. Berendes–Bridges–Good disease, after the authors who described it first,[811] and Landing–Shirkey disease,* in recognition of an independent observation published later in the same year,[812] have the disadvantages of eponymous nomenclature. The most frequently used terms are *'fatal granulomatous disease of childhood'*[813] and *'chronic granulomatous disease of childhood'*,[820] both of which are also applicable to cases of the wide variety of other granulomatous diseases that may occur in childhood. 'Progressive septic granulomatosis'[819] is also applicable to various other diseases. 'Congenital dysphagocytosis' has also been suggested,[815] but is

* Confusion between this disorder and the quite different condition known as ceroid storage disease (see page 767) resulted from the fact that the former—as indicated by Landing and Shirkey in the title of their paper (reference 812, page 877)—is associated with the presence of a yellow-brown pigment in macrophages in lymph nodes and elsewhere (see text). Because of this confusion, ceroid storage disease sometimes is known, incorrectly, as Landing–Oppenheimer disease.

K

unsuitable because the defect does not relate to phagocytosis but to the subsequent failure to kill the ingested bacteria.

Job's Disease.—Psychological disturbances affect a small proportion of patients with this leucocytic anomaly. Self-consciousness about the chronic, distressingly unsightly, perpetually discharging and malodorous, recurrent septic lesions of the skin may cause the patient—like Job smitten by Satan 'with sore boils from the sole of his foot unto his crown' (Bible, *Job* ii. 7)—to have feelings of guilt and to believe herself (the patient who develops this complication is usually a girl) despised and rejected by family and friends. The syndrome is one of several in the course of dermatological history that have been described as Job's disease or Job's syndrome.[821, 822]

'Lazy Leucocyte' Syndrome.[823]—The so-called 'lazy leucocyte' syndrome is quite distinct from the syndrome resulting from deficient bactericidal activity. It is characterized by persistent low fever and recurring infection of the mouth, throat and ears, with severe leucopenia. Examination of the bone marrow shows no abnormality. The fault is in neutrophil chemotaxis, with the result that this reaction to inflammatory stimuli is markedly deficient. The mechanism is not understood but evidently there is a failure to mobilize the neutrophils in the bone marrow.

Histology[820]

Although the diagnosis of granulomatous disease due to deficiency of the bactericidal activity of neutrophils can usually be suggested on the basis of the history and clinical picture, lymph node biopsy is quite commonly undertaken as a diagnostic procedure when the cause of the lymphadenitis is not immediately suspected. Unless the microscopist is familiar with the histological changes he may misinterpret the findings as simply indicative of a granulomatous lymphadenitis (Fig. 9.157): it may then be some time before the cause of this lesion is recognized. The clue to the diagnosis is the association of a necrotizing tuberculoid granuloma with the presence of pigmented macrophages. Neither alone is diagnostically helpful, and even their association is not pathognomonic, as it may occur in other circumstances: but in the presence of the typical clinical history the histological findings complete a clinicopathological triad that should indicate the diagnosis, which may be confirmed by relatively

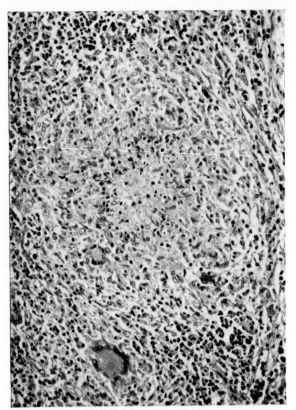

Fig. 9.157. Fatal granulomatous disease of childhood due to deficiency of bactericidal activity of neutrophils. Cervical lymph node biopsy showing a necrotizing tuberculoid granuloma, indistinguishable from tuberculosis and initially so diagnosed. Cultures of the same specimen yielded a heavy pure growth of a 'viridans' streptococcus that was also grown from the exudate from the surface of a small burn over the shoulder on the same side. Cultures for mycobacteria gave no growth. See also Fig. 9.158. *Haematoxylin–eosin.* × 160.

simple in-vitro tests of the ability of the neutrophils to inactivate bacteria.[813]

Pigmented Macrophages.—Pigmented macrophages are usually numerous in the lymph nodes. They are found both in the pulp and in the sinuses; in the latter they are often collected into small clusters. In general they are not particularly related to the granulomas, and indeed they may be completely absent from the vicinity of the latter. The pigment is yellow-brown in unstained sections and in haematoxylin–eosin preparations. In most of the cells it appears as a diffuse coloration of the entire cytoplasm, without the presence of granules. Other cells contain abundant, coarse particles of dark brown pigment, varying considerably in size. The diffusely coloured cells are liable to be overlooked in sections

stained with both haematoxylin and eosin; it can be very helpful to look at sections stained with haematoxylin alone. The pigment is Sudanophile, in paraffin wax sections as well as in frozen sections of fresh tissue. It gives a positive periodic-acid/Schiff reaction and it is variably acid-fast. It does not contain iron. In Giemsa preparations the cytoplasm of the diffusely pigmented cells is coloured a distinctive blue or greenish blue, an observation that led to comparable cells being described in another context as '*sea-blue histiocytes*' (see *Ceroid Storage Disease*, page 767). This peculiar staining is seen most strikingly in films or impression preparations of the cut surface of freshly excised, unfixed nodes. The particulate pigment has the same staining reactions as the diffusely pigmented cytoplasm of the macrophages, but usually gives an intenser result. With Romanowsky stains, particularly Giemsa's solution applied to paraffin wax sections, the particles are a greener blue than the 'sea blue' of the diffusely pigmented cells.

Although the pigmentation is so remarkable, its nature is still uncertain. The usual suggestions are that it is a lipochrome[812] or a ceroid. I have seen two cases in which 'Hamazaki–Wesenberg bodies' (see page 562) were present in considerable numbers in addition to the pigmented cells just described; the significance of the observation is questionable—the association could have been a chance one. Examination of the 'pigmented lipid histiocytes' with the electron microscope has shown no evidence that helps to determine their nature;[824] in particular, nothing has been found to suggest that the particulate pigment has a bacterial origin (such as has been found in the case of the periodic-acid/Schiff positive bodies in the cytoplasm of the macrophages in the bowel in Whipple's disease—see page 1084).

Tuberculoid Granulomas.—The tuberculoid granulomatous lesions of this disease closely resemble caseating tuberculous foci: indeed, they are distinguishable from tuberculosis only by the failure to demonstrate mycobacteria. There may be any stage in their formation from small epithelioid cell clusters through classic tubercles to extensive and confluent caseating masses (Fig. 9.157). In some instances it is possible to demonstrate bacteria (other than mycobacteria) in them, and it is possible to surmise that in this disease organisms that ordinarily provoke a tissue reaction in which neutrophils are conspicuous may, when the latter fail to control the infection, lead to a histiocytic response. It is notable that in some cases there is conspicuous phagocytosis of neutrophils by macrophages in the sinuses of the lymph nodes (Fig. 9.158) and sometimes also by those in the spleen and liver.

Plasma cells are usually numerous throughout those parts of the nodes that have not been destroyed by the granulomatous lesions.

Changes in Other Organs.—The pigmented macrophages are found in lymphoid tissue elsewhere in the body, most notably in the spleen. They may also be seen in the dermis, where they occur particularly at sites of active or healed septic dermatitis. They are often conspicuous in the portal tracts in the liver; the Kupffer cells are also pigmented and sometimes greatly swollen through accumulation in their cytoplasm of dark brown pigment granules. Small tuberculoid granulomas, with or without caseation, are often seen in the spleen; they are seldom found in the liver.

Storage Diseases

The lymph nodes are frequently enlarged in the storage diseases (lipidoses and comparable conditions). Sometimes, lymph node biopsy provides the

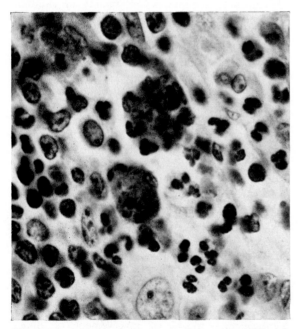

Fig. 9.158. 'Fatal granulomatous disease of childhood'. Another case. Phagocytosis of neutrophils by macrophages in a trabecular sinus of a cervical lymph node that elsewhere contained necrotizing tuberculoid granulomas similar to that illustrated in Fig. 9.157. The presence of neutrophils in macrophages, although not pathognomonic (it may be seen in some cases of simple sinus histiocytosis—see page 561), was a helpful clue to the correct diagnosis. *Haematoxylin–eosin.* × 1000.

first diagnostic evidence of the presence of the disease. These conditions are considered on page 757.

Tumours

Benign Tumours and Tumour-Like Conditions

Benign primary tumours of lymph nodes are so rare that they may be regarded as curiosities, with the exception only of the hamartomas that consist essentially of lymphoid tissue. The condition that has been referred to in this chapter as the *giant lymphoid hamartoma* ('angiofollicular lymph node hyperplasia') is described on page 544.

Occasionally, small encapsulate foci of lymphoid tissue are seen within otherwise normal lymph nodes (Fig. 9.159): these are thought to be hamartomatous, and may be analogous to the so-called 'intrasplenic spleniculi' (see page 739).

Apart from lymphoid hamartomas, the only benign tumour of a lymph node that I have seen was an encapsulate, moderately cellular, hyalinizing *fibroma*, 2 cm in its longest axis, and enclosed within the attenuated capsule of the node. The atrophic remains of the substance of the node were stretched over one aspect of the tumour, which was an incidental finding during a partial thyroidectomy for toxic goitre. In contrast, a macroscopically similar lesion in an axillary node removed 21 years after radical mastectomy for scirrhous carcinoma proved to contain a few very small islets of surviving carcinoma cells buried in dense, hyaline fibrous tissue; the carcinoma was discovered only when the specimen was sectioned at several deeper levels following the initial histological examination.

Malignant Primary Tumours

Lymphomas

The lymphomas are considered in a separate section of this chapter (see page 757).

Other Sarcomas

Apart from Kaposi's sarcoma (see below), sarcomas other than lymphomas occur exceptionally rarely in lymph nodes and need no particular mention.

Kaposi's Sarcoma [824a]*

Although first recognized among central European people, Kaposi's sarcoma has proved to be particularly prevalent among Africans. In Uganda, for

* The condition that Kaposi described as idiopathic multiple pigment sarcoma of the skin (Kaposi, *Arch. Derm. Syph.* [*Prag*], 1872, **4**, 265) has been given many other

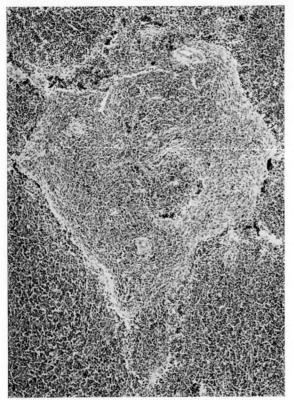

Fig. 9.159. This small, encapsulate focus of lymphoid tissue was an incidental finding in an inferior deep cervical lymph node excised in the course of a surgical search for a parathyroid adenoma in a case of hyperparathyroidism. It contains several conspicuous small blood vessels, some cut across and some cut lengthwise. Some of the latter enter a follicle-like structure, and present a picture reminiscent of that of the 'giant lymphoid hamartoma' (see Figs 9.20 to 9.22, pages 545 and 546). The condition is probably hamartomatous (see also Fig. 9.170, page 739). *Haematoxylin–eosin.* × 70.

---

names, ranging from multicentric cutaneous and visceral angiosarcoma to dysimmunogenic dysangioblastic preparalymphomatous fusicellular mesenchymoma. As its histogenesis is still unknown, although its sarcomatous nature is generally accepted, and as its original description is correctly attributed to Kaposi, Kaposi's sarcoma is currently the name of choice. None of the 15 other entries under this eponym in Jablonski's *Dictionary* (Jablonski, S., *Illustrated Dictionary of Eponymic Syndromes and Diseases and Their Synonyms*, pages 167–169; Philadelphia, London and Toronto, 1969) relates to any other neoplastic disease ('Kaposi–Spiegler sarcomatosis' is a synonym of 'Spiegler–Fendt sarcoid', which is a variety of lymphocytic granuloma and unrelated to sarcoidosis—see Chapter 39). It may be noted that xeroderma pigmentosum (see Chapter 39) is also one of 'Kaposi's diseases' (Kaposi, M., *Med. Jb.*, 1882, 619): it is a precancerous condition, but unlikely to be confused with Kaposi's sarcoma.

The identity of Kaposi Mór, Moritz Kaposi and Moritz Kohn is mentioned in a footnote in Chapter 39.

instance, it accounts for about 5 per cent of all malignant tumours.[824b] Outside Africa it has attracted more attention in North America than in Europe and Asia, and European doctors tend to think of it as an exotic disease: in fact, the disease is probably of worldwide distribution, although nowhere known to be so frequent as in Africa.

Involvement of lymph nodes by Kaposi's sarcoma requires more than cursory consideration in view of the importance and frequency of this disease, particularly in parts of Africa. Lymph nodes are affected more commonly than was recognized formerly, and their involvement may be the presenting manifestation.

It was long thought that Kaposi's sarcoma is essentially a cutaneous disease (see Chapter 39). Visceral lesions are now known to be present frequently, although seldom apparent clinically. Occasionally, a visceral lesion is the presenting manifestation. Lymph nodes are among the organs liable to be involved. There is a comparatively rare, rapidly progressive, form of the disease in which involvement of lymph nodes is the predominant feature:[824c] this unusually malignant manifestation of Kaposi's sarcoma occurs mainly in children, particularly girls, but sometimes in young adults,[824d] and may be manifested by generalized lymph node enlargement without accompanying lesions of the skin.[824e] In general, involvement of lymph nodes is found in about a third of adult African patients with the disease;[824b] occasionally it is their presenting symptom.[824b]

Among over 600 histologically confirmed cases of Kaposi's sarcoma in Uganda, little more than 5 per cent of the patients were female. The disease progressed more rapidly in women and presented earlier (about the middle of the fourth decade) than in men (about the end of the fifth decade).[824e]

In a series of 34 necropsies on Ugandan patients who died with the disease there were 18 instances of generalized lymph node involvement and 10 of involvement confined to nodes draining 'aggressive' local lesions.[824e] In contrast, a review of 47 published accounts of the post-mortem findings in white patients, mainly in North America, showed that there were three instances of generalized lymph node involvement and 18 of involvement of nodes draining local lesions.[824e] It seems that the disease in Uganda, or among Ugandans, is likelier to give rise to generalized involvement of lymph nodes; the significance of this impression remains to be assessed.

Histology of the Lymph Nodes.—There may be simple inflammatory changes in the superficial lymph nodes, the consequence of infection of the tumours in the skin. When the tumour itself is present in the nodes the histological picture (Fig. 9.160) is the classic complex of spindle-shaped cells and more or less well-formed vascular tissue (see Chapter 39).[824f] Pathologists accustomed to seeing biopsy specimens from cases of Kaposi's sarcoma have little difficulty in recognizing the disease when it is present in lymph nodes, but the characteristic picture may be perplexing to those whose experience has not previously brought them in contact with this problem. The specific changes may appear to develop first in the sinuses or, less often, in follicles.[824f] There may be heavy deposits of haemosiderin in the vicinity of the lesions, and haemorrhage may be a conspicuous feature. In a series of six cases seen in Britain in which lymph node involvement accompanied more or less extensive cutaneous lesions, the

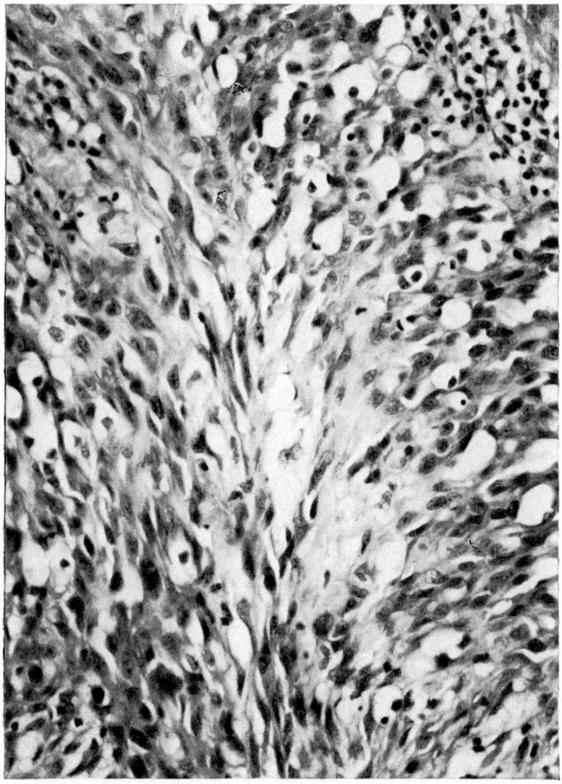

Fig. 9.160. Kaposi's sarcoma in an axillary lymph node. The patient was a Zulu with extensive involvement of the skin. The photograph shows the classic picture of spindle-shaped cells and vacuolate cells, the latter in places merging to form clefts lined by flat cells and containing red blood cells. The field is from the subcapsular region of the node: the sinus is obliterated by tumour tissue, which has replaced the adjoining lymphoid tissue, only a trace of which remains evident (top, right). *Haematoxylin–eosin.* × 220.

impression given by the histological picture in the nodes was more in keeping with metastatic invasion, with characteristic tumour tissue in lymphatics entering the nodes and in the sinuses, particularly the capsular sinus, but it would not be possible to exclude development of the disease *in situ.*[*807]

Lymphomatous and Lymphoma-Like Transformation in Lymph Nodes.—On the basis of a critical review, Kaposi's sarcoma is said to be associated with lymphoma—particularly 'follicular lymphosarcoma' and Hodgkin's disease—significantly oftener than would be accounted for by chance.[824g] It may precede or follow the first manifestations of the lymphoma. The association seems to be much rarer in African patients than in white patients, a difference that has led to the suggestion that the disease in Africa may not be identical with that elsewhere, particularly in North America: in spite of this striking and unexplained discrepancy, most observers regard the disease as a single entity.[824g]

In a few cases of Kaposi's sarcoma a peculiar lymphoma-like change has been noted in the lymph nodes.[824h] This is characterized by follicular hyperplasia with the formation of large germinal centres and a very notable increase in the number of small blood vessels in and between the follicles. There is a dense accumulation of plasma cells in some or all of the nodes that show this pattern. Enlargement of the spleen and liver and a polyclonal hypergammaglobulinaemia are other characteristics. The picture has been mistaken for a follicular lymphoma and for myeloma and immunoblastic lymphadenopathy (see page 703): the last of these being characterized by loss of the architecture of the nodes, it should not be confused with the lymphoma-like lymphadenopathy of Kaposi's sarcoma, in which the follicular pattern is well preserved. The diagnostic distinction presents a practical problem as Kaposi's sarcoma has on occasion been associated with a follicular lymphoma,[824g] myelomatosis[824i] and immunoblastic lymphadenopathy.[824j]

Oedema.—A limb affected by Kaposi's sarcoma is commonly oedematous. This has been explained as a consequence of obstruction to the flow of lymph through regional nodes involved in the disease.[824k] However, in most cases there is no dilatation of the lymphatic vessels of the oedematous part, as would be present if the condition were an obstructive

* Two of these six patients were Africans (a Yoruba and a Zulu), two were Asians (one from Guyana and one from Uganda) and two were Europeans (one from Iceland and one from Rhodesia). All were middle-aged men.

lymphoedema:[824f] the cause of the oedema remains unknown.

Nature of Kaposi's Sarcoma.—While it is clear that Kaposi's sarcoma is a malignant neoplastic disease, there is no certainty about the identity or origin of the spindle-shaped cells that are its most conspicuous element. Because of the associated vasoformative activity, ranging from the development of tissue that resembles a mature capillary haemangioma to ill-formed, immature vessels and clefts lined by flat or spindle-shaped cells, it has been assumed that the latter are angioblastic cells.

The occasional presence of hyperglobulinaemia,[824h] the occasional association with lymphomas (see above), and the occasional development of lymphoma-like follicular hyperplasia with a proliferation of small blood vessels and the presence of plasma cells and sometimes of 'immunoblasts'— a picture reminiscent of immunoblastic lymphadenopathy (see page 703)—suggest the possibility of a relation to certain diseases that are now recognized to have their origin in disturbances of immunological responses.[824m] A case is on record of multiple well-differentiated haemangiomas of the skin and viscera, including lymph nodes, with the development of hypergammaglobulinaemia and myelomatosis, and a slowly progressive course of 13 years to death:[824n] the condition was seen as possibly a form of Kaposi's sarcoma of relatively low malignancy, associated with an immunological disturbance.

Several recent reviews of Kaposi's sarcoma as it is seen in Africa have remarked on points of similarity to Burkitt's lymphoma (see page 824).[824m, 824p] Its particular frequency in certain regions of Africa, which overlap but do not exactly coincide with the regions of greatest frequency of Burkitt's lymphoma, the usually long course of the disease, its tendency to recur in previously unaffected sites after treatment, and the rapider progress and poor prognosis when there is lymph node involvement are features that Kaposi's sarcoma shares with Burkitt's lymphoma. Such common features suggest that there may be other, more fundamental discoveries to make from further study of these remarkable diseases.

The significance of the finding of a virus or viruses of the herpesvirus group in tissue cultures from Kaposi's sarcoma has not yet been assessed.[824q]

Leukaemia

The leukaemias are considered in Chapter 8 (pages 478 to 488).

Secondary Tumours

Involvement of the lymph nodes by extension of cancer arising in other organs or tissues is referred to on page 863 and in the accounts of the various primary tumours in the appropriate chapters. The first lymph nodes to be observed clinically to be

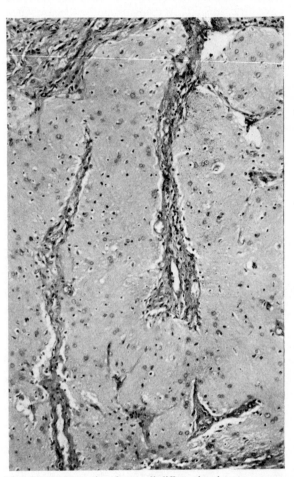

Fig. 9.161. Deposit of a well-differentiated astrocytoma replacing the substance of an inferior deep cervical lymph node. The patient was a young woman. The primary growth was in an otherwise typical 'dermoid cyst' (teratoma) of an ovary. The glioma had broken through the capsule of the teratoma, giving rise to multiple small deposits on the lining of the abdominal cavity, with extension through the lymphatics to the regional lymph nodes. The enlargement of the abdomen was thought to be a manifestation of the patient's obesity until the involved cervical node was found and excised. The histological appearances indicate that the glioma had been growing slowly in the node for a considerable time. This is a remarkable example of metastasis of a tumour that, arising in its usual site (central nervous system), does not gain access to lymphatic vessels. It is also an illustration of a secondary deposit, in a lymph node remote from the site of the primary growth, as the presenting manifestation of the disease. See also Fig. 9.282, page 864. *Haematoxylin–eosin.* × 100.

involved in cases of visceral cancer may be quite remote from the site of the primary growth (Fig. 9.161; and see Figs 9.282 and 9.283 on page 864). The classic instance of this is the presentation of a gastric or other abdominal carcinoma with enlargement of one or more of the inferior deep cervical nodes, usually on the left.[825] An involved node in this situation is variously known as a signal or sentinel node,* Virchow's node[826] and Troisier's node.[827, 828] The predilection for the left side is explicable by the anatomical relation between the nodes and the terminal part of the thoracic duct, which opens into the venous system at or near the confluence of the left internal jugular and subclavian veins.[828] Proven involvement of a node or nodes in this site is prognostically important and contraindicates radical surgical treatment of the primary growth. An involved node often can be found by careful deep palpation as a small, hard mass long before it becomes large enough to be immediately obvious on palpation or, later still, to cause a visible fullness in the root of the neck. Excision of the node or, less reliable, needle biopsy can be diagnostically invaluable in these cases; *both procedures are liable to be complicated by injury to the thoracic duct*, with the development of a lymph fistula that greatly adds to the patient's distress and accelerates the deterioration in his general condition.

As secondary tumour deposits in lymph nodes almost always are the outcome of carriage of cancer cells through the lymphatics, the earliest deposits are usually seen in the subcapsular lymph sinus, and it is here that the microscopist concentrates his search for evidence of beginning involvement of the nodes when examining specimens removed in the course of surgical treatment of cancer. However, obstruction of the efferent lymphatics may result in reversal of the lymph flow: the initial seeding of tumour cells may then be in the sinuses adjacent to the hilum. The malignant cells multiply and spread widely in the sinuses of an affected lymph node; in addition, they invade the adjacent medulla, and eventually a large part or the whole of the lymphoid tissue is replaced by the tumour, and the node may be enlarged to several times its normal size.

The occurrence of *sinus histiocytosis* in lymph nodes draining the site of a primary malignant tumour is mentioned on page 561. The *tuberculoid lymphadenitis* that is a rarer accompaniment of a

carcinoma or other primary tumour in the drainage area of the affected nodes is discussed on page 682.

LYMPH NODE BIOPSY

It has been said that the pathology of the lymphoreticular system is the pathology of lymph nodes. This aphorism, like so many of its kind, is no more than a half-truth, yet it makes a valid and important point. Lymphadenopathy occurs in such a large proportion of cases of these diseases that lymph nodes are of paramount diagnostic importance, and lymph node biopsy is in many cases the only certain means to accurate and complete diagnosis. Histological interpretation of lymph nodes can be difficult, largely because of the variety and intimate topographical relations of the component cells of the lymphoreticular system, their capacity to differentiate along various lines, and the consequent, often bewildering, variety of cytological and histological pictures that can be present under pathological conditions. Interpretation of pathological changes in the lymphoreticular system is, perhaps, oftener dependent on subjective impressions and inclination than is the case with diseases of other systems. No group of biopsy specimens in the whole field of clinical microscopy presents a greater problem than 'difficult' lymph nodes. Even under ideal conditions it may be impossible to distinguish between, for example, hyperplastic or inflammatory reactions and early malignant disease.

Technical Difficulties

Several avoidable factors add to the difficulty of histological diagnosis. These include the all too prevalent failure to provide adequate or even accurate clinical information about the patient, lack of care in choosing the site for biopsy, and damage to the specimen by surgical carelessness, improper fixation, or mishandling in the laboratory.

Choice of Node.—In cases of generalized lymphadenopathy, or when there is a choice of sites from which to take the specimen, it is desirable that inguinal nodes and cervical nodes (especially the upper cervical groups) should be avoided, as they are likely to show chronic inflammatory changes that modify the features of any associated disease and may confuse the interpretation. At operation it is essential to choose carefully the node that is to be removed: it is a frustrating experience, regrettably familiar to most histologists, to be sent a lymph node

---

* The enlarged lymph nodes draining the site of a syphilitic chancre have also been known as 'sentinel nodes' (see page 612).

half a centimetre in diameter when clinical examination has clearly shown the presence of nodes several times this size in the same region. This type of mistake not infrequently results from failure to brief the surgeon, who is simply told that a node is needed for biopsy; satisfactory lymph node specimens are relatively seldom obtained unless the surgeon and physician have discussed the individual case.

Surgical Artefacts.—The surgeon must know that crushing the specimen or traction on it during removal can so disrupt the tissues as to make accurate microscopical interpretation impossible, and may produce artefacts that can be mistaken for pathological conditions. He should also understand the need for prompt fixation or immediate delivery of the unfixed specimen to the laboratory. If he operates without immediate access to a laboratory and must therefore send the specimen elsewhere for examination, he should be familiar with the simple technique of initial fixation and cutting so that there is as little deterioration as possible in the tissues of the node (see below).

It is generally recognized that there is no satisfactory alternative to open biopsy and excision of the node intact within its capsule. Histological interpretation is properly based on examination of the whole extent of the node, so that changes in all parts and components may be seen in the contexture of their topographical relations. *Needle biopsy has no place in the diagnosis of lymphadenopathies*: for every occasion on which it clearly demonstrates the presence of sclerosing Hodgkin's disease or scirrhous carcinoma there are many in which it fails to provide material suitable for diagnosis, usually because the cylinder of tissue disintegrates, however carefully it is handled, or because the distribution, extent and full composition of the pathological changes cannot be assessed. In general, needle biopsy is practicable only in the examination of tissues with a close-knit connective tissue framework, such as that of the liver and kidneys, and of diffusely fibrosing lesions such as the exceptions mentioned.

Fixation.—It is quite exceptional for a laboratory to have such resources that it has complete control over biopsy specimens from the moment when the surgeon completes the excision. Without such control it is not possible to ensure the correct use of the particular methods of tissue fixation that are most appropriate for different classes of biopsy specimen. Personally, and notwithstanding the technical advantages of other fixatives, I believe it best that whatever fixative is found most generally suitable in the practice of a given laboratory should be the fixative used for lymph nodes.

Fixation must be begun without delay and, when possible, in such a way that its full effect may be obtained. This entails facilitation of penetration of the fluid throughout the node and at the same time care to avoid serious distortion through bulging of cut surfaces and the twisting effects of irregular shrinkage. The capsule of a lymph node is a barrier to the easy percolation of fixatives. For this reason, all but the smallest nodes should be bisected in their long axis (in the plane of the hilum, if this is identifiable) and nodes of over 0·5 to 1·0 cm in thickness should be cut in that plane into slices of appropriate thickness (0·3 to 0·4 cm, according to the size of the node). When a fresh node is bisected, the cut surface bulges: the extent to which this occurs may be reduced if the entire node is immersed in fixative for an hour before being cut.[829] When dealing with larger nodes, the halves of the bisected specimen may be fixed for a further hour to minimize the amount of warping that may follow slicing. Warping and 'dishing' of the slices makes it impossible to embed them flat in paraffin wax: marked distortion then makes it impracticable to cut sections that include the whole area of the slice.

Delay in fixation after excision may make a histological interpretation impossible because of autolysis throughout the node. Even when there is no delay, limited penetration of the fixative has the result that the tissues of the node are well preserved only to a depth of about 0·5 cm from the capsule while the central parts undergo autolysis (Fig. 9.250, page 840): this limits the proportion of the node that is usefully available for examination, and important changes—even, for instance, Hodgkin's disease—that are confined to the inadequately fixed zone may go unrecognized.

Other Histological Requirements.—From 10 to 20 per cent of the lymph node preparations that I am asked to review with colleagues are technically so poor that their inadequacy seriously limits or nullifies their diagnostic usefulness and might contribute directly to misinterpretation of the nature of the patient's disease. Diagnostic deductions are based too often nowadays on histological preparations of a standard that would have been unacceptable a generation back. It is surely perverse that laboratories that produce peerless sections, 2 μm thick, for histochemical or research purposes, and that maintain the highest standards in the preparation of material for electron microscopy, cannot make well cut, well stained, well mounted haematoxylin–eosin preparations of lymph node biopsy specimens.

It should not need to be stated that good staining of the sections is essential, yet too many pathologists try to interpret preparations that have been so leached of haematoxylin by overdifferentiation and so overstained with eosin that there is, for instance, no colour contrast between lymphocytes and epithelioid cell clusters. Sections thicker than 10 μm or so, which might not significantly hinder interpretation of a specimen of mammary tissue, may be impossible to read because of the compact cellularity and density of nuclear staining of lymphoid tissue. Lymph nodes, too, are particularly vulnerable to scratching and tearing by a defective knife edge and particularly prone to show the effects of knife chatter from faults in the tilt of the knife or from lack of rigidity of the knife or the block holder in their supports (see Fig. 9.243, page 834).[830]

Frozen Sections

The diagnosis of the nature of a chronic lymphadenopathy does not need to be made a matter of urgency. Yet sometimes a clinician, meeting a patient with lymphadenopathy for the first time, considers—say—Hodgkin's disease to be the likely diagnosis, and arranges for immediate excision of a node, which is sent to the laboratory with a request for a frozen section to be reported on at once so that a decision may be made whether to admit the patient to the wards for treatment. The pathologist soon learns that it is better for the patient, the clinician and himself that he resist the pressure to make a diagnosis on unsuitably prepared material and without time to reflect. The conventional frozen section, cut with the freezing microtome, and the section cut in the cryostat are unsuitable for the histological interpretation of lymph nodes. The former in particular is subject to artefact in consequence of the peculiar loose structure of lymph nodes, which predisposes sections to partial disintegration unless their constituents are held together (as they are when the tissue has been impregnated with paraffin wax); further, the thickness of the frozen section may completely obscure pathological changes, the mass of darkly stained lymphocytes making it impossible to see other cells clearly, and even hiding diagnostically important cells such as Sternberg–Reed cells. Necrotic foci, such as caseating tubercles, tend to collapse in frozen sections, so that a granulomatous lesion may be overlooked because the surrounding lymphoid tissue has by artefact come to overlie it. Sclerosing lesions will usually be recognized as fibrotic, but their nature is likely not to be identifiable: cellular foci that may be present within the fibrous tissue so often lose their identifying features in consequence of compression and distortion during preparation of frozen sections that it is seldom possible to decide whether they are composed of the cells of Hodgkin's disease, of a carcinoma, of a chronic inflammatory lesion, or of some other condition.

Most lymph nodes that are sent to the laboratory for immediate histological examination come from operations actually in progress, during which the surgeon needs to know—for instance—if given nodes are involved in the spread of the carcinoma that he is dealing with, or if a particular structure is one of the hyperplastic parathyroid glands that he is seeking or merely a lymph node. In such circumstances the rapid section is both appropriate and, often, informative. It is usually possible to identify a lymph node as such, even if it would not be practicable to recognize the details of its histology and cytology. The detection of metastatic carcinoma in frozen sections of lymph nodes is less certain: early invasion of the sinuses by carcinoma cells may not be distinguishable easily from swelling and proliferation of the endothelial macrophages, and it is these early stages that the surgeon is most concerned to detect. Nonetheless, he may—wisely—want confirmation of the nature of the enlargement of nodes that, while possibly involved in the cancer, may merely be large because of inflammatory or other benign reactive changes. The microscopist can usually, but not always, make this distinction by examining frozen sections (particularly sections cut in the cryostat).

Cryostat Microtomy.—In those rare circumstances in which it is justifiable to examine lymph nodes histologically without waiting for paraffin wax sections, there is no doubt that sections cut in the cryostat are very much more satisfactory than those cut with the simple freezing microtome. The regular use of the cryostat in place of paraffin wax microtomy is a different matter. It has not been my impression during short working visits to laboratories where all biopsy specimens are cut in the cryostat that this method produces sections of lymph nodes as suitable for diagnosis as conventional microtomy after embedding in paraffin wax. That this impression may not have been due to my inexperience in interpreting sections cut in the cryostat was suggested by the frequency with which the pathologists in these laboratories deferred giving a diagnostic opinion on lymph nodes until paraffin

K*

wax sections had been prepared from the half of the specimen that was set aside in case of such a necessity.

Other Methods of Investigation

Film Preparations ('Touch Impressions').—When excised lymph nodes are received in the laboratory promptly after the operation, and unfixed, it is possible to make film preparations by cutting off one pole of the node and pressing its cut surface on microscope slides ('touch impression' or 'imprint' preparations). Simple pressure of the node against the slide is preferable to pulling it along the glass surface to make a smear: the latter tends to result in distortion of some cells. In some conditions—Burkitt's lymphoma is the classic example (see page 832)—this procedure has diagnostic value. Specialists in lymph node pathology are using the method to study the practicability of cytological diagnosis of other lymphadenopathies:[831] at present most histopathologists rely still on histological study unassisted by this as yet incompletely assessed ancillary procedure.

Immunofluorescence.—Immunological methods are contributing to knowledge of the identification and role of different types of cell in the development of certain types of reaction of the lymphoreticular tissues. For instance, fluorescein-labelled anti-immunoglobulin antibody readily demonstrates immunoglobulin on the surface of B lymphocytes; in contrast, immunoglobulin is not ordinarily to be found on T lymphocytes.[832] Again, immunofluorescent staining can be used to verify a tentative diagnosis of systemic lupus erythematosus as the cause of changes in a lymph node biopsy specimen by specifically demonstrating complexes of nuclear antigens, immunoglobulin and complement. Microorganisms that are not otherwise demonstrable in sections may be shown by similar techniques, and their identity specifically indicated. In general, such studies require fresh unfixed specimens; these may, if necessary, be stored in the frozen state.

Electron Microscopy.—Electron microscopy as yet had made hardly any impact on the practical diagnosis of lymphadenopathies, but a great deal of research is in progress and will eventually bring diagnostic advances. Already it has been shown that ultrastructural observations may enable the pathologist to distinguish between lymphomas and other anaplastic tumours, to identify the cells of lymph-

omas more precisely and to indicate the degree of their differentiation.[833] Many other applications are developing.

Microbiological Investigation

It often seems to be very difficult for clinicians to organize the excision of a lymph node for biopsy in such a way that it is possible for the specimen to be used both for microbiological studies and for histological examination. So often, when it is clinically apparent that infection may be responsible for a lymphadenopathy and the need for microbiological investigation is recognized, the specimen is placed in fixative solution as soon as it is excised and the opportunity is lost. Alternatively, the fresh node is sent in its sterile container to the laboratory and then, the necessary samples for microbiological examination having been taken, its despatch to the histological department may be so long delayed that autolysis makes it valueless.

Standardized Systems of Reporting Histologically on Lymph Nodes

Histological interpretation is probably the most subjective field in the whole of laboratory diagnosis, and practising histopathologists have been slow, as a group, to try to standardize the presentation of their diagnostic opinions and of the observations that these are based on. To the scientists making remarkable advances in understanding of disease in terms of 'molecular biology', of ultrastructure, and of the functions and disorders of ultrastructural elements, the continuing failure of practitioners to apply the new knowledge is frustrating. It is more than frustrating when failure to apply this knowledges deprives the clinician in charge of the patient of information that might be useful in clinical assessment or in comprehension of the nature of a disease.

The World Health Organization published, in 1972, a concise and potentially valuable proposal to standardize the histological description of lymph nodes in relation to immunological function.[834] The implementation of such a system would add greatly to the intrinsic value of individual reports and to the store of information on lymph node pathology in those laboratories in which the system could be adopted. But the time involved, although perhaps not unrealistic, would be found only at the expense of other practical matters that demand the pathologist's attention while he is increasingly under pressure to provide more and more detailed and categorized information about a wide range of biopsy specimens. Shortage of funds and a shortage of pathologists are likely to militate against such imaginative innovations for a long time to come, and in most laboratories throughout the world.

Conclusion

The microscopist is wise to insist on deferring a final opinion on a biopsy specimen until additional information—whether from other laboratory investigations or from a period of further clinical observation—is available, rather than commit himself to a diagnosis of which he is not wholly convinced.

THE SPLEEN[835]

The spleen is the largest organized collection of lymphoid and reticuloendothelial tissue in the body. It is a secondary lymphoid organ (peripheral lymphoid organ) in the sense indicated on page 510. Its structure is well adapted for filtration of the blood that circulates through it. The reticuloendothelial cells take up particulate matter, certain normal and abnormal metabolites, effete blood cells and micro-organisms. Immunocompetent lymphocytes (see page 520), which are essential contributors to the antigenic functions of the spleen, migrate through the wall of the arterioles to enter the periarteriolar lymphoid sheath. The size of the spleen and the volume of the blood that passes through it in a given time are indices of its importance in the defensive and metabolic activities of the lymphoreticular system (see pages 520 and 530).

Normal Structure

Size

The spleen as seen at necropsy is appreciably smaller than in life, as a result of contraction of its elastic tissue and the tendency for the blood to be expressed into the veins of the portal system. Under these conditions the average weight of the spleen is about 150 g in young and middle-aged adults, with a range of 90 to 350 g.[836] In the elderly there is often considerable physiological atrophy of the organ, which in the most marked instances may then weigh no more than 40 to 50 g. As 'age atrophy' proceeds, the pulp becomes less abundant and the trabecular framework tends to collapse, forming white, fibrous streaks between which the remains of the pulp appear sunken and often very dark.

The weight of the normal spleen in life is estimated to be of the order of 25 per cent greater than its weight *post mortem*. Its spongy structure and the abundant elastic tissue of the capsule and trabeculae, possibly assisted by the small amount of smooth muscle in these parts, give the organ a considerable and rapidly variable distensibility; however, its role as a blood pool, or bank, is probably much less developed in man than in some animals, particularly those in which there is a large smooth muscle component in the splenic capsule and trabeculae (see page 720).

Histology[837]

The meshes of the splenic 'sponge' form the *red pulp* (often referred to simply as 'the pulp'). The *white pulp* consists of the periarteriolar lymphoid sheath and the adjoining splenic follicles (Malpighian bodies).

Red Pulp.—The red pulp consists of sinuses and 'pulp cords'. The *sinuses* are lined by endothelial macrophages (littoral cells) applied to a basement membrane formed of annular argyrophile fibres with lengthwise or obliquely oriented linking fibres.[838] Although the lining cells are closely apposed, electron microscopy has shown that they lack desmosomes and that they do not interdigitate:[839] blood can move easily from the pulp cords to the lumen of the sinuses by passing through the gaps between the rings of the basement membrane and between the lining cells.

The *pulp cords* are distensible spaces between the sinuses. Normally, they are sparsely cellular: the cells make up a pleomorphic collection, including reticulum cells and macrophages, lymphocytes and plasma cells, and occasional neutrophils, eosinophils and mast cells.

It is now agreed that there are two modes of circulation of the blood in the red pulp—'open' and 'closed'. Ultrastructural studies, by confirming that there is the anatomical pathway for each, resolved the argument about which mode operates. In the so-called *open circulation* the blood flows into the pulp cords—that is, into the interstices of the red pulp—from the capillary termination of the splenic arterioles after the latter have emerged from the follicles and divided to form the penicillary vessels.

It then passes through the fenestrate basement membrane of the wall of the sinuses and between the cells lining the latter to gain the lumen and so pass to the venous tributaries that lie in the trabeculae and drain the organ. In the so-called *closed circulation* the blood is channelled from the penicillary vessels directly into the sinuses and thence to the venous tributaries.

The 'open' and 'closed' modes of circulation have been known sometimes as the 'slow circulation' and the 'rapid circulation' respectively, but this terminology is now known to be misleading. The rate of circulation in the 'open' mode varies: this is because of the existence of a proportion of wide channels among the pulp cords that allow relatively rapid transfer of blood from the post-arteriolar capillaries to the sinuses.[839]

Abnormal and ageing red cells become sequestered in the pulp cords,[840] perhaps because they are less plastic than normal cells, or 'stickier', and cannot readily escape from the pulp cords by passing between the lining cells of the sinuses (see opposite). They may also be more readily ingested by the macrophages in the cords, a circumstance possibly related to abnormalities of their membrane.

The volume of the blood flow through the spleen and the existence of a splenic blood reservoir are considered below.

White Pulp.—The white pulp consists of the periarteriolar lymphoid sheath and the splenic follicles (Malpighian bodies). Topographically, the follicles are occasional enlargements of the sheath; they range from 0·25 to 1·5 mm across and they are usually disposed eccentrically in relation to the arteriole that traverses them and supplies them with blood through side branches. It may be noted that the arterioles in the spleen usually, at least in older adults, show well-marked hyalinization of their wall (see pages 134 and 183), apparently as an ageing phenomenon, although its genesis is still uncertain.

The splenic follicles commonly have a germinal centre. Their structure is, in general, that of lymphoid follicles wherever they occur (see page 512). The germinal centres and the lymphocytes surrounding them are 'bursa-equivalent'-dependent parts of the spleen (see page 515); the thymus-dependent tissue is the periarteriolar sheath.

Ageing is accompanied by a reduction in the size and number of the follicles, and in old age they may be lacking. The periarteriolar sheath also becomes less extensive with increasing age but it does not disappear completely.

It may be noted that lymphocytes are not confined to the sheath and follicles but are present also, usually in small numbers, in the cords of the red pulp (see above).

Blood Flow

The 'open' and 'closed' circulations within the spleen have been mentioned above. The blood flow through the spleen in health is said to be from 500 to 700 ml/min or, in terms of splenic weight, about 3 ml/g/min[841] (respectively, in *Système international* units, 0·008–0·012 l/s and 0·05 l/kg/s). These figures relate to a spleen weight of about 200 g (0·2 kg), and they were derived from studies in which measurements were made of the rate of extraction from the circulation of red cells labelled with radioactive chromium and—to promote their extraction by the spleen—rendered spherocytic by heating. They are of about the same order of magnitude as the figures for the blood flow through the kidneys and about thrice those for the liver.[841]

In cases of splenomegaly in which the spleen weighed from 2000 to 2500 g (2·0–2·5 kg), the blood flow through the spleen was from 1000 to 1200 ml/min[841] (0·017–0·02 l/s). This increase in the total flow was accompanied by a significant fall in the flow in terms of splenic weight (about 0·5 ml/g/min,[841] or 0·008 l/kg/s).

The Spleen as Blood Reservoir (Splenic 'Blood Pool').—Unlike many mammals, man has no significant splenic blood pool. It is said that the normal human spleen, in the adult, contains 20 to 70 ml of red blood cells, which represents about 1 to 5 per cent of these cells in the circulation:[842] this is an insignificant 'reserve' in comparison with the store of up to 20 per cent of the blood volume that is accommodated in the spleen of the dog or cat[843] and available for use in physiological conditions of need (hunting, flight and the like).

There is evidence that immature red cells (reticulocytes) are retained selectively in the splenic pulp cords in health,[844] probably because of the greater adhesiveness of their surface.[845] The purpose of this 'pooling' of reticulocytes may be to enable their maturation to be completed in the spleen (see page 723).

Abnormal red cells—particularly spherocytes, but also other deformed or deficient cells—also tend to accumulate selectively in the spleen. The metabolic effect on these cells of contact in the spleen with lymphocytes and reticuloendothelial cells, which have a much higher metabolic turnover, is to predispose them to lysis.[846] Spherocytes, for instance, show greater osmotic fragility when obtained from the spleen than when studied in the general circulation.[847] The sequestration of abnormal red cells in the spleen is probably attributable to changes in their shape, plasticity or surface adhesiveness that impede their movement within the pulp cords or their egress from the latter by passage between the cells lining the sinuses (see page 719).

Storage, or pooling, of blood platelets in the spleen is referred to below.

Functions of the Spleen

The functions of the spleen, in general terms, are the systemic functions of the lymphoid and reticulo-endothelial systems (see pages 520 and 530), together with particular functions relating to the blood and its cells.

Haemopoiesis in the Spleen

Erythropoiesis and, to a smaller degree, leucopoiesis (granulocytopoiesis) are most active in the spleen during the second to the sixth month of gestation and may still be evident until well into the first year of life.[848] Intrasplenic haemopoiesis accounts for an appreciably smaller proportion of the total output of blood cells during fetal life than intrahepatic haemopoiesis.

Splenic Haemopoiesis in Disease.—The spleen may resume haemopoietic activity at any time under pathological conditions. The most important of these are chronic haemolytic anaemia (see page 473) and, much less frequent, myelosclerosis (see page 462). Even in cases of longstanding and severe haemolytic anaemia—for instance, hereditary spherocytosis (see page 466)—the amount of compensatory erythropoiesis in the spleen is often very much less than that in other extramedullary sites, such as the liver.[849]

Lymphopoiesis in the Spleen

The former view that the spleen was a major site of active production of lymphocytes has been abandoned now that the circulation of lymphocytes has been recognized (see page 519). The lymphocytes of the periarteriolar lymphoid sheaths are long-lived cells that are continually circulating between lymph nodes and spleen, by way of the lymph and blood streams; their stay within the spleen is said to be, on average, from 4 to 6 hours.[850] These cells are T lymphocytes (see page 519) and, by analogy with

observations on animals,[851] they may account for 30 to 50 per cent of the lymphocytes in the spleen.

The short-lived lymphocytes of the 'bursa-equivalent'-dependent germinal centres and surrounding zone are partly of local origin and partly blood-borne; the latter come from bone marrow (see page 507).[852] Such lymphocyte formation as takes place in the spleen may largely result from antigenic stimulation.

'Pooling' of Blood Cells in the Spleen

As noted above, there is very little pooling of mature *red cells* in the spleen in health. *Platelets*, in contrast, are believed to form a splenic pool that may amount to 20 to 40 per cent of the total platelet mass;[853] it is possible, too, that platelets are rendered more adhesive during their retention in the spleen,[854] although splenectomy has also been observed to be followed by an increase in their adhesiveness.[855] *Polymorphonuclear leucocytes* do not tend to accumulate in the spleen in normal people;[856] in cases of chronic myeloid leukaemia it is readily shown that they do so.[857]

The Spleen and Medullary Haemopoiesis

The observation that anaemia, leucopenia and thrombocytopenia accompanying splenomegaly might become less severe, or be abolished, by splenectomy led to the concept of hypersplenism (see pages 441 and 724). Removal of the spleen because of its traumatic rupture, in the absence of disease, is followed by changes in the peripheral blood that may persist for a variable, and sometimes considerable, time after the operation: these changes may include neutrophil leucocytosis, eosinophilia, monocytosis and lymphocytosis,[858] reticulocytosis and showers of nucleated red cells,[859] and thrombocytosis.[860] Such changes do not necessarily indicate that the spleen produces humoral agents with inhibitory effects on the corresponding lines of haemopoiesis: while there may be such agents, the observed changes in the blood could be due to the removal, by splenectomy, of a main site of cell destruction and of a 'pooling' depot.[861]

Destruction of Effete Blood Cells

The spleen is only one site of disposal of ageing blood cells, this being a function of the reticuloendothelial system throughout the body (see page 532). Removal of the spleen has not been found to affect the life span of red cells[862] or platelets[863] in the otherwise normal individual, and it seems therefore that this disposal function is sufficiently subserved by the reticuloendothelial cells elsewhere. Increased destruction of platelets in other sites has been demonstrated following splenectomy.[864] Less is known about the role of the spleen in the disposal of effete polymorphonuclear leucocytes; this in part reflects the fact that these cells mainly function outside the circulation and are destroyed there or lost in the course of their defensive activities by diapedesis through the epithelial lining of the respiratory and alimentary tracts.[865]

Iron Metabolism.—Consequent on the breakdown of ageing red cells there is a constantly active turnover of iron in the spleen,[866] which accommodates a more labile store of the metal than the liver. Some of the ferritin derived from the red cells that have been ingested by the macrophages is stored; the greater part is released for carriage by plasma transferrin and eventual incorporation in the haemoglobin of another generation of red cells.

The Spleen and Coagulation of the Blood

Antihaemophiliac globulin (factor VIII) is believed to be synthetized throughout the reticuloendothelial system, including the spleen, and to be stored in the latter against short-term needs.[867, 868]

The Spleen and Immunity

Experimental evidence indicates that the spleen is most effectively stimulated to produce antibodies when antigen is present in the blood stream in a concentration that results from intravenous inoculation rather than from ingress by other routes.[869] Splenectomy generally has no remarkable effect on established immunity or on responsiveness to antigens, but it has been shown that the intravenous administration of heterologous red blood cells produces an abnormally low titre of haemolysin in patients who have lost their spleen.[870]

The spleen is a site of synthesis of immunoglobulin in association with its activity as an antibody-producing organ.[871] Studies after splenectomy suggest that, at least in children, it is particularly class M immunoglobulins (IgM) that are elaborated in the spleen.[872]

Effects of Splenectomy

It is remarkable that removal of the spleen—for example, when undertaken because of traumatic rupture—so often neither causes ill effects nor interferes with the capacity of the body to withstand subsequent infections: presumably the lymph nodes and the lymphoreticular tissue elsewhere are more than sufficient to carry out the functions performed by the spleen. However, it has lately become clear that we have been far too sanguine about the safety of splenectomy, particularly in childhood and in the presence of serious haematological disease. This change of attitude to splenectomy has been, in part, a consequence of the greatly increased frequency of the operation: the spleen is nowadays commonly removed as a diagnostic procedure in cases of splenomegaly, as a staging procedure in the clinical assessment of Hodgkin's disease in relation to the choice of therapeutic regimen, and as a matter of surgical convenience in the course of radical operations on other organs (for instance, total gastrectomy), in addition to its removal as a therapeutic procedure (for instance, in cases of hereditary spherocytosis, in some cases of chronic myeloid leukaemia, and so on).

The dangers of splenectomy are real and frequent. Predisposition to infection is by far the commonest and gravest of these. Haematological changes are also frequent, but with the rare exception of an increased liability to thrombosis they are of little practical significance. Complications that are rarer, in that they relate to splenectomy performed in the presence of particular diseases affecting the spleen, have a correspondingly limited practical importance, except to the individual patient and his surgeon: such complications include predisposition to rupture of oesophageal varices following splenectomy in cases of the congestive splenomegaly that accompanies portal hypertension, and the increased accumulation of lipid in other parts of the reticuloendothelial system following splenectomy in cases of splenomegaly due to certain storage diseases, particularly Gaucher's disease (see page 759).

Infections as Complications of Splenectomy

Adults.—Splenectomy for traumatic rupture of the spleen in otherwise healthy adults evidently carries little risk of an increase in the frequency or severity of infections.[859] Nonetheless, these individuals are not as well able to withstand some forms of infection as normal people, and this is most apparent during a period of 1 to 2 years after the operation. In particular, they are proner to develop severe manifestations of pneumococcal[873] and other forms of streptococcal sepsis. In areas where malaria caused by *Plasmodium falciparum* is prevalent, it is recognized that the person who has had a splenectomy before coming to the region—even many years before—is predisposed to rapidly fatal infection, particularly cerebral malaria. The relation between loss of the spleen and death in cases of the rare infection that is caused by species of the protozoon *Babesia* has been noted on page 668.

Adults who are already predisposed to infection by the effects of other diseases, including lymphoma, leukaemia and other blood disorders, and cirrhosis of the liver, become even likelier to develop serious, and commonly fatal, infection following removal of the spleen.[874] Although their underlying disease, or its treatment, predisposes particularly to the so-called 'opportunistic' infections that are caused by various moulds, species of candida, pneumocystis, and viruses (see page 362), it is notable that after splenectomy it is most frequently grave bacterial infections that occur. The bacterial infection is characteristically liable to be fulminant in its course, death sometimes resulting within 24 to 36 hours: in many instances an acute and extensive suppurative pneumonia or a very rapidly developing suppurative meningoencephalitis is evident at necropsy, although the clinical appearances are those of septicaemia or of toxaemia with circulatory collapse. The organisms most frequently noted by bacteriologists who have spoken with me about this hazard are *Streptococcus pneumoniae*, *Streptococcus pyogenes*, *Pseudomonas aeruginosa*, *Haemophilus influenzae* and *Nocardia asteroides*; rarer causes include *Neisseria meningitidis*, *Escherichia coli*, species of klebsiella and salmonella, and *Staphylococcus aureus*.

Children.—The risk of infection following splenectomy is very much greater in children than in adults.[875] The incidence and severity of this complication are greatest when the operation is performed during infancy.[876] Later in childhood the incidence of infection is less but the mortality of the infections that develop is still very high.[877] The liability to infection falls notably after a period of about 2 years has passed following the operation.[878]

Pathogenesis of Infection Following Splenectomy.— The explanation of the increased frequency of serious infection in patients who have lost their spleen is uncertain. It has been suggested that the spleen has an important role in the earliest stages of a septicaemic infection, when it efficiently extracts bacteria from the blood: this is probably in part an immunologically determined function as well as a manifestation of the phagocytic activity of its macrophages. Splenectomy in animals results in

deficient formation of 'opsonizing' class M immunoglobulins (IgM) during the primary response to an antigenic stimulus and of class G immunoglobulins (IgG) during a secondary response.[879] In man, the level of IgG seems usually to be normal following splenectomy;[880] the same is true of IgM in adults,[881] but in children there is a sustained fall in the level of IgM after the operation.[882] The role of such changes as have been observed is far from clear. It seems that other parts of the lymphoreticular system can compensate to a considerable extent, in adults, for the loss of the defences that the spleen offers against invasion of the blood stream by bacteria; in children this compensation is inadequately developed.

Changes in the Blood Following Splenectomy

Erythrocytes.—Quantitative changes affecting the red cells after splenectomy are generally seen only in cases in which the operation has had the purpose of modifying the effects of the disease of the blood for which it was undertaken. For instance, there may be erythrocytosis following splenectomy in cases of hereditary spherocytosis.[883]

Qualitative changes in the red cells include the invariable presence of Howell–Jolly bodies (see Fig. 8.9K, page 450),[884, 885] an increased proportion of target cells (see Fig. 8.9H, page 450), siderocytes (see page 449) and cells containing Heinz bodies (see Fig. 8.9, part 0, page 450), and a reduction in osmotic fragility (see page 466). *Howell–Jolly bodies** are seldom found in more than 2 per cent of the circulating red cells[886] and in some cases thousands of cells must be scanned in order to find one. Their confirmed absence from the blood of a patient who has had a splenectomy suggests that there is accessory splenic tissue (see page 726).[887] Howell–Jolly bodies consist of deoxyribonucleic acid and are of nuclear origin: it is uncertain whether their presence is due to the loss of a function of the spleen to remove the nucleus from circulating normoblasts, leaving these peculiar particles as the final residuum. They are also to be found in cases of congenital absence of the spleen (see page 725) and of splenic atrophy (see page 726), and in the presence of severe anaemia, particularly megaloblastic anaemias,[888] and in leukaemia.

Siderocytes—red cells that contain granules that

---

* The particles that are generally known as Howell–Jolly bodies were described by Howell in 1890 and by Jolly in 1923 (references 884 and 885, page 879). They were also described, in 1908, by Schur (Schur, H., *Wien. med. Wschr.*, 1908, **58**, 441).

give a positive Perls's reaction for iron—are now known to be present in normal blood and, in larger numbers, in various types of anaemia, in which similar granules are demonstrable in a proportion of nucleated red cells also. They are specially numerous in the blood of patients who have had their spleen removed, and it was in such cases that they first attracted serious attention.[889] It is probable that the spleen ordinarily removes 'free' iron from the reticulocytes while these cells are held in the pulp cords (see page 532).

Heinz bodies,[890] which consist of degraded haemoglobin,[891] result from the effect of excess of oxidants on the reducing potential of the red cell. They were originally observed following the action of phenylhydrazine and its derivatives on circulating red cells. Various other causes are now known, deficiency of glucose 6-phosphate dehydrogenase being the most familiar (see page 468).[892] They are seen in small numbers among the ageing red cells in the circulation of patients who have undergone splenectomy;[893] these older cells are abnormally sensitive to oxidation.

There may be a transient and usually slight reticulocytosis after splenectomy. Occasional normoblasts may be present in the circulating blood.

White Cells.[894]—Leucocytosis is often present within hours following splenectomy. The number of circulating white cells, mainly neutrophils, rises over a period of some days, and the total count then commonly remains between $10 \times 10^9/1$ and $15 \times 10^9/1$ for many weeks and sometimes for much longer periods. In some cases counts of well above $25 \times 10^9/1$ are found. There may be an absolute lymphocytosis or monocytosis in some cases, particularly when some weeks have elapsed since the operation. The number of circulating eosinophils and basiphils may also rise.

Platelets.—A notable but transient thrombocytopenia may occur during a period of some hours to a day or so after splenectomy.[883] Whether or not this initial fall in the platelet count takes place, there is a progressive rise in the count to a maximum some 10 to 15 days after the operation, when the count may reach and even exceed $1 \times 10^{12}/1$. The thrombocytosis tends to be severer and more persistent in cases in which there is chronic anaemia that has not been alleviated by the operation;[895] thrombosis may then develop, with consequences determined by its sites. Platelet adhesiveness is increased as a result of splenectomy.[855] Rarely, post-splenectomy thrombo-

cytosis is accompanied by spontaneous or uncommonly severe traumatic bleeding: in these cases there may be demonstrable abnormalities of the platelets, both morphological and functional, the condition being a variety of 'haemorrhagic thrombocythaemia'. However, it is doubtful whether this secondary state carries the grave prognosis that characterizes primary haemorrhagic thrombocythaemia, which is liable to develop into myelosclerosis (see page 462).

Hypersplenism

The *concept of hypersplenism*[896-898] rests on the assumption that the spleen produces a substance, or substances, that can inhibit the release of red cells, polymorphonuclear leucocytes and platelets from the bone marrow into the blood. The *syndrome of hypersplenism* comprises splenomegaly and a reduction in the number of cells in the blood, without the presence of any conspicuous number of circulating immature cells, and with normal marrow or—oftener—simple hyperplasia of those cells of the marrow that correspond to the type of cell, or cells, that are deficient in the circulation. The *diagnosis of hypersplenism* may not be accepted until all other causes of the observed changes in the blood have been considered and excluded.

The reduction in the number of cells in the circulation may involve the red cells, polymorphonuclear leucocytes and platelets together (*splenic pancytopenia*,[899] or splenic panhaematopenia[900]) or any one of these ('splenic anaemia',* splenic neutropenia[901] and splenic thrombocytopenia[902]). The return of the blood picture to normal after splenectomy, which may be observed in some cases, has been considered to support the hypothesis that the spleen produces humoral substances—sometimes referred to as *splenic hormones*—that inhibit the passage of cells from the marrow into the blood. However, some haematological disorders that are not related to hypersplenism respond to splenectomy—for example, hereditary spherocytosis, which is the manifestation of a congenital defect in the red cells. Similarly, while the reticulocytosis, leucocytosis and thrombocytosis that follow the removal of an otherwise normal spleen because of its traumatic rupture have been seen as evidence of the

---

* The term *splenic anaemia*, because of its traditional use as one of the synonyms of Banti's disease (Banti's syndrome, hepatolienal fibrosis or congestive splenomegaly—see page 731), has been eclipsed by the aversion of most non-Mediterranean pathologists from the concept of Banti's disease as an entity.

elaboration by the spleen of a humoral factor (or factors) that can retard the release of cells from bone marrow, there is an alternative view that these changes in the blood picture result from loss of the splenic pool and of the splenic capacity for destroying effete cells.[861] It has to be remembered also that splenomegaly may be accompanied by a moderate shortening of the life span of the red cells by the occurrence of pooling of red cells and by increased pooling of platelets, which contribute—but in limited measure only—to the severity of anaemia and thrombocytopenia respectively.

There is experimental evidence of both inhibitory[903] and stimulating[904] effects of the spleen on the formation and release of cells by the marrow.

Primary Hypersplenism.—In the comparatively rare primary form of hypersplenism the enlargement of the spleen has no evident cause and is described as 'idiopathic splenomegaly' or (to avoid confusion with the condition that commonly is referred to as tropical idiopathic splenomegaly—see page 743) as 'non-tropical idiopathic splenomegaly'.[905] The spleen often weighs about 2000 g, the range being from 500 to 5000 g. The histological findings in the spleen in this condition vary: the lymphoid follicles range widely in number and size and may or may not contain germinal centres; in some instances the white pulp occupies a substantially greater proportion of the spleen than usual and the picture may simulate that of a follicular lymphoma, particularly as there is often a high rate of mitosis in the follicles. In the red pulp the sinuses may be dilated and sometimes are markedly so. The pulp cords tend to be considerably more cellular than is normal but the cells are normal in type and in their relative proportions.

Secondary Hypersplenism.—In cases of secondary hypersplenism the splenomegaly is a manifestation of an identifiable disease that does not itself affect the release of cells from the marrow. The underlying disease accounts for the enlargement of the spleen, and the enlarged spleen then exerts an exaggerated effect on the blood picture. No doubt this is in part a manifestation of pooling and increased destruction of the blood cells, but it seems possible that other mechanisms are also at work, and these may well involve the action of substances that inhibit cell release in the bone marrow.

Among the causes of splenomegaly associated with secondary hypersplenism are various acute infections,[906] chronic infections (including tuberculosis,[907] brucella infection,[908] malaria,[909] kala azar[910] and amoebic 'abscess'[908]), schistosomiasis (Egyptian splenomegaly),[911] sarcoidosis,[912] rheumatoid arthritis (Felty syndrome—see page 690),[913] the tropical splenomegaly syndrome ('big spleen disease'—see page 743),[914] congestive splenomegaly (see page 730),[915] thyrotoxicosis,[916] lipidoses (particularly Gaucher's disease[917]), haemangioma,[918] hamartoma of splenic tissue ('intrasplenic splenoma' —see page 739),[919] lymphoma[920] and leukaemia.[920] It is apparent from this list that in some of these conditions hypersplenism may be a less likely cause of the changes in the blood picture than other effects of the diseases named. There is no doubt that the term 'hypersplenism' is too widely applied; nevertheless, some of the disrepute that it has consequently acquired is probably overstated.

Haemodilution Accompanying Splenomegaly

There may be a great increase in the plasma volume in cases of marked splenomegaly, whatever the cause of the latter. Its explanation is unknown. The consequent dilution of the blood tends to exaggerate the severity of any associated anaemia, whether due to hypersplenism or to the condition that caused the enlargement of the spleen ('haemodilution anaemia' —see page 430).

ABNORMALITIES OF THE SPLEEN

The spleen is involved in many of the conditions that have been described earlier in this chapter in the account of disorders that affect the lymph nodes. The pathological findings in the spleen in these diseases correspond in general to those in the lymph nodes, with allowance for peculiarities that are determined by the differences in the normal structure of the organs. In the following account of the pathology of the spleen attention is confined mainly to those conditions that are peculiar to the spleen or that present noteworthy features when they involve it.

Congenital Anomalies

Congenital Absence of the Spleen

Congenital absence of the spleen (asplenia, splenic aplasia, splenic agenesis) is a rare anomaly. It is almost always associated with other defects, particularly of the heart and great blood vessels (see page 79). Defects of the endocardial cushions are especially frequent (see page 87). There is often an accompanying transposition of the viscera; this is usually of the partial variety (see page 79).[921] There may be various anomalies of the lungs and of the duodenum and biliary tract (see page 80). The associated cardiac anomalies are generally incompatible with more than a year or two of life.

In some instances the spleen is represented by a number of spleniculi (see below).

Erythrocytic Anomalies.—Howell–Jolly bodies (see page 723) are found in some of the red cells in cases of congenital absence of the spleen.[922] Their demonstration, as an indication of the splenic anomaly, may be of practical significance since the association of absence of the spleen with congenital cardiovascular disease worsens the prognosis of the latter by predisposing to infection, including infection in the period following surgery for the correction of the circulatory anomalies.

Heinz bodies (see page 724) are said to be present in about 10 per cent of cases of splenic aplasia.[921] They are not pathognomonic, and they do not have the diagnostic significance of Howell–Jolly bodies. 'Target' cells and siderocytes may be numerous, as after splenectomy (see page 723).

Hereditary Splenic Hypoplasia[923]

This is a very rare condition in which the spleen is uncommonly small or rudimentary. Its functional effects are comparable to those of absence of the spleen, the most serious being the predisposition to infection, especially during infancy.

Lobation[924]

Lobation of the spleen is an occasional anomaly. It is usually associated with other malformations, particularly of the heart.

Accessory Splenic Tissue (Spleniculi)[925]

Speniculi (splenunculi), or accessory spleens, are found in about 10 per cent of people. Usually they occur in the hilum of the spleen, but occasionally they are found elsewhere, although generally in relation to the various peritoneal reflections about the spleen. About 15 per cent are situated within the tail of the pancreas. Very rarely, accessory splenic tissue is present in the scrotum (see Chapter 26); sometimes a spleniculus in this situation is large enough to be mistaken for a testicular neoplasm.

Accessory spleens are seldom more than 1·5 cm in diameter. The small ones may be buried from sight in the adipose tissue of the peritoneal folds or in the pancreas. They can usually be identified by the naked eye: they are darker than lymph nodes and generally more spherical. The larger ones usually project into the peritoneal cavity and have a complete serosal covering except at their hilum.

Spleniculi are important because if left behind at splenectomy they may undergo hyperplasia and grow to take the place of the spleen, with—in some cases—return of the symptoms for which the operation was performed (Fig. 9.162).

'Intrasplenic accessory spleens' are hamartomas. They are referred to on page 739.

Atrophy

Atrophy of the spleen as a natural accompaniment of ageing (see page 719) seems to have no demonstrable consequences. In contrast, pathological atrophy has haematological effects similar to those of splenectomy (see page 723). The conditions that are listed oftenest as causes of splenic atrophy are sickle cell anaemia, intestinal malabsorption and thrombocythaemia.

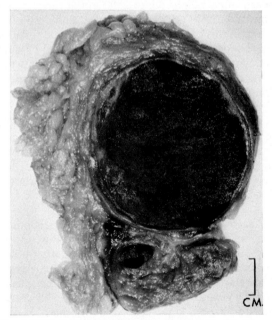

Fig. 9.162.§ Two accessory spleens (spleniculi). The larger, surrounded by a thick capsule, is in the retroperitoneal adipose tissue above the tail of the pancreas, which occupies the greater part of the width of the specimen at the bottom of the picture. The smaller accessory spleen is within the pancreas, just below a small haemorrhage between the latter and the larger spleniculus. The patient had chronic lymphocytic leukaemia. The normally situated spleen had been removed surgically some years before his death. The accessory spleens showed the usual splenic structure, with the changes of leukaemia superimposed.

Sickle Cell Anaemia and Splenic Atrophy[926, 927]

It is commonly said that atrophy of the spleen is a characteristic finding at necropsy in cases of sickle cell anaemia. In fact, this is oftener true in North America than in tropical Africa, where the co-existence of chronic malaria may somehow result in maintenance of some degree of splenomegaly. Where malaria is not endemic, atrophy of the spleen may become so marked that the organ is reduced to a siderotic nubbin of fibrous tissue no more than 2 to 3 cm across (Fig. 9.163).[928] This is the outcome of scarring as the sequel of the many episodes of ischaemic necrosis that result from the high viscosity of the abnormal blood. It is sometimes referred to as 'autosplenectomy'. It is always a late effect of the disease: it is not observed in young children, in whom splenic enlargement is usual, associated with sequestration of great numbers of sickle cells, which

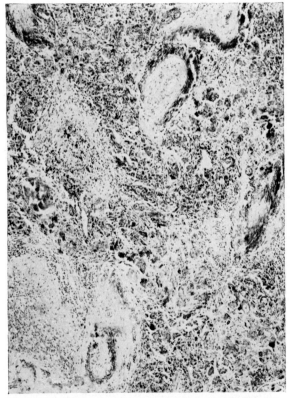

Fig. 9.163.§ Spleen in late stage of sickle cell anaemia. The spleen, from an adult, measured 3·5 cm in its longest dimension. The photograph shows shrinkage and heavy haemosiderosis of the red pulp, with extensive fibrosis, particularly of the trabeculae and white pulp. The trabeculae are approximated and the remains of their elastic tissue are impregnated with darkly stained salts of iron and calcium. There is no remaining lymphoid tissue. *Haematoxylin–eosin.* × 55.

cause striking distension of the pulp cords, even to the extent that they are much wider and more conspicuous than the sinuses (see page 719). In older children with sickle cell disease, the haematological changes that accompany loss of splenic function may be found while the spleen is still enlarged:[929] at this stage such changes are reversible, transfusion of normal blood being followed by the return of the blood picture to normal, and the functional failure is therefore thought to be due to the slowing of the flow of blood through the pulp because of its increased viscosity.

Intestinal Malabsorption and Splenic Atrophy[930]

Malabsorption syndromes, both primary and secondary (see page 1084), may be accompanied by marked atrophy of the spleen. The pathogenesis of the atrophy is quite obscure. The haematological effects of splenic atrophy—most notably, the presence of Howell–Jolly bodies (see page 723)—are evident on examination of the peripheral blood in 10 to 15 per cent of cases of malabsorption in adults. When patients with the most frequent form of malabsorption—gluten-sensitive enteropathy ('adult coeliac disease')—are subjected to examination by the sophisticated method of tracing the distribution of radioisotope-labelled spherocytes, it is found that practically all show splenic functional insufficiency.[931] Indeed, apart from splenectomy and sickle cell disease, the commonest cause of the haematological changes that indicate splenic deficiency is the presence of an intestinal malabsorption syndrome.[932, 933]

Thrombocythaemia and Splenic Atrophy

Although it is sometimes said that thrombocythaemia* is a cause of splenic atrophy, it is possible that the increase in the platelet count in cases of this association is a consequence of the atrophy rather than its origin (see page 724).[934] Primary (or essen-

---

* Thrombocythaemia and thrombocytosis are terms that different authorities use with different meanings. To some, thrombocythaemia is definable simply in quantitative terms —for instance, as a platelet count in the blood of $1 \times 10^{12}/1$ or more: any smaller increase over the normal range of $200–400 \times 10^9/1$ is designated thrombocytosis. Others limit the use of thrombocythaemia to those cases in which the circulating platelets include morphologically abnormal forms (misshapen or giant platelets particularly). Again, thrombocythaemia is often intended to imply specifically the primary state of excessive platelet production ('essential thrombocythaemia') that appears to be related to myelosclerosis and the 'myeloproliferative disorders' (see text).

tial) thrombocythaemia is associated with spleno-megaly, and tends to develop into myelosclerosis (of which splenomegaly is the most characteristic clinical feature): this would seem to support the view that an increase in the platelet count in associa-tion with atrophy of the spleen is secondary to the latter.

Rupture of the Spleen

Rupture of the Healthy Spleen

The healthy spleen may be ruptured by crushing of the abdomen, by the blast of explosions in water or air, or by kicks or blows, particularly jabbing blows with a truncheon or the butt of a gun. Rupture may also result from falls from a height, particularly when the body falls forcefully and is abruptly flexed, as may happen, for instance, when thrown from horse-back. If, as is usual, the capsule of the spleen is torn at the time of the injury, massive intraperitoneal haemorrhage results, and the clinical picture is that of severe internal bleeding. In other cases, the initial lesion is a closed intrasplenic haematoma; its rupture into the abdominal cavity may be delayed for up to several days, and the need to be on the lookout for this development, rare as it may be, puts a great responsibility on doctors working in casualty departments. In addition to the risk of delayed spontaneous rupture of the spleen, there is the hazard that palpation of a spleen that is the seat of a haematoma may cause it to rupture.

Rupture of the Diseased Spleen

Disease of the spleen increases its liability to rupture, and the rupture may occur 'spontaneously'—that is, there may be no history of injury, or a history only of a trivial knock or sudden movement. Among the conditions predisposing to this type of rupture are congestive splenomegaly (see page 730), infarcts, infections, amyloidosis (see below), cysts and pseudocysts, tumours and leukaemia. Indeed, it is probable that any enlarged spleen is likelier to be ruptured than the normal organ (see *Splenomegaly*, page 742). Infections that are specially prone to be complicated by rupture include infectious mono-nucleosis (see page 736), typhoid fever, brucella infection, leishmaniasis (kala azar) and malaria. In the case of malaria there is some evidence that rupture is likelier to affect those who acquire the disease for the first time as adults, either naturally, on visiting a malarious district, or—as was formerly practised in the treatment of neurosyphilis (parti-cularly general paresis) and sometimes of psychoses

—by therapeutic induction (the Wagner von Jauregg treatment[935, 936]).*

The splenomegaly that accompanies haemolytic disease of the newborn (erythroblastosis fetalis—see page 464) has been known to predispose to rupture during birth or during attempted resuscitation after birth.

The liability of the spleen to rupture is increased if it is bound to neighbouring structures by adhe-sions, the result of previous inflammation (see page 734).

Autotransplantation of Splenic Tissue[937]

Multiple foci of splenic tissue may be found any-where on the serosal lining of the abdominal cavity following rupture of the spleen. The condition is sometimes known as *splenosis*. The foci are distin-guished from accessory spleens by their number, irregular shape and wide distribution, and usually there is a history of trauma, maybe many years before. In one case, observed during laparotomy for acute appendicitis in 1976, the patient's only history of injury was in 1942, when he was exposed to the shock waves of depth charge explosions while swimming: he suffered severe abdominal pain at that time, but the symptoms subsided without surgery.

Sometimes the splenic foci cause complications, particularly intestinal obstruction by adhesions.

It has been said that autotransplantation does not follow rupture of a diseased spleen. This is not correct. I have known it to occur as a sequel of rupture of the spleen in infectious mononucleosis (two cases) and in malaria.

Amyloidosis

Secondary Amyloidosis

The spleen is one of the organs that are most fre-quently and most heavily involved in cases of secondary amyloidosis. In the early stages the deposition of amyloid is generally confined to the immediate vicinity of the walls of the small arteries. In more advanced cases two patterns of splenic involvement may be defined—focal and diffuse.

Focal amyloidosis is much commoner than diffuse

* While helping to lift a patient into bed in hospital, in Britain in the 1930s, a medical student collapsed from 'spontaneous' rupture of the spleen. It proved that he had benign tertian malaria (*Plasmodium vivax* infection): he was one of several people who were infected when mosquitoes carrying the organism were inadvertently released into the ward where patients were being treated by induced malaria.

amyloidosis. Innumerable, isolated, rounded deposits, 2 to 3 mm in diameter, are scattered through the pulp, replacing the splenic follicles (Fig. 9.164). In *diffuse amyloidosis*, confluent masses of amyloid replace the greater part of the organ, as a result of extensive involvement of the tissue between the sinuses: the deposition starts in relation to the basement membrane of the sinuses and encroaches progressively on the pulp cords. Sometimes, in the diffuse form, the splenic follicles are practically completely free from amyloid, although the periarteriolar lymphoid sheath may be wholly replaced by the deposition. In most cases of both patterns of secondary amyloidosis of the spleen the translucent waxy appearance of the amyloid material enables the condition to be recognized macroscopically: this impression can be confirmed by use of one of the iodine/sulphuric-acid methods of staining fresh specimens.

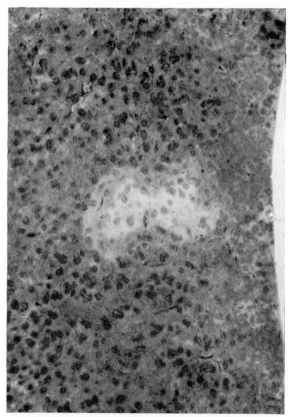

Fig. 9.164.§ Focal amyloidosis of the spleen. The dark, rounded foci are deposits of amyloid that have replaced the splenic follicles. Their dark appearance is due to staining by iodine solution applied to the cut surface of the organ in its fresh state. The pale area at the centre of the picture is an infarct. *Twice natural size.*

The spleen may weigh as much as 500 g in cases of either pattern. Rupture of the enlarged spleen is considered below.

Primary Amyloidosis

The spleen may also be involved in cases of primary amyloidosis—that is, when amyloidosis develops in the absence of any recognized predisposing disease. The splenic involvement is not as extensive as in cases of secondary amyloidosis. The amyloid is deposited mainly in the wall of the arterioles and is seldom visible to the unaided eye. It does not give specific staining reactions as regularly as the amyloid of secondary amyloidosis: the diagnosis—for instance, on examination of a spleen removed because of 'spontaneous' rupture—may have to rest on the morphological findings until confirmatory clinical evidence is obtained. It is not unusual in such circumstances that the amyloid in the wall of the vessels is mistaken for the hyaline material that so often characterizes the splenic arterioles (see page 732).

Rupture of the Amyloid Spleen

'Spontaneous' rupture—that is, rupture occurring from a degree of trauma that seems insufficient to have this effect—may complicate any type of amyloid disease of the spleen, and diffuse secondary amyloidosis in particular.

Rupture of the amyloid spleen is also a hazard of attempts to obtain material for histological examination by a percutaneous needle biopsy procedure. The presence of amyloid seems to make the spleen uncommonly friable, and the tear that may result from insertion of a needle is likely to necessitate splenectomy. In other instances, persistent oozing of blood from the puncture wound in the spleen may be a serious complication; it is due to failure of the tissues infiltrated with amyloid to retract and so seal the biopsy site.

Pigmentation of the Spleen
Endogenous Pigments

Haemosiderosis.—Any haemolytic condition is accompanied by haemosiderosis of the spleen as a manifestation of the activity of its reticuloendothelial component in the breakdown of the red cells and in storage of iron. In any chronic haemolytic anaemia the spleen is enlarged and of a colour noticeably darker than normal; a macroscopically striking Prussian blue reaction may be given by the fresh specimen. Similar appearances are seen in haemo-chromatosis (see page 1270). 'Iatrogenic' siderosis is mentioned below.

Melanin.—Melanin may be found in the spleen in cases of chronic exfoliative dermatitis and is presumably a spill-over from the lymph nodes (see *Dermatopathic Lymphadenitis*, page 686). The pigment is taken up by the macrophages. Splenic melanosis may also occur in cases of melanomatosis and may be quite heavy, even in the absence of secondary deposits of the tumour in the spleen: it is assumed to be the result of phagocytosis of melanin picked up by the blood as it circulates through tumour tissue or carried to the blood in the lymph.

Ceroid Bodies.—Ceroid bodies (Hamazaki–Wesenberg bodies—see page 562) appear not to have been observed in the spleen as frequently as in lymph nodes. In fact, however, they are quite commonly found in splenectomy specimens although comparatively rare in post-mortem specimens.[938] This discrepancy may be related to their tendency to undergo dissolution in dead tissues, as it is difficult otherwise to explain their frequency in spleens removed because of traumatic rupture and their rarity in material collected at necropsy. Their significance is still unknown. They are most frequent in the pulp cords and they may be found free or, less often, in the cytoplasm of macrophages.

Exogenous Pigments

Malarial Pigment.—Malarial pigment ('haemozoin') accounts for the characteristic slate purple colour of the spleen in chronic malaria. The unwary pathologist may attribute the pigmentation of the malarial spleen to haemosiderin, which is also present, and often in considerable quantity: the malarial pigment tends to be mistaken for *formalin pigment* (see page 667), which often develops in particularly large amounts in the spleen, probably because of the volume of blood that it contains. Pigment that is believed to be identical with malarial pigment accumulates in cases of heavy infestation of the portal venous bed by *Schistosoma mansoni*; it is less abundant in the spleen than in the liver.[939]

Carbon.—Carbon is the exogenous pigment that is most commonly found in the spleen. Some carbon is present in macrophages or interstitial tissue in the spleen of most town dwellers and it may be so abundant in some coal miners that the spleen is extensively mottled with black areas. The carbon in

these cases has escaped from the lungs and mediastinal lymph nodes to reach the blood and thence the reticuloendothelial cells elsewhere in the body. The heaviest pigmentation of the spleen is seen in those rare cases in which necrosis of anthracotic mediastinal lymph nodes has been followed by eruption of their contents into the circulation (see page 551).

Metals.—Other exogenous pigments found in the spleen include silver, in cases of *argyrosis*, and iron, in cases of excessive parenteral administration and as a result of repeated blood transfusion ('*iatrogenic*' *siderosis*).

Circulatory Disturbances Affecting the Spleen

The spleen has an unusual liability to *passive hyperaemia*. It is not only characteristically affected in states of chronic systemic venous congestion associated with congestive heart failure, but the fact that the venous blood from the spleen has normally to pass through the hepatic portal circulation before reaching the vena cava means that any hepatic cause of obstruction to the portal venous return—for example, cirrhosis—causes passive hyperaemia of the spleen.

The Spleen of Chronic Systemic Venous Congestion

The spleen in cases of simple passive hyperaemia of cardiac origin is little enlarged, 250 g being a usual figure; it is so rarely large enough to be palpable clinically that the finding of a palpable spleen in a patient with heart failure associated with valvular disease suggests the presence of a complicating infective endocarditis. The affected spleen has a curiously resilient hardness, and although engorged with blood it retains its shape when bisected, probably because of an increase in the amount of fine fibrous tissue in the trabeculae and pulp.

The Spleen of Portal Hypertension ('Congestive Splenomegaly')

When hyperaemia is due to obstruction of the portal circulation the spleen is considerably enlarged, commonly weighing from 500 to 1000 g; rarely its weight reaches several kilograms. It is very firm and its cut surface has a meaty red colour that is rather characteristic; the capsule is thickened and the trabeculae are conspicuous. The splenic vein is tortuous and may be sclerotic and show atheromatous changes in its intima; thrombosis is not uncommon. Often there is a sparse scattering of small, brownish, hard spots throughout the pulp: these are known as 'tobacco flecks', or Gandy–Gamma[939a, 939b] nodules (or bodies).* Microscopically, these nodules prove to be scars in which many of the collagen and elastic fibres are encrusted with iron and calcium (Fig. 9.165); some of the encrusted fibres have a curious greenish, glassy appearance, and may be segmented and appear to branch—they were formerly sometimes considered to be the mycelium of a fungus. The scars are the end-result of haemorrhages in the splenic follicles or adjacent to trabeculae.

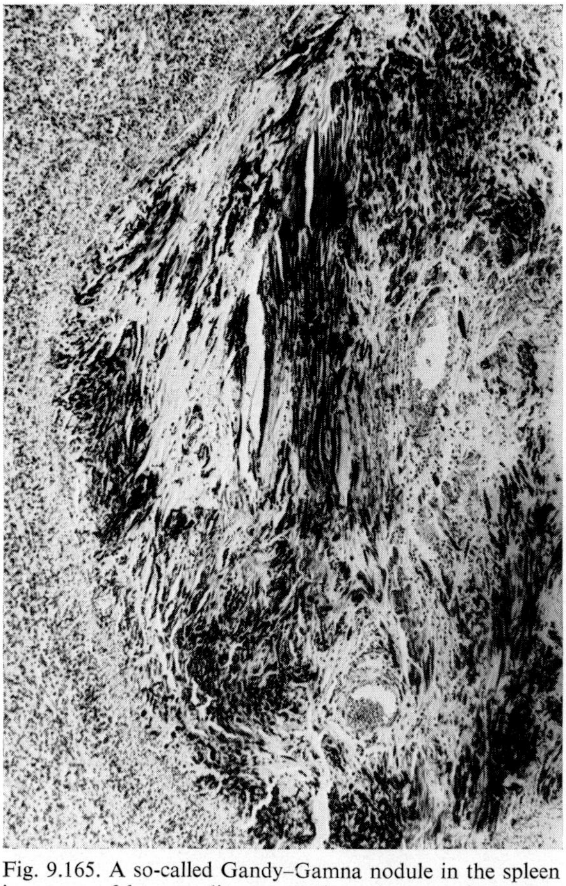

Fig. 9.165. A so-called Gandy–Gamna nodule in the spleen in a case of longstanding congestive splenomegaly accompanying cirrhosis of the liver. The fibrotic tissue of a scar is encrusted with iron and calcium salts, therefore staining intensely with haematoxylin. There is a patent blood vessel toward the centre of the fibrotic nodule. The nodules are considered to be the end result of haemorrhages within splenic follicles. *Haematoxylin–eosin.* × 60.

* The so-called Gandy–Gamna nodules were first described by Marini, three years before Gandy's account (Marini, G., *Arch. Sci. med.*, 1902, **26**, 105). They should not be confused with Gamna–Favre bodies of lymphogranuloma inguinale (see page 638).

Atrophy of the follicles and an increase in the amount of reticulin in the pulp are usual.

'*Banti's Disease*'.—Congestive splenomegaly, as just described, is typical of the condition formerly known as Banti's disease. It was thought that this started with splenomegaly and anaemia ('splenic anaemia'*) and was eventually complicated by the development of cirrhosis of the liver, ascites, and oesophageal varices.† There has been a continuing argument about the existence of Banti's disease.[940] It is clear now that in the cases in which cirrhosis of the liver is a feature, the hepatic disease is the cause of the portal hypertension and congestive splenomegaly: the enlarged spleen may then produce an inhibitory effect on the release of blood cells from the marrow into the circulation (see page 724). There remains only the very small proportion of cases in which splenomegaly that occurs without evident cause is associated with inhibition of cell release from the marrow: few would deny the occurrence of such cases (see page 725), but whether the eponymous designation should be retained is debatable.

Infarction

The spleen is particularly liable to infarction from embolism as a complication of infective endocarditis or of thrombosis within the chambers of the heart. Infarcts may also result from disease of the vasculature of the spleen itself: thrombosis complicating atherosclerosis of the splenic artery, polyarteritis (see below) and syphilitic arteritis are among these.

Infarcts are also seen in the spleen in many forms of splenomegaly (see page 742), and particularly in those conditions that give rise to the greatest enlargement, such as chronic myeloid leukaemia and Gaucher's disease. In some of these conditions it is possible to demonstrate thrombosis of intrasplenic

* The term *splenic anaemia* was long a synonym of 'Banti's disease' and is best avoided. It may be noted that Gaucher's disease, the cerebroside lipidosis (see page 759), was sometimes known as 'familial splenic anaemia' before its true nature was recognized.

† The name *Banti's disease* is said to be applicable only to those cases of 'idiopathic' splenomegaly with anaemia in which there is no hepatic cirrhosis. These are the cases that appear to correspond to the condition that Banti described in his earlier work on 'splenic anaemia' (Banti, G., *Dell' anemia splenica;* Firenze, 1882). The term *Banti's syndrome* is sometimes preferred when cirrhosis of the liver develops in association with splenomegaly and anaemia (Banti, G., *Sperimentale*, 1894, **48**, Sez. biol., 407): in the presence of so much other argument about the concept of Banti's disease (or syndrome), this seems a pointless semantic complication.

branches of the splenic artery; in other cases no obstructive lesions are found and it is presumed that infarction has then resulted from ischaemia due to inadequacy of an unimpeded blood supply to meet the circulatory needs of the progressively enlarging organ. Sickle cell anaemia is another condition in which functional ischaemia causes infarction (see below).

Torsion.—Splenic torsion is a rare occurrence and always associated with congenital anomalies of the peritoneal folds that connect the spleen to the stomach and the posterior abdominal wall. Partial or total haemorrhagic infarction results, and the infarcted spleen may rupture spontaneously.

Sickle Cell Anaemia.—Patients with the sickle cell trait (haemoglobin AS trait—see page 470), sickle cell anaemia (haemoglobin SS disease—see page 469) or 'haemoglobin SC disease' (see page 470) may suffer acute ischaemic episodes while flying at high altitudes unless the cabin pressure is enough to maintain the oxygen tension at a level that will not induce sickling. Splenic infarction[941] and infarction of bone (see Chapter 37) are the more frequent of these episodes. Similar splenic lesions are a frequent occurrence in the ordinary course of sickle cell anaemia: some are clinically silent and others are accompanied by pain over the spleen or in the region of the left shoulder, as a consequence of involvement of the serosa covering the splenic capsule, with the local development of fibrinous peritonitis. The eventual atrophy of the spleen that may result is referred to on page 727.

Polyarteritis

Polyarteritis is a cause of multiple foci of necrosis and of larger areas of infarction in the spleen. In some cases there is such extensive confluent necrosis that the appearances are those of one variety of the so-called 'speckled spleen' (*Fleckmilz*),[942, 943] which formerly was attributed to uraemia. The changes in the spleen are the result of ischaemia and are due to occlusion of vessels involved in the arteritis. The association with uraemia reflects the presence of the severe glomerulitis that may be a specific accompaniment of polyarteritis (see Chapter 24).

Polyarteritis may be associated with acute inflammation of the capsule and trabeculae of the spleen ('capsulitis' and 'trabeculitis').[944] The changes in the capsule usually do not extend to the overlying serosa. There is some degree of necrosis of the affected fibrous tissue, but this is generally liquefactive and without fibrinoid characteristics. The

cellular infiltrate consists of neutrophils, alone or with some admixture of eosinophils, and sometimes there is an epithelioid cell histiocytic reaction at the periphery (Fig. 9.166). As in lymph nodes (see page 693), there may be a curious granulomatous alteration of the splenic follicles (Fig. 9.167).[944] The folliculitis, like the inflammation of the capsule and trabeculae, may be the manifestation of lesions of the capillaries or of the connective tissue elements themselves; they are part of the pathological picture of polyartertis. Similar changes may be seen in some related diseases, particularly *anaphylactoid purpura*.

Wegener's Disease.—A variety of 'speckled spleen' that is characterized by the presence of many small necrotic foci, macroscopically somewhat resembling miliary tubercles, is seen in Wegener's disease (see page 214).

Acquired Peculiarities of Splenic Arterioles

Hyalinization.—Hyaline change in the walls of the small trabecular arteries and, more frequently and

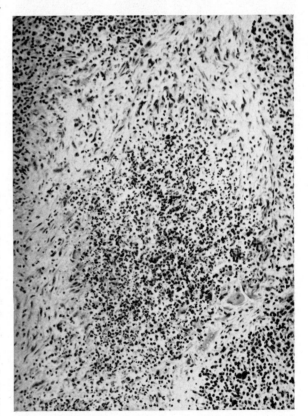

Fig. 9.166. Necrotizing splenic trabeculitis in a case of polyarteritis. There is an accumulation of neutrophils in the necrotic area. *Haematoxylin–eosin.* × 135.

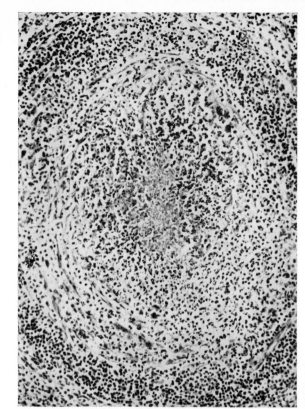

Fig. 9.167. Necrotizing splenic folliculitis in another case of polyarteritis. The necrotic centre of the follicle is surrounded by a zone of infiltration by neutrophils that merges into a peripheral zone of proliferation of histiocytes and fibroblasts. This lesion of polyarteritis develops in the connective tissue of the follicle and seems not to involve the central arteriole primarily. In some instances the arteriole remains patent and unaffected at the margin of the necrotic focus. *Haematoxylin–eosin.* ×135.

markedly, of the arterioles in the white pulp is invariably present in some degree in elderly people and is often conspicuous in the spleen of healthy young adults. Although the microscopical appearance of the vessels is very like that of the arteriolosclerosis of the benign phase of essential hypertension (see pages 134 and 175), there is no evidence that this change in the splenic vasculature has any relation to blood pressure.

Laminar Periarteriolar Sclerosis.—In *sarcoidosis,*[945] and more strikingly in *systemic lupus erythematosus* (Fig. 9.168),[946] a peculiar concentric fibrosis sometimes develops round the arteriole in the splenic follicles. This laminar or 'onion scale' periarteriolar sclerosis may be seen also round small arteries and arterioles in the lymph nodes and tonsils in these

diseases. In sarcoidosis, typically, the collagen fibres contributing to the sclerosis are uniform in appearance, hyaline, discrete and only lightly stained by eosin. The rest of the wall of the vessel shows no notable abnormality. In systemic lupus erythematosus the fibres are more variable in thickness and staining intensity, often showing patches of intense eosinophilia and the presence of fibrinoid material, with foci of necrosis. The rest of the vessel wall shows in varying degree the changes of a fibrinoid or necrotizing angitis. Similar changes are seen round splenic arterioles in some cases of *Felty's syndrome* (see page 690).[947]

Inflammatory Conditions of the Spleen
Perisplenitis

Perisplenitis is an accompaniment of many pathological states of the spleen.

Acute Perisplenitis.—Acute perisplenitis, with fibrinous exudate on the serosal surface, may occur in

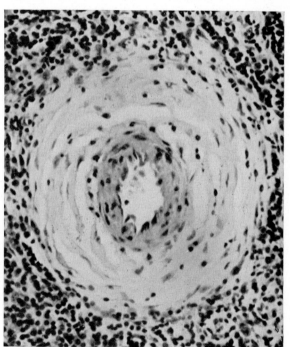

Fig. 9.168. Concentric fibrosis round the arteriole of a splenic follicle in a case of systemic lupus erythematosus. The lesion is quiescent, with little oedema and cellular infiltrate; the fibrous tissue is mature collagen and the fibroblasts are inconspicuous. The patient had been under treatment with corticosteroids for many weeks before her death from an intercurrent fungal infection. There had been a good clinical response to the treatment. *Haematoxylin–eosin.* ×245.

cases of the so-called 'acute splenic tumour' associated with acute septicaemic illnesses (see below). In a localized form, mainly confined to the serosa overlying the lesion, it is an accompaniment of infarcts and it is responsible for the pain that these may cause.

Adhesions.—Fibrous adhesions between the spleen and adjacent structures are common in association with any form of chronic splenomegaly, particularly when this is of infective origin. By restricting the mobility of the spleen they predispose to its rupture.

Chronic Perisplenitis.—A pearly white thickening of the splenic capsule, cartilaginous in consistency, may accompany almost any type of chronic splenomegaly. Its distribution may be patchy, or the entire serosal surface of the organ may be involved. The lesion consists of dense, hyaline, collagenous tissue; except where there are adhesions its outer surface is covered by normal serosal cells.

A similar condition of the spleen occurs as part of a more widespread hyalinization of the peritoneum —for example, in cases of polyserositis (see page 1184) and occasionally as an accompaniment of asbestosis (see page 383).

Generalized Infections and the Spleen

The filter-like function of the spleen in relation to the blood circulating through it commonly results in its involvement in generalized infections. In given circumstances, virtually any of the infections that are discussed in this chapter under the heading of lymphadenitis (see pages 572 to 669) may involve the spleen in the course of spread by the blood stream.

The Spleen in Acute Septicaemic Diseases

In cases of acute septicaemia the spleen may be twice to three times larger than normal. In spite of its size it is seldom palpable on clinical examination, being unusually soft. This type of splenomegaly used to be known as 'acute splenic tumour'. The pulp is dull greyish red, and often diffluent, so that gently squeezing the organ causes its substance to flow out as a thick, semifluid ooze.

Microscopically, the pulp is hyperaemic and very cellular. In most cases the reticulum cells and endothelial macrophages are swollen and increased in number, but the predominating cell type depends to some extent on the type of infection: thus, the spleen of *typhoid and paratyphoid infection* is packed with the mononuclear cells that are characteristic of the

enteric fevers (see page 575), while in *lobar pneumonia* and other cases of *infection by pyogenic bacteria* there are abundant neutrophils. Many of the cells show degenerative changes, but foci of necrosis are unlikely to be found except in typhoid fever and in the true suppurative splenitis of, for instance, staphylococcal septicaemia (pyaemia).

In *anthrax* the spleen is considerably enlarged, soft, and turgid with dark, often unusually viscous blood, and there is extensive haemorrhagic necrosis. The darkness of the blood and the frequent lack of post-mortem clotting are particularly characteristic, the colour accounting for the name, anthrax, and for its equivalents in several other languages, such as the French *charbon*. The German name for the disease, *Milzbrand*, and the former dialectal English milt-brand, both conveying the sense of a burning, inflammation, or gangrene of the spleen, represent the striking gross appearance of the spleen of anthrax. There is usually a marked perisplenitis, with the bacilli present in large numbers in the capsule and overlying exudate as well as throughout the intensely hyperaemic, fibrin-permeated pulp (Fig. 9.169).

The Spleen in Chronic Septicaemic Diseases

In the more chronic forms of septicaemic illness, such as subacute bacterial endocarditis and chronic meningococcal septicaemia, the spleen is palpably enlarged and firm. Its clinical enlargement in these conditions is of considerable diagnostic importance. Macroscopically, its colour is darker than normal, but there is usually sufficient hyperplasia of the lymphoid tissue for the follicles to be readily seen on the cut surface. Microscopically, lymphoid hyperplasia, with conspicuous germinal centres, an increase in the amount of reticulin in the pulp, and proliferation of large mononuclear cells—including immunoblasts—are the main features.

Acute and Chronic Forms of Granulomatous Bacterial Splenitis

Granulomatous splenitis may occur in a range of bacterial infections, including tuberculosis (see below) and the secondary and tertiary stages of syphilis. In exceptional cases of yersinial mesenteric lymphadenitis (see page 584), generalized yersinial infection develops: the spleen is involved regularly in these cases and shows lesions comparable to those in the nodes. Similarly, granulomatous foci are to be found in the spleen in cases of tularaemia (see page 586) and of the granulomatous form of brucella infection (see page 591).[948]

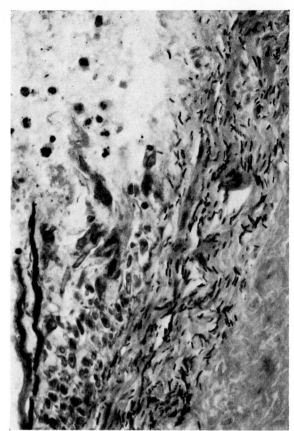

Fig. 9.169. Spleen in anthrax. The field is from the margin of the rupture in the capsule that was the immediate cause of death. The elastic lamella that underlies the serosa extends up the lower half of the left side of the picture. The rest of the fibroelastic tunic of the spleen has disintegrated toward the top of the field. Its deeper layers contain large numbers of anthrax bacilli. The substance of the spleen (below, right) is replaced by fibrin. Same case as Fig. 9.56, page 579. *Gram.* × 370.

Tuberculosis of the Spleen and Non-Infective Forms of Granulomatous Splenitis

The spleen is always involved in cases of generalized miliary tuberculosis. All other forms of splenic tuberculosis are rare. They include caseating splenitis as an accompaniment of generalized caseating tuberculous lymphadenitis (see page 601) and necrotizing splenitis as an accompaniment of acute non-reactive haematogenous tuberculosis (see page 602).

Tuberculous splenomegaly as the sole manifestation of tuberculosis has been described occasionally. It seems likely that most such cases may be instances of sarcoidosis (see page 747) or of the so-called Stengel–Wolbach sclerosis (see page 685): this is consistent with the fact that the histological picture is often described as 'non-caseating tuberculosis'. Very rarely, however, multiple, large and confluent caseous granulomas, from which tubercle bacilli have been isolated, have been found in the spleen in the absence of any evidence of active infection in other parts of the body. In one such case the patient, evidently a previously healthy man, died of rapidly developing tuberculous peritonitis following traumatic rupture of the caseous spleen.[949]

Infection of the Spleen by Actinomycetes and True Fungi

Any blood-borne fungus may set up infection in the spleen, but with few exceptions the resulting lesions are no more than incidental to the course of a generalized infection, whether that be a rapidly progressive 'opportunistic' complication of some other disease or the dissemination of an infection by a primary pathogen, such as *Histoplasma capsulatum*.

The pathological changes in the spleen, and the problems relating to the identification of the causal organism, are basically the same as in cases of infection of other parts of the body. These are considered in relation to the lungs in Chapter 7 (Volume 1, pages 346 to 360) and in relation to lymph nodes in this chapter (pages 616 to 630).

Infection by *Histoplasma capsulatum*, because in some cases it causes remarkable lesions in the spleen, may be referred to at greater length.

Histoplasmosis

Multifocal Calcification of the Spleen.—In some areas where there is a very high level of endemicity of infection by *Histoplasma capsulatum*, as in the Ohio-Mississippi Valley in the United States of America, where up to 90 per cent or more of the population react to the histoplasmin skin test, it is common to find foci of calcification in the spleen at necropsy.[950] These range from 0·1 to 5·0 cm across, although rarely larger than 1·0 cm. They are the end result of the benign, self-limiting, haematogenous dissemination of the infection that accompanies the development of the primary focus, or foci, in the lungs, most commonly in childhood.[951] While the infection is active there is no difficulty in detecting the histoplasmas within the cytoplasm of the macrophages, which soon form epithelioid cell aggregates that eventually undergo central caseation. As the foci enlarge they become encapsulate and ultimately they calcify. The histoplasmas may long continue to be demonstrable in the caseous core of these lesions; their detection commonly depends on the use of the hexamine (methenamine) silver procedure (see page 616), which shows the fungal cells well even when they are dead and no longer have an affinity for other stains. The condition is usually asymptomatic throughout its course.[952]

This type of multifocal splenic calcification resulting from histoplasmosis has to be distinguished from other conditions that may cause focal calcification in the spleen. These include tuberculosis, especially successfully treated miliary or submiliary tuberculosis, and sarcoidosis, brucella infection,[953] schistosomiasis and—although not as strikingly as in histoplasmosis—some other fungal infections, including cryptococcosis, 'North American' blastomycosis and paracoccidioidomycosis.

'Infantile' Disseminated Histoplasmosis.[954]—In the so-called 'infantile' form of rapidly progressive haematogenous dissemination of histoplasmic infection, the spleen is strikingly involved. It is markedly enlarged, and histological examination shows the red pulp, including the pulp cords, to be distended by great numbers of heavily parasitized macrophages. It can be difficult to make out cell boundaries or any landmarks of the original structure of the spleen. There is commonly extensive necrosis of the infected tissue. This form of the infection occurs mainly in infancy; exceptionally, it is seen in older patients, and then usually—but not always—when their resistance has been severely lowered by diseases that interfere with immunity or by treatment that has a comparable effect.[949]

Infectious Mononucleosis[955]

Splenomegaly is not a constant clinical finding in infectious mononucleosis (see pages 476 and 647). Specimens become available for examination only in the rare cases in which, as a result of the infection, 'spontaneous' rupture has occurred, generally in the 3rd or 4th week after the clinical onset of the disease. The reason for the predisposition to rupture is imperfectly understood, although usually attributed to weakening of the capsule by oedema and cellular infiltration.

In some cases the pulp cords and sinuses are stuffed with the pale, atypical cells that are characteristic of the disease (see page 650). The capsule and trabeculae are infiltrated also. In other cases the cytological picture is more complex, as there is a widespread accumulation in the pulp of normal-looking lymphocytes and of cells that may be variously interpreted as immunoblasts or reticulum cells. The splenic follicles are inconspicuous in most cases and germinal centres are usually lacking.

Protozoal Infections

Malaria

In the various types of *acute malaria* the spleen is moderately enlarged, due mainly to hyperaemia, together with some proliferation of macrophages, which are engaged in phagocytosis of the parasites.

In *chronic malaria* the spleen commonly weighs from 1 to 2 kg. It may even reach some 7 kg. It is characteristically slate-coloured, due to the presence of the haematin-like malarial pigment (see page 667). Its firm or hard consistency is associated with considerable friability, accounting for its proneness to rupture. There is a moderate increase in the amount of fibrous tissue throughout the organ. The greater part of its enlargement results from proliferation of macrophages in the pulp: these cells are packed with pigment derived from breakdown of the parasitized erythrocytes—the pigment is mainly the specific malarial pigment, but there is some admixture of haemosiderin.*

Leishmaniasis

Splenomegaly is so characteristic of visceral leishmaniasis (kala azar) that the disease was known formerly as 'tropical splenomegaly', a term that is used nowadays with other meanings (see page 743). Similarly, in Malta, where the disease is seen mainly in young children, the vernacular name, now obsolete, means 'splenic disease' (see page 661). However, the splenic involvement is but part of what is in fact a systemic infection of the lymphoreticular system (see page 658). Leishmaniasis is essentially a form of obligate intracellular parasitization of macrophages. The resemblance of the histological picture to that of histoplasmosis, the classic example of obligate intracellular parasitism among the fungal infections, can lead to confusion between the two diseases (see above and page 624).

---

* In one of the continuing sequence of cases of fatal, clinically unrecognized, cerebral malaria seen in recent years in north-western Europe among travellers returned from malarial regions, the striking slaty pigmentation (see page 1234) of the spleen, liver and lymph nodes was misinterpreted at necropsy, leading to a search for confirmation of a suggestion that the patient must have had ochronosis (alkaptonuria) or argyrosis. The correct diagnosis was made when the typical appearances in the small blood vessels in the brain were recognized on histological examination (as illustrated, for instance, in Fig. 34.55B in Volume 5).

Other Protozoal Infections

Trypanosomiasis.—Splenomegaly is among the manifestations of the acute phase of American trypanosomiasis (Chagas's disease—see page 665). It is commonly found at necropsy in cases of African trypanosomiasis: while causes other than trypanosomal infection may be responsible for the splenic enlargement in the African environment, proliferation of histiocytes and an accumulation of plasma cells in the pulp have been observed and are comparable to the changes in lymph nodes infected by the trypanosomes (see page 664).[956]

Toxoplasmosis.—There may be splenomegaly in cases of acute congenital toxoplasmosis. Rarely, the spleen is palpable in cases of the acquired infection in children and in adults (see page 653). In one instance, in an adult, splenectomy was performed as part of a 'staging' investigation (see page 772) following a histological misdiagnosis of toxoplasmic lymphadenitis as Hodgkin's disease: there were typical epithelioid cell clusters in the lymphoid tissue of the spleen, exactly comparable to those in lymph nodes infected by the toxoplasma.[949]

Metazoal Infestation and the Spleen

Nematode Infestation

Any of the nematodes that pass a phase of their life cycle within the tissues, migrating in the blood stream or directly traversing the substance of the viscera, may be found in the spleen. Very occasionally, the characteristic lesions of '*visceral larva migrans*' (see page 671) are seen in the spleen—for example, during the initial migration of the larvae in cases of ascariasis (page 671), toxocariasis (page 671), strongyloidiasis (page 671) and ancylostomiasis (see page 672).

Filariasis.—In cases of filariasis caused by *Wuchereria bancrofti* (see page 674), microfilariae may be found intact in the blood in the sinuses of the pulp. They may die, provoking the development of tuberculoid granulomas:[956a] these range in size from microscopical dimensions up to confluent nodules that may reach a few centimetres in diameter.[957] Microfilarial granulomas may also be found in the spleen in cases of occult filariasis (see page 675),[958] which may be associated with infestation by either *Wuchereria bancrofti* or *Brugia malayi*. In cases of filariasis caused by *Brugia malayi* the earliest stages in the formation of granulomas round microfilariae are seen most frequently within the pulp cords,[959] an observation that may mean no more than that it

is easier for the parasite to enter the cord in the circulating blood than to escape from it, with the result that it dies there.

Cestode Infestation

Although the occasional cysticercus may develop in the spleen in cases of widespread *cysticercosis*, the lesion is unlikely to be discovered other than by chance (see page 677).

Echinococcosis.[960]—The most frequent manifestation of cestodiasis in the spleen is the development of a *hydatid cyst* (see page 1238). This may be of any size up to 15 cm or so in diameter. Sometimes more than one cyst is present, and sometimes these are of different age, to judge from the wide variation in their appearance from typical, unilocular lesions containing innumerable brood capsules ('hydatid sand'), through those containing large numbers of daughter and granddaughter cysts to those that have become effete and appear as inspissated, shrunken, solid masses (see Fig. 21.39, page 1240) that may be in part calcified. Most hydatid cysts that develop in the spleen are of the simple unilocular variety.

The presence of a hydatid cyst predisposes to rupture of the spleen. This carries the hazard of dissemination of the infestation throughout the abdominal cavity. There is also the immediate danger of fatal anaphylactic shock.

Trematode Infestation

Schistosomiasis.—Splenomegaly is so characteristic a feature of many cases of infestation by *Schistosoma mansoni* that 'Egyptian splenomegaly' was long a familiar synonym of this type of schistosomiasis. It is now known that this species of fluke has a distribution far beyond the valley and delta of the Nile: it occurs throughout a vast area of tropical Africa and parts of southern Africa, and in large areas of Brazil and some other parts of tropical South America, with extension into some of the Caribbean islands. The enlargement of the spleen is a manifestation of portal hypertension (congestive splenomegaly—see page 730).

Once they have reached maturity in the liver, the adult forms of *Schistosoma mansoni* live mainly in the rectal and other intestinal veins, to which they migrate in the portal venous system, against the blood flow. Occasional adult pairs enter the splenic vein and, with care, may be recognized in the lumen of the larger tributaries of the main vein on examination of splenectomy specimens. This may explain the occasional finding of ova in the splenic trabeculae and their immediate vicinity, mainly in the hilar region of the spleen. Ova are found only seldom in the spleen, in contrast to the liver, to which they are carried in the portal blood stream.

Infestation by *Schistosoma japonicum* produces lesions of distribution and character similar to those caused by *Schistosoma mansoni* (see page 1237).

Schistosoma haematobium, which ordinarily is confined to the pelvic venous plexuses, with predominant involvement of the urinary bladder (see Chapter 25), is not a cause of splenic changes. It may be present in addition to *Schistosoma mansoni* in patients who have lived in those parts of Africa where both species are prevalent.

Liver Fluke Infestation.—Very rarely, a metacercaria of *Fasciola hepatica*, having reached the peritoneal cavity penetrates the capsule of the spleen instead of that of the liver (see page 1235). If this happens, the parasite dies, and its remnants may be found, particularly when splenectomy is performed in the course of surgical treatment of hepatic infestation.

Pentastomiasis

Larvae of *Linguatula serrata* and of *Armillifer* species may be found in the spleen (see pages 680 and 1242).

Other Non-Neoplastic Diseases of the Spleen

Many other conditions that have been considered in the section on lymph nodes earlier in this chapter—for example, hydantoin lymphadenopathy (page 697), immunoblastic lymphadenopathy (page 702) and primary macroglobulinaemia (page 706)—may cause splenomegaly and histological changes in the spleen that correspond to those in the lymph nodes. These need not be referred to further here.

Some lesions that are not appropriately dealt with elsewhere are described in this section.

Fibrotic Nodules

Fibrotic nodules, ranging from a few millimetres to a few centimetres in diameter, are sometimes found in the spleen at necropsy or in splenectomy specimens. Some of them may be healed granulomas, particularly if there is calcification: tuberculous and syphilitic lesions, lesions due to histoplasma infection or other mycoses, and the end result of a metazoal encystment (particularly in pentastomiasis) are among many diagnostic suggestions that may be put forward, often with little hope of confirmation. Localized ischaemic lesions are thought to account for some, particularly those that are continuous with the capsule, which may be indrawn in the shape of a cleft or funnel-like depression: such lesions may be the end result of organization of infarcts, and sometimes they are heavily pigmented with haemosiderin. In some cases of sickle cell disease pigmented nodules and more irregular scars are a feature of the progressive atrophy of the spleen that eventually converts it into a shrunken remnant (see page 727).

Siderofibrotic nodules that are much smaller than those of ischaemic origin, measuring no more than a few millimetres in diameter, are a typical feature of the spleen of portal hypertension ('congestive splenomegaly'). These are the so-called Gandy–Gamna nodules, which are the sequelae of haemorrhage from the arterioles in splenic follicles (see page 731). They contain a large amount of haemosiderin (see Fig. 9.165, page 731).

Unpigmented fibrotic nodules, ranging from a few millimetres to a centimetre or so in diameter, have been found in the spleen in almost 5 per cent of necropsies in some African communities, particularly in Uganda.[961] This incidence is considerably higher than in white people in the same environment The origin of these foci is uncertain.

Storage Diseases

Splenomegaly is one of the more constant clinical findings in cases of the various inborn errors of metabolism that result in the accumulation of lipids or other metabolites in the cytoplasm of reticuloendothelial cells throughout the body. These diseases are considered in the section beginning on page 757.

Cystic Lesions[962]

Cystic lesions are rare in the spleen. The most frequent are larval forms of metazoal parasites.

Parasitic Cysts.—Cystic forms of metazoal parasites that may be found in the spleen include hydatid cysts and cysticerci (see page 737) and pentastomid larvae (see page 680). Hydatid disease is the least rarely recognized of these conditions: it should be considered whenever any cystic lesion is found in the spleen—for instance, as an incidental observation at laparotomy.

Epithelial Cysts.—The epithelial cysts that may be found in the spleen are usually unilocular and solitary. They are generally lined by an epidermal type of epithelium and contain fatty, pasty debris such as is characteristic of *epidermoid cysts* in any situation. In a minority of instances the wall includes hair follicles and sebaceous glands: such cysts are classed as *dermoid cysts*. Very rarely, a unilocular cyst in the spleen is lined by a single layer of mucigenic epithelial cells: accidental rupture of such a cyst while performing a partial gastrectomy was followed by the gradual development of 'pseudomyxoma' of the peritoneal cavity (see page 1195).[963]

The origin of the epithelial cysts of the spleen is unclear. They have been attributed to developmental misplacement of epithelial tissue and to metaplasia (although what tissue is supposed to have become metaplastic is not certain).

Pseudocysts.—Liquefaction of splenic infarcts or of angiomas that have undergone extensive thrombosis leads to the development of cyst-like lesions containing opaque or cloudy, yellowish, semifluid or fluid material. These pseudocysts are often multiloculate. Some of them tend to enlarge progressively, possibly through osmosis, eventually reaching a diameter of 20 cm and more. They may rupture, especially the larger ones; this is sometimes a complication of haemorrhage into their cavity, in which case there may be catastrophic bleeding into the abdominal cavity.

Tumours of the Spleen

Benign Tumours and Tumour-Like Lesions[964]

Benign tumours of the spleen, including hamartomas, are rare.

Hamartomas of Splenic Tissue[965]

Hamartomas that are formed of splenic tissue are uncommon, but they are the least rare of the benign tumours and tumour-like lesions of the spleen. They are formed either of lymphoid tissue ('white pulp hamartomas') or of a complex of sinuses and structures that are equivalent to the pulp cords of normal splenic tissue ('red pulp hamartomas'); some are a mixture of both types of tissue (Fig. 9.170). They are quite well defined, but usually unencapsulate, rounded nodules, situated within the substance of the spleen and seldom outside the range of 2 to 4 cm in diameter. Occasionally there are two or more; when multiple, the hamartomas may represent both structural types.

These lesions are sometimes referred to by the

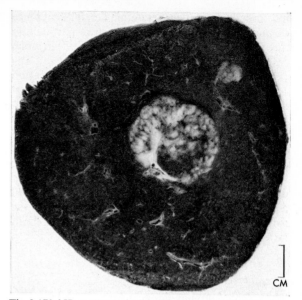

Fig. 9.170.§ Hamartomas in the spleen ('intrasplenic accessory spleens'). Two well-defined, pale masses stand slightly above the plane of the cut surface of the organ, one at its centre and one above and to the right. They are formed mainly of lymphoid tissue ('white pulp hamartomas'), although the larger has a substantial 'red pulp' component, which appears dark in the photograph because of its content of blood. The condition was an incidental post-mortem finding in a case of fatal coronary artery thrombosis.

term 'nodular hyperplasia of the spleen'. They are also called 'intrasplenic accessory spleens', splenomas, fibrosplenomas, splenadenomas, lienomas and 'benign lymphomas' of the spleen.

They have been associated with the syndrome of hypersplenism (see page 724).[919]

Haemangioma

The haemangioma is second in frequency to the hamartoma of splenic tissue among the benign tumours of the spleen. It is generally considered to be a vascular hamartoma.[966] Like the haemangioma of the liver (see page 1285), it is usually a small lesion, seldom exceeding 2 cm in any dimension, solitary, and found incidentally at necropsy or laparotomy. It is not encapsulate, and its vascular channels and caverns insinuate themselves between the surrounding splenic elements; their lumen communicates directly with that of the sinuses. Occasionally, a splenic haemangioma is so large that it occupies most of the organ, which may be sufficiently enlarged to become palpable. The larger angiomas may undergo thrombosis, and then— when the thrombus liquefies—become converted into pseudocystic, degenerate masses. The presence of multiple angiomas in the spleen is particularly rare; hypersplenism has been observed in such cases (see page 724).[918]

Thrombocytopenia associated with sequestration of platelets in splenic angiomas is referred to on the page opposite.

A haemangioma of the spleen may be associated with widespread haemangiomatosis, involving particularly the skin and the liver.[967] In one case a large cavernous haemangioma of the spleen was associated with hereditary telangiectasia (Rendu–Osler–Weber disease—see page 166) and multiple congenital aneurysms of the splenic artery;[968] aneurysms of the splenic artery were found in another case of hereditary telangiectasia.[969]

Lymphangioma

The splenic lymphangioma is rather rarer than the haemangioma. It is a hamartoma, like the latter, and in most instances is in continuity with the capsule or main trabeculae of the spleen, which accords with the view that lymphatics in the spleen are confined to these structures.

Other Benign Tumours and Tumour-Like Lesions

Fibromas, *chondromas* and *osteomas* have been said to occur in the spleen. Their nature is doubtful: some, at least, are the end result of scarring, with metaplastic formation of cartilage or bone—for example, following infarction.

Malignant Diseases of the Spleen

Lymphomas

Splenomegaly may be the first clinical manifestation of any of the lymphomas (see pages 784 to 850). It is exceptional for involvement of the spleen not to develop at some time in their natural course.

The role of diagnostic splenectomy in determining the extent of the disease in cases of Hodgkin's disease and of other lymphomas is considered on page 773.

Leukaemia and Polycythaemia

Splenomegaly is a regular feature of the leukaemias and of polycythaemia vera (see Chapter 8). The greatest enlargement of the spleen is seen in cases of myeloid leukaemia, in which its weight has been known to reach 15 kg.

Angiosarcoma

The spleen is one of the less rare sites of angiosarcoma. When this tumour arises in the spleen its development may be accompanied by macrocytic anaemia.[970] The explanation of this association is not known; it has been attributed to hypersplenism (see page 724), although this does not appear to explain the macrocytosis.

Secondary Tumours

Macroscopically evident secondary tumours are found in the spleen in about four[971] to eight[972] per cent of necropsies in cases of cancer (Fig. 9.171), and in about twice as many cases of widespread carcinomatosis if the spleen is thoroughly examined microscopically.[972] In this context, 'widespread' carcinomatosis is often defined as the presence of metastatic tumour deposits in at least one organ in both the thoracic cavity and the abdominal cavity,[973] and a 'thorough' microscopical examination entails sectioning at least ten blocks of splenic tissue in each case, selected at random.[972]

A formerly traditional view that the spleen is rarely the site of secondary tumours is not supported by such observations, although they do not necessarily dispose of the hypothesis—based on that

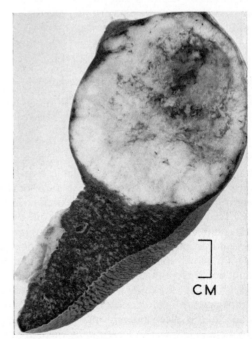

Fig. 9.171.§ A large metastatic deposit of carcinoma in a spleen. The primary growth was in the bronchial tree. Secondary tumours of such a size are particularly infrequent in the spleen.

belief—that there may be a splenic factor inimical to the establishment and growth of tumour deposits. The suggestion that there is an antitumour factor in the spleen has found theoretical support in the growing knowledge of the role of lymphocytes in immunity, including immune mechanisms that may be evident in certain types of cancer. However, no good evidence seems as yet to have been produced that supports this thesis demonstrably.

The primary tumours likeliest to give origin to secondary deposits in the spleen are melanoma, carcinomas of lung, breast and ovary, and chorio-carcinoma.

The Spleen in Non-Neoplastic Diseases of the Blood

The role of the spleen in certain blood diseases, including the *haemolytic anaemias* (see pages 462 to 473) and *thrombocytopenia* (see pages 491 to 494), is considered in Chapter 8. *Infectious mononucleosis* is considered on page 736 and—in relation to rupture of the spleen—on page 728. Some particular aspects of splenic pathology in relation to these and other non-neoplastic diseases of the blood may be considered in more detail here.

Sequestration of Deformed Red Blood Cells in Sickle Cell Anaemia and Other Diseases

Abnormal red cells—for example, spherocytes, elliptocytes and sickle cells (drepanocytes)—become sequestered in the pulp cords of the spleen. The explanation of this occurrence is uncertain. It may be that the deformed cells cannot readily pass from the cords to the sinuses, and they may be more liable to phagocytosis (see page 720). In some instances the accumulation of pathological red cells in the pulp cords not only leads to an extraordinary distension of the latter, with corresponding compression of the sinuses, but may cause the patient's death as a direct consequence of this internal loss of blood from the circulation. For example, a baby with haemoglobin SS disease developed pneumonia: the accompanying hypoxia caused exceptionally severe sickling, and it was estimated that half his red cell mass had become sequestered in the pulp cords of the spleen, death resulting.[974]

The characteristic sequence of changes in the spleen in typical cases of sickle cell anaemia, from enlargement to extreme atrophy, is described on page 727.

L

Splenic Histiocytosis in Blood Disorders

Proliferation of large, pale histiocytes may occur in the spleen in various conditions. This is, of course, characteristic of the various storage diseases (see page 757), such as Gaucher's disease and Niemann–Pick disease, and of some cases of Whipple's disease (see page 556): in these conditions there is histiocytosis throughout the reticuloendothelial system, and specific cytological and cytochemical features enable them to be identified. A somewhat similar histiocytosis is seen in the spleen following lymphangiography and results from access of the oily contrast medium to the blood (see page 567).

Sometimes, in the absence of any recognized cause, small collections of coarsely vacuolate histiocytes are seen in the pulp adjoining the splenic follicles.[974a]

A quite comparable, but less marked, histiocytosis occurs in the spleen in various disorders of the blood. In these cases the histiocytosis is usually confined to the spleen, which may be little, if at all, enlarged. It has been observed most frequently in cases of thrombocytopenia, both idiopathic[975] and secondary to sequestration of platelets within the vasculature of angiomas, particularly in cases of splenic angiomatosis[976] but also in association with the Kasabach–Merritt syndrome (thrombocytopenic purpura resulting from extensive platelet thrombosis in large haemangiomas in any part of the body—see page 493). Similar findings have been recorded in cases of haemolytic anaemia, particularly thalassaemia (see page 469),[977] and of hypoplastic anaemia (see page 460), the Felty syndrome (rheumatoid arthritis, splenomegaly and leucopenia) and acute leukaemia.[978]

In the form of splenic histiocytosis that accompanies blood disorders, the proliferating histiocytes range from 20 to 40 μm in diameter, have a single small nucleus and 'foamy' cytoplasm, and are distributed singly or in clusters in the red pulp (Fig. 9.172), where they are found in the sinuses or—more characteristically—in the pulp cords. They are rarely seen in the lymphoid tissue. They contain phospholipids, particularly sphingomyelin, and polysaccharides; the reason for their development is not known. It has been suggested that it is a result of the use of corticosteroids or their analogues in treating the blood disease, but this cannot be the only explanation as the same picture may be seen in the absence of this or other possibly significant medication. It is likely that the histiocytes contain breakdown products of the pathological blood cells or platelets.[976]

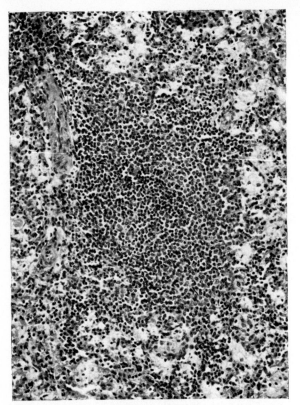

Fig. 9.172.§ Histiocytosis in the spleen in a case of idiopathic thrombocytopenic purpura. Most of the histiocytes have clear cytoplasm. They occur singly or in small clusters in the red pulp; they are not present within the follicle. A comparable picture may be seen in other diseases of the blood (see text). Splenic histiocytosis of this type must be distinguished from the histiocytosis of storage diseases (see Fig. 9.185, page 766). *Haematoxylin–eosin.* × 140.

Myelosclerosis[979]

In cases of myelosclerosis (myelofibrosis), the effects of progressive obliteration of the haemopoietic tissue of the bone marrow by fibrous tissue induces the re-establishment of extramedullary haemopoiesis, which normally ceases early in infancy (see page 721). The spleen may become greatly enlarged as this 'myeloid metaplasia' develops; it may weigh as much as 7 kg. It is friable, and prone to rupture through minor trauma (including aspiration biopsy —'splenic puncture'). Infarcts are commonly found but usually are silent clinically and have no functional consequences.

The pathological findings are modified by the nature of the associated haematological abnormalities, if any are present. Myelosclerosis may develop as a complication of polycythaemia vera, thrombocythaemia and, more rarely, chronic

myeloid leukaemia. Rather oftener it develops in the absence of these. It is rare before middle life, and most of the patients present in the 6th or 7th decade. Splenomegaly is sometimes the presenting manifestation.

Splenomegaly

With few exceptions pathological changes in the spleen lead to an increase in its size. Splenomegaly is consequently an important and frequent clinical finding, although its cause may be difficult to trace in individual cases. This is not the place to discuss the factors that may prevent an enlarged spleen from being palpable; it may be noted, though, that in an adult of average build, with normal abdominal musculature and no considerable excess of fat in the abdominal wall, a spleen of usual consistency weighing under 300 g is unlikely to be palpable.

An exhaustive list of causes of splenomegaly is not called for, as it is easy to compile one from knowledge of the diseases that affect the spleen. A skeleton classification into which the individual causes can be fitted may be considered instead.

Basic Classification of Splenomegaly

1. Splenomegaly associated with circulatory disturbances—
   (a) systemic venous congestion
   (b) portal hypertension ('congestive splenomegaly')
2. Splenomegaly associated with the accumulation of abnormal substances or of normal substances in abnormal amounts—
   (a) amyloidosis
   (b) storage diseases
3. Splenomegaly due to infection and other inflammatory states—
   (a) acute and chronic bacterial septicaemias (*e.g.*, coccal infections, including lobar pneumonia and meningococcal infection; subacute infective endocarditis; typhoid fever; tularaemia; and others)
   (b) tuberculosis; sarcoidosis; other tuberculoid granulomas
   (c) spirochaetal infections (*e.g.*, relapsing fever due to *Borrelia recurrentis* infection; relapsing fever due to *Spirillum minus* infection [Japanese rat-bite fever])
   (d) fungal infections (Fig. 9.99, page 628)
   (e) rickettsial infections (*e.g.*, Rocky Mountains spotted fever; typhus fever)
   (f) viral infections (*e.g.*, infectious mononucleosis)

(g) protozoal infections (*e.g.*, malaria, kala azar)

(h) metazoal infestation (*e.g.*, schistosomiasis —see page 678, and Fig. 9.131, page 679)

(i) lymphoid hyperplasia associated with arthritis (*e.g.*, Felty's syndrome)

4. Splenomegaly associated with diseases characterized by excessive destruction of the formed elements of the blood

5. 'Non-tropical idiopathic splenomegaly'

6. 'Tropical idiopathic splenomegaly'

7. Splenomegaly due to benign tumours (including hamartomas) and cysts

8. Splenomegaly associated with malignant diseases—

(a) malignant blood diseases (leukaemia; polycythaemia vera)

(b) systemic lymphomas

(c) primary cancer of the spleen (*e.g.*, angiosarcoma)

(d) metastatic tumours.

The commonest, and most important, causes of clinically detectable splenomegaly in most temperate countries include *leukaemia* and *subacute infective endocarditis*. Haematological examination must never be omitted in the case of any patient who is found to have an enlarged spleen, however clearly the associated clinical findings may seem to suggest some cause other than leukaemia. Likewise, the finding of splenomegaly in any patient known to have an abnormal heart valve—particularly if there is evidence of heart failure—should be considered to be due to the development of infective endocarditis until the contrary is proved beyond doubt.

Less urgently serious causes of splenomegaly, such as *infectious mononucleosis* (see page 736), *brucella infection* (see page 590) and *sarcoidosis* (see page 747), are frequent enough to require consideration in any case of splenomegaly. It is wise not to forget that the presence of a disease that is a recognized cause of splenomegaly does not necessarily mean that it is the cause in a particular case: I have seen the diagnosis of subacute infective endocarditis delayed because splenomegaly was considered to be a manifestation solely of coexistent Felty's syndrome in one instance and of coexistent sarcoidosis in another.

Splenomegaly in Hot Climates ('Tropical Splenomegaly')

Splenomegaly may occur in the tropics for any of the reasons that lead to its occurrence in other parts of the world. However, it is likelier to be due to the diseases that are peculiarly prevalent in the region: for example, malaria, leishmaniasis, trypanosomiasis or schistosomiasis may be the most usual cause of enlargement of the spleen in particular parts of the tropics and subtropics.

The term 'tropical splenomegaly' has no diagnostic connotation. It relates to different diseases in different regions. It has also been used, rather confusingly, as a synonym of 'tropical idiopathic splenomegaly' (see below).

Just as diseases that may each cause splenomegaly may coexist in temperate regions (see above), so in hot climates two or more causes may be present simultaneously. The possible combinations are almost unlimited: those that I have seen include chronic malaria with chronic meningococcal septicaemia and haemoglobin SC disease, visceral leishmaniasis with thalassaemia and massive caseating tuberculous splenitis, schistosomal portal hypertension with paracoccidioidomycosis and leukaemia, and brucella infection with chronic malaria. An atypical clinical picture or an uncharacteristic response to treatment should raise the question whether an observed splenomegaly might have more than one cause. For instance, it is said that about 10 per cent of patients with visceral leishmaniasis have a mild degree of cirrhosis of the liver following treatment with antimonial drugs, and that consequent portal hypertension may account for persistent enlargement of the spleen when the infection has been overcome.[980]

'Tropical Idiopathic Splenomegaly' ('Tropical Splenomegaly Syndrome')[981, 982]

This condition, which is known also as tropical cryptogenic splenomegaly and 'big spleen disease', occurs throughout tropical Africa.[982] Similar forms of splenomegaly are recognized in Algeria,[983] Yemen,[984] India[985] and Papua New Guinea,[986] and doubtless elsewhere: it is probable that a number of entities may be included among cases of different geographical distribution. The most characteristic clinical feature is splenomegaly, which is commonly of massive extent; it is not unusual for the spleen to weigh more than 2 kg, and it has been known to reach 6 kg. The liver is enlarged also. The diagnosis of idiopathic splenomegaly is excluded by the presence of any of the recognized causes of splenomegaly other than malaria (see below). Thus, the presence of cirrhosis of the liver has generally been considered to disqualify a case from inclusion in this

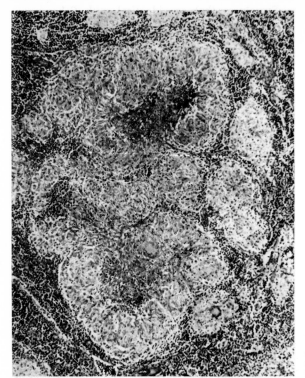

Fig. 9.177. Tuberculous lymphadenitis, for comparison with the pictures of sarcoidosis in Figs 9.174 and 9.175. The granulomatous foci are coalescent and there is considerable central necrosis. Multinucleate giant cells are present, but —contrary to the usual distinction between the two diseases— they are less conspicuous than those in the sarcoid granulomas in Fig. 9.175. The diagnosis of tuberculosis was confirmed by isolation of *Mycobacterium tuberculosis* from the specimen. *Haematoxylin–eosin.* ×65.

lies in a large and usually foamy-looking vacuole at the centre of a multinucleate giant cell or, exceptionally, of a large epithelioid cell. It is refractile but not anisotropic. Its core, and often—to a variable extent —its radiating processes, may show a considerable affinity for elastic tissue stains, an observation that has suggested that it may be derived from elastic fibres that have disintegrated as the granulomatous focus developed.[1024]

Asteroids may occur in any tuberculoid granuloma. They are found very much more rarely in some—such as tuberculosis and other infective lesions—than in others. Their presence in sarcoid lesions was described first by Winkler, in 1905.[1025] Generally, however, they are associated with the name of Wolbach, who observed them in a case of generalized giant cell granulomatosis, published in 1911:[1026] they are particularly numerous in this uncommon condition, which affects the spleen

predominantly and is of unknown aetiology, although possibly related to sarcoidosis—it is referred to sometimes as *Stengel–Wolbach sclerosis* (see page 685).

This type of asteroid has nothing in common with the morphologically somewhat similar, but extracellular, 'asteroids' of sporotrichosis and some other fungal infections (see Chapter 39) and should not be confused with them. Mycotic asteroids are particular instances of the *Splendore–Hoeppli phenomenon*[1027, 1027a]—the precipitation of antigen-antibody complexes on the surface of an antigenic foreign body that has evoked a local reaction with host immunoglobulin. The phenomenon was

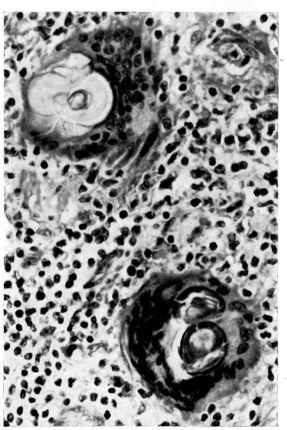

Fig. 9.178. Schaumann bodies surrounded by multinucleate giant cells in sarcoid granulomas in a lymph node. The brittleness of these bodies in indicated by the artefactual fissuring and displacement of the fragments, seen best in the haematoxyphile pair of bodies in the lower part of the field. The complexly shaped body in the upper giant cell shows little haematoxyphilia. Appropriate histochemical studies show that Schaumann bodies may be impregnated with iron or calcium or both: it is particularly these examples that stain intensely with haematoxylin. *Haematoxylin–eosin.* ×435.

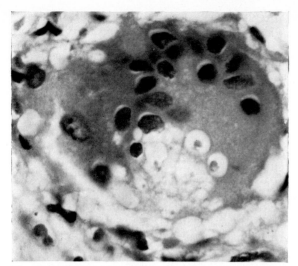

Fig. 9.179. Multinucleate giant cell in a sarcoid granuloma in a lymph node. There is a cluster of well-defined vacuoles in the cytoplasm at the lower pole of the cell. Most of these vacuoles contain a single, round or ovoid, opaque structure, varying considerably in size. These structures are so similar in appearance to certain parasites—particularly *Histoplasma capsulatum*, small cryptococci, small forms of *Paracoccidioides brasiliensis*, and leishmaniae—that the microscopist is commonly misled. Occasionally, they are birefringent, in whole or in part. It is possible that they may be an initial form in the development of Schaumann bodies or of asteroids (see Figs 9.178 and 9.180). They are eosinophile or amphiphile when stained with haematoxylin and eosin; they do not give a positive periodic-acid/Schiff reaction or blacken in Grocott–Gomori hexamine (methenamine) silver preparations. *Haematoxylin–eosin.* × 750.

described first in relation to *Sporothrix schenkii* (Fig. 39.179B, Volume 5).[1027] It may be associated with other fungi also, notably those that cause subcutaneous phycomycosis (see Chapter 39) and entomophthorosis (see page 208). It may be seen also round some bacterial colonies (see Fig. 9.70, page 596) and metazoal parasites, including dead larvae (see Figs 9.127A and 9.127B, pages 672 and 673) and, sometimes, ova.

Involvement of Other Organs and Tissues

The lesions of sarcoidosis are always most numerous in the lymphoreticular tissues. Involvement of lymph nodes and the spleen has been described above. The *tonsils* are said to be involved in from about ten[1028] to over sixty[1029] per cent of cases; they seem appreciably likelier to be affected in cases of sarcoidosis with other manifestations of the disease in the region of the head and neck[1030] (skin, nasal mucosa, pharynx, lymph nodes, cranium, meninges and brain).

A wide range of organs and tissues that are not primarily part of the lymphoreticular system may be involved in sarcoidosis. Some, like the lungs, are affected in a large proportion of cases; others, like the heart, are seldom affected yet may be the location of lesions that endanger life. These various seats of the disease may be noted here briefly.

Respiratory System

Respiratory Passages.—Sarcoid granulomas of the *nasal mucosa* and *nasal sinuses* are an infrequent finding;[1031] they may erode bone and occasionally are large enough to obstruct breathing. They are almost always associated with severe intrathoracic involvement. Sarcoidosis of the *larynx*[1032] and of the *trachea* and *bronchi*[1033] is rare, and seldom, if ever, seen in the absence of parenchymatous involvement of the lungs.

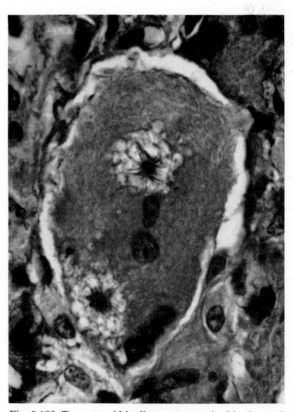

Fig. 9.180. Two asteroid bodies are present in this giant cell in a lymph node in sarcoidosis. They are eosinophile, often rather refractile structures, with a core from which many fine, curved, pointed rays project. Each asteroid lies in a seemingly multiloculate vacuole in the cytoplasm. *Haematoxylin–eosin.* × 750.

Lungs.—The lungs probably share with the lymph nodes the greatest frequency of involvement in sarcoidosis, but how frequent this involvement is cannot be said. Radiologically demonstrable changes in the lungs appear in perhaps 35 to 45 per cent of patients whose sarcoidosis is recognized at the stage of bilateral hilar lymphadenopathy without respiratory symptoms: these changes prove to be comparatively gross when the corresponding pathological specimen is seen alongside a specimen of a lung that is widely involved, yet not sufficiently so to have been in any way abnormal in a clinical radiograph.

The most important aspect of pulmonary sarcoidosis is the development of fibrosis of the diseased tissue (see page 372). If the lesions are in the prefibrotic stage the condition is still susceptible of spontaneous, complete resolution, with no sequelae. Once they enter the stage of fibrosis, the natural tendency is toward progressive deterioration of respiratory and circulatory function. Death may then result from respiratory insufficiency with or without accompanying cor pulmonale and cardiac failure (see page 283). Occasionally, caseating tuberculosis develops and is the cause of death.[1034]

Pleura.—Pleural involvement in sarcoidosis is very unusual. Those cases in which it is recognized are usually characterized by the development of pleural effusion, which may be bilateral.[1035] Spontaneous pneumothorax is an occasional manifestation.

Skin

Although the history of sarcoidosis began with the definition of various types of skin lesion—*lupus pernio, cutaneous sarcoids* and *subcutaneous sarcoids* —subsequent studies have shown that these are a feature of only a minority of cases (see page 745 and Chapter 39). It may be noted here that while the lesions just named are identifiable histologically by their characteristic sarcoid picture, a considerably larger proportion of patients with sarcoidosis presents with *erythema nodosum* than with specifically sarcoid lesions of the skin. The histological picture of erythema nodosum occurring in sarcoidosis does not differ from that of other cases of erythema nodosum (see Chapter 39):[1036] only in the most exceptional cases has sarcoid tissue been found.[1037]

The development of a *sarcoid granuloma in relation to foreign bodies* as a presenting manifestation of sarcoidosis is referred to on page 757 and in Chapter 39.

Skeletal Muscle

Symptomless granuloma formation may be common in the muscles in cases of active sarcoidosis: random muscle biopsy in 42 cases of the disease yielded sarcoid granulomas in 23 instances,[1038] a frequency that gives the procedure a potential diagnostic value when others fail. Rarely, a palpable granulomatous mass is found in a muscle.[1039]

Sarcoid Myopathy.—While sarcoid involvement of muscles is usually asymptomatic, a syndrome of progressive wasting and weakness of the musculature, reminiscent of chronic polymyositis (see Chapter 36), is an occasional effect, particularly in older women.[1040] Its relation to the presence of the granulomatous foci in the muscles is uncertain.

Bones and Synovial Structures

Sarcoid Osteitis.—Lesions are found in the bones of the hands or feet in from about 5 [1041] to about 15 [1042] per cent of cases of sarcoidosis. They are likeliest to be present in cases with sarcoid lesions of the skin.[1041] Other bones may be involved, including the cranium[1043] and sometimes the major long bones of the limbs.[1044] I have seen a 'pathological fracture' of a metacarpal bone as the result of a local granuloma in a case of generalized sarcoidosis. Vertebral collapse has been recorded.[1045]

Granulomas were identified in specimens of sternal marrow in 10 of 39 cases of known sarcoidosis.[1046]

Arthritis Accompanying Sarcoidosis.—Sarcoid arthritis has been demonstrated histologically in a few cases of recurrent polyarthritis affecting particularly the larger joints of the limbs.[1047]

Some patients whose sarcoidosis presents with erythema nodosum may have an accompanying febrile arthritis that possibly is non-specific in nature.[1048]

Tenosynovitis.—In the first recorded case of sarcoidosis—Besnier's patient with lupus pernio (see page 745)—there was tenosynovitis affecting several fingers.[999] Since then this manifestation has been seen only rarely.[1049]

Eyes

Sarcoidosis is a rare cause of *uveitis* (see Chapter 40): it was responsible for only 14 of 653 cases of the latter seen at the Institute of Ophthalmology in London (2 per cent).[1050] Uveitis occurs in 14 [1051] to

33 [1052] per cent of cases of sarcoidosis and is the presenting manifestation in 10 [1051] to 16 [1052] per cent.

Conjunctival sarcoidosis may be suspected clinically when minute, yellowish, translucent elevations are found in the conjunctiva, particularly of the inferior fornix. Lymphoid follicles have a similar appearance, and biopsy, usually necessitating preparation of serial histological sections, is essential for confirmation of the diagnosis. In this context it has to be remembered that similar histological lesions may occur in cases of rosacea involving the conjunctiva[1052] and of obstruction of the tarsal glands.[1053] Although it is said that conjunctival biopsy may be positive in 25 per cent of cases of sarcoidosis,[1054] the procedure is not suitable for general diagnostic use, requiring both specialized surgical experience and particular technical histological skills. Conjunctival involvement is present in only about a fifth of cases of intraocular sarcoidosis, which, indeed, can be identified only presumptively (on the grounds of the presence of confirmed sarcoid lesions in other parts of the body).

Heerfordt's Syndrome (Uveoparotid Fever).[1013]— This is one of the rarer presentations of sarcoidosis. The complete syndrome—uveitis, parotitis, fever and facial nerve palsy—accounted for 2 of 61 cases of sarcoid uveitis in ophthalmological practice[1052] but was not observed at all in a series of 275 patients in the practice of a chest physician.[1051]

Central Nervous System

Involvement of the central nervous system in the course of sarcoidosis is very rare, particularly in white patients.[1055] Among the cases recorded in the United States Armed Forces Institute of Pathology, in Washington, D.C., there was involvement of the meninges or brain in about 2·5 per cent of black patients but in none of the white patients; the latter made up about 40 per cent of the series.[1055]

Meningeal Infiltration.—The formation of sarcoid granulomas in the leptomeninges is the least rare manifestation of sarcoidosis in the central nervous system (see Chapter 34).[1056, 1057] It is usually accompanied by symptoms resulting from compression of cranial nerves or of the hypothalamus and infundibulum (pituitary stalk); occasionally, obstructive hydrocephalus develops. The meningeal involvement commonly leads to the formation of nodular foci of sarcoid tissue in the superficial parts of the brain, the result of extension of the granulomatous condition along the circumvascular space (Virchow–Robin space).

Granulomas in the Brain.—In addition to the multiple small foci that may be found in the brain as an accompaniment of meningeal sarcoidosis (see above), there may be larger granulomatous foci, usually solitary, that in their effects mimic neoplasms.[1058]

Spinal Cord.—Compression of the spinal cord by sarcoid granulomas, usually in the meninges, is a rare finding.[1059]

Endocrine Glands

Although an occasional sarcoid granuloma may be found at necropsy in any of the endocrine glands, involvement sufficient to interfere with the function of any part of the endocrine system is very rare.

Pituitary and Hypothalamus.—Diabetes insipidus is the least rare endocrine disorder to result from sarcoidosis. It is due to direct infiltration either of the gland itself[1060] or of the hypothalamic region.[1061] In some cases diabetes insipidus is accompanied by hypopituitarism in consequence of involvement of the anterior lobe of the pituitary (adenohypophysis) (see Chapter 29).[1062]

Adrenals.—There appear to be no cases on record of adrenal cortical insufficiency (Addison's disease) due to sarcoidosis. Caseous destruction of the adrenals that was found at necropsy in two cases of sarcoidosis[1063] proved on review of the histological material to be due to histoplasmosis (see Chapter 30).[1064]

Reproductive Organs

Sarcoid granulomas may be found in any of the reproductive organs, in both sexes, but very seldom attract attention. They have rarely been found in the endometrium:[1065] their presence—for instance, in curettings—is liable to be interpreted as evidence of tuberculosis, particularly as tubercles that form in the endometrium may not show caseation because the tissue is shed during menstruation before there has been time for its appearance (see Chapter 27).

Sarcoid granulomas may also be found in the uterine tubes.[1066] It may be very difficult to distinguish between sarcoidosis and tuberculosis in this situation, particularly in view of the unusual—and unexplained—frequency with which structures that are identical in appearance with Schaumann bodies may be found in the lesions of tuberculous salpingitis (see Chapter 27). Identical twins, who had been found to have sarcoidosis at the same time, were admitted to hospital in the same week with rupture of a uterine tube (the right in one case, the left in the other) at the site of an ectopic pregnancy associated with extensive sarcoid endosalpingitis; both sisters were pregnant for the first time.[1067]

Breasts.—The skin of the breasts may be involved in the cutaneous manifestations of sarcoidosis. Single cases have been recorded of sarcoid nodules presenting as palpable lumps within the substance of the breasts, simulating fibroadenomas or cancers, in patients with known sarcoidosis.[1068] In similar cases that I have seen, the sarcoid lesions were considered to have developed at the site of healing abscesses or in association with mammary duct ectasia in patients with sarcoidosis (see Chapter 28): the reaction may have been determined by the altered reactivity of the tissues in the presence of sarcoidosis and is possibly to be regarded as comparable to the sarcoid reaction to foreign bodies (see page 757).

Kidneys

The kidneys are among the organs least often and least extensively involved in the granulomatous process in fatal cases of sarcoidosis. However, they are commonly affected by the disturbance of calcium metabolism that so often accompanies sarcoidosis (hypercalcaemia and hypercalcaemic nephropathy —see Chapter 24).[1069] There is an accompanying liability to the formation of renal calculi.[1070] It is possible that the metabolic disorder reflects an unexplained over-sensitivity to vitamin D [1071] or to parathyroid hormone.[1072]

Alimentary Tract

Oesophagus.—A single case is on record of symptoms being associated with a sarcoid lesion of the oesophagus in a case of sarcoidosis.[1073]

Stomach.—Sarcoid granulomas have been found in gastroscopic biopsy specimens[1074] and in partial gastrectomy specimens in cases of peptic ulcer developing in the course of sarcoidosis.[1075] More rarely, a patient with sarcoidosis has developed pyloric or prepyloric obstruction because of the formation of a mass of granulomatous tissue in the mucous membrane.[1076]

Intestines.—Apart from a possible case of sarcoid appendicitis necessitating appendicectomy as an emergency procedure,[1077] the presence of granulomas in the bowel of patients with sarcoidosis seems not to have been responsible for clinical manifestations. Some published instances of supposed sarcoid involvement of the small bowel may be identified in retrospect as Crohn's disease (regional enteritis) (see page 1073); it is no longer believed that Crohn's disease and sarcoidosis are related.[1078]

Peritoneum.—Involvement of the peritoneal serosa and the development of ascites has been observed in rare cases.[1079]

Liver

Liver biopsy shows sarcoid granulomas in about a third of cases of sarcoidosis, in the absence of any hepatic symptoms.[1080] In the great majority of cases of sarcoidosis with hepatic involvement there is no notable abnormality of liver function. Jaundice and liver failure are very rare.[1081] When granulomas are found in a liver biopsy specimen it is necessary to keep in mind the possibility that they are due to conditions such as infectious mononucleosis (see page 1226), brucella infection (see page 1229) and tularaemia (see page 1229).

Heart

Although other forms of granulomatous myocarditis tend to be misinterpreted as manifestations of sarcoidosis (see page 47), sarcoidosis itself involves the heart, directly or indirectly, in the great majority of fatal cases of this disease. Sarcoid granulomas may be the cause of sudden death, usually through heart block (Stokes–Adams syndrome),[1082] although complete recovery has been known in some cases in which the latter has been due to this disease.[1083]

The most frequent cardiac complication of sarcoidosis is progressive myocardial failure, usually as a consequence of fibrosis of the pulmonary granulomas (cor pulmonale—see page 283) and rarely because of infiltration of the myocardium itself by granulomatous tissue. Various arrhythmias may develop, adding to the burden on the heart muscle.

Diagnosis

Biopsy.—Biopsy may be performed when there are lesions of *skin* or *bone*, and *liver* or *lung* tissue may be examined when appropriate. However, in any case in which there is enlargement of accessible lymph nodes, the most regularly helpful procedure is *lymph node biopsy*. In cases of the bilateral hilar lymphadenopathy syndrome, when there may be no lesions that are macroscopically identifiable outside the chest, liver biopsy and 'random' biopsy of skeletal muscle—for instance, a gastrocnemius—may be the means to confirm the diagnosis: in such circumstances *liver biopsy* may be positive in up to 80 per cent of cases,[1084] although the interpretation of the histological findings is not always straightforward (see page 1229); random *muscle biopsy* may give positive results in up to about half the cases investigated, particularly in the earlier stages of the disease (for example, when the only recognized manifestation is the bilateral hilar lymphadenopathy syndrome—see page 746). *Biopsy of a scalene node* and *mediastinoscopy biopsy* are advocated by some clinicians in cases of asymptomatic intrathoracic disease without lesions elsewhere. If there is radiological evidence of lesions in the lungs in such cases, *lung biopsy* through a small thoracotomy incision may prove diagnostic, if the slight but real risk to the patient is thought to be justified by the information that may be obtained. *Conjunctival biopsy* is mentioned on page 753.

Whatever the tissue examined, the most that can be deduced from the findings is that they are consistent with the diagnosis of sarcoidosis. However typical, the histological picture is not by itself sufficient grounds for the diagnosis of sarcoidosis, which requires confirmatory support from the clinical picture and the results of other investigations.

Supporting Evidence.—Supporting evidence may include absence of demonstrable skin sensitivity to tuberculin (or, more usually, a positive reaction only when the test is carried out with a concentration of tuberculin appreciably higher than is required by the average positive reactor). In areas where histoplasmosis or coccidioidomycosis is very prevalent, as indicated by a high proportion of positive reactions to the histoplasmin or coccidioidin skin test, the patient with sarcoidosis may show a comparably marked diminution of sensitivity to the fungal extract as to tuberculin: the change is due to relative deficiency of cell-mediated immune reactions in these patients, and it is not, of course, pathognomonic. Neither are the changes in serum chemistry—such as hypercalcaemia and hypergammaglobulinaemia—that are often present at some stage in the course of the disease, nor the occasional monocytosis or lymphocytosis in the blood.

Kveim Test.—Although the Kveim test,[1085] sometimes known as the Nickerson–Kveim test [1086, 1087] or Kveim–Siltzbach test,[1088, 1089] is said to be the most specific diagnostic procedure that is available for investigation of possible cases of sarcoidosis, its application is not straightforward. It is not a substitute for formal biopsy of the natural lesions of the disease; fortunately, there are few cases in which the diagnosis turns upon its result.

The test entails intradermal injection of a reagent—often loosely referred to as 'Kveim antigen'—that has been prepared from known sarcoid tissue, and histological demonstration of the occurrence at the site of inoculation of a granulomatous reaction. The granuloma may not develop until several weeks have elapsed. Interpretation of the histological picture is a matter for the microscopist who is expert in this often difficult and admittedly subjective assessment (see page 373).

Materials prepared by different methods or derived from active lesions of different patients may vary considerably in value as the test reagent. Standardization *in vivo*, by comparison with known preparations in known reactors, is essential.[1090] Quite apart from the occasional difficulty in deciding whether a given reaction should be interpreted as positive, it must be kept in mind that a frankly positive result is occasionally seen in other diseases—for example, in some cases of tuberculosis,[1091] sometimes following immunization with bacillus Calmette–Guérin (BCG),[1092] and in some cases of histoplasmosis,[1093] coccidioidomycosis[1093] and Crohn's disease (regional enteritis—see page 1073).

The Nature of Sarcoidosis

Both the nature and the causes of sarcoidosis are unknown. Few common diseases have been the subject of so extensive and varied a literature of aetiological speculation and argument as sarcoidosis. It has been regarded as an unusual form of tuberculosis, leprosy or syphilis, a viral infection, a fungal infection, a manifestation of allergy to bacterial or other antigens, a result of metazoal infestation, a form of zirconium poisoning, and even a 'collagen disease' and a multicentric neoplasm. The various theories are dealt with in accessible monographs[995, 997, 998, 1094, 1095] and need not be discussed in detail here. The most favoured concept of the disease today is that it is the manifestation of an inborn or acquired, immunologically determined, change in the quality of the body's reaction to a variety of extrinsic agents. There is abundant evidence, but no incontrovertible proof, that in many cases—possibly a large majority of cases—the extrinsic agent is *Mycobacterium tuberculosis*. Some authorities have been so convinced of the tuberculous nature of sarcoidosis that they have preferred to avoid aetiologically non-committal terms and to call the disease 'non-caseating tuberculosis'.[1096]

Attempts to demonstrate tubercle bacilli in the lesions of sarcoidosis have been almost invariably unsuccessful: indeed, the absence of organisms is so regularly a feature that the cases in which they have been found tend to be looked on as cases of tuberculosis, not of sarcoidosis. It has been said, for instance, that the distinction between sarcoidosis and 'chronic hyperplastic tuberculosis', which is characterized by granulomatous tissue with little or no necrosis, is the presence of the mycobacteria in the lesions of the latter.[1095] Specific chemical substances in sarcoid tissue have been identified with residues of mycobacteria:[1097] they include alpha-epsilon-diaminopimelic acid and mycolic acid, compounds that are foreign to mammalian tissue and that occur in some bacteria, particularly *Mycobacterium tuberculosis*. However, acid-fast lipids and an amino acid similar to diaminopimelic acid are found in the pollen of pine trees, and these produce epithelioid cell granulomas in guinea-pigs that have been sensitized to tuberculin:[1098] this observation led to the suggestion that sarcoidosis may be a consequence of exposure to pine pollen, at least among those patients who have lived in regions where there are pine forests.[1099] In fact, it is now recognized that there is no regular association of sarcoidosis with pines:[1100] the disease is frequent in some coniferous forest lands in parts of North America and Scandinavia and infrequent in comparable regions elsewhere (in Europe and in Japan and Uruguay). It may be that pine pollens, and possibly other pollens, are among factors that may contribute to a change in tissue reactivity, with the consequence that exposure to some other factor—conceivably, tubercle bacilli—is followed by a sarcoid response instead of the response that this other factor ordinarily would evoke.

In the past, much stress was placed on the importance of the observation that the patient with sarcoidosis reacts to an intradermal tuberculin test only when the concentration of tuberculin is much greater than is necessary for a positive result in the average reactor. It is now recognized that this finding in patients with sarcoidosis is a manifestation of the general deficiency in their ability to show the delayed type of hypersensitivy response (see page 520). It does not indicate a specifically tuberculous cause of the disease. A comparable relative failure of the delayed hypersensitivity responses is seen in some cases of Hodgkin's disease and of leukaemia. As in these conditions, there is a predisposition in sarcoidosis to the occurrence of certain infections, including cryptococcosis,[1101, 1102] and to the generalization of dormant infections, including histoplasmosis,[1103] coccidioidomycosis[1104] and listeria infection (see page 577).

An equivocal development in the course of sarcoidosis is the appearance of frank tuberculosis with the readily demonstrable presence of *Mycobacterium tuberculosis*.[1105] The tuberculous lesions may appear in the lungs, differing in no significant way from pulmonary tuberculosis arising in the absence of sarcoidosis. Tuberculous meningitis,[1106] miliary tuberculosis and generalized tuberculous lymphadenitis with extensive caseation[1067] are other, less frequent, manifestations of this sequence. It seems likely that in some instances the tuberculous infection is a straightforward infective complication of sarcoidosis, and the result of its resistance-lowering effects; but in other cases—for instance, with the development of generalized caseating lymphadenitis —there is at least the possibility that the overt tuberculous condition is a transformation of the sarcoid lesions. If the latter explanation should be correct, the tubercle bacillus presumably has been present in some inapparent form: there is no evidence that supports such speculation, and the factual explanation of these cases remains unknown. What is well attested, if infrequent, is that a patient with cutaneous or other manifestations of sarcoidosis may develop classic tuberculous lesions elsewhere—for example, cavitation of the lungs.[1107] In such cases, the overt tuberculosis may be the result of lowering of immunity by widespread sarcoidosis interfering with the defensive functions of the lymphoreticular system, the sarcoidosis itself not necessarily being of tuberculous origin; alternatively, the tuberculous disease may have presented initially as sarcoidosis, later assuming its more usual form as a consequence of changes in the immune state of the patient. In some of these cases the development of florid tuberculosis is followed by reappearance of cutaneous sensitivity to tuberculin, and when this occurs the cutaneous sarcoids may disappear.[1108]

In sum, the relation between sarcoidosis and tuberculosis remains undecided. A continuous spectrum of histological findings links the classic picture of epithelioid cell granulomatosis, without necrosis and without any demonstrable mycobacteria, to the classic picture of caseating tuberculosis demonstrably caused by *Mycobacterium tuberculosis*. At the middle of the spectrum are the cases of non-caseating, discrete or confluent, epithelioid cell granulomatosis in which *Mycobacterium tuberculosis* is present. The available evidence suggests that most cases of sarcoidosis in Britain are of tuberculous origin.[1109] Equally, the evidence does not exclude the possibility that some cases have a different cause, and that these may range from mycobacteria other than *Mycobacterium tuberculosis* through other types of micro-organisms, such as fungi, to non-infective antigenic factors.

Genetic and Ethnic Factors. — A considerable number of observations of sarcoidosis in identical twins is on record (see page 754, for instance).[1109] Among dizygotic twins, in contrast, it is exceptional for the twin of a patient with sarcoidosis to develop the disease: there are relatively more numerous instances of sarcoidosis among other siblings and near relatives. The fact that almost all reports of the disease affecting both members of a pair of twins relate to monozygotic twins suggest a genetic influence rather than exposure in common to an environmental factor.

The considerable preponderance of black patients among those with sarcoidosis in the United States of America[1110] is sometimes put forward in support of the view that there may be a racial predisposition. In contrast, while tuberculosis is prevalent in Africa, sarcoidosis is rarely seen, and particularly so among Africans, although it has been reported among miners in Zambia.[1111] Indeed, the disease is infrequent in the tropics in general.[1112] Such observations support an interesting speculation that sarcoidosis may be a manifestation of tuberculosis in the late stages of an 'epidemic' of that disease that has continued throughout many successive generations of a given population.[1109]

Sarcoidosis Heralded by a Sarcoid Reaction to Foreign Bodies

Whatever its nature, sarcoidosis is accompanied by a liability to the formation of sarcoid granulomatous tissue round various foreign bodies in the tissues. The first indication of the incipient development of sarcoidosis may be the appearance of a sarcoid granuloma at any site where foreign material, particularly siliceous material and unabsorbed surgical sutures, has lain dormant in the tissues, maybe for very many years. This type of delayed sarcoid granuloma, of which Shattock's 'pseudotuberculoma silicoticum' (see Chapter 39)[1113] is the best known example, is not always associated with or followed by sarcoidosis; nevertheless, the sequence is sufficiently common to require that every patient with such a sarcoid reaction to foreign bodies should be kept under observation for signs of incipient sarcoidosis.[1094, 1114, 1115]

The fact that a sarcoid reaction occurs at the site of foreign bodies in these patients suggests that the presence of sarcoidosis, or liability to its eventual florid development, is accompanied by an alteration in the reactivity of the tissues such that the sarcoid type of granuloma is evoked rather than the usual, simple, foreign-body type of giant cell reaction. In the case of the simple type of foreign-body granuloma the reaction is confined to the immediate vicinity of the foreign substance. In the case of the sarcoid reaction, the granulomatous foci extend widely into the tissue surrounding the site of the foreign body: a single knot of suture material, perhaps less than a millimetre in diameter, may be found at the centre of a granulomatous nodule a centimetre or more across. The explanation of the extent of the lesion is unknown.

LIPIDOSES AND OTHER STORAGE DISEASES

The so-called storage diseases ('thesauroses') are characterized by progressive accumulation of normal or abnormal metabolites in the tissues. Typically, the accumulation is intracellular and leads to enlargement of the affected cells and, when the reticuloendothelial cells are involved, to their widespread hyperplasia. When the distended cells die their contents are liberated into the interstices but do not collect there, being removed either in the lymph flow or by phagocytes, presumably by pinocytosis (see page 524). It has become customary to include metachromatic leucodystrophy (see Chapter 34) among the storage diseases: this seems inappropriate, as the metachromatic material that is characteristic of the condition accumulates mainly in the interstitial substance of the brain and spinal cord, such relatively minute amounts as are found within the Hortega cells (cerebral histiocytes) being there in consequence of the phagocytic activity of these cells and not through any disorder of their metabolic functions.

The cells in which 'storage' takes place are generally those that normally are involved in the metabolism of the substance (or substances) concerned in the particular disease. The exceptions to this general condition are the rare *secondary storage diseases*, in which phagocytes—mainly macrophages—take up a metabolic product that is present in excess in the blood as a consequence of some recognized disease: the type example is secondary lipidosis, which develops as an accompaniment of the hypercholesterolaemia of, for example, diabetes mellitus (see below). The *primary storage diseases* are the manifestations of a variety of inborn errors of metabolism that relate to deficiency of particular intracellular enzymes. Some of these deficiencies are of enzymes that are located in lysosomes: this prompted the suggestion that the corresponding storage diseases might be designated *lysosomal diseases*.[1116]

The most familiar storage diseases are the lipidoses and the glycogenoses. The clinical manifestations of most of the *lipidoses* are due to the accumulation of lipid in the cells of the reticuloendothelial system, and for this reason it is appropriate to consider them in this chapter.[1117, 1118] The reticuloendothelial system is also involved in some rarer storage diseases—*mucopolysaccharidoses*,[1119] of which Hunter–Hurler disease (Hurler–Pfaundler disease)[1120–1122] is the best known (see Chapter 34), and *ceroid storage disease*.[1123] In both these rarer forms there is an accumulation of sphingolipids in addition to the substances that have given their names to the diseases. In contrast, the various *glycogen storage diseases*—with one exception (see below)—are not accompanied by any important changes in the reticuloendothelial system: each affects the particular organs and tissues that normally are the site of the enzyme that is congenitally deficient in the disease (see pages 44 and 1276).[1124, 1125] The exception is the very rare type IV glycogenosis (Andersen's amylopectinosis,[1126] or 'branching enzyme' deficiency—see page 1277), in which splenomegaly occurs: however, the latter is not a manifestation of accumulation of the abnormal polysaccharide but an accompaniment of portal hypertension secondary to cirrhosis of the liver, which is the main feature of the disease.

THE LIPIDOSES[1117, 1118]

Lipidoses may be primary (the manifestation of congenital enzyme deficiency) or secondary (a result of hyperlipidaemia that is symptomatic of another disease, such as diabetes mellitus). The level of lipids in the plasma may be within normal limits in cases of primary lipidoses (for example, in the sphingolipidoses and in the normocholesterolaemic cholesterol lipidoses, of which Hand–Schüller–Christian disease is the best known). Alternatively, there may be hyperlipidaemia (for example, in idiopathic familial hypercholesterolaemia) or hyperlipaemia (an increase in the amount of neutral fat in the circulation, as in idiopathic hyperlipaemia—the Bürger–Grütz syndrome[1127]). These various conditions are described below.

A classification of primary lipidoses according to whether there is an increase in the amount of lipid in the blood or not (hyperlipidaemic and normolipidaemic lipidoses) is less generally useful than the alternative, which is to base classification on the chemical identity of the material that accumulates in the affected tissues. In cases of secondary lipidosis the material stored is cholesterol.

Primary Lipidoses

The primary lipidoses result from congenital enzyme deficiency. They may be classified into sphingolipidoses and cholesterol lipidoses, with a subordinate category for the very rare lipidosis of the idiopathic hyperlipaemia syndrome.

Sphingolipidoses

The sphingolipids, or 'ceramides', are fatty acid amides of sphingosine. Each sphingolipid has its own characteristic structural component, which is attached to a particular site on the molecule by an ester or glycoside bond. The sphingolipids involved in the various forms of sphingolipidosis are shown in Table 9.1. All known sphingolipidoses are primary lipidoses: most, if not all, of the enzymes that are congenitally deficient in sphingolipidoses are lysosomal enzymes and the corresponding diseases may therefore be classed as lysosomal diseases (see above).

The sphingolipidoses that involve the reticuloendothelial system predominantly are Gaucher's disease and Niemann–Pick disease (often referred to respectively as cerebrosidosis and sphingomyelinosis, although other sphingolipids—gangliosides—are also involved in both diseases). They are considered in more detail below.

Other sphingolipidoses typically involve the central nervous system, or the central nervous system and the eyes, predominantly, but may be

Table 9.1. *Composition of Sphingolipids in Various Lipidoses*

Sphingolipidosis	Sphingolipid involved	Enzyme deficiency responsible
Gaucher's disease	Glucose cerebroside (kerasin); also gangliosides	Glucocerebrosidase
Niemann–Pick disease	Sphingomyelin; also gangliosides	Sphingomyelinase
Tay–Sachs disease and other forms of amaurotic familial idiocy	Gangliosides	Galactose-transferring enzymes; possibly fructose 1-phosphate aldolase
Hunter–Hurler disease	Gangliosides (*note:* mucopolysaccharides also accumulate)	?
Fabry–Anderson disease (angiokeratoma corporis diffusum)	Ceramide hexosides	?

accompanied by clinically evident involvement of the reticuloendothelial system in some cases (splenomegaly, or hepatosplenomegaly, and very occasionally enlargement of lymph nodes). The least rare of these, as a group, are the various forms of *amaurotic familial idiocy*, of which Tay–Sachs disease is the type example (see page 1280 and Chapters 34 and 40): the material that accumulates—mainly in neurons in the retina and brain, but also in macrophages in both situations—is a ganglioside, its identity depending on the particular enzyme deficiency. Other essentially neuronal lipidoses include *Hunter–Hurler disease* (Hurler–Pfaundler disease),[1120–1122] in which a mixture of various gangliosides[1128] and acid mucopolysaccharides[1129] accumulates (see page 1280 and Chapter 34).

In cases of *Fabry–Anderson disease*[1130, 1131] ('angiokeratoma corporis diffusum', or hereditary dystopic lipidosis—see Chapters 24, 34 and 39), ceramide hexosides accumulate in neurons of the hypothalamus and thalamus and of some other parts of the brain, as well as in cells of the autonomic nervous system and in the skin, heart and kidneys. In some cases there is considerable storage of the specific sphingolipids throughout the reticuloendothelial system.[1132] In *Krabbe's disease*[1133] (globoid cell leucodystrophy—see Chapter 34), a cerebroside similar to kerasin (the sphingolipid

characteristic of Gaucher's disease), if not identical with it, distends the cytoplasm of cells in the white matter and elsewhere in the brain. The cells are probably Hortega cells (cerebral histiocytes).[1134] In exceptional cases of Krabbe's disease the cerebroside accumulates also in reticuloendothelial cells in the spleen, lymph nodes, lungs and elsewhere.[1135] Conversely, in some cases of *Gaucher's disease* (see below), but only in the comparatively rare infantile and juvenile forms, there may be involvement of the central nervous system (see Chapter 34): in the infantile form there may be accumulation of the cerebroside (kerasin) in a proportion of the cells, but widespread neuronal degeneration is more characteristic;[1136] in the juvenile form there may be very conspicuous neuronal cerebrosidosis.[1137] Neuronal sphingomyelinosis and gangliosidosis may be found in some cases of *Niemann–Pick disease* (see below); most patients with this lipidosis die before there is any notable involvement of the central nervous system (see Chapter 34).

Metachromatic leucodystrophy (see Chapter 34) is often grouped among the other sphingolipidoses that may affect the central nervous system. It differs from them in one important aspect—the sphingolipid that collects in the brain and spinal cord, a sulphatide, is essentially extracellular, and this distinguishes the condition from all the other lipidoses, whether they affect the nervous system primarily or not.

Gaucher's Disease[1138]

Gaucher's disease (Gaucher–Schlagenhaufer disease,[1139, 1139a] cerebroside lipidosis, cerebrosidosis, or kerasinosis) is the least rare of the sphingolipidoses. When Gaucher, a French physician, described the first case, in 1882,[1138] he considered the condition to be a primary epithelial neoplasm of the spleen because of the preponderant involvement of that organ and the likeness to epithelial cells of the large, pale cells that had replaced much of its normal structure. Because anaemia may be a notable feature, and the disease runs in families, the name 'familial splenic anaemia' had some currency, relating the condition to 'Banti's disease' (see page 731). Schlagenhaufer recognized it to be a systemic disease of the lymphoid and haemopoietic tissues.[1139] Although it was suggested by Marchand, in 1907,[1140] that the peculiar cells contain an unusual substance, it was not until 1924 that this was identified as a cerebroside, kerasin.[1141, 1142] Gangliosides are now known to be present also, at least in some cases.[1143]

Histopathology.—In adolescents and adults, the spleen, liver and bones, and—to a smaller degree—the lymph nodes are affected most frequently and conspicuously. The spleen generally weighs from 2 to 4 kg, but it is sometimes enormously enlarged: a specimen formerly in the Surgical Museum of the Queen's University of Belfast weighed 13·5 kg. The cut surface of the affected organs is firm and pale. There are usually infarcts in the spleen. In the infantile and juvenile forms of the disease the brain is characteristically affected (see above, and Chapter 34); involvement of the central nervous system is very rare in adult patients.

Microscopically, the *Gaucher cells* are pathognomonic (Figs 9.181 and 9.182). They are reticuloendothelial cells, modified by the presence of the sphingolipids. Ultrastructural studies have supported this interpretation of their nature.[1144] They are uncommonly large cells, usually ranging from 20 to 50 μm in diameter. Singly, they are round or oval; when crowded, as usually they are, their shape

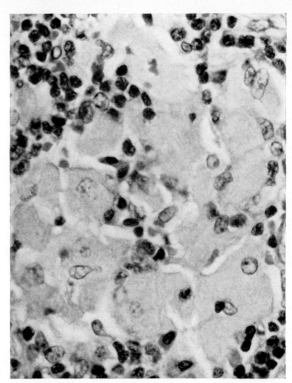

Fig. 9.182. Gaucher's disease. Another case. The cytoplasm of the Gaucher cells has a characteristically ground-glass-like appearance. In a few of the cells it is possible to make out faint traces of linear streaking of the cytoplasm. *Haematoxylin–eosin.* × 600.

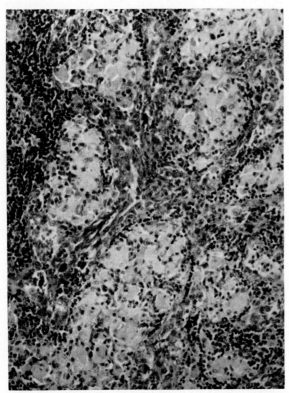

Fig. 9.181. Gaucher's disease. The opacity of the cytoplasm of the clustered histiocytes in this lymph node biopsy specimen is characteristic. See also Fig. 9.182. Compare with the picture of other forms of histiocytosis illustrated in Figs 9.49, 9.50, 9.81 and 9.172 (pages 569, 569, 609 and 742). *Haematoxylin–eosin.* × 140.

is irregular. Most of the cells contain one or two nuclei; some have as many as a dozen, and these multinucleate forms may be up to 100 μm in diameter. The nucleus of the Gaucher cell is peripherally situated, oval or round, and relatively small (5 to 7 μm across). The cytoplasm has an appearance like ground glass; its most characteristic feature is striation by fine, slightly wavy, parallel, linear striae, which may be abundant, criss-crossing the cytoplasm, or sparse. The material in the cytoplasm does not stain with Sudan dyes. Chemical analysis shows it to contain a large proportion of the cerebroside, kerasin, which often is of an abnormal type, being a glucose cerebroside and not a galactose cerebroside. Gangliosides are present also.[1143] There is marked acid phosphatase activity[1145] in a large proportion of the cells, an observation that corresponds to the presence of increased levels of an unusual form of acid phosphatase in the serum.[1146]

It is the great accumulation of Gaucher cells that accounts for the main clinical features of the disease—enlargement of the spleen, liver and lymph nodes and destructive skeletal lesions. The lower end of the femora and the bodies of the vertebrae are the parts of the skeleton most heavily affected (see Chapter 37). Replacement of bone marrow by Gaucher cells may result in anaemia, leucopenia and thrombocytopenia.

Other Findings.—Patchy overpigmentation of the skin and melanosis of the bulbar conjunctiva are often found. Fever is common, and when it accompanies episodes of acute pain that are associated with the lesions in bones, particularly the femora, acute suppurative osteomyelitis may be diagnosed in error: there is no accompanying leucocytosis, and this may be of diagnostic help.

Aetiology and Prognosis.—The disease is hereditary and not infrequently is present in different generations of a family. It is more frequent in Jews than in other people, but no ethnic group is exempt. It occurs in two age groups particularly. A relatively acute form occurs in infants and ends fatally within a year or so: there is severe disease of the central nervous system in these babies (see above, and Chapter 34) and, because of the rapid progress, other organs—including those of the reticuloendothelial system—are much less heavily affected than in older children and adults. The more chronic form, which occurs in older patients, commonly begins to manifest itself clinically toward the end of the first decade, although the diagnosis may not be made until well into adult or even middle life. The earlier the disease becomes evident, the worse the prognosis: if its presentation is delayed until the third or fourth decade, its further progress may be slow, with little or no disability over a period of 20 to 30 years.

Splenectomy.—The spleen has been removed in some cases of Gaucher's disease, because its size and friability have predisposed to rupture, or in order to relieve the patient of the discomfort or pain resulting from its enlargement, or as a diagnostic procedure. In a considerable proportion of the patients who have been submitted to the operation, its aftermath has been a notable increase in the rate of development of lesions elsewhere, and particularly in the skeleton.[1147] It seems clear that the spleen is ordinarily the main site for storage of the excess of cerebrosides and other sphingolipids, and that its removal promotes accelerated storage in other parts of the reticuloendothelial system. It is a corollary of this observation that the excess of sphingolipids does not result merely in their storage in the cells that elaborate them: they enter the circulation and are then taken up by the reticuloendothelial cells,

which undergo hyperplasia as the need for progressively more storage increases.

Diagnosis.—Examination of the serum for cerebrosides has given conflicting results, although the more sophisticated chemical methods now available tend to show some elevation above the small amounts that are present normally.[1148]

Morphologically characteristic Gaucher cells may be demonstrable in the blood[1149] or bone marrow or in aspirates from the spleen, liver or enlarged superficial lymph nodes. Aspiration biopsy of the spleen carries a risk of haemorrhage and has been known to be followed by 'spontaneous' rupture of the organ within a few days, with a fatal outcome.[1150] Lymph node biopsy is preferable, although it is not always possible to find nodes that are obviously enlarged. If the nodes are relatively lightly involved the Gaucher cells may be sparse and difficult to distinguish from other histiocytes; however, if the typical cytoplasmic striae are found the diagnosis may be made with some confidence. Chemical analysis of a biopsy specimen may clinch the diagnosis.

Deficiency of glucocerebrosidase may be demonstrable in leucocytes in the blood.[1151]

Niemann–Pick Disease

Niemann–Pick disease[1152, 1153] (sphingomyelin lipidosis, sphingomyelinosis) is considerably rarer than Gaucher's disease. The substances that accumulate in the tissues—mainly in reticuloendothelial cells—are sphingomyelin, a phospholipid, which is the predominating constituent, and gangliosides.[1128] The disease has a more marked familial incidence than Gaucher's disease, and the proportion of the patients who are Jewish is greater. It occurs much more frequently in infancy than at other ages. Almost all the affected babies die from involvement of the brain (see Chapter 34),[1154] death occurring at about the end of the second year of life. Although usually apparently healthy at birth, the baby is likely to show the first manifestations of illness a week or so later.

The disease has been recognized exceptionally rarely in adults. The prognosis is less serious, although the expectation of life is considerably shortened. Involvement of the central nervous system is slight or lacking in adult patients; splenomegaly or hepatosplenomegaly, and sometimes pulmonary involvement, with progressive fibrosis, are the main manifestations.[1155] In some adult cases the disease has dated from early childhood (but not from infancy) and progression has been slow, and compatible with a fairly active life.[1156]

Histopathology.—At all ages, enlargement of the spleen, and often of lymph nodes, is conspicuous, although much less marked than is usual in Gaucher's disease. In general, there is proportionately more enlargement of the liver than of the spleen. The increased size of these organs is due to the great proliferation of the so-called Niemann–Pick foam cells. These are modified histiocytes, on average rather smaller than Gaucher cells (see page 760) although with much the same range of size (20 to 50 μm). They differ from Gaucher cells in having a foamy-looking cytoplasm and no cytoplasmic striae. They never contain more than one or two nuclei. The foamy appearance in paraffin wax sections is due to the presence of innumerable minute vacuoles from which the lipid contents have been dissolved in the course of histological processing. These cells are found in practically every organ and tissue, but particularly in the spleen, liver and lymph nodes (Fig. 9.183), and in bone marrow and the lungs.

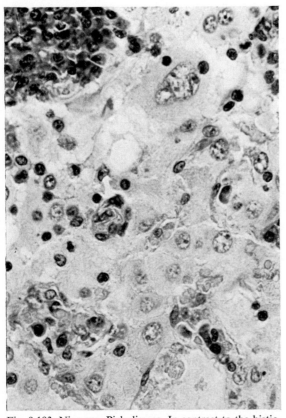

Fig. 9.183. Niemann–Pick disease. In contrast to the histiocytes in Gaucher's disease (Fig. 9.182), those of Niemann–Pick disease have a very finely vacuolate cytoplasm, which gives them a foamy appearance. The field is from the cortex of a lymph node; remarkably little lymphoid tissue remained. *Haematoxylin–eosin.* × 600.

Other Findings.—In some cases, in infancy, a 'cherry red' spot is seen in the macular region of the retinae on ophthalmoscopy, as occurs more typically in certain forms of amaurotic familial idiocy, such as Tay–Sachs disease (see Chapter 40). The latter group of diseases is characterized by accumulation of gangliosides in the affected tissues, and it is notable that these compounds may also be found in association with the predominant sphingomyelin in cases of Niemann–Pick disease,[1128] which, in infancy, is often regarded as a variety of amaurotic familial idiocy.

The baby's skin and sometimes the buccal mucous membrane may be blotched with areas of excessive melanin pigmentation. The so-called 'Mongolian spot'—a slate-coloured macule in the skin of the sacral or lumbosacral region, formed of 'mesodermal melanocytes' (see Chapter 39)—is present much oftener in cases of Niemann–Pick disease than in other infants;[1157] multiple blue naevi (Jadassohn–Tièche naevi—see Chapter 39) were present in three of five patients with Niemann–Pick disease in two generations of an affected family.[1150]

Diagnosis.—There is no abnormality of the amount of sphingomyelin in the serum. Vacuolate cells are demonstrable in bone marrow and other aspirated specimens; their demonstration in the marrow is a valuable pointer to the diagnosis, and may be possible even before other manifestations of the disease become evident.[1154]

Lymph node biopsy, taking the opportunity for chemical analysis of the tissue as well as examining histological sections, is often diagnostic. In the absence of facilities for chemical study the histological findings alone may justify a presumptive diagnosis, depending on such considerations as the clinical picture and family history for support.

If splenectomy is performed, the spleen may be analysed for its lipid content. As in Gaucher's disease, it is possible that the operation is contra-indicated, except as an emergency procedure following rupture of the organ: in the case of an adult with Niemann–Pick disease, splenectomy was followed by a marked acceleration in the development of pulmonary lesions, with fibrosis, and of lesions in the bones, with severe anaemia of leuco-erythroblastic type (see page 462).[1150]

Generalized Gangliosidosis

The most familiar forms of gangliosidosis are the various diseases that are grouped under the heading of amaurotic familial idiocy (see Chapters 34 and 40). Gangliosides form a small proportion of the sphingolipids that accumulate in the tissues in Niemann–Pick disease, in which the bulk of the stored material is sphingomyelin (see above). A very small number of instances of generalized gangliosidosis has been recognized in which only these substances are present in excess:[1158] the liver, kidneys and spleen are most notably involved. The histological picture in the spleen is similar to that of Niemann–Pick disease.[1159]

Such cases of generalized gangliosidosis underline the growing recognition that many, if not all, of the sphingolipidoses involve both the central nervous system (including the eyes, and predominantly so in cases of the classic forms of amaurotic familial idiocy) and the tissues of other parts of the body, particularly the reticuloendothelial system.[1160] There is a tendency for the central nervous system to be more heavily affected in those sphingolipidoses that are manifested very early in life, particularly in infancy, and for the reticuloendothelial system to be predominantly affected in older patients.

Cholesterol Lipidoses*

The lipidoses that are characterized by accumulation of cholesterol may be primary or secondary. The *primary cholesterol lipidoses* are divided into two groups—those in which the level of cholesterol in the serum is within normal limits (the normo-cholesterolaemic cholesterol lipidoses, of which Hand–Schüller–Christian disease is the best known) and those in which the level of cholesterol in the serum is above normal (the hypercholesterolaemic— or hyperlipidaemic—cholesterol lipidoses, which include idiopathic familial hypercholesterolaemia). *Secondary cholesterol lipidosis* develops as an accompaniment of hypercholesterolaemia of known causation. It is usually accompanied by the formation of so-called xanthomas in the skin (see Chapter 39). Some of these conditions may be considered in more detail here.

Hand–Schüller–Christian Disease

Hand–Schüller–Christian disease[1161–1166] (normo-cholesterolaemic primary cholesterol lipidosis)

* By analogy with the naming of other lipidoses, the term *cholesterolosis* has sometimes been used as a synonym of 'cholesterol lipidosis'. It is best avoided, in this sense, in view of its use in other contexts in which it does not relate to a lipidosis—for example, cholesterolosis of the gall bladder (see page 1321), pulmonary cholesterolosis as a synonym of 'cholesterol pneumonia' (see page 374) and cholesterolosis as a synonym of cholesterol granuloma complicating nasal polyps (see page 199) or arising in the middle ear (see Chapter 41).

occurs with much the same frequency as Gaucher's disease. It has no special familial or racial incidence. Most of the patients are young children, but the disease occurs in adults also. The clinical triad of exophthalmos, diabetes insipidus and deformity due to osteolytic defects in bones, particularly the flat bones of the skull, is diagnostic: however, in a significant proportion of cases the triad is not complete.[1167] The disease is insidious, and generally progressive, death resulting from intercurrent infection in many instances, after a course of from 3 to 30 years. Other causes of death include pulmonary involvement, with fibrosis and 'honeycomb' change (see page 369),[1168] and eventually cor pulmonale. In some cases leucoerythroblastic anaemia or pancytopenia result from exceptionally extensive involvement of bone marrow. Occasionally there is spontaneous regression of some lesions.

The manifestations of the disease are due to accumulation of cholesterol and its esters in histiocytes,[1169] which become aggregated to form tumour-like masses that occupy the orbits, displace or compress the pituitary and hypothalamus, and destroy bone. Proliferation of these cholesterol-laden cells occurs in other parts of the body also, and particularly in the spleen and lymph nodes, and in the liver, although these organs do not become as heavily involved as in the sphingolipidoses (see above). Xanthomas of various clinical forms are commonly present in the skin (see Chapter 39).

Histopathology.—The lipid-filled histiocytes are conspicuous by reason of their size and the pallor of their relatively abundant cytoplasm. The latter may be opaque or clear. The cells are from 15 to 30 μm in diameter and are round or ovoid, or moulded by the pressure of adjoining cells. In biopsy material they are particularly large and closely packed, and their cytoplasm is likely to be clear (Fig. 9.184). The nucleus is relatively small (usually within the range of 8 to 12 μm), vesicular and somewhat ovoid, and central in the cell or displaced toward its periphery. Binucleate and multinucleate cells are not uncommon.

In the earlier stages lipid is not demonstrable in the proliferating cells. In lymph node biopsy specimens the picture is that of an increased number of macrophages in the sinuses with the development of small clusters of similar, opaque, discrete cells in the interfollicular tissue and, often, in the follicles. This so-called proliferative phase merges into what has been described as the granulomatous phase, in which there is more marked clustering of the macrophages, the development of multinucleate cells and a variable infiltration by eosinophils and, sometimes, neutrophils.[1169] By this stage it is possible to show that lipid is present in small amounts in the cytoplasm of some of the macrophages. The accumulation of lipid increases, and the macrophages become vacuolate; the cytoplasm of many of the cells is clear or foamy-looking in paraffin wax sections. In frozen sections the lipid is birefringent and often disposed in the form of microcrystals, which may be scanty or densely packed: the cytoplasm is coloured green to blue by Schultz's method for staining cholesterol,[1170] and the presence of cholesterol and cholesterol esters can be confirmed by chemical analysis of the specimen. Later, the xanthoma-like picture is gradually replaced by the development of fibrosis. These various stages in the histological progression of the lesions

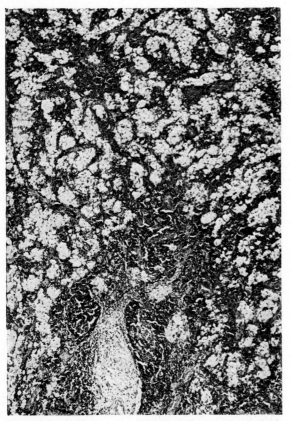

Fig. 9.184. Hand–Schüller–Christian disease. A relatively early stage is seen in this lymph node from a child, aged 8 years. The lipid-laden histiocytes contrast strikingly with the lymphoid tissue. The picture at this magnification is very like that in the cases of lepromatous leprosy and silicone lymphadenopathy illustrated in Figs 9.81 (page 609) and 9.50 (page 569) respectively. The diagnosis will clearly depend on other observations. *Haematoxylin–eosin.* ×45.

may coexist, either in different parts of the body or in a single organ.[1169]

The presence of eosinophils is demonstrable at some stage in almost all cases (see above). They may be dispersed rather uniformly among the histiocytes or aggregated into dense clusters within the histiocytic foci or at their margin. They may be very numerous in one biopsy specimen and absent from an otherwise identical specimen obtained a few weeks later.[1171]

Minute foci of necrosis are found in some specimens but often there is no such change. More extensive necrosis may be seen in the spleen or in bone marrow, and seems then to be related to ischaemia.

Nature.—Some regard Hand–Schüller–Christian disease as a lipidosis resulting from a deficiency of an enzyme system that relates to the metabolism of cholesterol and its esters; no such defect seems yet to have been identified. Others have suggested that the lipid is the result of breakdown of dead tissue in the necrotic foci:[1172] however, as the amount of cholesterol and its esters in the affected tissues may be 10 to 20 times greater than in the corresponding normal tissue it is difficult to accept that so much lipid could be released from the small foci of necrosis that are found.[1173]

Relation to Letterer–Siwe Disease and to Eosinophil Granuloma of Bone.—It is commonly maintained that Letterer–Siwe disease (see page 858) is a malignant, rapidly progressive manifestation in infancy of the same basic disturbance that presents in rather later childhood as Hand–Schüller–Christian disease and in adults, typically, as solitary eosinophil granuloma of bone (see Chapter 37). Together, these three conditions have been designated '*histiocytosis X*'.[1174] The main evidence in support of this thesis is twofold—the accumulation of cholesterol-containing histiocytes in association with eosinophils, and the observation of rare cases of transition from one form to the other. Transition between Letterer–Siwe disease and Hand–Schüller–Christian disease has been recorded in a small number of instances.[1175] Similarly, cases of solitary eosinophil granuloma of bone have been observed in which multiple similar lesions have developed eventually,[1169] with, it is said, the features of Hand–Schüller–Christian disease.

Differential Diagnosis.—Although the clinical picture ordinarily indicates the possibility of Hand–Schüller–Christian disease, there are conditions that must be considered in the differential histological diagnosis. The possibility of mistaken interpretation is greatest when the biopsy specimen is accompanied by inadequate or inaccurate clinical information: in the case of lymph node biopsy specimens two categories of misdiagnosis are possible—mistaking the picture for that of other forms of histiocytic lymphadenopathy (lepromatous leprosy, for instance, and other conditions that are characterized by an accumulation of large, pale histiocytes—see pages 608 and 569), and mistaking it for other forms of lymphadenopathy in which eosinophils may be a conspicuous component of the cellular reaction (see page 688).

Repeated biopsy may be necessary before histological evidence is found that supports a diagnosis of Hand–Schüller–Christian disease. Analysis of the tissues for their lipid content may be specially helpful. In contrast, there is no abnormality of the level of lipids in the serum.

Idiopathic Familial Hypercholesterolaemia[1176]

This condition, which is known also as essential hypercholesterolaemic xanthomatosis, or Thannhauser–Magendantz disease,[1177] is inherited through an autosomal dominant gene.[1176] The constant feature is hypercholesterolaemia: the total cholesterol level in the serum is usually within the range of 8·0–13·0 mmol/l (310–500 mg per 100 ml) and rarely exceeds 16 mmol/l (620 mg per 100 ml). A proportion of the patients show no visible lesions as evidence of their metabolic anomaly; however, at least some of these develop acute or chronic ischaemic lesions—myocardial and cerebral infarction, and gangrene of the limbs—as a consequence of thrombosis complicating the precocious development of atherosclerosis (see page 131). Oftener, there are overt clinical manifestations in the form of xanthomatosis of the skin (including xanthelasma of the eyelids) and tendon sheaths (see Chapters 38 and 39). Clinically evident accumulation of lipid in the reticuloendothelial system is exceptionally rare, but histological examination of the spleen and lymph nodes, marrow, liver, lungs and other tissues usually shows the presence of 'xanthoma cells', either isolated or in small clusters. Most of these cells in the viscera have a single nucleus. Sometimes, characteristic multinucleate 'Touton cells' are found, as in the lesions in the skin. The cytoplasm of the cells has a foamy appearance and contains both Sudanophile fat and cholesterol and cholesterol esters.

Idiopathic Hyperlipaemia[1178]

Perhaps not surprisingly, there has been considerable verbal confusion clinically and in the literature between the *hyperlipidaemias* in which cholesterol and its esters are present in excess in the blood (hypercholesterolaemia) and those in which the excess consists of neutral fat (*hyperlipaemia*).

Idiopathic Hyperlipaemia in Children.—Idiopathic hyperlipaemia (essential hyperlipaemic xanthomatosis, or Bürger–Grütz disease[1127]) is a very rare condition. It is usually recognized in childhood but occasional cases are found among adults (see below). A familial incidence has been observed only exceptionally.[1178] The main clinical features in children are cutaneous xanthomatosis and enlargement of the liver and spleen. A history of recurrent attacks of severe abdominal pain, often with acute collapse, has been a feature of about half the few published cases. The cause of this complication is not usually apparent: laparotomy has seldom been reported—it showed no abnormality other than a small excess of free fluid in the peritoneal cavity in one case[1178] and a fresh splenic infarct in another.[1179]

The serum has a milky appearance. Its total lipid content has been known to reach 95 mmol/l (9500 mg per 100 ml),[1127] the normal range being of the order of 4·0–7·0 mmol/l (400–700 mg per 100 ml).[1180] When the lipids in the blood are above about 20 mmol/l (2000 mg per 100 ml) the appearance of the fundus of the eyes, particularly alongside the retinal blood vessels, has been described as creamy looking and the condition can be recognized ophthalmoscopically (*lipaemia retinalis*). The size and extent of the xanthomas and the size of the liver and spleen vary as the degree of lipaemia varies: a diet that is very low in fat (20–30 g a day), if maintained, may bring the lipid content of the blood to within the normal range, and the manifestations of the disease may disappear.

Idiopathic Hyperlipaemia in Adults.[1117]—In adults, the hyperlipaemia is seldom as severe as in childhood cases. Xanthomatosis is infrequent, and the condition is often discovered by chance during an examination of the blood. The liver and the spleen are little, if at all, enlarged, and there is no tendency to suffer from acute abdominal symptoms. In contrast to the affected children, adult patients may have slight hyperglycaemia and glycosuria: these do not respond to insulin but disappear while the patient is on a low-fat diet.

Histopathology.—Few pathological studies have been made. It is said that there is little evidence of accumulation of lipids in the tissues of the viscera, only a small scattering of 'foam' cells being found in the spleen and liver.[1181] There are similar cells in the bone marrow also. The xanthomas, in contrast, show the histological structure seen in the comparable cutaneous lesions of diabetes mellitus (see Chapter 39).

There seems to be no particular predisposition to atherosclerosis.

'Mixed Hyperlipidaemia'[1118]

There is a group of conditions in which both neutral fat and cholesterol are present in excess in the blood. The clinical and pathological manifestations combine the features of idiopathic hypercholesterolaemia with those of idiopathic hyperlipaemia (see above). In particular, hepatosplenomegaly, xanthomatosis and the precocious development of atherosclerosis and its complications are found, and there may be diminished glucose tolerance and episodes of acute abdominal pain.

Refsum's Disease[1182]

Refsum's disease[1183, 1184] ('heredopathia atactica polyneuritiformis', or phytanic acid storage disease) is a familial condition with autosomal recessive inheritance. The main findings are retinitis pigmentosa, parenchymatous polyneuropathy (see Chapter 35) and an increase in the amount of protein in the cerebrospinal fluid. An excess of phytanic acid (tetramethylhexadecanoic acid, a fatty acid) is found in the plasma and in the liver, kidneys, peripheral nerves, muscle and adipose tissue. There is no evidence that the reticuloendothelial system is involved.

Secondary Lipidosis

Lipidosis may be described as secondary when it represents the accumulation of a lipid that is present in increased amounts in the blood as a consequence of a recognized metabolic disorder, such as diabetes mellitus and other conditions noted below. In these conditions it is predominantly cholesterol and its esters that are present in increased concentration in the blood and that accumulate in the tissues, particularly in the reticuloendothelial cells. For practical purposes, therefore, secondary lipidosis is synonymous with secondary cholesterol lipidosis, although usually other lipids, such as phospholipids and neutral fats, are also present in excess in the blood and accumulate along with cholesterol in reticulo-

endothelial cells. These other lipids make up only a relatively small proportion of the total amount of lipid in both situations.

Secondary Cholesterol Lipidosis

Hypercholesterolaemia, usually with hyperlipaemia (that is, hypertriglyceridaemia), is a frequent accompaniment of diabetes mellitus (see page 1340), hypothyroidism (see Chapter 31) and the nephrotic syndrome (see Chapter 24). It may also occur in cases of type I glycogenosis (von Gierke's disease—

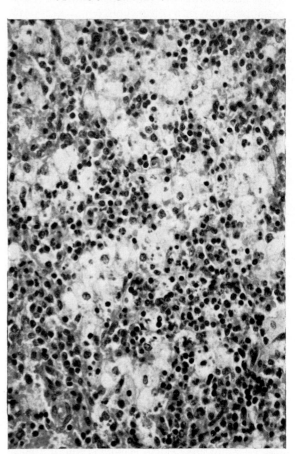

Fig. 9.185. Ceroid storage disease. The cytoplasm of the histiocytes illustrated in this photomicrograph of a splenectomy specimen was yellowish brown when seen in unstained sections and in sections stained with haematoxylin alone. Eosin, unless used very delicately, tends to obscure the pigmentation. When stained with Giemsa's solution the cytoplasm of many of the ceroid-laden histiocytes took on the 'sea blue' colour that is a striking characteristic in this disorder. In the half-tone reproduction the brown pigment appears grey. Under the microscope the colour of the cytoplasm of the histiocytes makes the distinction between this form of histiocytosis and, for instance, that illustrated in Fig. 9.172 (page 742) much simpler than can be appreciated from a comparison of the two figures. *Haematoxylin.* × 250.

see page 1276), presumably as an effect of the disordered glucose metabolism. Particularly high levels of cholesterol and its esters are found in the serum in cases of primary biliary cirrhosis (xanthomatous biliary cirrhosis—see page 1267).

In any of these conditions there may be some degree of histiocytosis in the reticuloendothelial system, with the formation of 'foam cells' laden with lipid. This secondary lipidosis never reaches an extent comparable to the primary cholesterol lipidoses, particularly Hand–Schüller–Christian disease (see page 763).

CEROID STORAGE DISEASE

Ceroid is an acid-fast, yellowish brown, autofluorescent pigment that is considered to be a mixture of substances and to belong to the group of lipofuscin compounds,[1185] of which 'wear-and-tear pigment' in ageing or atrophying tissues is a familiar instance. It is seen in a variety of pathological conditions in man and animals and, without suggesting that the deficiency has any part to play in its occurrence under natural conditions, it has been a conspicuous feature in skeletal muscle and in the brain of animals deprived of vitamin E.[1186]

Ceroid storage disease (Oppenheimer–Andrews syndrome;[1186a*] the 'syndrome of the sea-blue

* Ceroid storage disease is sometimes referred to as 'Landing–Oppenheimer disease': this is a misnomer (see footnote on page 709).

histiocyte';[1186b] Silverstein's syndrome;[1186b] idiopathic ceroid histiocytosis[1123]) is a rare condition, recognized comparatively recently.[1186a] It is sometimes confused with other conditions in which the so-called 'sea-blue histiocytes' are found: these include the fatal granulomatous disease of childhood that is associated with deficiency of the bactericidal activity of the neutrophils (see page 708). It occurs at any age and in both sexes, and is sometimes familial. Its pathogenesis is unknown. The histological picture has the features of a storage disease, with proliferation of histiocytes in the lymphoid tissues and elsewhere. These cells contain ceroid, their cytoplasm appearing yellowish brown in paraffin wax sections stained with haematoxylin and eosin (or, preferably, with haematoxylin alone) and a striking blue or greenish blue in Giemsa preparations (see page 710). Splenomegaly (Fig. 9.185), hyperlipaemia and involvement of the bone marrow are practically constant features,[1123] and there may be enlargement of lymph nodes. Other findings have included thrombocytopenia and purpura, changes in the fundus of the eyes (a white ring in the macula, surrounding the fovea centralis), motor disabilities of central origin, mental retardation, fibrosing infiltration of the lungs and cirrhosis of the liver:[1186c] these are associated with accumulation of ceroid-containing histiocytes in the corresponding tissues.

The disease progresses very slowly, as a rule, and its prognosis is believed to be relatively good.

LYMPHOMAS

When the first edition of this book was published, just over 10 years ago, this section of the corresponding chapter was headed, *The Malignant and Potentially Malignant Diseases Arising in the Lymphoreticular System*. It is an advance that this awkward phrase may now be replaced by the one word, *Lymphomas*. The change reflects capitulation on two points—namely, that all these diseases are malignant, and may therefore be referred to by the term that is now generally conceded to indicate a malignant tumour arising in the lymphoreticular tissues, and, second, that Hodgkin's disease is as much a neoplastic condition as is, for example, a lymphocytic lymphoma.

These diseases will be considered in two main categories—Hodgkin's disease, and the lymphomas other than Hodgkin's disease. Some observations

that are relevant to the lymphomas in general will be mentioned first.

Aetiology

Frequency

The Registrar General's statistical review of England and Wales for the year 1973 showed that the number of deaths from Hodgkin's disease was 776 and from other neoplasms of lymphoid tissue 1780 (see Table 9.2).[1187] In that year the population of the two countries together was estimated to be just under 49·25 million and 121 297 of these died from neoplastic disease.[1187] The number of deaths from cancer arising in selected parts of the body is shown in Table 9.3 as an indication of the frequency of

Table 9.2. *Number of Deaths from Lymphoma in England and Wales in 1973**

Disease	Males	Females	Total
Hodgkin's disease	450	326	776
'Lymphosarcoma and reticulum cell sarcoma'	735	654	1389
Follicular lymphoma	14	10	24
Mycosis fungoides	14	9	23
Other neoplasms of lymphoid tissue	171	173	344
All lymphomas	*1384*	*1172*	*2556*

* From: *The Registrar General's Statistical Review of England and Wales for the Year 1973*, Part 1(A); London, 1975.

Table 9.3. *Number of Deaths from Lymphoma and Other Cancers in England and Wales in 1973 (in Order of Frequency of the 24 Most Frequent Sites or Types of Cancer)**

Order of frequency	Primary cancer (site or type)	Males	Females	Total
1	Trachea, bronchi and lungs	26 032	6144	32 176
2	Large intestine, including rectum	7412	8856	16 268
3	Stomach	7114	5077	12 191
4	Breasts	67	11 428	11 495
5	Pancreas	2780	2559	5339
6	Prostate	4236	—	4236
7	Urinary bladder	2788	1179	3967
8	Uterus	—	3815	3815
9	Ovaries	—	3429	3429
10	Oesophagus	1782	1432	3214
11	Leukaemia	1707	1338	3045
12	*Lymphoma*	*1384*	*1172*	*2556*
13	Brain ('malignant neoplasm'—primary or secondary not specified)	1035	802	1837
14	Kidneys	978	628	1606
15	Myelomatosis	576	579	1155
16	Gall bladder and extrahepatic biliary ducts	415	695	1110
17	Larynx	609	161	770
18	Melanoma of skin	263	335	598
19	Liver	340	209	549
20	Bone	297	221	518
21	Skin, other than melanoma (see above)	271	214	485
22	Thyroid	119	296	415
23	Tongue	216	143	359
24	Testes	265	—	265

* From: *The Registrar General's Statistical Review of England and Wales for the Year 1973*, Part 1(A); London, 1975.

these cancers relative to that of cancer of the lymphoreticular system.

In fact, public records must be recognized to be an imprecise guide to the real frequency of lymphomas, although they may be accepted as a rough index of their frequency relative to that of other cancers. The reason for this unreliability includes lack of uniformity in nomenclature and erratic standards of diagnostic accuracy of death certificates and other records. Comparable difficulties thwart attempts to correlate figures of the numbers of cases of different types of lymphomas in different published series.[1188] If an agreed classification can be developed, and if reasonable accuracy of categorization of individual cases within that classification can be achieved in the practice of general pathologists as well as in diagnostic reference centres, such problems will be overcome: that time is not in sight. The division of the lymphomas into Hodgkin's disease and lymphomas other than Hodgkin's disease, and the prospect of devising a practical classification of the tumours that make up the second of these groups, will lead to improvement of this situation. However, it is practically impossible to compare most older published series with those that are based on the newer systems of classification: most of the material that made up those series is no longer available, because of dispersal, lack of storage facilities, borrowings or simple lack of foresight. Some of the recent series include a proportion of cases previously published in terms of outdated classifications and now re-categorized, but, in general, the newly formulated classifications have not been in use for long enough for many large series to be presented in accordance with their principles (see page 783).

Age and Sex Incidence

Any of the lymphomas may be seen at any age. I have seen Hodgkin's disease in a baby of 9 months and in a man aged 107 years. Hodgkin's disease has its greatest incidence in the first half of adult life; other lymphomas have their greatest incidence well beyond middle age (Figs 9.186 and 9.187).

In general, there is a preponderance of male patients, but this becomes less marked after middle life; in the seventies and upward the majority of patients are women. The greater frequency in men has been interpreted as evidence that endocrine or occupational factors may have a part in the aetiology of these diseases, but this remains speculative. It used to be said that Hodgkin's disease occasionally was exacerbated by pregnancy, and might regress

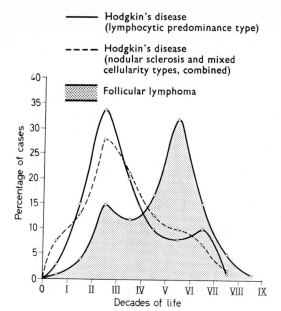

Fig. 9.186.§ Graphs of the comparative incidence, by decades, of the lymphocytic predominance histological type of Hodgkin's disease (continuous line) and the nodular sclerosis and mixed cellularity histological types of Hodgkin's disease (grouped together—interrupted line). The incidence of follicular lymphoma is shown for comparison (continuous line enclosing stippled area). See also Fig. 9.187.

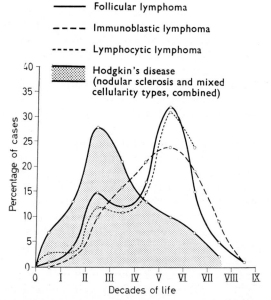

Fig. 9.187.§ Graphs of the comparative incidence, by decades, of follicular lymphoma (continuous line), immunoblastic lymphoma ('reticulum cell sarcoma') (interrupted line) and lymphocytic lymphoma (dotted line). The combined incidence of the nodular sclerosis and mixed cellularity histological types of Hodgkin's disease is shown for comparison (continuous line enclosing stippled area). See also Fig. 9.186.

after childbirth in these cases, but there are now many reports—including reviews that cover hundreds of instances of pregnancy in association with Hodgkin's disease—that indicate that neither condition has any deleterious effect on the other.[1189] The same seems to be true of pregnancy in association with other lymphomas, although this is a much less frequent occurrence in consequence of the substantially greater proportion of the patients with lymphomas other than Hodgkin's disease who are beyond the age of child-bearing when their symptoms first develop.[1189]

Miscellaneous Aetiological Factors

In general, the cause of lymphomas is unknown. In the case of Burkitt's lymphoma the association with the Epstein–Barr virus presents a recognized aetiological factor that is without parallel in relation to all other lymphomas (see page 827). Some other observations are of potential, but not yet assimilable, aetiological importance in relation either to particular varieties of lymphoma or to lymphomas in general: these may be considered briefly.

Association with Predisposing Diseases and with Immunodeficiency

Autoimmune Diseases.—It has long been known that there are some diseases that seem to predispose to the development of lymphomas, and particularly to well-differentiated lymphocytic lymphomas. The association is always rare, but it has been frequent enough to become well known. Among the conditions that carry this occasional liability are long-standing hyperthyroidism,[1190] Hashimoto's thyroiditis (see Chapter 31),[1191] the so-called 'benign lymphoepithelial lesion' of salivary glands (Sjögren's syndrome—see page 952),[1192] chronic ulcerative colitis (see page 1117),[1193] rheumatoid arthritis[1194] and systemic lupus erythematosus.[1194] Such observations must be assessed very carefully before it is accepted that they represent a causal association between the two diseases. For instance, it can be difficult to distinguish between Hashimoto's disease and lymphocytic lymphoma of the thyroid; rarely, the lupus-erythematosus-cell phenomenon ('LE cell' formation—see page 693) may be observed in cases of lymphoma in the absence of clinical and pathological evidence that might confirm the co-existence of systemic lupus erythematosus,[1195] while the lymphadenopathy of the latter (see page 691) has been mistaken for Hodgkin's disease and other lymphomas.[1196]

It is notable that all the diseases just mentioned as possible antecedents of lymphomatous change have an autoimmune element.[1197] This becomes of particular interest in relation to advances in knowledge of the immunological functions of the lymphoreticular system, the identification of certain types of lymphoid cell with particular immune functions (see page 520) and the observation that tumour cells of corresponding functional types may be recognizable.[1198]

Immunodeficiency States.—Lymphomas occasionally develop as a complication of various congenital and acquired states of immunodeficiency. They have occurred in some cases of hypogammaglobulinaemia, both congenital[1199] and acquired,[1200] of 'ataxia-telangiectasia' (Louis-Bar's syndrome—see page 902) and of the Wiskott–Aldrich syndrome (see page 902).[1201] Primary macroglobulinaemia is occasionally complicated by the development of a rapidly progressive lymphocytic or undifferentiated lymphoma (see page 707).

Therapeutic Immunosuppression Predisposing to Lymphoma.—Patients who have received an organ allograft have a significantly greater liability to develop cancer than other people.[1202] This is attributed—in part, at least—to immunosuppressive therapy, particularly with azathioprine and prednisone. Other measures, such as thymectomy and splenectomy, and administration of antilymphocyte serum or antilymphocyte globulin, are likely to be contributory factors if, as seems clear, it is the state of induced immunodeficiency that determines the increased incidence of malignant tumours. In a series of 149 consecutive patients who received a renal allograft and survived the operation for not less than 4 months there were 10 who developed cancer (6·7 per cent, a figure 115 times greater than that for the corresponding general population): seven of the tumours were superficial carcinomas (six in the skin and one in the uterine cervix) and three were lymphomas.[1202] Lymphomas, usually described as reticulum cell sarcomas, have been particularly frequent among such patients; it is notable that most of the patients are well below the age at which such lymphomas are most frequent, and a further peculiarity of the tumours is that they commonly involve tissues that are not conspicuously often affected when histologically comparable growths arise in patients who have no immunodeficiency.[1202] The prognosis of these lymphomas is very poor: they are a much more serious complication than the seemingly more numerous epithelial tumours, which usually are of a type and in a situation that gives good hope of successful eradication.

The Role of Immunological Disturbances

It is evident that immunological disorders of various sorts predispose to the development of lymphomas, although the evidence does not justify the conclusion that this is a factor in the causation of all these tumours or even of most of them. Two main explanations have been put forward—that the immunological state permits infection by oncogenic viruses or facilitates their proliferation and spread,[1203] and that immunodeficiency limits the effectiveness of the 'surveillance' by which the immunologically competent normal cells recognize and destroy or inhibit mutant and potentially neoplastic cells.[1204] There are other possibilities. The particular frequency of highly malignant lymphomas ('reticulum cell sarcomas') among patients who are under immunosuppressive therapy following organ transplantation has been explained tentatively as a result of accelerated malignant change in cells continuously exposed to antigenic stimulation by the presence of the graft: however, the observation that a comparable mechanism may produce lymphomas in mice[1205] is not necessarily related to the occurrence of tumours in patients with allografts. Other possibilities have been suggested: for instance, a graft-against-host reaction, due to the presence of lymphoid tissue transferred to the patient with the grafted organ,[1206] might predispose to lymphomatous change in the host's lymphoreticular tissues; the relevance of the development of lymphomas in animals with a chronic graft-against-host reaction[1207] is uncertain. There appears to be no evidence that therapeutically administered immunosuppressive agents have any direct oncogenic activity.

The causation of lymphomas in the absence of such artificial circumstances as surround their development in patients with an allograft is speculative. The possible role of infective agents and the hypothesis of antigenic overstimulation with consequent neoplastic change and the eventual development of a tumour-against-host reaction is referred to briefly in the account of Hodgkin's disease (see page 813).

Drug-Induced Lymphomas

The possible indirect role of immunosuppressive drugs in the development of lymphomas in patients with renal or other allografts has been mentioned above. It probably has no relation to the still unknown manner in which some other drugs, particularly the hydantoin anticonvulsants, are involved in the pathogenesis of lymphoma-like and lymphomatous changes. These conditions are considered on page 696.

Prognosis[1208, 1209]

The natural tendency of the lymphomas is to progress to death. In general, survival is longest in cases of Hodgkin's disease with lymphocytic predominance and in cases of follicular lymphoma, and shortest in cases of undifferentiated and anaplastic lymphomas. Again, the less extensive the disease the less grave the outlook. Lymphomas arising in organs that are not primarily part of the lymphoreticular system tend to have a worse prognosis than those arising in, say, lymph nodes. Involvement of the mediastinum,[1208] the retroperitoneal tissue, the kidneys,[1210] the lungs (see page 407)[1211] and the central nervous system, is particularly serious. But these generalizations may be upset in individual cases and by many circumstances. For instance, inadequate treatment, especially in the early stages of the disease, may result in prolonged and recurrent illness, and eventual death, when effective initial treatment might be curative. Or, occasionally, a lymphoma that histologically is highly malignant may present while the disease is confined to one part of the body: in some such cases the patient may then be treated successfully. The prognosis in any case of lymphoma is worsened, and may be seriously so, by such factors as the coexistence of other diseases or the development of particular complications of the lymphoma itself. The age and sex of the patient may have prognostic significance: the results in some centres suggest that women respond to treatment rather better than men,[1208] and very young and aged patients of either sex fare worse than others.

Some of these factors may be considered here in more detail.

Complications of Lymphomas

Some of the complications of lymphomas are those that may be associated with any cancer. These include pressure effects of tumours and leucoerythroblastic anaemia resulting from replacement of the marrow by lymphomatous tissue.

Neurological complications, including paraplegia, may be due to direct involvement of nervous tissue in the extension of the lymphoma. In other cases they are manifestations of any of the varieties of encephalopathy, myelopathy and peripheral neuropathy that occur in the course of various types of cancer, including lymphomas[1212] (see Chapters 34 and 35). For instance, multifocal leucoencephalopathy is a demyelinating disease of the brain that is associated with leukaemia and lymphomas, particularly Hodgkin's disease, oftener than with other predisposing diseases.[1213, 1214] Similarly, various forms of myopathy may occur (see Chapter 36). Rapid clinical deterioration may accompany these 'neuromyopathies'.

Other complications are more specifically related to the lymphoma that they accompany. Thus, while leucoerythroblastic anaemia has been mentioned above as a manifestation of displacement of haemopoietic marrow by tumour tissue, some other haematological disturbances are associated with lymphomas oftener than with other cancers. These include haemolytic anaemia and thrombocytopenia with an autoimmune basis, especially in cases of Hodgkin's disease.[1215] Leucopenia (granulocytopenia) and lymphocytopenia[1216] also occur. Macroglobulinaemia may complicate a lymphoma (secondary macroglobulinaemia—see page 707), and amyloidosis develops in the course of a small proportion of cases of Hodgkin's disease.[1217] Resistance to infection may be seriously affected (see page 774), and intercurrent infection—or activation of dormant infection—is the commonest immediate cause of death.

Complications of Diagnostic Procedures and of the Treatment of Lymphomas

Splenectomy is increasingly frequently undertaken in the course of diagnostic laparotomy, the primary purpose of which is to establish the staging of the individual patient's disease (see page 772). The potential hazards of splenectomy have been mentioned earlier in this chapter (page 722). In a series of 1558 cases of splenectomy in the presence of lymphoma, collected from published records, there were 18 deaths attributable to the operation (1·2 per cent).[1218]

The chemotherapy of lymphoma inevitably lowers resistance to infection because it interferes with the activity and supply of the cells that are concerned in defence—neutrophils, macrophages and lymphoid cells. This adds to the predisposition already established by the presence of a lymphoma, particularly Hodgkin's disease, which may notably diminish the body's capacity to inhibit invasion by certain types of organism (see page 774). Radiotherapy has a comparable effect, and the effect is further enhanced when corticosteroids or their synthetic analogues are given—for instance, in the treatment of an accompanying haemolytic anaemia.

Chemotherapy and irradiation disturb haemopoiesis, with consequent anaemia, leucopenia, thrombocytopenia or pancytopenia. Other occasional side effects of irradiation may endanger the patient's life, immediately or more remotely. Hypothyroidism may follow irradiation of the neck, particularly when a dose level of about 3500 rads is considerably exceeded.[1219] Hyperuricaemia and consequent acute renal failure[1220] may result from the destruction within a short period of the nuclei of great numbers of tumour cells. Constrictive pericarditis is an occasional late complication of irradiation of the mediastinum;[1221] the extent and toughness of the fibrous tissue that forms may make surgical relief of the condition very difficult.

Clinical Staging

Whatever the histological type of a lymphoma, widespread disease is less likely to be satisfactorily controlled by treatment and therefore has a poorer prognosis than localized disease. The extent of the disease at the time of initiating treatment is recognized to be both of great prognostic significance and, from the practical point of view, of cardinal importance in planning the treatment. This led to the introduction of a system of clinical staging that facilitates the precise recording of the recognized extent of the disease in individual patients in such a way that the course of the illness and the response to treatment can be accurately compared, not only among the patients under care in particular centres but between as many centres as understand and accurately follow the discipline of the staging system. The system that has become most widely used is often known as the *Ann Arbor staging classification*, as it was formulated in Ann Arbor, Michigan, in 1971.[1222] It was based on an earlier classification, the work of a conference in Rye, New York, in 1965.[1223] The Rye conference also recommended a histological classification of Hodgkin's disease (see page 787),[1224] and—sometimes confusingly—each has been referred to as the 'Rye classification'; since the staging classification was revised at Ann Arbor the earlier eponym is currently applied only to the histological classification.

Staging was introduced in relation exclusively to Hodgkin's disease. More recently, it has begun to be applied, and advantageously, to the lymphomas other than Hodgkin's disease.[1225] The Ann Arbor classification comprises four stages of increasingly widespread distribution of the disease: it is summarized, in simplified form, in Table 9.4. The full classification, which is primarily of use for clinical purposes, and particularly in planning treatment, may be consulted in various texts.[1222, 1225, 1226]

Table 9.4. *Clinical Staging of Hodgkin's Disease (Ann Arbor Staging Classification)**

Clinical stage	Extent of disease
I	Involvement of a single lymph node region [that is, involvement confined to a single anatomical region, such as one side of the neck, or one axilla, although nodes in more than one named group within the single region may be affected]
	or, involvement of a single 'extralymphatic' organ or site†
II	Involvement of two or more lymph node regions on the same side of the diaphragm
	or, localized involvement of an 'extralymphatic' organ or site† and of one or more lymph node regions on the same side of the diaphragm
III	Involvement of lymph node regions on both sides of the diaphragm, which may be accompanied by localized involvement of an 'extralymphatic' organ or site,† or by involvement of the spleen, or by both
IV	Diffuse or disseminate involvement of one or more 'extralymphatic' organs or tissues† [for example, liver, ‡ lung,§ pleura,§ bone marrow, bone or skin], with or without associated lymph node enlargement

* This classification (Carbone, P. P., Kaplan, H. S., Musshoff, K., Smithers, D. W., Tubiana, M., *Cancer Res.*, 1971, **31**, 1860) has been adopted also in relation to lymphomas other than Hodgkin's disease (Moran, E. M., Ultmann, J. E., Ferguson, D. J., Hoffer, P. B., Ranniger, K., Rappaport, H., *Brit. J. Cancer*, 1975, **31**, suppl. 2, 228). Amplification of some details in the original published version has been added [in brackets] for greater clarity.

† The 'extralymphatic' organs and tissues are those organs and tissues that are not 'lymphatic structures'. For the purposes of this classification, the latter are said to comprise the lymph nodes, spleen, thymus, Waldeyer's ring [of fauciopharyngeal lymphoid tissue], the appendix and Peyer's patches [the aggregated lymphoid follicles of the small intestine].

‡ Involvement of the liver is always regarded as 'diffuse' and therefore requires that the disease be classified as Stage IV.

§ Multiple nodules limited to one lobe of one lung are considered to constitute 'localized extralymphatic disease'; so too is juxtahilar extension associated with hilar lymphadenopathy on the same side. Unilateral pleural effusion with hilar lymphadenopathy, whether with or without involvement of the lung, is also regarded as 'localized extralymphatic disease'.

The clinical staging according to this scheme is supplemented by *pathological staging*, which indicates by means of letters representing organs and tissues, and associated positive or negative signs, whether microscopical examination has or has not shown the disease to be present in specimens other than that of the initial diagnostic biopsy (see below).[1226]

Determination of Staging in Individual Cases

Simple clinical examination alone provides at best an unreliable assessment of the formal clinical stage that the disease has reached. Sophisticated investigations, some of them free neither from apprehension and discomfort on the part of the patient nor from risk to his life, provide the means to assess 'staging' objectively and with a remarkable degree of accuracy. The procedures include lymphangiography[1227] and other radiological investigations, and, in appropriate circumstances, laparotomy, isotope scanning,[1228] mediastinoscopy and other biopsy procedures. The purpose of laparotomy is to disclose the extent of involvement of the organs and tissues of the abdominal and pelvic cavities, and particularly, by splenectomy, to find out whether there is gross or microscopical involvement of the spleen:[1218] a palpably enlarged spleen is not necessarily affected by the tumour, nor is an involved spleen necessarily palpable or the presence of tumour in it always disclosed by scintigraphy.

The importance of accurate staging once the diagnosis of lymphoma has been made is threefold. In two respects it is significant from the point of view of the individual patient, providing an index of prognosis and—more pertinent—being a determining factor in relation to the choice of treatment to be adopted, and particularly in the selection of fields for irradiation. The third role of staging is the advantage it brings in terms of communicability of clinical experience between different medical centres, with reference particularly to the results of different schemes of therapy.

Pathological Staging and Histological Diagnosis

Pathological Staging.—The Ann Arbor staging classification, in its published form,[1222, 1226] includes a system of pathological staging, dependent on the extent of the disease as disclosed by microscopy (see above). The present situation seems to be that pathological staging adds to the total of information that can be encoded in the documentation of individual patients' cases and of series of cases; there is no good evidence that it provides information that leads to modification of the clinical assessment provided by clinical staging.

Histological Diagnosis.—In general, the extent of the disease has more practical significance than its histological type. At the same time, the outlook in individual cases in which the disease is of comparable extent is generally related to the histological diagnosis. Among cases of Hodgkin's disease, determination of the histological type—for instance, as currently categorized in the Rye classification (see page 787)—has an essential purpose in assessing the likely prognosis and longterm response to treatment. Similarly, among the lymphomas other than Hodgkin's disease the outlook is broadly equatable to the histological variety and to the degree of differentiation of the tumour.

The prognosis in any case of lymphoma is affected unfavourably by histological progression of the disease from a less malignant type to a more malignant type (see note below Table 9.5, page 778). Such progression is likeliest to occur in cases of Hodgkin's disease (see page 803).

Treatment as a Factor in Prognosis

The advances that have been made in the last two decades by pathologists and clinical diagnosticians specializing in the study of lymphomas have been paralleled by the continuing development of effective methods of treatment. The result is the remarkable improvement in outlook for the patient in terms of greatly prolonged survival, eventually in circumstances that some regard as a return to normal enjoyment of life. The incentive to study these diseases in detail may be attributed in part to the achievements of the earlier radiotherapists and the resulting need for preciser knowledge of the pathological changes and their relation to the choice and effectiveness of treatment. The development of effective chemotherapy has underlined the importance of such studies.

It is salutary to remember that before the days of treatment with X-rays the patient with Hodgkin's disease lived, on average, for 20 months after the diagnosis was made.[1229] Very few patients were known to live significantly much longer. The first indications of a more hopeful outlook came during the 20 years from 1917 to 1937, mainly through the work of Gilbert, in Geneva.[1229] Although Pusey, in Chicago, Illinois, had used X-rays in the treatment of Hodgkin's disease in 1901,[1230] it was Gilbert who showed the possibility of a longterm response of the

M

disease to such treatment, more than doubling the average period of survival from 20 months in 1917 to 42 months by 1937, with some patients alive 6 years and more after being treated. Since then, advances in irradiation technology and in the techniques of radiotherapy, and the introduction of modern chemotherapy, particularly in the 1960s and 1970s, have transformed the outlook for patients with lymphoma. Even patients with the prognostically most unfavourable clinical stage of Hodgkin's disease may have a 27 per cent survival rate at 7 years after diagnosis, and those with the least malignant histological types and the least extensive disease have a survival rate of better than 90 per cent at 5 years.[1208]

Good therapeutic results depend on many factors. Among these are accuracy and completeness of diagnosis, and to approach this ideal closely it is essential that the pathologist be a member of the clinical team and involved throughout the diagnostic study, appraisal and reappraisal of each patient.

Predisposition to Infection[1231]

Patients with malignant lymphomas have a notably greater liability than other individuals to certain types of infection. These infections include certain mycoses, tuberculosis and various other bacterial infections, and viral and protozoal infections. Their manifestations are often unusual, they often run an unusually rapid course and have a considerably heightened mortality, and they are often the immediate cause of death or among its major contributory factors. Other diseases that involve and destroy a considerable part of the lymphoreticular system—for example, the leukaemias and sarcoidosis—are also liable to be complicated by such infections. Treatment given for the lymphoreticular disease also predisposes to infection (see below) and this greatly increases the hazard of overwhelming microbial invasion of the body. It is highly significant that infection in these patients commonly develops so rapidly and with so little direct evidence of its presence that death results without this immediate cause being recognized before the post-mortem examination. Indeed, in some instances—particularly of mycotic infection—the condition is first discovered when the tissues are examined histologically after death.

In some cases the infecting organisms are such as ordinarily are of only limited pathogenicity, if indeed they cause infection at all in the absence of predisposing conditions. The disease that they cause in patients with a lymphoma comes therefore into the category of the so-called opportunistic infections (see page 262, volume 1), and this term is often also applied to the fatal generalization of infections, such as cryptococcosis and even tuberculosis, that in other circumstances would not become disseminate and progressive. Lymphomas predispose to obtrusive and serious manifestations of infections that are widely prevalent in subclinical form. Thus, in parts of the world where brucellosis is endemic, patients with systemic lymphomas, such as Hodgkin's disease, are particularly liable to have overt illness due to the infection (see page 591). Similarly, where mycoses such as histoplasmosis, coccidioidomycosis or 'North American' blastomycosis are endemic, a significant proportion of the rare, fatal, disseminate forms of the infection is found among patients with lymphoma, particularly Hodgkin's disease: these cases present a striking contrast to the benign subclinical course that ordinarily is characteristic of these mycoses. Sarcoidosis has a comparable predisposing role (see below).

Some other complicating infections may be considered separately.

Cryptococcosis

Unlike histoplasmosis and the other mycoses just noted, cryptococcosis has no known endemic or subclinical form, and in the greater proportion of recognized cases the infection is progressive and, in the absence of treatment, fatal. It is noteworthy that as many as a sixth, and more, of the patients in some series of cases of generalized or meningocerebral cryptococcosis developed the infection during the course of Hodgkin's disease[1232] or sarcoidosis.[1233] In a series of 166 cases of cryptococcosis, from various parts of the world and mostly unpublished, 34 (20 per cent) were associated with Hodgkin's disease, 11 (6·6 per cent) with sarcoidosis and one (0·6 per cent) with immunoblastic lymphadenopathy:[1234] these 46 cases represent 39 per cent of the 119 cases of progressive disseminate infection; none of the 47 cases of successfully treated, isolated manifestations of cryptococcosis in this series was associated with any systematized lymphoreticular disease. Whatever the nature of the deficiency that predisposes patients with these diseases to progressive cryptococcosis (see below), the need for early diagnosis of the complication is imperative if the infection is to be treated successfully and without disabling sequelae, such as meningeal adhesions following meningoencephalitis. Patients with Hodgkin's disease and sarcoidosis are particularly vulnerable to the hazard of infection by cryptococci in the environment, particularly where bird droppings have provided a natural medium for the growth of the fungus.[1235, 1236]

The lymphomas that have a more rapidly progressive course—that is, those other than Hodgkin's disease, and the more malignant types of Hodgkin's disease itself (see Table 9.12, page 788)—are rarely complicated by cryptococcosis. It is possible that this indicates that the failure of immunity may have to be of longer duration, or may develop only when there is more complete replacement of the normal lymphoreticular tissues than is usually the case with the more rapidly progressive lymphomas.

Bacterial Infections

Tuberculosis.—Although it is now recognized that the association of tuberculosis with Hodgkin's disease may have been overstated in the past, through misinterpretation of the epithelioid cell aggregates in some cases of the latter,[1237] there is no doubt that the association exists, even if its frequency has fallen in some parts of the world in correspondence with the fall in incidence of tuberculosis in the population.[1238] Pulmonary, meningeal or miliary tuberculosis[1239] may be the immediate cause of death in cases of Hodgkin's disease, and even today tuberculosis is a greater—and commoner—risk to patients with Hodgkin's disease than some doctors realize. Such manifestations of tuberculosis as lupus vulgaris may be reactivated as Hodgkin's disease progresses, with consequent generalization of the infection.[1240]

A rare and remarkable distribution of tuberculous lesions is seen in exceptional cases of Hodgkin's disease, only the organs of the lymphoreticular system being involved. Lymph nodes, and sometimes the spleen and bone marrow, are converted into masses of necrotic tissue in which tubercle bacilli may be exceptionally numerous, both in the necrotic matter and, particularly, in the surrounding histiocytes. The microscopical picture is comparable in some respects to that of lepromatous leprosy, at least in the areas that are not necrotic, and the term 'lepromatous tuberculosis' has understandably, but rather unfortunately, been applied.[1241] In this form of tuberculosis, which is essentially that described as generalized non-reactive tuberculosis (see page 602), it may be difficult to find recognizable traces of the predisposing disease *post mortem* in spite of unequivocal biopsy evidence prior to the tuberculous infection becoming manifest: however, the more extensive the histological study, the less likely it is that the underlying disease will elude confirmation.

Similar apparent obliteration of a lymphocytic lymphoma by the development of disseminate histoplasmosis has been reported.[1242]

Other Bacterial Infections.—Patients with lymphomas are also predisposed to the development of acute bacterial infections. These have a notable tendency to take the form of a rapidly progressive septicaemia[1243] and the organisms responsible range from *Streptococcus pyogenes* and *Staphylococcus aureus* through klebsiellae, species of proteus and other coliform bacilli to those, such as corynebacterial species, that otherwise are rarely, if ever, observed as the cause of such infection. Salmonella infection, in the form of severe enteritis,[1243] or of fulminating septicaemia[1244, 1245] caused by organisms that ordinarily are responsible for bacterial 'food poisoning' (see page 575), is particularly serious in these patients. Septicaemia, meningitis or meningoencephalitis from infection by *Listeria monocytogenes* is also particularly frequently associated with lymphomas (see page 577).[1246, 1247]

Viral Infections

Predisposition to overt infection by cytomegalovirus, with widespread microscopical evidence of the disease at necropsy, is probably the best known manifestation of the increased susceptibility of patients with a lymphoma or leukaemia to develop serious viral infections.[1248, 1249] However, other viral diseases may occur in a rapidly progressive, fatal form in such patients. Generalization of herpes simplex (infection with *Herpesvirus hominis*), with fatal involvement of viscera, particularly the brain, is among these.[1243, 1250] Patients with Hodgkin's disease who harbour *Herpesvirus varicellae* are liable to repeated attacks of herpes zoster, with or without a generalized eruption characteristic of varicella, and in some cases accompanied by visceral disease, particularly encephalitis.[1251] Similarly, patients who are vaccinated against smallpox while suffering from a lymphoma or leukaemia are liable to develop progressive vaccinia, again with visceral involvement, particularly pneumonia and encephalitis.[1252] Indeed, immunization with live viruses is contraindicated by the presence of a lymphoma or of leukaemia because of the significant risk that a progressive infection may be established—vaccination with yellow fever virus is another example of this danger.[1253]*

* For the same reason, administration of bacillus Calmette–Guérin (BCG) is contraindicated. In a recent case, BCG was given to a child at school, the school doctor being

Pneumocystis Infection

The frequency with which infection by *Pneumocystis carinii* accompanies generalized infection by cytomegalovirus justifies including it at this point (see page 324, Volume 1). The continuing uncertainty whether the organism is a fungus or a protozoon has been mentioned on page 630. Pneumocystis pneumonia and the much rarer infections of other tissues (see page 630) are seen in adults most frequently as a complication of a lymphoma, particularly Hodgkin's disease, and particularly when treatment with corticosteroids is necessary.[1253] The pneumonia may be so extensive that it endangers the patient's life, and its recognition is the more important as the infection may respond to treatment, provided the contributory predisposing role of other drugs can be interrupted.[1254] It may be possible to detect the organism in sputum or, preferably, in material aspirated from the trachea or bronchi.

Protozoal Infection

Toxoplasmosis is of peculiar importance in relation to lymphomas as it may occur in the form of a severe and potentially fatal infection complicating the latter;[1255] in other instances, toxoplasmosis is itself mistaken for Hodgkin's disease (see page 655).[1256] While the prognosis of toxoplasma infection in otherwise healthy adults is good, apart from the risk of transmission of the disease to the fetus if the patient is pregnant, the prognosis of toxoplasmosis developing as a complication of a lymphoma or leukaemia may be very grave. The importance of recognizing its presence in such cases is reflected in the necessity for starting appropriate treatment with as little delay as possible if irreversible damage to the brain and, less frequently, other organs, including the heart, is to be avoided. Acute destructive encephalitis or meningoencephalitis, myelitis and acute myocarditis are the usual fatal manifestations. Rapidly progressive, fatal toxoplasmic peritonitis has been described as a complication of Hodgkin's disease.[1257]

Treatment of Lymphoma and Predisposition to Infection

Apart from the predisposing role of a lymphoma or of other diseases that involve the lymphoreticular

system extensively, such as leukaemia and sarcoidosis, treatment that is given for these conditions contributes in several important ways to the occurrence of infection. Radiotherapy, chemotherapy and corticosteroids and their analogues all interfere with the defences against infection. Reduction in the capacity of the bone marrow to produce neutrophils, destruction of lymphoid tissue and consequent deficiency of antibody responses, and interference with the phagocytic activity of the reticuloendothelial cells and with their capacity to proliferate are among the more obvious effects of these therapeutic agents. It is likely that they also act in ways that are not yet evident, for there is some degree of specificity in the kinds of infections that particular types of drug predispose to: for instance, corticosteroids seem to encourage the development of pneumocystis infection and of infection by *Nocardia asteroides*, the former possibly representing activation of a dormant endogenous infection while the latter is believed to be always exogenous. Cytotoxic (immunosuppressant) drugs of all types share a liability to permit the establishment of progressive visceral and haematogenous infection by moulds, particularly species of aspergillus and the various phycomycetes. In general, however, it is impossible in a given case, or even from consideration of series of cases, to indicate which drug or other agent is responsible for a particular infection, and the likelihood is that they act more or less together to lower resistance to the wide range of organisms that are known to cause these so-called 'opportunistic infections'. Similarly, it is not possible to determine to what extent the underlying disease and the treatment respectively contribute to the occurrence of infection.

In most instances the source of the infecting organism is not determinable. The moulds are generally considered to be of exogenous origin; in contrast, *Candida albicans*, and possibly other species of candida, may usually be endogenous and part of the patient's personal flora, although in some cases it may be that the organism comes from the mouth and throat of those looking after him.

Sometimes changes in intestinal flora resulting from the administration of broad spectrum antibiotics enables an organism such as a candida or *Geotrichum candidum*, or an antibiotic-resistant strain of *Staphylococcus aureus*, to proliferate in the intestine and thence gain access to the tissues, as through the surface of an ulcer: once the tissues are invaded, rapid dissemination throughout the body is encouraged by the state of immunodeficiency induced by other drugs.

---

unaware that the child was under treatment for Hodgkin's disease: disseminated infection resulted, but was treated successfully.

Pathogenesis of Infections Complicating Lymphomas

Remarkably little is known about the mechanisms that underlie the acquired immunodeficiency that characterizes certain types of lymphoma. It is clear that an acquired defect in cell-mediated immunity is present in many cases of Hodgkin's disease (as also in sarcoidosis), with the result that skin tests are negative when in fact they should indicate delayed hypersensitivity to, for instance, tuberculin or histoplasmin in individuals who are known to have overcome a past infection by the corresponding organism. It is this deficiency in cell-mediated immunity that accounts for the activation of dormant infection and the rapid progression of the resulting disease. This means that there is a failure in the function of the T lymphocytes (see page 520). In cases of Hodgkin's disease there is little or no evidence of any disturbance in the production of circulating antibodies, or of complement, or in the capacity of passively sensitized tissues to react;[1258] the infective complications of Hodgkin's disease are therefore usually caused by organisms that ordinarily evoke a cell-mediated response. Eventually, the immunodeficiency becomes very complex,[1259] and this complexity to some extent is bound up with effects of the various therapeutic agents.[1243]

In contrast, it has been shown that in cases of chronic lymphocytic leukaemia (or at least in the majority of cases—those in which the leukaemic cells are of the B cell series) the deficiency is in the formation of humoral (circulating) antibodies, with hypogammaglobulinaemia.[1259a] Bacterial infections are frequent in these cases and are caused by the types of organisms that ordinarily evoke this variety of antibody response.

From the practical point of view, these disturbances add gravely to the danger to the patient's life. The risks were strikingly illustrated in an extreme and unprecedented example. A middle-aged man with Hodgkin's disease (initially with lymphocytic predominance and later of mixed cell type) developed haemolytic anaemia and, terminally, acute leukaemia as complications. He was treated with X-rays, various cytotoxic drugs and corticosteroids. He survived an acute episode of non-reactive tuberculosis with generalized necrotizing lymphadenitis, followed by cryptococcal meningitis. Eventually he died, with six distinct varieties of terminal haematogenous infection (staphylococcal pyaemia, candidosis, aspergillosis, phycomycosis, cryptococcosis and cytomegalovirus infection); there was also pneumocystis pneumonia.[1260]

Classifications

(Tables 9.5, 9.6 and 9.7)

The diagnosis and differential diagnosis of lymphomas, and particularly their distinction from benign conditions, are among the most frequent and most difficult problems in the practice of the general pathologist. A part of the difficulty that we experience is directly a consequence of the changing tenor both of classification and the bases of classification. Debate and argument about new and sometimes conflicting classifications and their modifications and variations, particularly in relation to lymphomas other than Hodgkin's disease, have not yet led to the generally acceptable, practical system of nomenclature and categorization that is so widely called for. In some centres that I have visited recently, in Europe as elsewhere, it has been disquieting to find different terminology and classifications in use by different groups of individuals, all of whom are concerned in the care of the same patients. The possibility that confusion or misunderstanding may arise, to the detriment of the patients, is not fanciful. For such reasons, any drafts of further new classifications, or of modifications of existing ones, would best be restricted initially to circulation between experts who are in a position to assess whether the innovations are well found, in keeping with general experience of these diseases, and advantageous.

It is not surprising that some general physicians, and some pathologists, are confused and exasperated by the number and complexity of the 'modern' classifications, which seem so often to be phrased in terms that are novel in themselves in addition to expressing novel concepts and novel interpretations of the identity and function of cells, tissues and body systems. The practising clinician gladly accepts and applies the advances made by his more research-minded colleagues when they are reasonably clearly expressed, and identifiable in terms of his own experience. But, fundamentally, he requires of the laboratory an expression of opinion whether the biopsy specimen from a given patient shows evidence that amounts to, or at least may lead to, a diagnosis of the latter's illness: the clinician wants to know, in simple and familiar terms, whether the patient has a lymphoma or some other disease, and, if it is a lymphoma, whether it is of a type likely to respond to treatment. Rightly or wrongly, he is not particularly interested in the terminology: his interest is in his patient's condition and in what is to be done to improve it. He may also recognize—and sometimes better than his

Continued an page 783

Table 9.5. *The Henry Rappaport Classification of Malignant Lymphomas**

Rappaport classification	Earlier synonymous terms	Notes
Undifferentiated lymphoma (consists of cells 15 to 35 μm in diameter, with pale, often scanty cytoplasm and no evident cell borders; the nuclei are twice to 4 times as large as those of lymphocytes and are oval or round, with a distinct membrane, delicate chromatin and a single, small nucleolus; reticulin fibres are scarce and probably are the remains of pre-existing stroma)	Stem cell lymphoma; reticulum cell sarcoma; syncytial reticulum cell sarcoma; undifferentiated reticulum cell sarcoma; undifferentiated reticulosarcoma; immature form of retothelial sarcoma	Rappaport, because of the predominance of undifferentiated cells, classified Burkitt's tumour tentatively as an undifferentiated lymphoma rather than as a poorly differentiated lymphocytic lymphoma (see reference [*] below, page F8–99)
Histiocytic lymphoma (consists of cells that vary much in appearance, in accordance with their differentiation: size, amount of cytoplasm, staining intensity, and presence or absence of phagocytic activity — *e.g.*, ingested nuclear debris—are among the variable features; cell borders are distinct in the better differentiated tumours, and this is accentuated by the intercellular reticulin fibres, which are a characteristic in these cases; nuclei may be indented, like those of monocytes, or oval, like those of epithelioid cells in granulomas, or elongated, like those of fibroblasts; nucleoli are prominent, and larger than in undifferentiated lymphomas	Clasmatocytic lymphoma; reticulum cell sarcoma; dictyocytic reticulosarcoma; dictyosyncytial reticulosarcoma; fibrillary reticulosarcoma; differentiated reticulosarcoma; reticuloendothelial sarcoma; mature form of retothelial sarcoma	A pleomorphic, giant-celled form of lymphoma, formerly included in the category 'Hodgkin's sarcoma' (pleomorphic reticulum cell sarcoma), was classified by Rappaport as a variant of the histiocytic lymphoma. He retained the category 'Hodgkin's sarcoma' for those pleomorphic, giant-celled lymphomas that include cells with the features of Sternberg–Reed cells. See reference [*] below, pages F8–101 and F8–160.
Mixed cell (histiocytic-lymphocytic) lymphoma	Reticulolymphosarcoma	
Poorly differentiated lymphocytic lymphoma (consists of cells that are larger than mature lymphocytes and smaller than histiocytes; their nucleus is round or, less often, of irregular shape, and the chromatin is coarse; there is usually marked mitotic activity)	'Lymphoblastic' lymphosarcoma;† 'lymphoblastic' reticulosarcoma†	
Well-differentiated lymphocytic lymphoma (consists of cells that have the appearances of mature lymphocytes; there is little, if any, variation in the size and shape of the nuclei)	Lymphocytic lymphosarcoma	
Hodgkin's disease: Hodgkin's paragranuloma Hodgkin's granuloma Hodgkin's sarcoma		'Hodgkin's sarcoma': see *Note* opposite 'histiocytic lymphoma' (above)

During their natural course some lymphomas may change their histological type. For instance, occasional undifferentiated lymphomas become differentiated and develop the cytological characteristics of the histiocytic type or of the poorly differentiated or well-differentiated lymphocytic type; mixed cell lymphomas may develop into the histiocytic or poorly differentiated lymphocytic type; the well-differentiated lymphocytic lymphoma may acquire the characteristics of the poorly differentiated lymphocytic lymphoma, and the latter may become transformed into the histiocytic type; and Hodgkin's disease may become transformed into a histiocytic lymphoma (but see *Note* opposite the latter in the body of the table).

The Rappaport classification explicitly indicates also that any type of malignant lymphoma may occur in two patterns—'nodular' ('follicular') and 'diffuse' ('non-follicular'). It does not recognize the occurrence of any variety of follicular lymphoma as an entity.

* From: Rappaport, H., *Tumors of the Hematopoietic System* (Atlas of Tumor Pathology, sect. 3, fasc. 8), pages F8–97 to F8–161; Washington, D.C., 1966.

† 'Lymphoblastic' in this context refers to cells that at the time were regarded as the immediate precursors of lymphocytes. The concept of the transformed lymphocyte, which is known sometimes as a 'lymphoblast' as well as by the more usual term 'immunoblast', is of more recent date (see page 517).

Table 9.6. *The Lukes–Collins Classification of Malignant Lymphomas Other than Hodgkin's Disease**†

Lukes–Collins classification	Nearest correspondence to categories of the Rappaport classification (see Table 9.5)*
U cell lymphoma (undefined cell lymphoma)‡	Undifferentiated lymphoma
T cell lymphomas [tumours of thymus-dependent lymphocytes]	
1. Mycosis fungoides and Sézary's syndrome§	——
2. Lymphoma of convoluted lymphocytes‖	Undifferentiated lymphoma; poorly differentiated lymphocytic lymphoma
3. Immunoblastic sarcoma of T cells¶	Histiocytic lymphoma
B cell lymphomas [tumours of 'bursa-equivalent'-dependent lymphocytes]	
1. Lymphoma of small lymphocytes (chronic lymphocytic leukaemia is the leukaemic manifestation of this tumour)	Well-differentiated lymphocytic lymphoma
2. Lymphoma of plasmacytoid lymphocytes**	——
3. Lymphomas of follicular centre cells (follicular; diffuse; follicular and diffuse; sclerotic)††	
(a) Lymphoma of small cells with cloven nucleus	Poorly differentiated lymphocytic lymphoma; well-differentiated lymphocytic lymphoma
(b) Lymphoma of large cells with cloven nucleus	Histiocytic lymphoma; mixed cell (histiocytic-lymphocytic) lymphoma; poorly differentiated lymphocytic lymphoma
(c) Lymphoma of small cells with non-cloven nucleus	Undifferentiated lymphoma; poorly differentiated lymphocytic lymphoma
(d) Lymphoma of large cells with non-cloven nucleus	Histiocytic lymphoma
4. Immunoblastic sarcoma of B cells¶	Histiocytic lymphoma
Histiocytic lymphoma‡‡	Histiocytic lymphoma‡‡
Unclassifiable lymphomas§§	——

The following footnotes relate specifically to this table and are intended to explain some aspects of the classification, including the cytological terminology adopted in its categories.

* From: Lukes, R. J., Collins, R. D., *Brit. J. Cancer*, 1975, **31**, suppl. 2, 1.

† The Lukes–Collins classification is described as a 'functional classification'—that is, it attempts to relate the varieties of lymphoma to the function of the non-neoplastic cells that are considered to be the analogues of the tumour cells.

‡ The 'U cells' (undefined cells) are so-called because they lack discriminative membrane markers and cytochemical indicators. They cannot be identified with T cells or B cells, which have specific immunological membrane markers and, in certain circumstances, pyroninophile cytoplasm, or with histiocytes, which may be identifiable by certain enzyme systems (Yam, L. T., Li, C. Y., Crosby, W. H., *Amer. J. clin. Path.*, 1971, **55**, 283). The U cells are known also as 'null cells'. Lukes and Collins described them as 'essentially hypothetical' (reference [*] above).

§ See page 853 and Chapter 39, Volume 5.

‖ The 'convoluted lymphocytes' appear to be peculiar to this variety of lymphoma, which is characterized by the association of a mediastinal tumour with acute lymphoblastic leukaemia, usually in adolescence (Barcos, M. P., Lukes, R. J., in *Conflicts in Childhood Cancer: An Evaluation of Current Management*, edited by L. F. Sinks and J. O. Godden, page 147; New York, 1975). They are so-called because their nucleus is patterned by fine linear divisions amounting in effect to a convolutional (gyriform) subdivision or lobation (it is only the nucleus that is convoluted, not the cell as a whole). The arrangement of the divisions has been likened to the footprints of chickens and the cells are sometimes referred to as 'chicken foot cells'. The nucleus retains a rounded outline, as—generally—does the cell itself. Only the larger cells of the tumour show this nuclear convolution; these cells are described as ranging up to the size of a 'reactive histiocyte' [that is, a macrophage such as may be seen with ingested nuclear debris in a germinal centre in a lymphoid follicle—about 25 μm in diameter]. The smaller cells range upward from the size of the nucleus of a small lymphocyte; they have an unconvoluted, round nucleus. All the cells, irrespective of size and nuclear configuration, are discrete ('non-cohesive'); their nuclear chromatin is finely dispersed, there may be a small, central nucleolus, and mitotic figures are usually numerous.

¶ The 'immunoblastic sarcomas' are considered to be tumours of transformed lymphocytes ('immunoblasts'—see page 517), which almost always are B cells. They are highly malignant. They complicate longstanding diseases that are characterized by immunological disorder, including rheumatoid arthritis, systemic lupus erythematosus and macroglobulinaemia, and it is possible that what has previously been regarded as a 'reticulum cell sarcoma' arising as a complication of Sjögren's syndrome (see page 952) or of immunosuppressant therapy in recipients of grafts (see page 770), or in association with alpha heavy chain disease (see page 847) and congenital immunodeficiency states (see page 770), is in fact an immunoblastic sarcoma. It has been suggested, therefore, that this is a tumour that 'may develop in abnormal, damaged or even senescent immune systems following chronic antigenic stimulation' (reference [*] above). The tumour cells are large, with abundant cytoplasm, which is pyroninophile and of irregular outline. Their nucleus is large and, in many cells, oval; the chromatin is finely dispersed and one or more prominent nucleoli are present. Some of the cells are plasmacytoid.

** The lymphoma with plasmacytoid lymphocytes is usually composed mainly of small lymphocytes, but includes a variable proportion of plasmacytoid lymphocytes, which have an eccentric nucleus of lymphocytic type. Some of the cells may contain an intranuclear inclusion that gives a positive periodic-acid/Schiff reaction: this inclusion is

Notes continued on next page.

identical with that occasionally found in the lymphocytes in primary macroglobulinaemia (see page 706).

†† The lymphomas of follicular centre cells are formed of cells that correspond to the cells with cloven (cleaved) nucleus or to those with pyroninophile cytoplasm and non-cloven (non-cleaved) nucleus [these cells, with the 'stainable body' macrophages (see page 512) and the dendritic reticular cells (see page 514), constitute the follicular centre ('germinal centre'—see page 512)]. Large cell and small cell varieties are distinguished. The cleavage of the nucleus may be more marked than in the normal cell. The larger cells with cloven nucleus tend to be cohesive and have a small amount of pyroninophile cytoplasm; the smaller cells appear non-cohesive and their cytoplasm is scanty or inapparent. Mitosis is rare among the smaller cells and less so among the larger. The cleavage of the nucleus of the latter may be so extreme that the appearance simulates a multinucleate cell and may be taken for a Sternberg–Reed cell. Tumours of follicular centre cells with non-cloven nucleus are designated as of the small cell type when the nucleus in most of the cells is smaller than that of the 'stainable body' macrophages, which are commonly present in these tumours; they are designated as of the large cell type when the nucleus of most of the tumour cells is as large as or larger than that of the macrophages. The cells with non-cloven nucleus have conspicuously pyroninophile cytoplasm that varies in amount;

neighbouring cells tend to be cohesive. The smaller cells have a round nucleus with fine chromatin and small nucleoli. The large cells have an oval nucleus with fine chromatin and one large or 2 or 3 smaller nucleoli, often situated on the nuclear membrane. Mitotic figures are numerous. The Burkitt lymphoma is assigned to the category of follicular centre cell lymphoma of small cells with non-cloven nucleus (reference [*] above).

‡‡ The histiocytic lymphoma of this classification is difficult to distinguish from the follicular centre cell lymphoma of large cells with non-cloven nucleus, unless fresh material is available for investigation of enzyme activity and of immunological membrane markers (reference [*] above). It is a tumour of macrophages or identifiable reticulum cells (that is, cells demonstrably containing alpha-naphthol acetate esterase [or that have other cytochemical or immunological characteristics that distinguish them from the other cells with which they may be confused, particularly lymphoma cells of the B-cell series]). The histiocytic lymphoma is very much rarer than the tumours formerly referred to as reticulum cells sarcomas (or by such synonyms of this term as reticulosarcoma, retothelial sarcoma, reticuloendothelial sarcoma and stem cell sarcoma).

§§ The unclassifiable lymphomas are those that cannot be categorized because, for technical reasons, their cytological features cannot be distinguished.

Table 9.7. *The Kiel Classification of Malignant Lymphomas Other than Hodgkin's Disease*[*][†]

Kiel classification	Nearest correspondence to categories of the Rappaport classification (see Table 9.5)	Nearest correspondence to categories of the Lukes–Collins classification (see Table 9.6)
LYMPHOMAS OF LOW-GRADE MALIGNANCY		
Lymphocytic lymphomas		
1. Chronic lymphocytic leukaemia (B cell type)	Well-differentiated lymphocytic lymphoma (see below also)	B-cell lymphoma of small lymphocytes
2. 'Hairy cell' leukaemia (?)‡	——	——
3. Mycosis fungoides and Sézary's syndrome		T-cell lymphomas: mycosis fungoides and Sézary's syndrome
4. Chronic lymphocytic leukaemia (T-cell type)§	——	——
5. T-zone lymphoma‖	——	——
Lymphomas of immunoglobulin-secreting cells	These tumours were considered by Rappaport apart from the lymphomas: he classed them as 'proliferative diseases with dys-proteinaemia' (pages F8–207 to F8–237 of reference [*] in Table 9.5)	
1. Lymphoplasmacytic/lymphoplasmacytoid lymphoma (lymphoplasmacytoid immunocytoma)	——	B-cell lymphoma of plasmacytoid lymphocytes
2. Plasmacytic lymphoma (plasmacytoma¶)	——	——
Lymphomas of germinal centre cells		
1. Centrocytic lymphoma (germinocytoma, centrocytoma)**	Well-differentiated and poorly differentiated lymphocytic lymphomas; mixed cell (histiocytic-lymphocytic) lymphoma; histiocytic lymphoma	B-cell lymphoma of follicular centre cells with cloven nucleus (diffuse type)

Table 9.7 continued on next page.

Table 9.7 (*continued*)

Kiel classification	Nearest correspondence to categories of the Rappaport classification (see Table 9.5)	Nearest correspondence to categories of the Lukes–Collins classification (see Table 9.6)
2. Centroblastic/centrocytic lymphoma (germinoblastoma):**†† follicular follicular and diffuse diffuse with or without sclerosis	Well-differentiated and poorly differentiated lymphocytic lymphomas; mixed cell (histio-cytic-lymphocytic) lymphoma; histiocytic lymphoma	B-cell lymphoma of follicular centre cells with cloven nucleus
LYMPHOMAS OF HIGH-GRADE MALIGNANCY *Centroblastic lymphomas* (germinoblastic sarcomas)**†† 1. Primary [*i.e.*, arising without relation to a pre-existing tumour] 2. Secondary [*i.e.*, arising from a centro-blastic/centrocytic lymphoma, or arising in the presence of such a tumour but in another site]	Histiocytic lymphoma; undifferentiated lymphoma	B-cell lymphoma of large follicular centre cells with non-cloven nucleus
Lymphoblastic lymphomas (lymphoblastic sarcomas, including acute lymphoblastic leukaemia)‡‡ 1. Burkitt lymphoma§§	Undifferentiated lymphoma; poorly differentiated lymphocytic lymphoma Burkitt's tumour was classed by Rappaport as an undifferentiated lymphoma (see Table 9.5)	B-cell lymphoma of small follicular centre cells with non-cloven nucleus As above
2. Lymphoma of convoluted cells [*i.e.*, cells with 'convoluted' (gyriform) nucleus] (lymphoma of acid-phosphatase-containing lymphoblasts)‖‖ 3. Unclassified lymphoma¶¶	Undifferentiated lymphoma; poorly differentiated lymphocytic lymphoma Poorly differentiated lymphocytic lymphoma	T-cell lymphoma of convoluted lymphocytes [*i.e.*, lymphocytes with 'convoluted' (gyriform) nucleus] U-cell ('undefined cell') lymphoma; unclassifiable lymphomas
Immunoblastic lymphomas (immunoblastic sarcomas):*** with plasmablastic/plasmacytic differentiation (derived from B cell series) without plasmablastic/plasmacytic differentiation (derived from B cell series or T cell series) (*a*) Leukaemic variant (immunoblastic leukaemia)	Histiocytic lymphoma	Immunoblastic sarcoma of B cells; immunoblastic sarcoma of T cells

The following footnotes relate specifically to this table and are intended to explain some aspects of the classification, including the cytological terminology adopted in its categories.

*This table represents the Kiel classification as modified in the monograph (in English) by Professor Lennert and his colleagues (reference 1264 on page 884), which he generously made available to me in typescript in August 1976. The modification is derived from the first published version of the classification (reference 1265 on page 884).

† The Kiel classification, like the Lukes–Collins classification (Table 9.6), relates to the functional characteristics of the cells that constitute the tumours. It does not include tumours of reticulum cells (that is, of cells that are demonstrably reticulum cells—see footnote [‡‡] of Table 9.6), and so it has no category corresponding to the histiocytic lymphoma of the Lukes–Collins classification.

M*

‡ See page 861.

§ The Sézary syndrome accounts for many cases of chronic lymphocytic leukaemia of the T-cell type and is characterized by erythroderma, generalized enlargement of lymph nodes and the presence of peculiar lymphocytes ('Lutzner cells', or 'Sézary cells'—see page 856) in the blood and lymph nodes. In contrast to the majority of cases of chronic lymphocytic leukaemia, which are of B cell type, the cells of the leukaemia accompanying Sézary's syndrome are of T cell type. Exceptionally, chronic lymphocytic leukaemia of T cell type, even when accompanied by erythroderma, is characterized by cells that morphologically distinguish the condition as distinct from Sézary's syndrome.

‖ The so-called T-zone lymphoma is characterized by

Notes continued on next page.

neoplastic proliferation of T cells in the T cell region (deep cortex, or 'paracortical area') between the lymphoid follicles of lymph nodes. The follicles or their remnants are often to be found among the collections of tumour cells. The tumour is regarded as relatively well differentiated and as the T cell region analogue of the follicular lymphoma, which is the correspondingly differentiated tumour of the B cell region of the follicles (germinal centres).

¶ 'Plasmacytoma' [that is, myeloma] in this context refers only to those tumours that arise outside bone marrow (extramedullary myelomas).

** Centroblasts and centrocytes are the proliferating cells of germinal centres and correspond to the follicular centre cells that respectively have a non-cloven ('non-cleaved') nucleus and a cloven ('cleaved') nucleus as described by Lukes and Collins (see footnote [††] of Table 9.6).

†† The follicular type and the follicular and diffuse type of centroblastic/centrocytic lymphoma correspond to the tumour that is still generally understood by the term 'follicular lymphoma' (see page 835).

‡‡ The term 'lymphoblastic lymphoma' is applied to all lymphomas that consist of small to medium-sized 'blast cells'. The designation 'lymphoblastic' is not used as an indication that the proliferating cells are precursors of lymphocytes, 'lymphoblasts' in this sense no longer being considered to exist (lymphocytes are considered to proliferate and regenerate through immunological stimulation, which causes transformation of B lymphocytes into centroblasts and of T lymphocytes into T immunoblasts, which divide to produce a fresh generation of respectively B lymphocytes and T lymphocytes). Instead, it is said to be used in the 'haematological sense' and to indicate that the tumour consists of atypical lymphocytes with basiphile cytoplasm and the capacity for mitosis. These cells are further said to differ from the 'lymphoblasts' of chronic lymphocytic leukaemia, which are regarded as 'underdeveloped B immunoblasts'.

§§ Burkitt's tumour is composed of cells that resemble small centroblasts and is regarded as a lymphoblastic lymphoma (in the sense indicated in footnote [‡‡] above), the tumour cells being 'lymphoblasts' of the B cell series.

‖‖ The cells with convoluted (gyriform) nucleus (see footnote [‖] of Table 9.6) are regarded as 'lymphoblasts' in the sense relative to the 'lymphoblastic lymphomas' (footnote [‡‡] above). They are considered to be of the T cell series.

¶¶ The unclassified lymphoblastic lymphomas are those that have not been clearly identified as tumours of either the B cell series or the T cell series.

*** It is not always easy to draw the distinction between immunoblastic lymphomas and centroblastic lymphomas and between immunoblastic lymphomas and lymphoplasmacytic/lymphoplasmacytoid lymphomas. Confusion with centroblastic lymphomas results from the fact that immunoblasts and centroblasts are closely related and both cells may be present in a single tumour: as immunoblasts show differentiation toward plasma cell formation, and as any tumour should be classified according to the highest degree of differentiation that it attains, such tumours are regarded as immunoblastic lymphomas. Confusion between immunoblastic lymphomas and lymphoplasmacytic/lymphoplasmacytoid lymphomas results from the occasional dedifferentiation of the latter and their consequent transformation into the former.

Table 9.8. *Malignant Lymphomas Described in This Chapter and Their Percentage Incidence in a Series of 1403 Cases**

Disease	Number of cases (total 1403)	% of 1403 cases
Hodgkin's disease (see page 784)	652	46
		% of 652 cases
Type: lymphocytic predominance	104	16
nodular sclerosis	261	40
mixed cellularity	196	30
lymphocytic depletion	91	14
Lymphomas other than Hodgkin's disease (see page 819)	740	53
		% of 740 cases
Lymphocytic lymphoma (lymphosarcoma†) (page 821) well differentiated poorly differentiated plasmacytoid	280	38
Follicular lymphoma (page 835)	111	15
Immunoblastic lymphoma (immunoblastic lymphosarcoma†) (page 849)	263	36
Undifferentiated lymphoma, including pleomorphic anaplastic lymphoma (page 850)	83	11
Histiocytic lymphoma (reticulum cell sarcoma)‡ (page 851)	3	0·4
Lymphomas in association with 'heavy chain diseases', and similar conditions		
Malignant histiocytosis and similar conditions	11	1

* This is not intended as yet another formal classification. It is simply a personal list of those lymphomas that it has seemed practicable and useful to distinguish in a general biopsy practice. The list is based as closely as possible on the Rye classification of Hodgkin's disease (Table 9.10) and the Lukes–Collins classification of the lymphomas other than Hodgkin's disease (Table 9.6, page 779). The conditions listed are referred to in more detail in the text. The series of 1403 cases has not been published but it includes the 1067 cases tabulated in the first edition of this book (Symmers, W. St C., in *Systemic Pathology*, edited by G. Payling Wright and W. St C. Symmers, vol. 1, chap. 5, page 247, table 5.1; London, 1966). Necessarily, the categorization of all these cases is open to criticism on the grounds of the unavoidable element of subjective interpretation.

† The term 'lymphosarcoma' has been dropped, reluctantly, in an attempt to conform to the current practice of the majority of diagnostic histopathologists.

Notes continued on next page.

‡ The diagnosis of reticulum cell sarcoma has been made, for the purposes of this tabulation, only when there is demonstrable evidence that the tumour cells have features that are said to be specific to reticulum cells (see page 852). For various reasons, not necessarily discreditable, the conditions under which a biopsy service is provided in a general laboratory are seldom such that the specific methods for identifying reticulum cells can be used. Some reticulum cell sarcomas are therefore likely to be included among the lymphomas classified as 'undifferentiated'. The term 'histiocytic lymphoma' is used synonymously with reticulum cell sarcoma in the contemporary sense of the latter term; it is also applied to those rare tumours that consist in part of cells that are demonstrably phagocytic.

colleagues in the laboratory—that the clinical usefulness of any classification of lymphomas may be limited both by the variability in the behaviour of lymphomas that are classified pathologically as of the same type and by the occasional change in type that may be evinced in the course of a patient's illness.

Current Classifications

In preparing this chapter the Rye classification of *Hodgkin's disease* has been followed (see page 787).[1224] Classification of other lymphomas has been more difficult, as witness the number of systems that are currently mooted and the embarrassment of many general pathologists by the resulting uncertainties. There are three classifications of the *lymphomas other than Hodgkin's disease** that have a present following that justifies their consideration outside the pages of an encyclopaedic monograph: these are the Henry Rappaport classification (sometimes known as the Washington—or Armed Forces Institute of Pathology—classification),[1261, 1262] the classification of Lukes and Collins[1198] and the Kiel classification of Lennert and his associates.[1263-1265] The lack of general acceptance of any of the classifications evolved up to now is seen in the number of other schemes that have been put forward latterly;[1266-1268] it is small wonder that this situation has provoked exasperation, confusion and criticism.[1269-1271] It is not desirable to compare and contrast these and other classifications here: within limits this task has been carried out in some of the relevant original publications.[1198, 1262-1265] The three classifications named above are summarized in Tables 9.5, 9.6 and 9.7.

* The lymphomas other than Hodgkin's disease are frequently known at present as the 'non-Hodgkin's lymphomas', a phrase of its time that has been appropriately described as inelegant (Lennox, B., *Lancet*, 1976, **2**, 1140).

Ambiguous terms, idiosyncratic literary style and poor translation from one language to another are among important minor factors that delay better understanding of what the experts are trying to explain.

If any particular statement epitomizes the practical divergence of views that separates the clinician and the laboratory worker in this field of pathology it is the apposite, but at first sight startling, verdict that the Rappaport classification 'was clinically very useful but scientifically incorrect'.[1271] A whole changing philosophy of Medicine is contained in that aphorism. Its corollary, later in the same paper, is equally remarkable, and may prove to be more than thought-provoking:

> 'What is needed is a cytologically founded, consistent classification which also agrees with the results of modern experimental immunological research. Such a scientifically correct classification will also be clinically relevant, whether one recognizes it now or not'.[1271]

The scientific advances that have been made already in the field of lymphoma research point to some of the ways toward understanding of the aetiological and pathogenetic mechanisms. Sooner or later there will be parallel advances in the ability to recognize and treat lymphomas more effectively, in the light of increasing knowledge of their causation; eventually, the means to limit their occurrence may be found. Meantime, the scientific classification of these tumours is already ahead of clinical requirements, and this situation is not without some danger to today's patients. To hold this view is not to underestimate clinicians' need for precise and detailed diagnostic information: but clinical requirements are not met by information, however scientific, that is not comprehensible to the recipient. So many new terms are included in the new classifications of lymphomas that the credibility of biopsy reports is undermined by their injudicious and unexplained use. This is particularly so when pathologists feel themselves obliged to adopt this or that innovation and to phrase their reports in terms that may not yet be generally understood and, worse, that they may not themselves understand clearly enough to use correctly. Premature attempts to put new classifications into use may increase resistance to the eventual introduction of an agreed classification. However, there is no doubt that an agreed classification will be evolved as the advantages and weaknesses of the present classifications are recognized and respectively consolidated and corrected. The development of an accurate system of classification can be regarded properly as a research undertaking and should not impinge on the day to day work of clinicians, whose diagnostic needs can continue to be met without recourse to tentative or controversial innovations.

Malignant Lymphomas Described in This Chapter

The malignant lymphomas that are described in the following pages are listed in Table 9.8. It must be stressed that this list is not intended to be a system of classification: it is a series of headings that have proved to be of use to one pathologist in his practice and that seem to make sense to most of his clinical colleagues.

'Methodological Developments'

In most medical centres the general histopathologist, and therefore most of his clinical colleagues, will continue for some time to rely for diagnosis on the use of conventional histological preparations, stained by everyday methods, and examined under the light microscope. The use of imprint preparations from the cut surface of fresh specimens will become more general only as authoritative atlases become available.

Methods for the identification of membrane-bound immunoglobulin and of specific immunoglobulins in cytoplasm, and other techniques for the identification of T lymphocytes, B lymphocytes and histiocytes, although not particularly complicated are beyond the resources of the average laboratory at present. Maybe, too, they have yet to establish their practical importance in terms of what is necessary to the clinician so that he may give his patients the best care.

The electron microscope will undoubtedly have an important diagnostic role in the future. For the present, this role is only beginning to be outlined: it is encouraging that much of this work is being undertaken by pathologists who are closely in touch with the practice of their clinical colleagues and with the paramount importance of the patient's interests.

Malignant Diseases of the Lymphoreticular System in Animals[1272]

Neoplastic diseases that have been described as lymphosarcoma, lymphatic leukaemia and 'reticulum cell sarcoma' have been observed in many species of animals, both domestic and wild. They are, in general, more frequent in cats,[1273] dogs[1274] and cattle[1275] than in other animals.[1276] In addition, there are various less well-defined types of primary malignant disease of the lymphoreticular tissues in animals. The terms 'lymphomatosis' and 'leucosis' are commonly used to indicate any generalized lymphoma, irrespective of its histological appearances and whether or not there is an accompanying leukaemia. 'Lymphosarcoma' is the name often used for tumours of lymphocytes that are macroscopically confined to a single group of lymph nodes or at most to adjoining groups, although the term tends then to be retained when it becomes apparent that other organs, such as the spleen and liver, have become involved. Follicular lymphoma, sometimes corresponding histologically to the classic follicular lymphoma of human pathology (see page 835), is occasionally seen, mainly in dogs and cats. In contrast, a disease that corresponds closely to Hodgkin's disease is, it is said, unknown in animals; the tumours of pigs[1277] and of dogs that are sometimes regarded as of the same general histological pattern are not, in fact, convincingly similar, although there may be exceptions (Fig. 9.188).

Hodgkin's Disease[1278]

Introduction

The first detailed account of diseases originating in the organs of the lymphoreticular system rather than involving them secondarily was given in 1832 by Thomas Hodgkin, of Guy's Hospital, London.[1279] It is likely that such cases had been observed by many early morbid anatomists, as Hodgkin himself remarked, and a commonly cited example is mentioned briefly by Malpighi in a work published in Bologna in 1666.[1280] In his paper, 'On Some Morbid Appearances of the Absorbent Glands and Spleen', Hodgkin wrote,

> 'As far as could be ascertained from observation, or from what could be collected from the history of the cases, this enlargement of the glands appeared to be a primitive affection of these bodies, rather than the result of irritation propagated to them from some ulcerated surface or other inflamed texture through the medium of their inferent vessels.' [1279]

His seven cases—the first collected series of cases of these diseases—provide the first instance of the difficulty of defining their variety, for later appraisals of his account of the clinical and post-mortem findings have indicated the unlikelihood that all the cases were of the same sort. Specimens from three of Hodgkin's cases are still in the Gordon Museum at Guy's Hospital: two show the microscopical

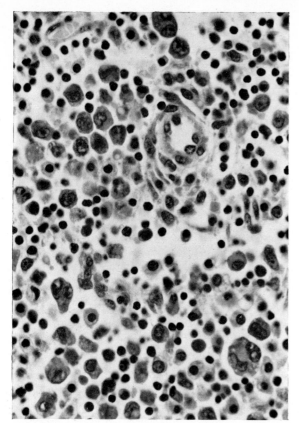

Fig. 9.188. Section of one of several considerably enlarged lymph nodes in the neck of an 18 years old golden Labrador dog that had spent all its life in a farming region of Norfolk, England. The histological picture is comparable to that of the reticular form of the lymphocytic depletion type of Hodgkin's disease in man (compare with Fig. 9.221, page 810): atypical reticulum cells, some of which are binucleate or multinucleate, are seen, including some that are reminiscent of Sternberg–Reed cells. There was involvement of mediastinal and lumbar nodes also, and of the spleen and bone marrow. Post-mortem specimen. *Haematoxylin–eosin.* × 400.

appearances that are now recognized as characteristic of the disease that has commonly been known as *Hodgkin's disease* since Samuel Wilks, also of Guy's Hospital, introduced that name in 1865 (see Fig. 9.189);[1281] the third specimen is probably a lymphocytic lymphoma, but the poor state of preservation of the tissues makes interpretation uncertain.[1282]*

It is now generally accepted that Hodgkin's disease is neoplastic and may be classified as a lymphoma

* Professor Keith Simpson, when Curator of the Gordon Museum, and the late Professor G. Payling Wright generously allowed me to see their histological preparations from these three cases.

(see page 813). The characteristics that most persuasively indicate its malignant neoplastic nature are its progressive involvement and destruction of the tissues and its inevitably fatal outcome in the absence of appropriate treatment. Its various histological types share certain specific features that relate them to one another and that are not present in other lymphomas: this distinction has led to the basic division of lymphomas into the two main categories, *Hodgkin's disease* and *lymphomas other than Hodgkin's disease* (see page 783). The specific histological features are described below (see *Histology*, page 794). It is easy to understand why a disease with the histological picture that is characteristic of the classic type of Hodgkin's disease (the type now described as of 'mixed cellularity') was formerly thought to be closer akin to the chronic infective granulomas than to any form of neo-

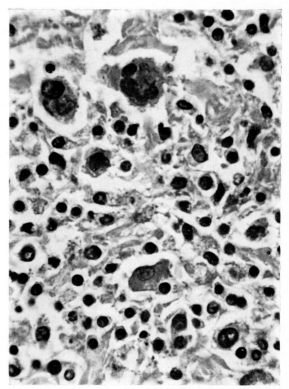

Fig. 9.189.§ Hodgkin's disease. Section prepared in 1958 from a lymph node from one of Dr Thomas Hodgkin's patients (Hodgkin, T., *Med.-chir. Trans.*, 1832, **17**, 68 [Case 2]). The specimen is preserved in the Gordon Museum, Guy's Hospital, London. Permission to make and reproduce photomicrographs of the histological preparations was given by Professor Keith Simpson, when Curator of the Museum, and the late Professor G. Payling Wright, Guy's Hospital Medical School, London. Compare with Fig. 9.215, page 807. *Haematoxylin–eosin.* × 600.

plasm. And it is ironical that, after a century of unsuccessful search for the infective agent that it was thought should be the cause of a granulomatous disease, the accumulation latterly of epidemiological evidence for the possibility that a viral or similar infection may be a factor in the occurrence of Hodgkin's disease has come at a time when it is no longer regarded as idiosyncratic to consider that some forms of neoplasia may have an infective cause (see page 814).

The history of Hodgkin's disease has recently been definitively reviewed.[1282a]

Classification

The proliferation of classifications of lymphomas, including classifications of Hodgkin's disease, has been a phenomenon of the 1960s and 1970s that leaves the definitive system yet to be developed (see pages 777 to 784). However, one classification of Hodgkin's disease has emerged that, in its current modified form, has become widely accepted throughout much of the world. This is the classification that was introduced in 1963 by R. J. Lukes, working in Los Angeles, California:[1283] it proved at once to meet a much needed requirement, that of relating prognosis—including response to treatment—to named histological pictures that are distinctive and recognizable, and therefore a basis for intelligible and potentially accurate comparison. Previously, the only classification to achieve any real measure of support on a national and international level was that of Jackson and Parker (see below).[1284]

Classification of Jackson and Parker

Jackson and Parker, in 1947, working in Boston, Massachusetts, proposed a classification of Hodgkin's disease into three types—paragranuloma, granuloma and sarcoma.[1284] This classification was based on the premise that the disease in most cases is an inflammatory process, only the comparatively rare Hodgkin's sarcoma being neoplastic. There was a considerable international following for this system, but its inherent aetiological commitment was far from generally acceptable, and the search for a universally satisfying classification continued, with an increasing trend toward regarding all forms of Hodgkin's disease as neoplastic.

Original Version of the Lukes Classification

The original Lukes classification (1963) comprises six categories (Table 9.9).[1283] An aspect that particularly attracted many practising pathologists, and

Table 9.9. *Original Version of the Lukes Histological Classification of Hodgkin's Disease* (superseded by the Rye Classification)*†

Type	Histological characteristics
1. Lymphocytic and/or histiocytic nodular	Mature lymphocytes predominate Epithelioid histiocytes may be present, usually in very small clusters Abnormal reticulum cells and Sternberg–Reed cells always sparse and may be difficult to find Reticulin fibres form coarse mesh; occasional thicker fascicles divide the abnormal tissue into nodule-like aggregates that usually are apparent only in silvered preparations No collagenous bands or thickening of capsule of lymph nodes
2. Lymphocytic and/or histiocytic diffuse	In general, as in lymphocytic and/or histiocytic nodular type (above), but without nodularity Epithelioid histiocytes prominent in about half the cases; they may form clusters mimicking toxoplasmosis (see page 654) or tubercle-like foci with multinucleate cells of Langhans type (as in tuberculosis) Abnormal reticulum cells and Sternberg–Reed cells less sparse
3. Nodular sclerosis	Collagenous thickening of capsule of lymph nodes; fibrous extensions traverse node, eventually separating nodular foci of cellular tissue Reticulin fibres form irregular mesh, mainly in cellular areas Very wide variation in proportions of lymphocytes, abnormal reticulum cells and Sternberg–Reed cells; 'lacunar cell' variant of Sternberg–Reed cell, with indented outline from cytoplasmic retraction, particularly characteristic of some cases (see page 796)
4. Mixed cellularity [classic Hodgkin's disease]	Characteristically mixed cytological constitution, lymphocytes no longer predominating, epithelioid cells rare, and abnormal reticulum cells and Sternberg–Reed cells correspondingly more numerous Eosinophils, neutrophils, plasma cells and fibroblasts in varying proportions Variably dense reticulin framework, often with a proportion of collagen
5. Diffuse fibrosis	Extensive collagenous fibrosis without intervening cellular nodules Relatively sparse cellularity, with abnormal reticulum cells and Sternberg–Reed cells predominating, although not always easy to recognize in the fibrotic mass; few lymphocytes

Table 9.9 continued on next page.

Table 9.9 (continued)

Type	Histological characteristics
	Fibroblasts often numerous; eosinophils sometimes numerous; epithelioid histiocytes lacking
6. Reticular	Conspicuously dense reticulin, maybe with associated collagen formation
	Abnormal reticulum cells and Sternberg–Reed cells predominate; lymphocytes sparse; 'tumour giant cells' of bizarre types may be present
	Eosinophils and fibroblasts vary in numbers

The nodular sclerosis type is distinct and does not tend to merge with the other types. The latter are not clear-cut entities and therefore there is considerable possibility of differences of opinion on the categorization of individual cases (see Table 9.11). For instance, there is a continuous histological variation from the 'lymphocytic and/or histiocytic diffuse type' to the 'mixed cellularity type' and from the latter to the 'reticular type'. Often the diagnostic decision rests on a subjective assessment of the amount of fibrosis or the proportion of atypical reticulum cells and of Sternberg–Reed cells.

* Lukes, R. J., *Amer. J. Roentgenol.*, 1963, **90**, 944.

† This classification is sometimes known as the Lukes–Butler classification (Lukes, R. J., Butler, J. J., *Cancer Res.*, 1966, **26**, 1063).

that therefore encouraged serious consideration and eventual adoption of this classification and of the Rye modification of it (see below), was the inclusion of the category of Hodgkin's disease with nodular sclerosis, which for the first time specifically recognized a form in which nodules of cellular tissue with the picture characteristic of Hodgkin's disease are enclosed by extensive zones of dense fibrotic tissue, a variety familiar to all histopathologists from their own practice and yet not represented clearly in earlier classifications.

By 1965 the original Lukes classification had been revised and simplified.[1224] This version has become known as the Rye classification (see below).

Rye Classification

The Rye classification was formulated by a committee under the chairmanship of Dr Lukes and was published at a symposium in Rye, New York, in 1965.[1224] Its relation to the earlier Lukes classification and to the classification of Jackson and Parker is shown in Table 9.10. A decade of experience with this classification in many centres has convinced those with particular interest and responsibility in relation to the diagnosis and treatment of Hodgkin's disease that a good level of correlation between histological type and prognosis has been achieved. Accurate use of the Rye classification provides a significant advance in the reliability of prognostication in cases of Hodgkin's disease, particularly when used in conjunction with the prognostic information that is provided by determining the extent of the disease by clinical staging at the time of beginning treatment (see page 772). However, as shown in Table 9.11, there is considerable variation in the proportion of cases allocated by various authorities to the different categories of Hodgkin's disease defined in the Rye classification, and this seems to indicate some degree of difficulty in achieving uniformity of interpretation of the histological findings in different large series of cases. Such variation may in part result from such factors as differences in the age and sex of the patients in different series, as these may affect the relative proportions in which the four histological types are represented. For instance, the nodular sclerosis type is rather commoner in female patients, both children and adults, whereas the other types are distinctly commoner in males. Again, geographical differences in the incidence of the different types have to be taken into account: the mixed cellularity

Table 9.10. *Rye Classification of the Histological Types of Hodgkin's Disease**

Rye classification	Correspondence to categories of the original version of the Lukes classification (see Table 9.9)	Correspondence to categories of the Jackson and Parker classification (see text, page 786)
1. Lymphocytic predominance type	Lymphocytic and/or histiocytic types (*both* nodular *and* diffuse)	Hodgkin's paragranuloma
2. Nodular sclerosis type	Nodular sclerosis type	——
3. Mixed cellularity type	Mixed cellularity type	Hodgkin's granuloma
4. Lymphocytic depletion type	Diffuse fibrosis type *and* reticular type	Hodgkin's sarcoma

* Lukes, R. J., Craver, L. F., Hall, T. C., Rappaport, H., Ruben, P., *Cancer Res.*, 1966, **26**, 1311.

Table 9.11. *Percentage Distribution of Different Histological Types of Hodgkin's Disease (Rye Classification) among 4285 Patients Included in 10 Series of Cases*

Type	Range of percentage distribution in 8 series* (totalling 2452 patients) (from tabulation by C. V. Harrison†)	Series of Lennert and Mohri‡ (1181 patients)	Personal series § (652 patients)	Average for the 10 series
Lymphocytic predominance	From 5% (series of 176 cases) to 30·5% (series of 674 cases)	31%	16%	17%
Nodular sclerosis	From 21% (series of 149 cases) to 52% (series of 176 cases)	34%	40%	38%
Mixed cellularity	From 21% (series of 559 cases) to 54% (series of 149 cases)	25%	30%	31%
Lymphocytic depletion	From 6% (series of 176 cases) to 23% (series of 559 cases)	10%	14%	14%

* (1) Lukes, R. J., *Amer. J. Roentgenol.*, 1963, **90**, 944 [377 cases]; (2) Franssila, K. O., Kalima, T. V., Voutilainen, A., *Cancer (Philad.)*, 1967, **20**, 1594 [97 cases]; (3) Keller, A. R., Kaplan, H. S., Lukes, R. J., Rappaport, H., *Cancer (Philad.)*, 1968, **22**, 487 [176 cases]; (4) Landberg, T., Larsson, L.-E., *Acta radiol. Ther. Phys. Biol.*, 1968–69, **8**, 390 [149 cases]; (5) Andersen, A. P., Brincker, H., Lass, F., *Acta radiol. Ther. Phys. Biol.*, 1969–70, **9**, 81 [179 cases]; (6) Hamann, W., Oehlert, W., Musshoff, K., Nuss, A., *Germ. med. Mth.*, 1970, **15**, 509 [559 cases]; (7) Mackenzie, D. H., *personal communication to C. V. Harrison* (reference in footnote [†] below) [674 cases]; (8) Bennett, M. H.,

Farrer–Brown, G., Harrison, C. V., *personal observations* (cited in reference in footnote [†] below) [241 cases].

† Harrison, C. V., in *Recent Advances in Pathology*, No. 9, edited by C. V. Harrison and K. Weinbren, page 73 [table 2, page 74]. Edinburgh, London and New York, 1975.

‡ Lennert, K., Mohri, N., *Internist (Berl.)*, 1974, **15**, 57.

§ Includes 486 cases referred to in the first edition of this book (Symmers, W. St C., in *Systemic Pathology*, edited by G. Payling Wright and W. St C. Symmers, vol. 1, chap. 5, page 247, table 5.1; London, 1966).

and lymphocytic depletion types have proved to be more frequent among children in some tropical and subtropical regions, including parts of South America and Africa,[1285] in contrast to the greater proportion of cases of the lymphocytic predominance and nodular sclerosis types in childhood in temperate climates.

The Rye Classification and Prognosis.—The real usefulness of the Rye classification as an index of prognosis has been shown in the results of many centres in different parts of the world (Table 9.12). It is also evident that the histological types that have the better outlook are the types that present with the disease still at the more favourable clinical stages (see page 772 and Tables 9.4 and 9.12).[1286]

Other Classifications

The classification proposed by R. M. Cross, at the Royal Air Force Institute of Pathology and Tropical Medicine, Halton, Buckinghamshire, in 1969, also provides a good correlation between histological appearances and prognosis.[1287] Although attractive and practical, it is unlikely to compete with the Rye classification, if only because the latter is already so widely and well established internationally.

Table 9.12. *Prognosis and Clinical Staging in Relation to Histological Types of Hodgkin's Disease (Rye Classification)*

Type	Mean survival*	Clinical staging at time of diagnosis:† percentage of patients in stages—		
		I	II or III	IV
Lymphocytic predominance	About 7 years	70	20	10
Nodular sclerosis	About 4½ years	35	35	30
Mixed cellularity	About 20 months	35	40	25
Lymphocytic depletion	About 10 months	10	35	55

* Figures based on data from: (1) Lukes, R. J., *Amer. J. Roentgenol.*, 1963, **90**, 944; (2) Franssila, K. O., Kalima, T. V., Voutilainen, A., *Cancer (Philad.)*, 1967, **20**, 1594; (3) Landberg, T., Larsson, L.-E., *Acta radiol. Ther. Phys. Biol.*, 1969, **8**, 390; (4) Symmers, W. St C., *personal observations*.

† See Table 9.4 (page 772).

Synonyms

Classic Form of Hodgkin's Disease

The synonyms of the classic form of Hodgkin's disease (which consists mainly of the mixed cell histological type of the Rye classification and—as it was for long not distinguished from the latter—the nodular sclerosis type also) may be mentioned first as this is the form in which the disease has longest been recognized as an entity. Many names have been used, and some are still current and therefore should be noted, although several of these are rarely seen nowadays. In chronological order, they include Bonfils' disease[1288] (though it is doubtful if the patient described by Bonfils had Hodgkin's disease), lymphadenoma (or lymphadenoma verum),[1289] Hodgkin's disease itself (so named by Wilks[1281]), malignant lymphoma[1290] (still sometimes used with the intention of referring to Hodgkin's disease, in spite of the common contemporary practice of implying by this term any variety of malignant disease arising in the lymphoreticular system), malignant granuloma[1291] (now liable to cause confusion with the non-healing nasal granulomas of unknown cause, which also are often known by this term—see pages 212 to 217, Volume 1), lymphogranuloma[1292] (a persistent cause of international misunderstanding—see footnote on page 635) and lymphogranuloma malignum, lymphoblastoma and scirrhous lymphoblastoma,[1293] lymphomatosis granulomatosa,[1294] fibromyeloid medullary reticulosis[1295] and Hodgkin's granuloma.[1284]

Lymphocytic Predominance Type of Hodgkin's Disease

Since its first clear description by H. Jackson, in 1937, as 'early Hodgkin's disease',[1296] this type has successively acquired several names. These include Hodgkin's paragranuloma,[1284] lymphoreticular medullary reticulosis,[1297] benign Hodgkin's disease[1298] (the disease is not benign), reticular lymphoma[1299] and indolent Hodgkin's disease[1300] ('indolent' has been criticized on etymological grounds, its meaning by derivation being 'painless' and not 'persistent' or 'slowly progressive', as had been intended).

Clinical Manifestations

Age and Sex

Age.—Most patients with Hodgkin's disease are seen first in early adult life. The age-specific incidence curve is bimodal (Fig. 9.186, page 769), with the major peak at 25 to 30 years and a second peak in the 7th decade. The second peak is least evident—and may be absent—in series of cases of the nodular sclerosis histological type, the incidence of which falls gradually from its peak in the 3rd decade to reach its steady lowest level at about 70 years.

Sex.—In general, the incidence of Hodgkin's disease is lower in girls and women than in boys and men. However, the sex incidence of the nodular sclerosis type is equal or reversed.

Presenting Manifestations

The commonest of the first clinical manifestations, whatever the histological type of the disease, is enlargement of a group of superficial lymph nodes, most frequently in the neck. Except in the lymphocytic depletion type the clinically detectable involvement is usually unilateral at this stage. Other manifestations draw attention to the disease in some cases—for instance, fever, splenomegaly, haematological disturbances or the chance radiological finding of a mediastinal shadow. The nodular sclerosis type is particularly frequently found to originate in the mediastinum. Rarely, Hodgkin's disease presents with involvement of an organ that is not primarily part of the lymphoreticular system: among the more frequent of such visceral sites are the stomach (Figs 9.190A and 9.190B),[1301] small intestine[1302] and rectum,[1303] a lung,[1304] the brain[1305] or a breast.[1306] In one such case the disease was accidentally implanted in the skin during gastrectomy:[1307] this is possibly the only instance on record of surgical implantation of Hodgkin's disease.

Course

When the patient is first examined there is commonly some involvement of parts other than those affected in the presenting manifestation. Eventually, in most cases, the disease involves groups of lymph nodes throughout the body, and the spleen, the liver, bone marrow, the thymus and sometimes other organs, particularly the lungs. The extent of the disease is recorded in terms of clinical staging (see page 772 and Table 9.4).[1308]

Delayed Progression and Spontaneous Regression.—The course of the disease may be interrupted by periods of inactivity and even of spontaneous regression. Correspondingly, the enlargement of affected lymph nodes may be progressive, or it may reach a certain stage and then increase no further, or there may be alternating periods of enlargement and of maintenance of a given extent or even shrinkage. Occasion to observe such fluctuation is rare because, ordinarily, the natural course of the

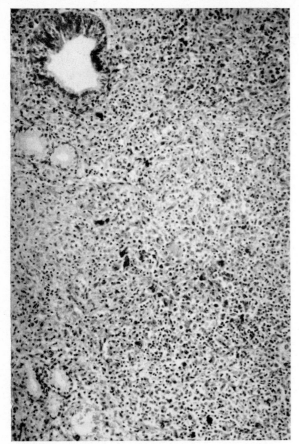

Fig. 9.190A.§ Hodgkin's disease presenting with involvement of the stomach. There is widespread infiltration of the sub-mucosa of the pyloric antrum by the proliferating cellular tissue. See Fig. 9.190B. *Haematoxylin–eosin.* × 100.

disease is interrupted by treatment once the diagnosis has been established. There have been cases in which the interval between the initial, competently confirmed, histological diagnosis and a further biopsy, showing the same appearances, has been from one to 10 years,[1309] with freedom from obvious progression of the disease during this period although the patient received no treatment. In a unique case the interval was 25 years.[1310]

In some cases, shrinkage of affected nodes in the absence of treatment is a manifestation of their fibrosis as part of the natural trend of the nodular sclerosis and mixed cellularity types. It may require a meticulous and wide-ranging search to reveal cellular areas that show the diagnostic histological picture.

When recovery from Hodgkin's disease appears to have taken place without conventional treatment, and is maintained, the usual presumption is that the diagnosis has been wrong, and in a large proportion of cases this presumption is confirmed on reviewing the histological evidence. The same is true of a proportion of instances of 'cure' following treatment. Nevertheless, although the range of benign and malignant conditions that may be misinterpreted histologically as Hodgkin's disease is remarkable (see page 817), it must not be assumed that such errors account for all cases of recovery. The standard of histological diagnosis in centres specializing in the treatment of lymphomas is so high that the chance of serious error is very small. It is prior to referring the patient from other hospitals to the treatment centre that misdiagnosis usually occurs; however infrequent these mistakes may be, it is this circumstance that justifies the insistence of the therapist that biopsy diagnosis be reviewed by specialists before treatment is planned.

Persistence of Clinically Silent Disease after Treatment.—Most patients who live for many years without symptoms or signs after treatment for unequivocal Hodgkin's disease may be regarded as cured, and in fact have been freed of the disease by

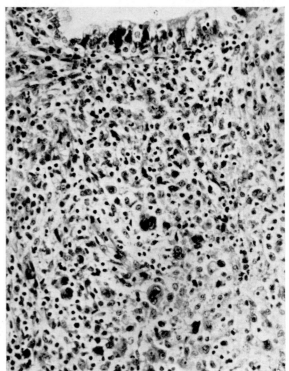

Fig. 9.190B.§ Same specimen as in Fig. 9.190A, showing more detail, including multinucleate and other atypical reticulum cells. *Haematoxylin–eosin.* × 360.

the treatment that they have had. In contrast, there is the occasional instance in which clinically silent disease is found unexpectedly in patients long after treatment, perhaps during surgery for some other condition or at necropsy following death from an unrelated cause.[1311] It may be that the patients in this rare category have become able, through treatment, to live asymptomatically in the presence of the residuum of their disease, the latter itself persisting but no longer progressive. Such observations must maintain interest in the peculiar nature of this disease, which has so many facets that are remarkably unlike the characteristics of other forms of cancer.

Complications

Hodgkin's disease may be complicated by the direct effects of the pathological tissue on the affected or adjoining parts of the body, by indirect effects of the disease on the function of various body systems, and by side effects of treatment.

Direct Effects.—The most important and most frequent direct effects are compression of the spinal cord by extradural foci, obstruction of the venae cavae, particularly the superior vena cava, and obstruction of hollow viscera, including the trachea and bronchi, the oesophagus and the ureters. Pathological fracture may result from the presence of foci in long bones; vertebral collapse is a rare manifestation, due to involvement of vertebral bodies. Thrombocytopenia, leucopenia or leuco-erythroblastic anaemia may occur if there is uncommonly extensive involvement of bone marrow.

Ulceration through the skin or through a mucous membrane leads to infection locally and may provide a portal through which bacterial or other infection of the blood stream takes place. Haemorrhage may complicate ulcerative lesions.

Indirect Effects.—Infection needs to be mentioned under this category, but with reference also to the lowering of resistance that is an effect of both radiotherapy and chemotherapy (see also pages 774 to 777). Patients with Hodgkin's disease are liable to reactivation of dormant infections, such as tuberculosis, histoplasmosis and zoster: indeed, any endogenous or exogenous bacterial, fungal, viral or protozoal infection may escape from the controlling influences of the body's defences. The whole range of so-called 'opportunistic' infections (see page 362,

Volume 1) is a potential threat to the patient who is under treatment for Hodgkin's disease. As mentioned elsewhere, there is a particular association between cryptococcosis and Hodgkin's disease (see page 774).

In a different category of indirect effects is the peculiar recurrent fever (Murchison's fever,[1312] Pel–Ebstein fever[1313, 1314]) that accompanies the disease in some cases; it is neither frequent nor pathognomonic. Peripheral neuropathy (see Chapter 35),[1315] which may antedate the clinical appearance of Hodgkin's disease,[1316] and other types of degenerative disorder of the nervous system (see Chapter 34), such as multifocal leuco-encephalopathy[1213] and subacute cerebellar degeneration,[1317] may occur, although they are rarer than in cases of carcinoma, particularly bronchial carcinoma; they develop in perhaps 2 per cent of cases of malignant disease arising in the lympho-reticular system.[1212] Similarly, any of the disorders of skeletal muscle that may accompany other forms of cancer (see Chapter 36) may complicate Hodgkin's disease.[1212]

A wide range of non-specific changes may occur in the skin; they are less rare than direct cutaneous involvement by lesions of Hodgkin's disease.[1318] Pruritus and consequent traumatic excoriation are among the most frequent. Erythroderma and frankly exfoliative dermatitis, crops of pruriginous papules, herpetiform dermatitis, ichthyosiform lesions and increased pigmentation are also frequent. It is likely that most of these cutaneous complications are a manifestation of autoimmunization.

Haemolytic anaemia of some degree is common among patients with Hodgkin's disease. It has been said to occur in 80 per cent of cases in which the disease is widespread,[1215] but it is seldom severe. Changes in the osmotic fragility of the red cells[1319] and the development of autoantibodies[1320] are among suggested explanations. Chemotherapy with alkylating agents, such as cyclophosphamide and other drugs of the nitrogen mustard group, is said to increase the frequency of haemolytic anaemia; whether these drugs produce this effect by acting as a hapten or by disturbing the balance of the immunity system is debatable.[1321] In some cases the onset of autoimmune haemolytic anaemia dates back months or even a few years before the appearance of any other manifestation of Hodgkin's disease.[1322]

Side Effects of Treatment.—Some of these are mentioned in the immediately preceding paragraphs; others are noted on page 771.

Hodgkin's Disease and Pregnancy

A study of 82 pregnancies among 56 women with Hodgkin's disease suggested that the occurrence of pregnancy at an early stage of the disease, before treatment, may exacerbate the disease and is associated with significantly shorter survival than pregnancy in the patient who has been treated.[1323] Pregnancy in the patient who has been treated, and who appears well, may precipitate a relapse, particularly when conception takes place early in the state of remission.[1323] There seems to be comparatively little risk to the fetus, but this depends on avoidance of combination chemotherapy, wide field irradiation and certain staging procedures, such as lymphangiography.[1323]

Other authorities are less dogmatic about the possible hazards of pregnancy.[1324]

Morbid Anatomy*

Lymph Nodes

Affected lymph nodes vary considerably in size: their longest dimension is generally from 2 to 3 cm. They have a characteristic resilience, like hard rubber. The nodes generally remain discrete (Fig. 9.191). Their cut surface is off white and of uniform appearance. Older lesions are fibrotic: in cases of the mixed cellularity type the eventual fibrosis is patchy or diffuse and in the latter instances has a whorled pattern that may be evident to the naked eye; in cases of the nodular sclerosis type the fibrotic

---

* Three of Robert Carswell's paintings shown on the occasion of Hodgkin's original presentation of his paper (see page 536) have been reproduced in colour (Dawson, P. J., *Arch. intern. Med.*, 1968, **121**, 288). They illustrate cervical and axillary lymph nodes *in situ*, abdominal nodes and the spleen.

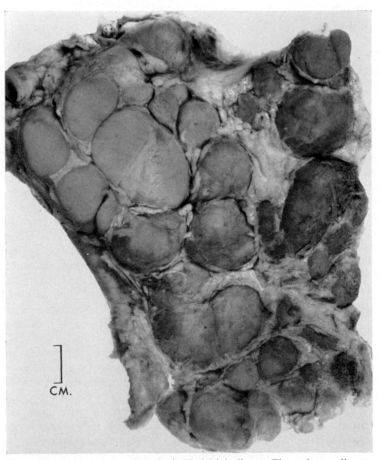

Fig. 9.191.§ Mesenteric lymph nodes in Hodgkin's disease. The nodes are discrete, and their cut surface is homogeneous. Compare with the appearances of tuberculous lymphadenitis in Fig. 9.71 (page 598).

patterning of the cut surface is coarser, and softer areas of yellowish or pinkish colour indicate the larger foci of surviving cellular tissue. When fibrosis is extensive there is often firm fusion of the capsule of adjacent nodes, although they are still fully recognizable as distinct structures.

Spleen

Occasion to examine the spleen in cases of Hodgkin's disease has become much more frequent since the introduction of laparotomy and splenectomy (Fig. 9.192) for purposes of clinical staging (see page

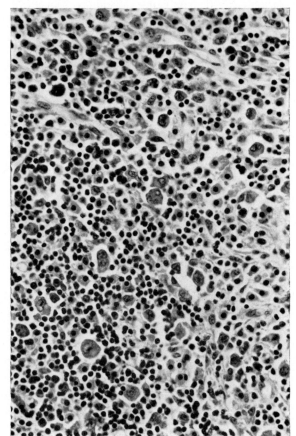

Fig. 9.192. Hodgkin's disease of the spleen. The patient presented with enlargement of a single lymph node in the neck. Biopsy showed this to have the histological picture of the mixed cellularity type of Hodgkin's disease. There was no clinical evidence of disease elsewhere. The results of lymphangiographic studies were normal. Laparotomy showed no macroscopical abnormalities. The spleen was removed. It weighed 135 g. There was no indication of disease in 13 out of 16 blocks examined histologically: the picture illustrated is typical of the findings in a small proportion of the splenic follicles in the other three blocks. The disease was progressive and the patient died within 2 years. *Haematoxylin–eosin.* × 250.

773).[1325] In consequence, it has become known that the extent of involvement of the spleen varies considerably and, in particular, that the foci of the disease may be of only microscopical proportions. About 50 per cent of spleens obtained for staging purposes prove to be involved.[1326, 1327] When no macroscopical abnormality is found on examination of thin slices (about 3 mm apart) of the well-fixed spleen, blocks of tissue including the largest splenic follicles should be taken for sectioning as experience has shown that it is such follicles that are likeliest to be the site of early involvement.[1327]

At necropsy in advanced cases the degree of splenic involvement varies considerably. Even when weighing as much as 700 g or so the spleen may contain no foci of the disease; conversely, a spleen that is smaller than normal may be affected microscopically or even macroscopically. The involved spleen may weigh as much as 3 kg, but in most instances is of the order of 500 g (the weight of the involved spleen obtained at laparotomy, during staging, is of the order of 300 g[1327]). The cut surface shows a remarkable range of appearances. In the most characteristic form (Figs 9.193A and 9.193B) there is a variegate pattern of more or less sharply outlined foci of pathological tissue, irregular in size and shape, their pallor contrasting with the hyperaemic intervening pulp: these are the appearances that have been likened to porphyry. In other cases the appearances of the cut surface are reminiscent of a regularly distributed follicular hyperplasia (Fig. 9.194), or they may simulate miliary tuberculosis, sarcoidosis or metastatic tumour deposits (Fig. 9.195). For descriptive purposes these various patterns have been designated the paucinodular, multimicronodular (Fig. 9.194), multimacronodular and massive tumourous (Fig. 9.195) forms.[1326]

Infarcts may be present, as in any enlarged spleen (see page 731).

Liver

The liver is commonly enlarged in cases of advanced Hodgkin's disease; its weight seldom exceeds about 2 kg. Its substance may be fairly evenly studded with irregular masses of tumour tissue, or the disease may be confined to one lobe, usually the right lobe. Sometimes the pathological tissue is found only in the larger portal tracts: the cut surface then resembles that in cases of the so-called 'pipe stem' form of hepatic fibrosis in schistosomiasis (see page 1237).

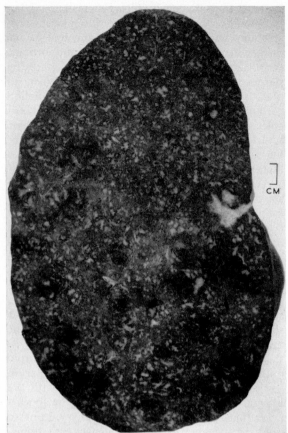

Fig. 9.193A.§ Spleen in Hodgkin's disease: typical, variegate appearance. The irregularly outlined, whitish foci consist of the pathological tissue. They are enclosed by the red pulp. See Fig. 9.193B.

Bone Marrow

The naked-eye appearances of involved bone marrow may be indistinguishable from those of carcinomatosis, especially in bones that have a fine carcellous structure, such as the vertebral bodies; the bone trabeculae often remain largely intact. The disease seldom extends through periosteum or articular cartilage: when there is such extension from affected vertebrae, the tumours that form in the vertebral canal compress the spinal cord and often its nerve roots and the spinal nerves themselves.

Histology

The histological diagnosis of Hodgkin's disease depends on the demonstration of three features that are essential to the recognition of the disease, whatever its histological type in terms of the Rye or any

other classification. These features are the presence of Sternberg–Reed giant cells, the presence of abnormal reticulum cells, and the replacement of the normal structure by pathological tissue with the accompanying appearance of a reticulin pattern that is distinct from the normal. Few pathologists today demand the presence of eosinophils as a criterion for the diagnosis; those who do are mistaken in their insistence on this feature.

The pathological changes may not affect the whole of a diseased organ. In affected lymph nodes they commonly do so—in the spleen and bone marrow there is always normal tissue in association with the pathological. If there is incomplete involvement of lymph nodes, it is usually at the periphery that the unaffected tissue persists.

Before describing the changes that characterize the different histological types it is appropriate to give an account of the cells that are the main distinctive feature.

Cytology of Hodgkin's Disease

Sternberg–Reed Cells.—Giant cells of various types may be seen in the lesions of Hodgkin's disease. It is

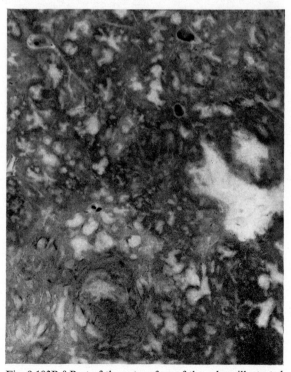

Fig. 9.193B.§ Part of the cut surface of the spleen illustrated in Fig. 9.193A, magnified to almost twice the natural size to show the appearance of the diseased foci in more detail.

It has at least two nuclei and usually four or five; sometimes there are as many as 10 or more. The nuclei commonly overlap, even when there are only two, and they tend to vary in size and intensity of staining. They are usually ovoid but may be round or of irregular shape. Their position is central and the plentiful cytoplasm can usually be seen readily, although sometimes it stains palely and is not

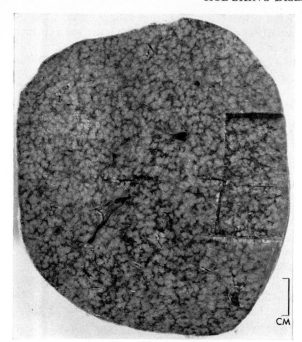

Fig. 9.194.§ Spleen in a case of Hodgkin's disease of the mixed cellularity histological type. The macroscopical appearances could be mistaken for those of sarcoidosis or of other types of miliary granuloma. In the fresh state, the picture may be indistinguishable from that of follicular lymphoma (see Fig. 9.245B, page 837): when the spleen has been fixed well, and is uniformly hardened, the cut surface in cases of follicular lymphoma lacks the clear contrast between the tumour 'follicles' and the pulp; the lesions of Hodgkin's disease tend to be as obvious in the fixed organ (as illustrated here) as they are in its fresh state.

practically impossible now to be sure of the identity of the giant cells that were mentioned by the pioneer microscopists in their accounts of Hodgkin's disease. Such cells were found by W. S. Greenfield, in Edinburgh, in 1878 [1328] and, in the same year, by H. G. Sutton and E. C. Turner of the London Hospital[1329] and by Sidney Coupland of University College Hospital, London.[1330] Carl Sternberg of Vienna described them in 1898[1331] and Dorothy Reed (Mrs Mendenhall) of Baltimore, Maryland, in 1902,[1332] the year of an account of them by F. W. Andrewes of St Bartholomew's Hospital, London.[1333] It has become traditional to refer to the most familiar giant cell of Hodgkin's disease as the Sternberg–Reed cell; other names that have some currency still are 'Hodgkin's cell' and 'lymphadenoma cell', both of which, confusingly, have also been used as terms for the atypical mononuclear reticulum cells (see below).

The Sternberg–Reed cell may range from 15 to 50 μm in its longest dimension (Figs 9.196 and 9.197).

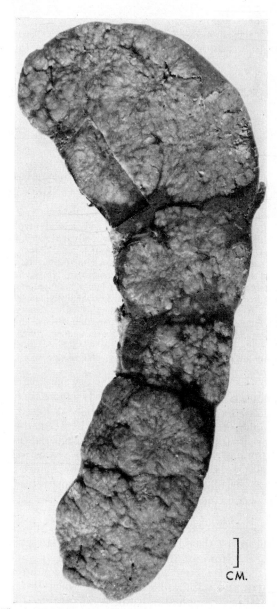

Fig. 9.195.§ This spleen was removed surgically in a case of Hodgkin's disease of the mixed cellularity type. The macroscopical appearances suggest secondary deposits of carcinoma or a massive granulomatous condition rather than Hodgkin's disease. The microscopical findings were characteristic.

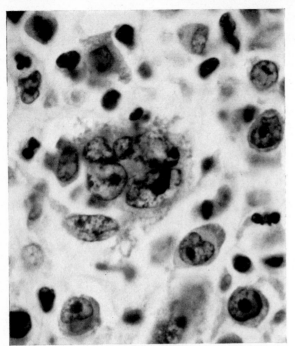

Fig. 9.196. A Sternberg–Reed cell and several atypical reticulum cells, lymphocytes and neutrophils are seen in this field. From a needle biopsy specimen of hepatic tissue: the biopsy was undertaken as the only procedure ('interference') that the patient would permit. Generalized lymph node enlargement (including the so-called 'bilateral hilar lymphoma syndrome'—see page 746), with splenomegaly, nodular lesions of the skin and markedly diminished sensitivity to tuberculin had led to a clinical presumption of sarcoidosis. The patient refused treatment, and the subsequent course of her illness was that of progressive Hodgkin's disease, eventually confirmed at necropsy. *Haematoxylin–eosin.* × 1000.

immediately evident. Sometimes, when there are two nuclei they are almost symmetrically disposed in relation to an imaginary plane between them, forming the so-called 'mirror image' giant cell (Figs 9.198 and 9.199). The nuclei contain one or more relatively large, oval or round, eosinophile nucleoli. The nucleoli often lie in a clear area of nucleoplasm. They are commonly attached to the nuclear membrane by fine haematoxyphile filaments.

Sternberg–Reed cells are the most distinctive feature of the histological picture of Hodgkin's disease. However, they—or cells remarkably similar to them—are found occasionally in other conditions, particularly infectious mononucleosis[1334] and hydantoin lymphadenopathy (see page 697),[1335] but also rarely in lymphocytic lymphomas,[1336] chronic lymphocytic leukaemia,[1336] rubella and a variety of other conditions.[1337]

It has generally been considered that Sternberg–

Reed cells are derived from reticulum cells, particularly as abnormal forms of the latter are a further essential constituent of the diagnostic picture of Hodgkin's disease. Others interpret them as malignant histiocytes.[1338] It has been suggested that a likelier explanation is that they are polyploid transformed lymphocytes (immunoblasts).[1334]

'Lacunar Cells'.—The so-called lacunar cell (Figs 9.200 and 9.201), or lacuna cell, is commonly said to be peculiar to the nodular sclerosis type of Hodgkin's disease. In fact, it may be seen also in the mixed cellularity type. It is a variety of Sternberg–Reed cell, differing from the usual forms in that its cytoplasm has a characteristically recessed outline, the points between the recesses being attached to neighbouring cells by tenuous cytoplasmic filaments. It usually contains from two to five nuclei and these are often rather smaller than is typical of Sternberg–Reed cells and have smaller, less markedly eosinophile nucleoli and less clarity of the nucleoplasm surrounding the nucleoli.

Other Giant Cells.—The 'mirror image' binucleate cell, mentioned above, is sometimes regarded as a distinct type of abnormal cell. In fact, it is probably no more than a rather striking variant of the Sternberg–Reed cell.

Another form of giant cell is sometimes described

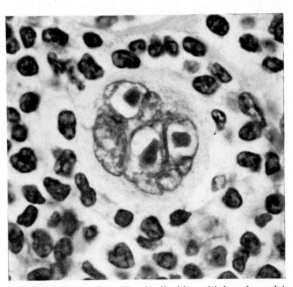

Fig. 9.197. A Sternberg–Reed cell with multiple pale nuclei. In three of the nuclei there is a very large nucleolus with a surrounding clear zone in the karyoplasm. These nucleoli are markedly eosinophile in the original preparation. From the field illustrated in Fig. 9.214 (page 806). *Haematoxylin–eosin.* × 1000.

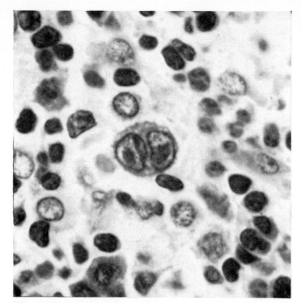

Fig. 9.198. A 'mirror image' giant cell, so called because its two nuclei have a somewhat symmetrical setting on opposite sides of an imaginary plane through the cell. The nuclei of the cell illustrated—from a case of Hodgkin's disease of the mixed cellularity type—have a rather coarse membrane, finely dispersed chromatin and large nucleoli that are eosinophile in the original preparation: these are the nuclear appearances of the atypical reticulum cells of Hodgkin's disease (see Fig. 9.196). Compare with Fig. 9.199. *Haematoxylin–eosin.* × 1200.

as megakaryocytoid because it has a single but strangely contorted, multilobate nucleus that is reminiscent of the nucleus of a megakaryocyte (Fig. 9.202).

Other multinucleate giant cells include some with the nuclei arranged in a ring (Figs 9.202 and 9.203). Some of these are variants of the Sternberg–Reed cell and their nuclei have the characteristics of the nuclei of the latter. Others are histiocytic giant cells, more or less resembling the Langhans giant cell of tuberculosis and having pale nuclei with nucleoli that are small, round and haematoxyphile (Fig. 9.204).

Atypical Reticulum Cells.—These are large mononuclear cells with a relatively small amount of pale cytoplasm (Fig. 9.196). The nucleus is of the type that is seen in Sternberg–Reed cells (see above) and ranges moderately in size and shape; it may be pale or intensely hyperchromatic. These cells have been regarded as malignant histiocytes.[1338] Others might interpret them as atypical transformed lymphocytes (immunoblasts), in keeping with the comparable speculation on the immunoblastic nature of the

Sternberg–Reed cell (see above). Since their nature remains undecided they may continue to be referred to here as reticulum cells.

Epithelioid Histiocytes.—Histiocytes are frequently present in the lesions of Hodgkin's disease (Figs 9.204 and 9.205). They may be distributed without any tendency to become clustered, or they may form small groups such as are seen in toxoplasmosis (see page 654) or even develop into tuberculoid foci (Fig. 9.206). The clusters may be so conspicuous that the picture is regarded as a distinct variant (see page 806). It is particularly in relation to the tuberculoid foci that the occasional Langhans type of giant cell may be seen (see above).

Tuberculoid granulomas may be seen in some cases of Hodgkin's disease in tissues, including lymph nodes, that are not the site of the histologically specific lesions of the latter (Fig. 9.207).[1339] It is important to note that these granulomatous foci are not evidence of involvement of the affected tissue by

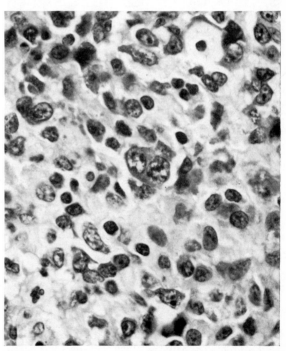

Fig. 9.199. A 'mirror image' giant cell in another case of Hodgkin's disease of the mixed cellularity type. The characteristics of its nuclei are less like those of the atypical reticulum cells of Hodgkin's disease (compare with the binucleate cell in Fig. 9.198): instead, they are naggingly reminiscent of the nucleus of the 'immunoblasts' of immunoblastic lymphomas (the former 'reticulum cell sarcomas')—see Fig. 9.265 on page 851, for example. *Haematoxylin–eosin.* × 630.

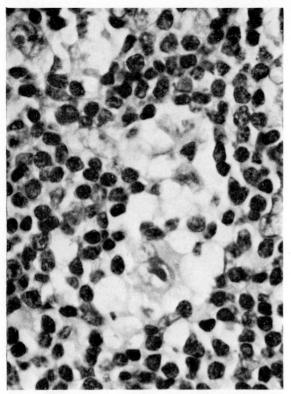

Fig. 9.200. 'Lacunar cells' in Hodgkin's disease of the nodular sclerosis histological type. There are parts of several of these cells in this field, which otherwise consists mainly of lymphocytes. The wide, curved recesses at the cytoplasmic edge, with filamentous prolongations of cytoplasm stretching across to link with processes of neighbouring cells, are seen well in the binucleate lacunar cell that occupies the middle of the lower half of the picture. See also Fig. 9.201. *Haematoxylin–eosin.* × 750.

Hodgkin's disease:[1340] their development is probably akin to that of similar changes in lymph nodes draining the site of a carcinoma (see page 682). On their own they must be neglected when determining the stage of Hodgkin's disease (see page 773).

Histology of the Lymphocytic Predominance Type of Hodgkin's Disease

It is convenient in this section (and in the succeeding sections that deal with the other histological types of Hodgkin's disease) to describe the histological appearances as they are seen in lymph nodes, as these are the commonest biopsy specimens. The findings in other lymphoid organs are essentially the same. In organs and tissues that are not basically part of the lymphoreticular system the findings are more or less modified by the variation in the normal

histological structure on which the pathological changes are imposed.

The normal structure of the affected nodes is more or less extensively, and often totally, replaced by the pathological tissue (Fig. 9.208). It is characteristic that the normal reticulin framework is replaced by a sparse spongework of fine fibres that are disposed in an irregular fashion (the 'diffuse lymphocytic and/or histiocytic type' of the original Lukes classification—Table 9.9, page 786) or, less often, with the formation of occasional circles that define nodule-like aggregates of cellular tissue (the 'nodular lymphocytic and/or histiocytic type' of the original Lukes classification—Table 9.9, page 786). The space enclosed within the ring of reticulin fibres is occupied predominantly by mature lymphocytes. Simple histiocytes and epithelioid histiocytes are present: they are usually sparse in the nodular instances and quite numerous in the diffuse form. The epithelioid cells tend to form small clusters in some cases (see Fig. 9.224, page 812): the picture can be confused with that of toxoplasmosis and other conditions in which comparable clusters of epithelioid histiocytes occur

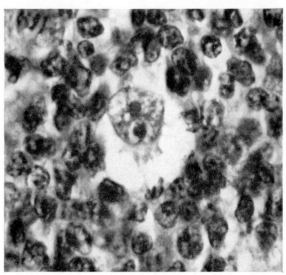

Fig. 9.201. Another lacunar cell, also in a case of Hodgkin's disease of the nodular sclerosis type. In this instance the amount of cytoplasm is less and the characteristic outline is correspondingly less immediately recognizable than in Fig. 9.200. Attention is drawn to the cell by the clear space about it, contrasting with the close arrangement of the lymphocytes and other cells. If the lacunar appearance is an artefact, it is nonetheless significant, as it indicates a peculiarity of the cell, and the cell with this peculiarity is so frequently seen in the nodular sclerosis type of Hodgkin's disease that the finding of such cells in an equivocal biopsy specimen may be of help in coming to a diagnosis. *Haematoxylin–eosin.* × 1000.

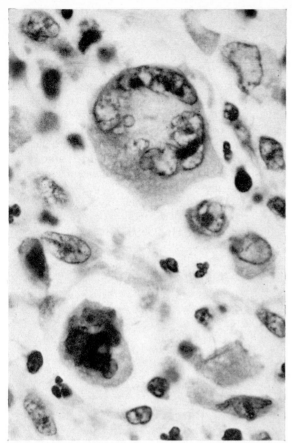

Fig. 9.202. Two varieties of giant cell are included in this field in a lymph node in a case of the mixed cellularity type of Hodgkin's disease. The upper cell is a Sternberg–Reed cell in which the nuclei are arranged in a circle toward the periphery ('ring' cell). The cell at the lower left of the picture has a single, much contorted and partly hyperchromatic nucleus: that the nucleus is solitary can be demonstrated only under the microscope, when focusing with the fine adjustment permits the entire thickness of the cell to be studied. This is a variety of giant cell that is described as megakaryocytoid, because of its supposed resemblance to the megakaryocytes of bone marrow. *Haematoxylin–eosin.* × 1000.

(see pages 654 and 656). In the nodular form epithelioid clusters are rare, and when they are present they are usually confined to the centre of the nodular collections of lymphocytes (Fig. 9.209). Sometimes multinucleate giant cells of Langhans type are found in relation to the epithelioid cells: in exceptional cases the picture is confused with that of tuberculosis.

Abnormal reticulum cells and Sternberg–Reed cells are relatively sparse in most cases of the lymphocytic predominance type of Hodgkin's disease (Figs 9.210 and 9.211). They may be so few, particularly the Sternberg–Reed cells, that a long search is necessary before they are found.

The capsule of the nodes is not notably thickened in this type of the disease and there is no increase in the amount of collagen in their substance. Necrosis does not occur.

Histology of the Nodular Sclerosis Type of Hodgkin's Disease

The substance of a lymph node affected by the nodular sclerosis type of Hodgkin's disease is traversed by more or less broad bands of collagen (Figs 9.212 and 9.213). The bands extend from the capsule throughout the node; the capsule is uniformly fibrotic, measuring up to 3 mm in thickness. The nodularity that is indicated by the term nodular sclerosis consists of the cellular tissue that is enclosed by the interconnected bands of sclerosing collagenous tissue. The cellular tissue varies in composition. When it is predominantly lymphocytic there are comparatively few reticulin fibres within the nodules; when the cellularity is more mixed the amount of reticulin is greater, and this relates to the presence of many abnormal reticulum cells and, often, classic Sternberg–Reed cells (Fig. 9.214).

Lacunar cells are a characteristic component of the cytological picture of the nodular sclerosis type of Hodgkin's disease (Figs 9.200 and 9.201, opposite). They are present in both the predominantly lymphocytic and the mixed cellularity type of nodular focus. In some cases the collagenous bands are thin and indistinct and the diagnosis may be in doubt:[1341] the observation of characteristic lacunar cells is then the essential clue to the diagnosis. Such incompletely developed cases are not rare; their recognition—or failure to recognize them—may account for the variation in the proportion of cases

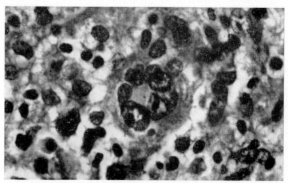

Fig. 9.203. Another 'ring' form of Sternberg–Reed cell in a lymph node in a case of the mixed cellularity type of Hodgkin's disease. *Haematoxylin–eosin.* × 500.

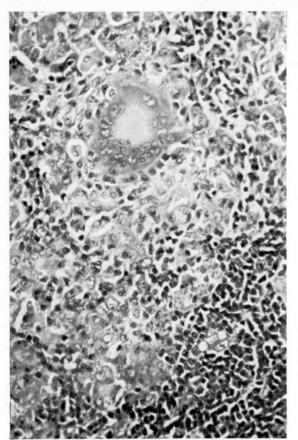

Fig. 9.204. Epithelioid histiocytosis in a lymph node in a case of Hodgkin's disease of the lymphocytic predominance type. The field includes a histiocytic giant cell with multiple, peripherally disposed nuclei. *Haematoxylin–eosin.* × 300.

of this type of the disease in different series (from about 20 to over 50 per cent—see Table 9.11, page 788).

Necrosis is seen in some of the cellular nodules in occasional cases. It is almost always of small extent.

Histology of the Mixed Cellularity Type of Hodgkin's Disease

The mixed cellularity type of Hodgkin's disease is commonly referred to as the 'classic' type of the disease.* Abnormal reticulum cells appear to

* The histological picture that came to be known conventionally as 'classic' Hodgkin's disease was not described until many years after Hodgkin's death. The cases that were put in this classic category included some that now would be regarded among the histologically more variegate examples of the lymphocytic predominance type of the disease; they also included cases of the nodular sclerosis type and some of the less undifferentiated cases of the reticular form of the lymphocytic depletion type.

predominate over lymphocytes, and there are many Sternberg–Reed cells (Figs. 9.215 and 9.216). Mitotic figures are common. Eosinophils, neutrophils, plasma cells and fibroblasts are usually present. Epithelioid cells are infrequent and practically never form conspicuous clusters. There is abundant reticulin, forming a meshwork that varies considerably both in the number of fibres in a given area and in the thickness of the fibres and in their number in the bundles into which in places they are collected. Strands of collagen may be interspersed among the reticulin fibres. There may be some necrosis; its extent is always small.

Microscopists differ in their assessment of where to place the arbitrary distinction between the mixed cellularity type of Hodgkin's disease, the lympho-

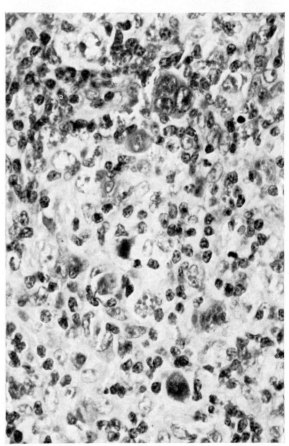

Fig. 9.205. Histiocytosis in a lymph node in another case of Hodgkin's disease of the lymphocytic predominance type. The histiocytes are without the notably epithelioid characteristics of those in Fig. 9.204. They are scattered among lymphocytes and abnormal reticulum cells, including a Sternberg–Reed cell (above). It is mainly the pallor and the abundant cytoplasm of the histiocytes that draws attention to their presence. *Haematoxylin–eosin.* × 440.

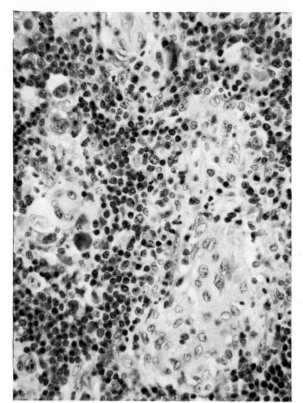

Fig. 9.206. Histiocytosis in a lymph node in another case of Hodgkin's disease of the lymphocytic predominance type. Some of the histiocytes have undergone epithelioid metamorphosis and clustering, with the formation of foci comparable to those seen in toxoplasmic lymphadentis. Compare with Figs 9.116B (page 655) and 9.224 (page 812). The presence of atypical reticulum cells in the field of this photograph is the clue to the diagnosis of Hodgkin's disease, which was confirmed by the presence of extensive, histologically characteristic changes elsewhere in the specimen. However, it has to be remembered that toxoplasmosis itself may cause lesions that simulate Hodgkin's disease (see Fig. 9.119, page 657). *Haematoxylin–eosin.* × 350.

cytic predominance type (see above) and the reticular form of the lymphocytic depletion type (see below): these three types form a continuous sequence (Figs 9.217 and 9.218). The observation most important in determining the categorization of a given case is the number of Sternberg–Reed cells, which is relatively very small in the lymphocytic predominance type and large in the reticular form of the lymphocytic depletion type.

Histology of the Lymphocytic Depletion Type of Hodgkin's Disease

Two distinct histological pictures are grouped under the heading of the lymphocytic depletion type of Hodgkin's disease. They are Hodgkin's disease characterized by diffuse fibrosis and the reticular form of Hodgkin's disease: both were included separately in the original version of the Lukes classification (Table 9.9, page 786) and brought together in the Rye modification (Table 9.10, page 787). It is in some ways difficult to accept that they should now be classified together: in most cases they differ so strikingly in histological appearance that they might more logically have been kept apart, with benefit to diagnostic accuracy. The justification for

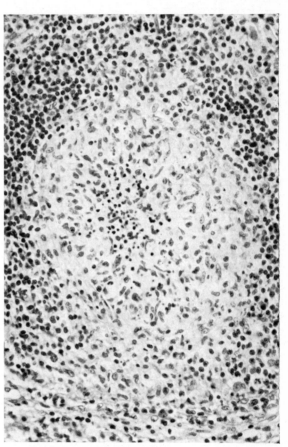

Fig. 9.207. Tuberculoid granuloma in a lymph node that was one of several dissected from the neck. Some of the other nodes showed changes of the mixed cellularity type of Hodgkin's disease. Similar necrotizing tuberculoid granulomas—all of comparable dimensions—were present in other nodes that were free from recognizable lesions of Hodgkin's disease and also in the otherwise normal part of one of the nodes that was only partly destroyed by the latter. No micro-organisms could be demonstrated in the sections (culture was not practicable). The cause of the tuberculoid reaction is not known: infection cannot be excluded, but it is possible that such granulomas form as a consequence of the presence of Hodgkin's disease (see text). *Haematoxylin–eosin.* × 250.

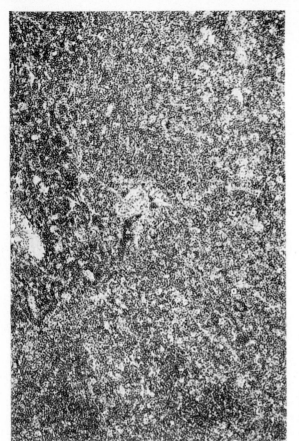

Fig. 9.208. Lymphocytic predominance type of Hodgkin's disease. The coarse 'nodularity' of the pathological tissue in this lymph node is readily seen at this low magnification. The relative pallor of the nodular areas is due partly to slightly less crowding of the lymphocytes and partly to the greater proportion of large mononuclear cells among them. The silvered preparations of adjoining sections showed these areas to be outlined by a fine but distinct, if incomplete, boundary of reticulin fibres. *Haematoxylin–eosin.* × 65.

grouping them together is that it is not very unusual to see cases in which the histological picture combines features of both (see Figs 9.222A and 9.222B).

Lymphocytic Depletion: (a) *Diffuse Fibrosis.*—The striking feature of this type of Hodgkin's disease is replacement of the normal tissue by diffuse collagenous fibrosis (Fig. 9.219). The fibrous tissue is not broken into strands that enclose cellular foci, as in the nodular sclerosis type of Hodgkin's disease, but is spread uniformly throughout the node. Abnormal reticulum cells and Sternberg–Reed cells are present in the interstices of the fibrous tissue (Fig. 9.220), but their recognition may require a long search (even, in exceptional cases, the examination of

many serial sections). Cells with one or more unusually large hyperchromatic nuclei may be present and sometimes mislead the histologist into making a diagnosis of poorly differentiated fibrosarcoma or of rhabdomyosarcoma. Reticulin fibres may be demonstrated in relation to some of these cells but otherwise are sparse. Epithelioid cells are lacking; fibroblasts, in contrast, may be numerous. Lymphocytes are outnumbered by the other cells. Eosinophils may be plentiful, infrequent or absent.

Some degree of necrosis is present in most cases. Its extent ranges from foci of microscopical size to large confluent areas. Fibrinoid material may be conspicuous in these foci, especially those of moderate size. Sometimes there is an accumulation of neutrophils, with or without eosinophils, in the necrotic parts.

Lymphocytic Depletion: (b) *Reticular Form.*— Abnormal reticulum cells and Sternberg–Reed cells

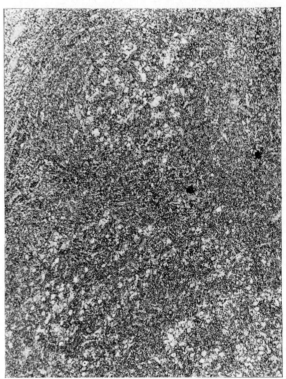

Fig. 9.209. Lymphocytic predominance type of Hodgkin's disease. The normal structure of the lymph node is largely replaced by proliferating lymphocytes, among which single large mononuclear cells (reticulum cells) are rather sparsely scattered, accounting for some of the small, clear areas. There is also a scattering of histiocytes; under higher magnifications it was seen that some of the histiocytes were clustered in very small groups. See also Figs 9.208, 9.210 and 9.211. *Haematoxylin–eosin.* × 50.

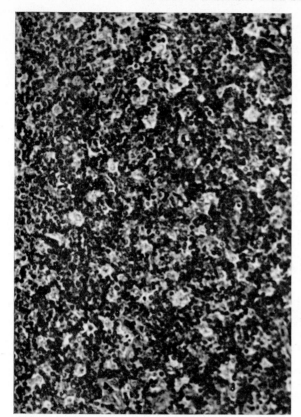

Fig. 9.210.§ Lymphocytic predominance type of Hodgkin's disease. Higher magnification, showing the distribution of the lymphocytes and reticulum cells in a lymph node in another case. *Haematoxylin–eosin.* ×275.

life, presenting clinically with enlargement of a single node in the neck, usually in one of the upper deep cervical groups. Examination during the operation for excision of this node may show that there is some enlargement of adjacent nodes, though of less degree, and if these are also removed for histological study they may or may not show the changes of Hodgkin's disease: if they do, it is of the same type as in the largest node.

Subsequent biopsy investigations may show the same picture as in the original specimens, or there may be a change in the type of the disease. In the

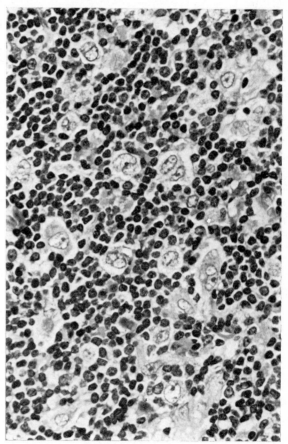

Fig. 9.211.§ Lymphocytic predominance type of Hodgkin's disease. The large mononuclear cells are conventionally assumed to be pathological reticulum cells. Their nucleus is vesicular and contains a nucleolus that usually is solitary and of moderate size. The cytoplasm is mostly opaque. They are rather evenly distributed among the lymphocytes. A few of the reticulum cells are binucleate and in some the nucleus is pyknotic. No strikingly abnormal forms are included in this field. Compare with the reticulum cells of other types of Hodgkin's disease (for example, in Figs 9.196 on page 796 and 9.217 on page 808). *Haematoxylin–eosin.* ×400.

predominate in this form of Hodgkin's disease (Fig. 9.221); lymphocytes are only scanty. Mitotic figures are frequent among the reticulum cells and a proportion of them are atypical. Bizarre, pleomorphic giant cells with multiple hyperchromatic nuclei are sometimes a feature, as in the form with diffuse fibrosis (see above). Fibroblasts may be present. There is a marked degree of reticulin formation, the fibres often running in fascicular groups. Collagenous fibres may form, particularly where the production of reticulin has been most conspicuous (Figs 9.222A and 9.222B). Necrosis is usually present (Fig. 9.223), as in the cases of diffuse fibrosis (see above).

Transformation and Evolution of the Histological Types of Hodgkin's Disease

Lymphocytic Predominance Type

The lymphocytic predominance type is most frequently seen first in late adolescence or early adult

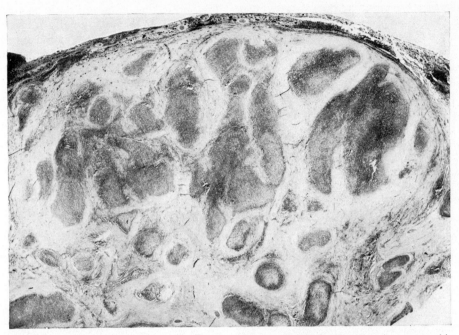

Fig. 9.212A. Nodular sclerosis type of Hodgkin's disease. Zones of dense fibrosis traverse this lymph node, surrounding the more darkly stained foci of cellular tissue. The capsule is also fibrotic, and the node is inseparably bound to its neighbours. The darker parts of the cellular foci consist mainly of small lymphocytes; the rather lighter areas include a notable proportion of large lymphocytes and reticulum cells, including lacunar cells (see Figs 9.200 and 9.201, page 798). See also Fig. 9.212B (same case). *Haematoxylin–eosin.* ×6.

latter event it is usually the picture of the mixed cellularity type that develops (Fig. 9.217); occasionally, the change is toward the lymphocytic depletion type, either in its reticular form or, less frequently, in the form of diffuse fibrosis.

The disease may spread to other superficial groups of lymph nodes and eventually to the abdominal nodes and, sometimes, those in the pelvis. Involvement of mediastinal lymph nodes in cases of the lymphocytic predominance type of Hodgkin's disease is always rare.

Mixed Cellularity Type

The mixed cellularity type usually presents toward the end of the third decade, and most frequently with enlargement of a group of nodes in the neck. In contrast to the lymphocytic predominance type, several contiguous nodes are commonly found to be involved clinically as well as microscopically when the patient is first examined. Extension to mediastinal nodes is not seen as frequently as involvement of abdominal and pelvic nodes but is not as rare as in the lymphocytic predominance type of the disease.

As the disease progresses collagenous fibrosis may become conspicuous in affected nodes. It is typically of irregular distribution and lacks the broad extent and characteristic tendency to enclose cellular foci that are seen in the nodular sclerosis type of the disease. It seldom predominates, except in those rare cases in which the disease evolves into the lymphocytic depletion type with diffuse fibrosis.

If the mixed cellularity type of Hodgkin's disease changes its histological picture significantly it usually develops into the reticular form of the lymphocytic depletion type (Fig. 9.218).

Lymphocytic Depletion Type

The patient who presents with Hodgkin's disease of the lymphocytic depletion type is usually a man, and usually in the 5th decade or older. There is often fairly uniform involvement of many nodes throughout the body at the time of diagnosis, and it is unusual for the nodes to be more than a little enlarged. The disease progresses quite rapidly, with fever and other general symptoms. Death occurs within a few months, cachexia and eventually intercurrent infec-

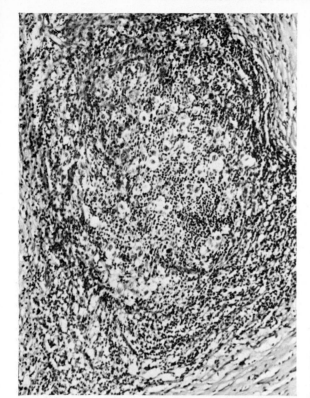

Fig. 9.212B. Higher magnification of a cellular focus from the specimen illustrated in Fig. 9.212A. A zone of small lymphocytes intervenes between the central collection of large lymphocytes and lacunar cells and the surrounding fibrous tissue. Even at this magnification the lacunar cells stand out by reason of the clear area round the cell body (see Figs 9.200 and 9.201, page 798). Compare with Figs 9.213A, 9.213B and 9.214. *Haematoxylin–eosin.* × 90.

tion generally being more evident features than the lymphadenopathy, which often remains of very moderate degree, although generalized.

Nodular Sclerosis Type

It is characteristic of the nodular sclerosis type of Hodgkin's disease that it remains histologically true to its type throughout its course and that it commonly affects the mediastinum. The amount of fibrosis may vary in successive biopsy specimens, being less or more abundant; this may simply indicate that the disease is at different stages in different groups of nodes at any particular time. In general, however, the tendency is for the fibrosing state to become more developed. The cellular component may become progressively more pleomorphic.

It is mainly a disease of young people, particu-

larly adolescents and young women. Its presentation after the 3rd decade is unusual, but it may set in at any age. The nodes first involved are commonly in one of the lower cervical groups, the disease spreading to the other side of the neck and then to other groups of superficial nodes. Mediastinal nodes are affected in about three quarters of the cases.

The preponderance of female patients, the lack of a secondary peak in incidence in older age groups (see page 789), the frequency of mediastinal involvement (which is very much greater than among cases of the other histological types of Hodgkin's disease) and the lack of transition to other histological types make up a set of distinctive features that together may indicate that the nodular sclerosis type is an entity distinct from other types of Hodgkin's disease. This possibility is one of the unanswered questions that relate to our continuing uncertainty

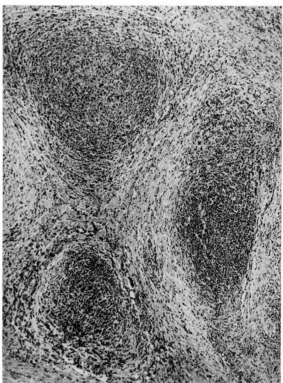

Fig. 9.213A. Nodular sclerosis type of Hodgkin's disease. In this example it is again possible to see at low magnification that the cellular foci are of varied composition, comprising lymphocytes, which predominate, and an obvious proportion of larger cells. The larger cells are dark and most lack the clear zone about them that is characteristic of the lacunar cell (compare with Fig. 9.212B). See also Fig. 9.213B. *Haematoxylin–eosin.* × 55.

N

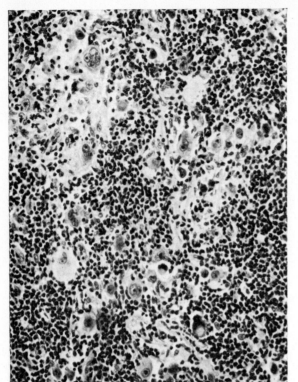

Fig. 9.213B. Higher magnification confirms that the abnormal reticulum cells in this case are not lacunar cells but represent the pathological forms that are characteristic of all histological types of Hodgkin's disease—bizarre mononuclear cells, binucleate 'mirror image' cells and Sternberg–Reed cells. See also Fig. 9.214. *Haematoxylin–eosin.* × 190.

as to the nature and cause of Hodgkin's disease (see below).

Histological Variants

There are numerous accounts of supposed variants of Hodgkin's disease, but most differ in such relatively small details from the range of commonly accepted histological pictures covered by contemporary classifications that they can be placed in accepted existing categories without real difficulty. This is probably true also of the currently most familiar variant, 'Hodgkin's disease with constantly high content of epithelioid cells',[1342] which some would include in the lymphocytic predominance type of the Rye classification, which includes other forms of Hodgkin's disease in which epithelioid histiocytes are conspicuous. However, the interest in this variant and its differential diagnostic importance are enough to warrant its separate consideration.

Hodgkin's Disease with Extensive Epithelioid Cell Clusters (Hodgkin's Disease with Constantly High Content of Epithelioid Cells)

Clusters of epithelioid histiocytes are so abundant throughout large areas of the affected lymphoid tissue in this variant of Hodgkin's disease that the descriptive term 'epithelioid cell granulomatosis' is appropriate for this component of its histological picture (Fig. 9.224). The epithelioid cell clusters in fact present a picture that is common to a considerable range of pathological conditions affecting the lymphoid tissue, and lymph nodes in particular: the picture is exemplified in toxoplasmosis (see page 654). This is the more important in view of the fact that a picture reminiscent of Hodgkin's disease is seen in a very small proportion of cases of proven

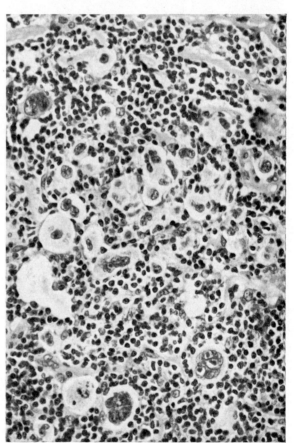

Fig. 9.214. Nodular sclerosis type of Hodgkin's disease. This field shows something of the range of appearances that may be found among the pathological reticulum cells, which here include 'mirror image' binucleate cells and a number of different varieties of Sternberg–Reed cells. A few cells show karyorrhexis or karyolysis. See also Fig. 9.197. *Haematoxylin–eosin.* × 250.

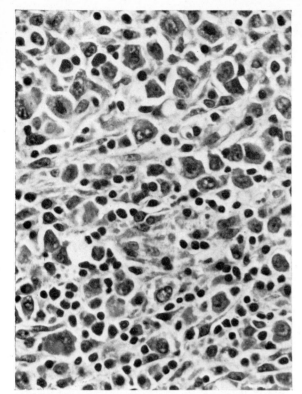

Fig. 9.215. Mixed cellularity type of Hodgkin's disease. Atypical reticulum cells are the most striking feature of the changes in this lymph node. They vary much in size and shape and in the intensity of staining of both nucleus and cytoplasm. Some have two or more nuclei, and in the more vesicular nuclei it is possible to make out one or more relatively large nucleoli. Lymphocytes, an occasional neutrophil and eosinophil, and fibroblasts are present also. There is intercellular fibrosis. See Figs 9.216 and 9.217. See also Fig. 9.189 (page 785), which is a photomicrograph of one of Thomas Hodgkin's original cases, and Figs 9.190A and 9.190B (page 790), 9.192 (page 793), 9.196 to 9.199 (pages 796 and 797) and 9.202 and 9.203 (page 799). *Haematoxylin–eosin.* × 360.

toxoplasmic lymphadenitis (see page 655 and Fig. 9.119). What distinguishes those cases that are regarded as instances of Hodgkin's disease is the presence elsewhere in the specimen of Sternberg–Reed cells and atypical reticulum cells of the kinds that characterize the latter. Both types of cell are present only sparsely, and often must be carefully sought; they are said not be be precisely identical with the corresponding cells of unequivocal Hodgkin's disease,[1342] but the significance of this view has to be defined more fully before making the presumption that the cytological details are sufficient to preclude the interpretation that these are cases of Hodgkin's disease. There is often a slight or

moderate increase in the amount of reticulin; collagenous fibrosis does not occur. There is no necrosis. The normal structure of the affected tissue is usually replaced completely; rarely, small parts persist, mostly at the periphery of the affected node or tonsil.

The patients are usually past middle age and there is possibly a small preponderance of men. Any superficial group of lymph nodes may be the starting point, the cervical nodes being those oftenest affected. The fauciopharyngeal lymphoid tissue is involved in some 5 to 10 per cent of cases.

This condition has acquired several names. It has been called the Lennert lymphoma,[1343] in recognition of its description by K. Lennert in 1963 [1344] and of his later studies.[1342] It has also been named after a patient in whose biopsy specimens Robb-Smith first recognized the condition in the late 1930s.[1345] Most of the names have been descriptive, and unavoidably wordy, and this has encouraged its designation either by the eponymous terms or as 'epithelioid cell lymphogranulomatosis'. The latter

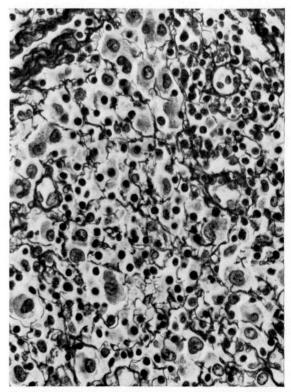

Fig. 9.216. Mixed cellularity type of Hodgkin's disease. Lymph node from another case. The section has been impregnated with silver to show the fine reticulin fibres between the cells. Compare with Fig. 9.215. *Robb-Smith modification of Foot silver method.* × 360.

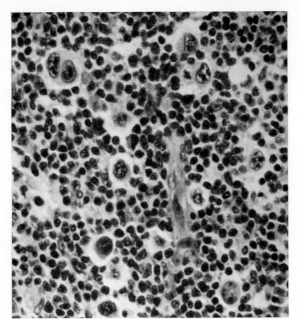

Fig. 9.217. Field in a lymph node from a case of the lympho-cytic predominance type of Hodgkin's disease with transition to the mixed cellularity type. As in Fig. 9.211 the pathological reticulum cells are still solitary, but some are binucleate and in others the nucleus is hyperchromatic or can be made out to contain several nucleoli. There are occasional eosinophils, neutrophils and plasma cells among the lymphocytes. *Haematoxylin–eosin.* × 330.

was proposed in the English summary of a paper written in German,[1342] and the English-speaking reader sometimes fails to appreciate what is implicit in the original German text, and what in fact is indicated by the English subtitle, that 'lympho-granulomatosis' is used as a synonym of Hodgkin's disease.

Effects of Treatment on the Histological Picture

Remarkably little seems to have been written about the changes that take place in the affected tissues as a result of treatment. The immediate effects are rarely seen. They include marked reduction in the number of lymphocytes, even to an extent that the histo-logist, particularly if unaware that the patient has had treatment, may take the appearances for those of a rapidly progressive lymphocytic depletion type of Hodgkin's disease (Fig. 9.225) The atypical reticulum cells and Sternberg–Reed cells may show marked swelling of both cytoplasm and nuclei, with lysis and, often, karyorrhexis (Fig. 9.226). This is accompanied in some instances by an accumulation of macrophages with ingested nuclear debris

(Flemming's stainable bodies—see page 512); in other cases it seems that the activities of the macro-phages are inhibited by the treatment. Sometimes considerable numbers of neutrophils accumulate. Necrosis of tissue is seldom extensive and may be absent. Thrombosis of small blood vessels and fibrinoid change in their wall and vicinity are occasional results of irradiation.

The late effect of treatment is the more or less extensive replacement of the diseased tissue by fibrosis, often with marked hyalinization. The fibrotic tissue is often only sparsely cellular. In other cases there may be recognizable foci of Hodgkin's disease or of regenerating but essentially normal-seeming lymphoid tissue.

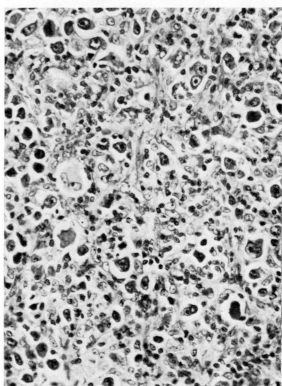

Fig. 9.218. Field in a lymph node from a case of the mixed cellularity type of Hodgkin's disease with transition to the reticular form of the lymphocytic depletion type. Sternberg–Reed cells, 'mirror image' binucleate cells and the usual range of mononuclear reticulum cells predominate, lympho-cytes being sparse. Earlier biopsy specimens from the patient had shown a picture characteristic of the mixed cellularity type of the disease: this had persisted throughout a period of 6 years, during which the response to treatment had been reasonably satisfactory between successive recurrences. The change in histological picture illustrated was accompanied by early recurrence following further courses of treatment, and death within 8 months. *Haema-toxylin–eosin.* × 250.

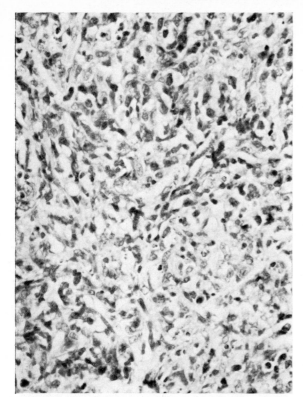

Fig. 9.219. Lymphocytic depletion type of Hodgkin's disease (diffuse fibrosis form). In this field, from a lymph node, it would not be possible to identify the condition as Hodgkin's disease, most of the cells being fibroblasts and none of the specific cell forms being apparent. A long search was necessary to find proof of the diagnosis (see Fig. 9.220). *Haematoxylin–eosin.* × 250.

Leukaemic and Sarcomatous Transformation of Hodgkin's Disease

'Hodgkin's Sarcoma'.—Before considering the development of leukaemia and sarcoma as complications of Hodgkin's disease, it is pertinent to refer to the old concept of Hodgkin's sarcoma, which reached its peak of acceptance as a histological diagnosis with the establishment of the Jackson and Parker classification of Hodgkin's disease (Table 9.10, page 787).[1284] The most malignant of the three types of the disease that this classification comprised was designated 'Hodgkin's sarcoma': the presence of Sternberg–Reed cells was considered to be essential to the diagnosis, the tumour being regarded as a 'reticulum cell sarcoma' in their absence. In fact, most of the cases that pathologists would have categorized under the heading of 'Hodgkin's sarcoma' at that time would now be regarded as belonging to the reticular form of the lymphocytic

depletion type in the Rye classification (see page 802). These cases are characterized by their particularly pleomorphic cytology, with conspicuous, bizarre, multinucleate 'tumour giant cells'. These cells have very large, irregular, often intensely hyperchromatic nuclei and are quite distinct from Sternberg–Reed cells, although doubtless related to them. It is now usual to place such cases under the lymphocytic depletion heading of the Rye classification (see page 801 and Table 9.10, page 787).

The term 'Hodgkin's sarcoma' should be avoided for the further reason that, long before the introduction of the Jackson and Parker classification, it was applied to the more anaplastic or pleomorphic varieties of so-called 'reticulum cell sarcoma'. Most of these tumours would now be regarded as pleomorphic examples of the immunoblastic or histiocytic lymphomas of the Lukes–Collins classification of the lymphomas other than Hodgkin's disease (see Table 9.6, page 779, and also the note relating

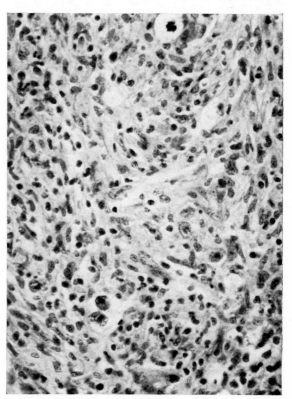

Fig. 9.220. Lymphocytic depletion type of Hodgkin's disease (diffuse fibrosis form). The presence of a binucleate reticulum cell and a scattering of atypical mononuclear reticulum cells indicate the diagnosis. Many fields in this lymph node lacked such specific elements altogether. See also Fig. 9.219. Compare with Fig. 9.225 (page 812). *Haematoxylin–eosin.* × 300.

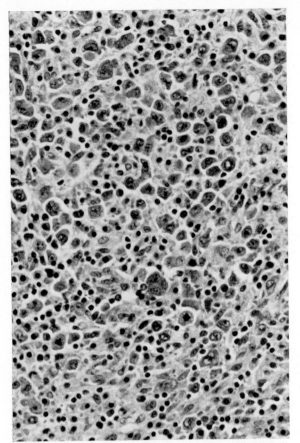

Fig. 9.221. Lymphocytic depletion type of Hodgkin's disease (reticular form). Abnormal reticulum cells predominate and lymphocytes are relatively sparse. There is some intercellular fibrous tissue, but fibrosis is inconspicuous in contrast to its extent in the diffuse fibrosis form of lymphocytic depletion (see Figs 9.219 and 9.220). See also Figs 9.222A, 9.222B and 9.223. *Haematoxylin–eosin.* × 250.

to Rappaport's category of 'histiocytic lymphoma' in Table 9.5).

Leukaemia and Hodgkin's Disease

Leukaemia and Hodgkin's disease are rarely associated. Monocytic leukaemia, which is usually acute, acute myeloblastic leukaemia and chronic lymphocytic leukaemia have been reported. The first is the rarest,[1346] and some of the cases were probably instances of acute myeloblastic leukaemia. The latter seems almost always to occur in patients whose Hodgkin's disease has been treated by irradiation; while rare, the association is commoner than would arise by chance.[1347] The interval between irradiation and the appearance of leukaemia has ranged from 9 months to 18 years.[1348] Chronic lymphocytic

leukaemia, in contrast, is almost always recognized prior to the overt development and recognition of the accompanying Hodgkin's disease.[1349] Acute lymphoblastic leukaemia[1350] and chronic myeloid leukaemia[1351] are so rarely associated with Hodgkin's disease that their occurrence is possibly coincidental.

Sarcomatous Change in Hodgkin's Disease

The concept of 'Hodgkin's sarcoma' has been mentioned above (page 809). The development of sarcomatous change in association with Hodgkin's disease is quite distinct. It is also a great rarity. The tumour is sometimes known as Yamasaki's sarcoma,[1352] but this is based on acceptance of a published account of sarcomatous change complicating Hodgkin's disease that, more critically reviewed, is unconvincing; the eponymous term should not be used. I have seen three instances of unequivocal histological evidence of the development of distinctive sarcomatous change in the mixed

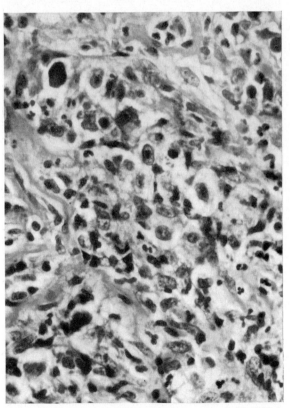

Fig. 9.222A. Lymphocytic depletion type of Hodgkin's disease (reticular form). Fibrosis is conspicuous in this lymph node. Abnormal reticulum cells and some neutrophils and scanty lymphocytes and plasma cells are present in the interstices. See Fig. 9.222B. *Haematoxylin–eosin.* × 360.

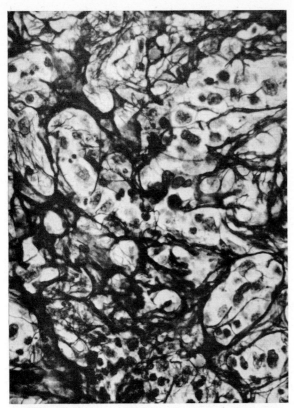

Fig. 9.222B. Same specimen as Fig. 9.222A, impregnated with silver to show the reticulin fibres. Compare with Fig. 9.216, which shows the much finer reticulin pattern in a case of the mixed cellularity type of Hodgkin's disease. *Robb-Smith modification of Foot silver method.* × 360.

cellularity type of Hodgkin's disease:[1234] a well differentiated lymphocytic lymphoma (without leukaemia), a very anaplastic and pleomorphic tumour formed predominantly of syncytial masses of undifferentiated cells, and a well differentiated fibrosarcoma. The fibrosarcoma was confined to the spleen and appeared to have arisen from one of the several large foci of Hodgkin's disease; both the other tumours were widely disseminated, for the most part involving tissues also involved by Hodgkin's tissue, the two types of lesion being so intimately associated that the origin of the second form of tumour from the longstanding lesions of Hodgkin's disease seemed a reasonable histological assumption.

'Extranodal' Hodgkin's Disease (Primary 'Extranodal' Hodgkin's Disease)

What has come to be known as 'extranodal' Hodgkin's disease—that is, Hodgkin's disease arising in tissue other than lymph nodes—is seen relatively rarely. It is to be expected that any site of lymphoreticular tissue might be the starting point of Hodgkin's disease, as of other lymphomas, and the infrequency with which this expectation is realized is surprising.

Strangely, in view of the large proportion of cases in which it is eventually involved, the *spleen* is seldom the first affected site, but this is in keeping with the rarity of other primary lymphomas of the spleen. I know of no unequivocal published report of Hodgkin's disease presenting with splenic involvement in the absence of evidence of the disease elsewhere. A student whose disease presented in 1939 with progressive splenomegaly was found to have no clinical, radiological or surgical evidence of lesions elsewhere, and remained in apparently good health for almost 2 years after splenectomy, without

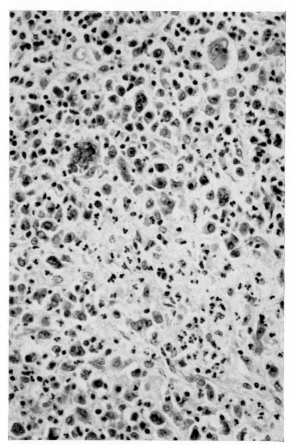

Fig. 9.223. Lymphocytic depletion type of Hodgkin's disease (reticular form). The picture in this field is generally similar to that in Fig. 9.221, except for the small area of necrosis, which is sparsely infiltrated by neutrophils. *Haematoxylin–eosin.* × 250.

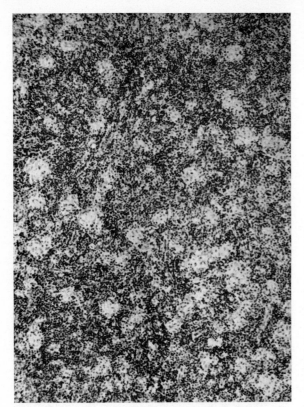

Fig. 9.224. Hodgkin's disease with extensive epithelioid cell clusters. This variant of the histological picture of the lymphocytic predominance type of the disease is liable to be mistaken for other conditions, particularly toxoplasmosis (see page 654 and Figs 9.116A and 9.116B, page 654). See also Fig. 9.206, page 801. The small aggregates of epithelioid histiocytes among the proliferating lymphocytes may be distinguishable from those of toxoplasmosis only by the loss of the normal structure of the node and the presence of atypical reticulum cells of the varieties that are characteristic of Hodgkin's disease. The rare coincidental coexistence of Hodgkin's disease and toxoplasmic lymphadenitis, and the very occasional development in cases of the latter of lesions simulating Hodgkin's disease (see Fig. 9.119, page 657), may make the differential diagnosis difficult. *Haematoxylin–eosin.* × 85.

other treatment; she was killed then in an air raid.[1353]

The *liver* may be affected alone,[1354] or appear to be so (in one such case involvement of abdominal lymph nodes was found when the patient died 2 months after the initial diagnosis[1355]).

Hodgkin's disease arises much less often than other lymphomas in the *fauciopharyngeal lymphoid tissue* (Waldeyer's ring).[1356] In a consecutive series of 2200 specimens of surgically removed tonsils (palatine tonsils, with or without the nasopharyngeal tonsil) there were six instances of clinically un-

suspected malignant lymphoma (two of well differentiated lymphocytic lymphoma, two of poorly differentiated lymphocytic lymphoma, an immunoblastic sarcoma and Hodgkin's disease of mixed cellularity);[1234] in one further case in this series the histological finding of Hodgkin's disease of the tonsil (mixed cellularity) led to the discovery that the child—during the period of over two years that had passed before her turn for admission from the waiting list for tonsillectomy—had been attending another hospital for treatment of Hodgkin's disease, diagnosed elsewhere.

Some *other organs* that may be the primary site of Hodgkin's disease are noted on page 789. Probably, however, the most frequent of all extranodal sites is the *thymus*; Hodgkin's disease accounts for some cases of the so-called 'granulomatous thymoma'

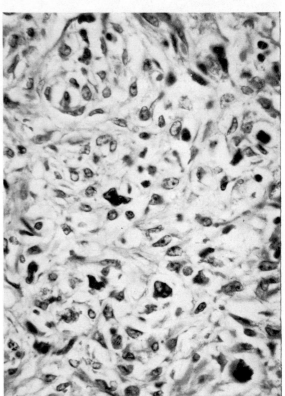

Fig. 9.225. Simulation of the picture of the diffuse fibrosis form of the lymphocytic depletion type of Hodgkin's disease as a consequence of radiotherapy and chemotherapy in a case of the mixed cellularity type of the disease. Apart from a small number of abnormal reticulum cells the field is wholly occupied by developing fibrous tissue with many fibroblasts. Biopsy 9 weeks after completion of a course of treatment. Five months later there was recurrent active disease of lymph nodes in the same region; the histological picture of the recurrent lesions was identical with that prior to the treatment. *Haematoxylin–eosin.* × 400.

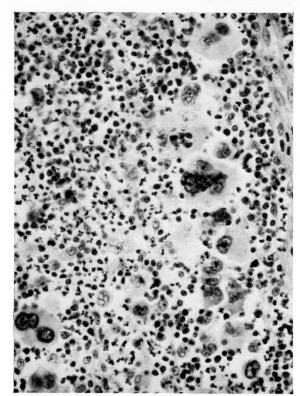

Fig. 9.226. Changes in the histological appearances of the mixed cellularity type of Hodgkin's disease in a lymph node excised 8 days after the start of a course of treatment with mustine (mechlorethamine), vincristine, procarbazine and prednisone. Compared with the picture in a lymph node examined a week before the treatment began, the cytoplasm of the Sternberg–Reed cells and mononuclear reticulum cells is swollen and more opaque, and some of the cells show karyorrhexis, pyknosis or karyolysis. Similar changes have affected the lymphocytes. The tissue has become infiltrated by neutrophils. *Haematoxylin–eosin.* × 250.

(see page 911), and it is probable that a proportion of those cases that are simply described as involving the mediastinum may have originated in thymic tissue. Indeed, the thymus was considered to be a major source of Hodgkin's disease in one large series;[1357] more recent figures indicate that its real frequency as the primary site of the disease is low.[1358, 1359]

Spread

It remains arguable whether the development of specific lesions of Hodgkin's disease in lymph nodes other than those initially involved, and eventually in other tissues, is a manifestation of metastasis or of multifocal origin of the disease. The appearances suggest the latter, particularly in lymph nodes, in which early lesions are not centred on the sinuses, where metastatic tumour tissue is to be seen first, but within the pulp. Multifocal origin of the disease has sometimes been denied on the grounds that there is successive involvement of different groups of lymph nodes and other structures: this could be explicable as a manifestation of the spread of a causal agent from an established focus of the disease, the passage of time between the appearance of successive clinical manifestations corresponding to the period in which the agent produces its effect at a given site and there establishes itself sufficiently to replicate and eventually pass to other sites. Such an agent might be carried free in lymph or blood or within cells that likewise may pass along lymphatic or blood channels to reach other potential centres of the disease.

Knowledge of the pattern of spread from site to site is as essential to the therapist[1360] as precise knowledge of the extent of the disease in the body.[1361] Familiarity with the patterns of spread and the likely situation of successive lesions permits some selection of fields for irradiation; definition of the extent of the disease in the individual patient, through meticulous staging procedures (see page 772), determines the minimal extent of the body that must be irradiated if the risk of leaving diseased parts untreated is to be as small as is practicable and possible.

Extent of the Disease at Necropsy.—The distribution of the lesions of Hodgkin's disease at necropsy in a small series of cases is indicated in Table 9.15 (page 831).

Nature

The argument whether Hodgkin's disease is inflammatory or cancerous is rarely heard nowadays: it is generally considered to be neoplastic, and most discussion now concerns its pathogenesis and the possibility of identifying its causes. In common with other lymphomas,[1362] Hodgkin's disease has come to be regarded as a neoplastic disease arising from cells of the lymphoreticular system specifically in relation to the immunological functions of the system. The view most widely held at present is that it is the manifestation of neoplastic proliferation of cells concerned in cell-mediated immunity (thymus-dependent lymphocytes—T cells): this proliferation is thought to be the outcome of prolonged or abnormal stimulation, predisposed to by inherited or, oftener, acquired anomalies of the immune system.[1363] Among acquired factors that may contri-

N*

bute to the causation of Hodgkin's disease—and of other lymphomas—are repeated antigenic stimulation through exposure to micro-organisms, autoimmune disease, thymectomy, and administration of immunosuppressant drugs, corticosteroids and antilymphocyte serum. Stimulation of immunocompetent cells in the normal course of interaction between the body and exogenous antigenic matter would not be likely alone to precipitate the neoplastic transformation and proliferation of these cells. Their contact with an oncogenic agent, whether living or chemical, might effect this transformation, establishing a mutation characterized perhaps by loss of one or more histocompatibility antigens: such cells would react destructively with normal cells that contain these antigens. The sustained antigenic stimulation would perpetuate and reinforce the proliferation of the abnormal cells, facilitating progressive neoplastic growth.[1364] Alternatively, the establishment of a chronic reaction of 'graft-against-host' type, requiring the continued proliferation of host cells to make good the associated loss of cells, might lead to malignant transformation of the reacting host cells.[1364] Equally, any alteration in the surface antigens accompanying infection of lymphocytes by an oncogenic virus would render such cells a target for uninfected immunocompetent cells. Hindrance of the functions of the latter through the operation of any variety of immunosuppressive agency would permit the infected cells to proliferate and eventually establish a neoplastic state.

It seems that the role of an oncogenic virus in the pathogenesis of Hodgkin's disease might be either to transform infected cells into tumour cells or to provoke neoplastic change in uninfected host cells reacting to sustained antigenic stimulation by the infected cells. Such hypotheses remain conjecture. It seems that the interaction between oncogenic agents and the immunological reactions of the body must be complex and subject to a series of facilitating and inhibiting effects (this is referred to again in the account of Burkitt's tumour—see page 828).

Infective Agents as a Factor in the Causation of Hodgkin's Disease

Many varieties of micro-organisms have been isolated in cases of Hodgkin's disease and proposed as its cause. None has withstood critical examination. It is only comparatively recently that published observations of small 'outbreaks' of Hodgkin's disease, relating individual patients through recognizable opportunities for personal contact with one another or with a potential 'carrier', have encouraged speculation on the existence of a specific infective agent—presumably a virus or virus-like agent.[1365]

'Epidemics' (Case Clusters) of Hodgkin's Disease.— These collections of cases are not of the conventional nature of epidemics. Rather, they are retrospectively identified groupings—'case clusters'—of small numbers of cases of Hodgkin's disease that seem to have been related through community of residence or occupation.[1366] No infective agent has been identified. In the largest series to be studied, 34 patients with a malignant lymphoma—Hodgkin's disease in 31 of the cases—were found to be linked, 9 of them through case-to-case association and 25 through the intermediary of common contacts. Attention was drawn to this series by the observation that there had been several cases of the disease among students at a high school in Albany, New York: investigation disclosed the occurrence of the 34 linked cases in the period from 1948 to 1970, the patients ranging in age from 14 to 74 years. There were instances of all the histological types of Hodgkin's disease. These and later observations suggested that the disease is infective, may be associated with a carrier state and has a long incubation period (up to 12 years, the median being 3 years).[1367] Other observers, studying smaller case clusters, have put the 'incubation' time at 2 to 6 months.[1368] Clustering of cases has not been recognized in studies in Britain (for instance, in the Manchester region over the period 1962–68).[1369]

More recent investigations in the United States of America have provided data that may indicate that the occurrence of a case of Hodgkin's disease in a school is liable to be followed by further cases, and that the number of these is slightly but definitely greater than would accord with the incidence of the disease in the corresponding age group of the population of the area in general.[1367] The incidence of the disease has been found to be higher among school teachers than among other adults in the State of Washington:[1370] this does not necessarily indicate an occupational exposure to an infective agent—its explanation may include factors such as the relatively low mortality of teachers from other causes, and their status, Hodgkin's disease being notably more frequent among the socially less deprived members of the community.[1371]

An obvious question is that of the frequency of Hodgkin's disease among the medical profession. Figures for upstate New York seem to show that the disease is significantly less rare in doctors than in dentists and in the general population.[1372] In Britain, in contrast, doctors seem not to be likelier than other adults to develop the disease.[1373] There is no evidence that radiotherapists, who may be expected to have an uncommonly high rate of professional contact with the disease, have a higher rate than others in medicine.[1373]

Family Incidence.—It is said that a near relative of a patient with Hodgkin's disease is about thrice as likely to develop the disease as an individual of the same age who has no family history of its occurrence.[1374] The disease has been recognized in several sets of siblings,[1375] including three of five children in one family found to have the mixed cellularity type of the disease within a period of 3 years (the age of the affected siblings in this family ranged from 4 to 11 years at the time of diagnosis of the illness).[1234] A few instances of the disease in husband and wife have been recorded.[1376]

Congenital Hodgkin's disease has been demonstrated in a baby of $4\frac{1}{2}$ months whose mother had the disease at the time of the birth.[1377] The child had enlarged lymph nodes at birth.

Familial cases of Hodgkin's disease are probably as likely to result from common exposure to environmental factors as from inheritance. However, a relation between particular histocompatibility antigens and susceptibility to the disease has been reported, and an inherited predisposition cannot be excluded (see page 817).

Seasonal Incidence. — Several reports that the incidence of Hodgkin's disease is related to season[1378, 1379] and others that there is no such relationship[1380] have still to be evaluated. Such observations are open to error in that their accuracy depends on the reliability of the individual patient's estimate of the date of the first sign of the disease. A seasonal factor would indicate a climatic or infective agency. For instance, it is said that in parts of the United States of America an unexpectedly high proportion of boys who develop the disease are born in July and August and that this suggests that these children are exposed to a seasonal aetiological factor, possibly sex-related, operating early in life.[1381]

Association with Known Viral Infection.—High titres of antibodies to the Epstein–Barr virus have been found in some series of cases of Hodgkin's disease, with the highest figures in cases of the lymphocytic depletion histological type,[1382] in which the level may be comparable to that in cases of Burkitt's lymphoma (see page 828) and of naso-

pharyngeal carcinoma.[1383] The findings were not considered to distinguish between an aetiological significance of the virus and a 'passenger' state.[1382] Other investigators have found no significant differences in the frequency and titre of antibodies to this virus and to other herpesviruses in patients with Hodgkin's disease when compared with controls of corresponding ages.[1384]

However, patients who have had infectious mononucleosis have been found to have a significantly greater liability to develop Hodgkin's disease subsequently than other individuals. There were 17 patients who developed Hodgkin's disease among 17 073 people in Denmark who had had a positive Paul–Bunnell reaction (see page 476) during a period of 30 years:[1385] the expected number was six. The explanation and significance of this observation are uncertain. In itself it does not demonstrate a causal relation between the Epstein–Barr virus and Hodgkin's disease.

Deprivation of Lymphoreticular Tissue and the Incidence of Hodgkin's Disease.—Attempts have been made to relate the development of Hodgkin's disease in some cases to loss of lymphoid tissue—that is, of tissue with a protective immunological role that ordinarily may prevent a postulated agent of low virulence from successfully establishing itself in the tissues in the vicinity of its portal of entry. Appendicectomy[1386] and tonsillectomy[1387] have been considered to increase the liability to Hodgkin's disease. For instance, the risk of developing the latter has been said to be 2·9 times greater among individuals up to the age of 40 years who have had tonsillectomy than among those who have not;[1387] removal of the tonsils was considered to facilitate invasion of the tissues by the presumptive virus.[1388] Support for this view was seen in a number of other observations.[1389] For instance, the fact that both tonsillectomy[1390] and Hodgkin's disease[1391] are more frequent among the higher income groups in the United States of America is potentially significant in this context. The possibility that an infective agent of the disease might most frequently enter the body through the upper part of the respiratory tract or the mouth or throat may relate to the frequency of cervical lymph node involvement as the initial clinical manifestation.

A further argument in favour of a protective function of the fauciopharyngeal lymphoid tissue is that the mortality of Hodgkin's disease is commonly seen to rise steeply at about the 11th year of age, which—allowing for a usual survival period of about 3 years—corresponds to initiation of the disease in the 8th or 9th year, the time when physiological regression of the lymphoid tissue begins.[1392] It may be reasoned also that the second peak in the frequency of the disease, later in life, is related to the time when continuing regression of lymphoid tissue has levelled off.[1389]

Conclusions.—It is possible, but unproven, that Hodgkin's disease has a viral cause. If so, the virus appears to be slow to manifest its effects. Various factors—immunosuppression by drugs or by irradiation, for instance, or thymectomy—might activate an oncogenic virus already latent in the tissues; oftener, there is no evidence that such identifiable disturbances are at work, and more elusive factors, such as predisposition through the possession of particular histocompatibility antigens, may be responsible for the overt consequence of Hodgkin's disease.

The overall incidence of Hodgkin's disease in the population is relatively so low—of the order of 4 in 100 000 [1393]—that even if the occurrence of cases in a school means that other cases may appear among the close associates of the patients, or of their close contacts, the risk that any individual child (or adult) will develop the disease is still very small. Some reassurance may properly be given to parents, and others, concerned.[1393]

It seems likely that the agent ultimately responsible for Hodgkin's disease will prove to be widely distributed, and that it can cause the disease only when other factors increase the vulnerability of the cells of the lymphoreticular system to its action.

Immunological Aspects of Hodgkin's Disease

Immunological processes are an integral part of the pathogenesis of Hodgkin's disease, if current views of the nature of the disease are correct (see page 813). At the same time, the pathological changes that characterize Hodgkin's disease themselves result in disturbances of immunological functions, with consequent development of certain autoimmune phenomena (for instance, some cases of haemolytic anaemia complicating Hodgkin's disease—see page 791) or a predisposition to serious infections. Other autoimmune phenomena may be advantageous in so far as they are to some extent aimed at eliminating the tumour cells. The field is vast, complicated and potentially rich in information that will lead to understanding of the disease, its causation and its prevention or control.

Immunodeficiency.—Depression of cellular immunity may be evident quite early in the course of Hodgkin's disease but is most characteristic of advanced disease, particularly in the lymphocytic depletion histological type. 'Anergy' to tuberculin, with failure to react to its intracutaneous inoculation, was observed by Dorothy Reed in 1902.[1332] Since then this depression of delayed hypersensitivity reactions has become familiar, and it has been recognized that the patient's capacity to react may return when a remission of the Hodgkin's disease develops.[1394] The reaction is depressed rather than abolished: if there is no reaction to a given amount of antigen a larger amount may lead to a reaction; alternatively, the reaction may occur but only after a delay of some days, a negative result being observed after 2 days and a positive reaction after 5 days.[1395]

The practical importance of depression of the delayed hypersensitivity reaction is that the deficiency determines a fall in the ability to combat infection by organisms that ordinarily are resisted by means of cell-mediated immunity. It is particularly organisms that tend to become intracellular parasites, especially of reticuloendothelial cells, that evoke the cell-mediated immune response and that therefore most commonly endanger patients with Hodgkin's disease (or with other diseases accompanied by depression of cellular immunity): these organisms include the tubercle bacillus and other mycobacteria, brucellae, listeria, *Cryptococcus neoformans*, histoplasma and other fungi that occur in the tissues in a yeast-like form, *Herpesvirus varicellae* (causing zoster), toxoplasma and various others. It is important to remember that radiotherapy and treatment with immunosuppressant drugs—and splenectomy as a staging or therapeutic procedure[1396]—also interfere with cell-mediated immunity, and probably account for this form of immunodeficiency oftener than the disease by itself.[1397]

Humoral antibody responses are usually normal until the disease is very advanced;[1259] even then they are never as depressed as cell-mediated immunity. Hypogammaglobulinaemia is uncommon,[1398] in contrast to its frequency in cases of chronic lymphocytic leukaemia:[1399] usually, immunoglobulin of class M (IgM) is reduced most and IgA less so, while IgG is within the normal range or rather increased.[1400] Most patients with Hodgkin's disease produce normal amounts of antibody to bacterial and viral antigens[1401] and have normal levels of isoantibodies to blood group antigens.[1402] If there is an impairment in the production of humoral antibodies it is usually attributable to malnutrition and the poor general state of the patient's health.[1403] Splenectomy may appreciably lower the amounts of

IgM and IgA in the circulation; this needs to be kept in mind as a potentially dangerous sequel of the operation.[1404]

From the practical point of view, it is above all the patient with the lymphocytic depletion type of Hodgkin's disease who is most vulnerable to the effects of immunodeficiency, which in general is not sufficiently marked in the other histological types to endanger life, at least until the disease is very widely disseminated.[1405]

One other effect of immunodeficiency in these patients that needs mention is their increased liability to develop other forms of malignant disease, including leukaemia (see page 810) and carcinoma.[1406] The development of a second cancer, and sometimes of multiple further cancers, may be related to an inhibitory effect of immunosuppressive therapy on the body's immunological defences against neoplasia rather than to any tendency for Hodgkin's disease to induce immunodeficiency, which ordinarily is a late complication and unlikely to be survived.

Heritability of a Predisposition to Hodgkin's Disease

Although, as suggested above (page 815), the occurrence of familial cases of Hodgkin's disease may be explicable as an effect of sharing common environmental hazards, evidence is beginning to accumulate that susceptibility to the disease is higher in those individuals who have inherited particular histocompatibility antigens. For instance, the presence of certain HL-A antigens is apparently associated with predisposition to the disease:[1407] antigen A5 is increased in frequency among patients with the nodular sclerosis type, regardless of the duration of the disease, and A1 and A8 are increased in those with lymphocytic predominance or mixed cellularity, the rise in the amount of A1 being independent of the duration of the disease whereas A8 becomes high only when the disease has been present at least 5 years. It is thus possible that the histological type of Hodgkin's disease may be influenced by the patient's HL-A phenotype.

Other Factors

So much consideration is given nowadays to the possibility of finding an infective cause of Hodgkin's disease that there may be a tendency to neglect other possibilities. If, or when, an infective agent is eventually and unequivocally demonstrated, it is very unlikely that it will prove to be alone capable of causing the disease (or any type of the disease, for it may well be wrong to assume that all the histological types of Hodgkin's disease are varieties of a single pathological entity). Other factors are likely to be involved. Some, like immunodeficiency states, are already recognized (see opposite). Some may not yet have been considered. For instance, it has been noted that men who are chemists have a higher death rate from cancer, particularly malignant lymphomas and pancreatic carcinoma, than men in the population as a whole.[1408] This observation in the United States of America prompted a study of chemistry graduates in Sweden that suggested that practical chemists, particularly those working in organic chemistry, are significantly likelier than comparable groups of the male population in general to die of leukaemia or of a malignant lymphoma, particularly Hodgkin's disease.[1409] Clearly, such a possibility has to be studied very carefully before it may be regarded as of practical significance: nevertheless, it is a pointer toward the value of a constant watch for clues to the aetiology of Hodgkin's disease and related conditions.

Diagnosis

Histological Examination

Histological investigation is essential for the diagnosis of Hodgkin's disease. In most cases the appearances are sufficiently characteristic to enable the disease to be recognized and placed in its appropriate histological category without difficulty. The commonest mistake, in fact, is to suggest a diagnosis of Hodgkin's disease on inadequate histological grounds: doubt about the nature of a given histological picture in a lymph node biopsy specimen often leads to reporting the appearances as 'atypical Hodgkin's disease' when the condition proves eventually not to be Hodgkin's disease, and in an appreciable proportion of such cases not even to be a malignant condition. The pathologist faced with the not infrequent problem of the difficult lymph node is liable to be misled by the presence of some proliferation of large mononuclear cells, perhaps with some fibrosis and the presence of eosinophils, and to interpret these findings as indicative of Hodgkin's disease or of something supposedly akin to it: as always, circumspection is necessary before suggesting so serious a diagnosis when the observed details are not typical.

In a review of 600 cases of lymphadenopathy in which the initial histological diagnosis was Hodgkin's disease it was found that this interpretation could be confirmed in only 317 cases.[1410] Of the remaining 283 cases, 69 were considered to be instances of other malignant diseases, including 34 'reticulum cell sarcomas' and 29 metastatic tumours, and 192 were considered to be inflammatory or other non-neoplastic conditions, including 89 examples of chronic non-specific lymphadenitis.

In a remarkable study in Chicago, Illinois, it was shown that three competent histologists of differing length of experience did not agree often enough in their separate interpretation of the same series of biopsy sections from untreated cases of Hodgkin's disease for the results to be scientifically useful.[1411] When the same three pathologists worked together, comparing opinions and producing a 'consensus finding', the resulting histological data were considered to be more accurate than any one of the three might have achieved alone, and of significantly better quality as a basis for studies of the disease that would be appropriate to the assessment of therapeutic trials.

Another aspect of the same problem is the consistency of interpretation of histological findings by any individual. In one such study there was a 95 per cent concordance between the original classification of a large series of cases of Hodgkin's disease and the same pathologist's review of the series 6 months afterwards, with safeguards to ensure against disclosure of the earlier interpretation before the review categorization was effected.[1412] Such a measure of excellence would not be universally attained.

Epithelioid Cell Clusters.—One of the more difficult histological distinctions is that between the form of Hodgkin's disease with extensive epithelioid cell clusters (see page 806) and the various other pathological conditions that present a similar histological picture. Early tuberculosis, early sarcoidosis and—most characteristically—toxoplasmosis are among the diseases that may take this form (see page 656 and compare Figs 9.74, 9.116A and 9.173 with Fig. 9.224). The finding of frankly abnormal reticulum cells and Sternberg–Reed cells is an important observation because, when unequivocal, it generally indicates the presence of Hodgkin's disease: failure to demonstrate such cells after a most careful search is usually evidence that the lymphadenopathy is not a manifestation of Hodgkin's disease, and it then becomes imperative to determine the cause of the reaction by means of the investigations appropriate to the causes listed on page 657.

Until the cause has been proven, the prognosis must be guarded.

Drug-Induced Lymphoma-Like Lymphadenopathies.—The special diagnostic difficulties posed by some cases of drug-induced lymphadenopathy, particularly the lymphadenopathy that may accompany anticonvulsant therapy (hydantoin lymphadenopathy) are referred to and illustrated earlier in this chapter (see page 698).

Brucella Infection.—In very rare instances the histological picture in lymph nodes in cases of brucella infection so closely reproduces that of the mixed cellularity type of Hodgkin's disease that only the passage of time may provide the correct answer (see page 591). In this context is is proper to mention again that the coexistence of Hodgkin's disease and brucella infection is bound to be observed from time to time in regions where the latter is prevalent.

Simulation of Hodgkin's Disease Following Treatment of Leukaemia

A pleomorphic histological picture, closely resembling that of the reticular form of the lymphocytic depletion type of Hodgkin's disease (see page 802), has been seen in lymph nodes following chemotherapy in cases of chronic leukaemia (Fig. 9.227). It has been observed both in chronic myeloid leukaemia and in chronic lymphocytic leukaemia.[1413] The condition has been interpreted as a non-neoplastic reaction occurring in the terminal stage of treated leukaemia and, alternatively, as the development of Hodgkin's disease as a terminal complication: neither suggestion is immediately persuasive and the significance of the association remains quite uncertain. Such cases probably account for a proportion of instances in which the development of Hodgkin's disease has been recorded as an accompaniment of leukaemia.

Gordon's Test

The Mervyn Gordon test for Hodgkin's disease[1414] is now recognized to have no specific diagnostic value. The encephalitis that it caused in rabbits (following intracerebral inoculation with a suspension prepared from a lymph node biopsy specimen) is now considered to result from the presence of eosinophils or other non-specific constituents of the inoculum.[1414a] Surprisingly, physicians of all generations still occasionally ask for the test to be carried out.

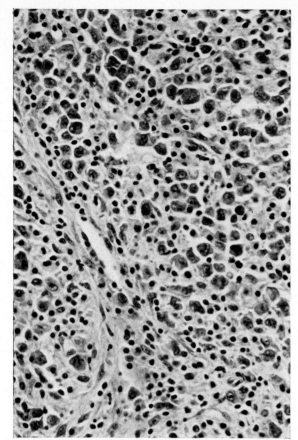

Fig. 9.227. This histological picture, so closely similar to that of the reticular form of the lymphocytic depletion type of Hodgkin's disease, was found at necropsy in the case of a patient who had been having chemotherapy for chronic myeloid leukaemia over a period of almost 4 years. The leukaemic condition was in every respect typical, and there was nothing in the clinical picture to suggest the development of Hodgkin's disease. The changes illustrated were found only in lymph nodes, although many blocks of tissue from the spleen and bone marrow, and from the liver and other organs, were examined. The explanation of this rare finding is unknown (see text). *Haematoxylin–eosin.* × 250.

Lymphomas Other than Hodgkin's Disease* 1415

Only the diagnostically more important features of the main groups of the lymphomas other than Hodgkin's disease will be dealt with here (see Table 9.8, page 783). Various aspects of their aetiology (page 767), prognosis (page 771) and classification (page 777) are considered earlier in this chapter; some comments on their histology are

* The tumours considered in this section are now commonly referred to as the *non-Hodgkin's lymphomas*, an intrusive jargonic phrase (see footnote on page 783).

included in Tables 9.5, 9.6 and 9.7 (pages 778 to 782).

Terminology.—Although the attempt is made here to avoid using the once universally familiar terms, lymphosarcoma and reticulum cell sarcoma, it is fair to remark that both are still widely current, and reasonably understood by clinicians and pathologists. The view has been expressed that the pathologist who uses such terminology today, except to condemn others for doing so, is a danger to his clinical colleagues and their patients: I cannot believe that such a stricture is justified. Advances that are being made by scientifically oriented pathologists are guiding the rest of us toward better understanding of the cytogenesis, nature and control of the lymphomas and related conditions: these advances will prove to have been of cardinal importance, even if further knowledge necessitates fundamental revision of the concepts that today are fresh and stimulating, and even revolutionary. Meantime we do not all feel obliged to advocate the immediate adoption of nomenclature and of concepts that, however interesting and persuasive, are novel and not yet accepted in detail by all who are qualified to judge them, let alone by those who can no more than try to comprehend the problems and the explanations in the light of their own experience in diagnostic practice.

Prognosis.—The new classifications of lymphomas other than Hodgkin's disease have not been in use for long enough, and probably are not yet accurately enough applied in diagnostic practice in general, for particular prognostic deductions to be based on the corresponding categorization of an individual patient's tumour. These classifications have not yet achieved the prognostic value of the Rye classification of Hodgkin's disease (see Table 9.12, page 788). In general, prognosis—as might be anticipated—is better when the tumour is relatively well differentiated and distinctly unfavourable when it is poorly differentiated.1416 Similarly, prognosis is related to the extent of the disease as disclosed by clinical staging.1417 Tumours with a follicular pattern are prognostically more favourable than those with a diffuse pattern.1418 Whether the tumour arises in lymph nodes or is initially extranodal (as it may be in up to 25 per cent of cases of lymphomas other than Hodgkin's disease), the outlook is closely related to the clinical staging of the disease at the time of its first recognition, whatever its histological type.1419

'Extranodal' Lymphomas

Like Hodgkin's disease (see page 789), other lymphomas—apart from Burkitt's lymphoma (see page 828)—arise most frequently in lymph nodes but may originate in organs and tissues elsewhere. It is often impossible to be sure of the identity of lymphomas described in published case reports, and most series refer to 'lymphosarcomas' and 'reticulum cell sarcomas'. For this reason it is better to refer here to such 'extranodal' lymphomas, both primary and secondary, rather than attempt to separate the histological types and consider their extranodal manifestations under the headings of the different tumours. Some particular instances of visceral involvement will be mentioned when considering Burkitt's lymphoma (see page 829) and follicular lymphoma (see page 836).

Other Lymphoreticular Organs.—Splenomegaly, with or without hypersplenism (see page 724), may be the presenting manifestation of any lymphoma.[1420] At necropsy splenic involvement is found in at least half the cases.[1421]

The fauciopharyngeal lymphoid tissue (Waldeyer's ring), particularly the palatine tonsils, is by no means rarely involved and may be the site first involved.[1422] It is important to recognize that patients who present with symptoms of a lymphoma apparently confined to a part of Waldeyer's ring are often found to have occult involvement of abdominal tissues, particularly retroperitoneal lymph nodes (as disclosed by lymphangiography)[1423] and the stomach.[1424]

Lungs.—Primary lymphomas of the lungs may be difficult to distinguish from the so-called 'benign lymphoma' (pseudolymphoma), which some regard as a chronic inflammatory condition (see Volume 1, page 391), others as a benign tumour[1425] and others as a malignant lymphoma (see Volume 1, pages 391 and 407).[1426] Unequivocally malignant primary lymphomas arise relatively rarely in the lungs.[1427] It should be noted that a mediastinal shadow in the chest radiograph may be the first evidence that a patient has a lymphoma.[1428]

Gastrointestinal Tract.[1429]—Lymphomas may arise primarily in the stomach (see page 1049),[1430] the small intestine (see page 1095)[1431] or the large intestine (see page 1148), particularly the rectum.[1303] The familiar benign lymphoid polyps of the rectum and anal canal (see page 1147) are, occasionally, difficult to distinguish histologically from malignant lymphomas.[1432] Lymphomas of the small bowel are particularly frequent in the Middle East,[1433] where they are the main feature of the syndrome of the so-called 'Mediterranean lymphoma' (see page 845).

Liver.—Primary lymphomas of the liver are rare. Their primary nature is difficult to establish unless there is no evidence of involvement of other organs.[1434] Exceptionally, a tumour confined to part of the liver has been resected successfully, with long survival.[1435] In a series of 1269 cases of 'lymphosarcoma' clinical examination had shown the liver to be palpable in 46 per cent of the patients: at necropsy, tumour was found histologically in the liver in only 57 per cent of the cases in which the organ had been detectably enlarged during life.[1421]

Bones.—The long bones, particularly the femora, may be the site of a primary lymphoma. The disease is rare as a primary manifestation, occurs mainly in young adults and in most cases has been interpreted as a 'reticulum cell sarcoma'.[1436] In cases of lymphoma originating outside the skeleton there is demonstrable involvement of the bones in about 10 to 15 per cent of cases (see Chapter 37, volume 4).[1421, 1437]

Central Nervous System.—Primary 'reticulum cell sarcoma' of the brain has been recognized on many occasions[1438] and there has been controversy whether it should be regarded as a tumour peculiar to the central nervous system ('microglioma')[1439] or as a lymphoma comparable to lymphomas arising elsewhere in the body (see Chapter 34, volume 4). In the great majority of cases the disease remains confined to the central nervous system; in the other instances the tumours in the brain and those elsewhere in the body usually have the same histological appearance and correspond to familiar types of lymphoma.[1440]

The primary intracerebral lymphoma is one of the commoner lymphomas to develop as a complication of longterm immunosuppressive therapy following organ transplantation.[1441]

Lymphomatous infiltration of the leptomeninges may develop as a rare complication of a lymphoma originating elsewhere in the body.[1442] The tumour is usually of an undifferentiated or pleomorphic type.

Eyes.—Lymphomas may arise primarily in the region of an eye, sometimes on both sides simultaneously, and may involve the conjunctiva,[1443] lacrimal apparatus, orbital tissue or uveal tract.[1444]

Other Organs and Tissues.—The breasts,[1445] testes,[1446] ovaries,[1447] uterus (usually the cervix,[1448] but often involving the body[1449]), thyroid,[1450] adrenals[1451] and any other organ or tissue may be the site of a primary lymphoma. There is commonly an association between lymphomas of the thyroid and similar tumours of the stomach or, oftener, of the small intestine (see Chapter 31, volume 3).[1452]

The heart is quite often involved in the course of dissemination of lymphomas, sometimes by direct extension from foci in the mediastinum and sometimes by metastasis. The frequency of cardiac involvement has been estimated at about 30 per cent in cases of 'reticulum cell sarcoma' and about 20 per cent in cases of 'lymphosarcoma';[1453] the lesions are demonstrable histologically twice as often as macroscopically.[1454] Evidence of disorderly function of the heart is seldom observed in cases that prove to show myocardial involvement by the tumour.[1454]

Extent of the Disease at Necropsy

The distribution of lymphomatous tissue at necropsy in a small series of cases is indicated in Table 9.15 (page 831).

Lymphomas as a Complication of Therapeutic Immunosuppression[1202, 1455]

The development of a lymphoma in the course of immunosuppressive treatment of patients who have received an organ transplant is referred to on page 770. The peculiar tendency for the tumour in such cases to arise in the central nervous system is mentioned above.

Lymphocytic Lymphomas

The lymphocytic lymphomas were first described in 1863, by Virchow,[1456] and, independently, in 1891, by Dreschfeld,[1457] but it was not until Hans Kundrat, of Vienna, published his paper 'On Lympho-Sarcomatosis',* in 1893,[1458] that they began to be

recognized widely.* The tumours that now are referred to as lymphocytic lymphomas include those that formerly were generally known as lymphosarcomas ('lymphocytic lymphosarcomas' and so-called 'lymphoblastic lymphosarcomas') and also follicular lymphoma and Burkitt's tumour. The two last have characteristics that make their separate consideration expedient (they are described on pages 835 and 824 respectively). It is important to note that the distinction between chronic lymphocytic leukaemia and those cases of lymphocytic lymphoma in which some tumour cells enter the circulating blood is not made easily (see page 487) and may be impossible. Both the Lukes–Collins classification and the Kiel classification of lymphomas include chronic lymphocytic leukaemia, the former as the leukaemic manifestation of the B cell lymphoma of small lymphocytes (Table 9.6, page 779) and the latter as separate categories of chronic B cell leukaemia and chronic T cell leukaemia under the general heading of lymphocytic lymphomas (Table 9.7, page 780). Sézary's syndrome accounts for many cases of chronic lymphocytic leukaemia of T cell type (see page 856).

Histopathology

The lymphocytic lymphomas may arise in any group of lymph nodes, or in a tonsil, the spleen or thymus, or in other organs or tissues (see opposite). Lymph nodes are by far the commonest site of their origin; the invasive growth of the sarcoma leads to fusion and coalescence of affected nodes and their adherence to adjacent tissues, which may be deeply penetrated by the tumour.

Microscopically, the normal structure of the affected tissues is obliterated by masses of closely packed tumour cells. In many cases the cells cannot be distinguished from normal small lymphocytes (Fig. 9.228) or large lymphocytes (Fig. 9.229). Tumours that are believed to be formed of immunoblasts (transformed lymphocytes—see page 522) are considered separately under the heading of 'immunoblastic lymphomas' (see page 849).

The cells of any given tumour are usually uniform in type. Occasionally, a well-differentiated tumour that consists predominantly of small lymphocytes may be found to include areas in which the cells are

---

* In my father's manuscript book of notes on the histological preparations in the class in practical [pathological] histology in the University of Aberdeen in 1886–87, when he was a student there, a section of a 'round cell sarcoma of lymphatic glands' is described. 'Lymphosarcoma' is mentioned as the alternative term, and is attributed to Professor D. J. Hamilton (who occupied the chair of pathology in Aberdeen from 1882 to 1908).

* Lymphosarcoma, or lymphosarcomatosis, is still occasionally referred to as Kundrat's disease. The term Kundrat's disease is also applied sometimes to the presence of any major congenital defect of the limbic system ('rhinencephalon'), such as Patau's trisomy-13 (see page 75, Volume 1) (Kundrat, H., *Wien. med. Bl.*, 1882, **5**, 1395).

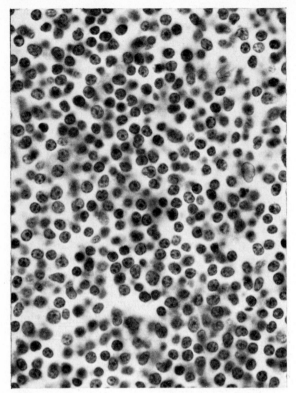

Fig. 9.228. Lymphocytic lymphoma composed of small lymphocytes. *Haematoxylin–eosin.* × 630.

larger lymphocytes (Fig. 9.230); more rarely, pleo-morphic areas are seen. In some instances, the second element in such tumours of composite structure may be composed of cells that have the morphological characteristics now regarded as those of immunoblasts (Fig. 9.231). Whatever the type of cell, lymphocytic lymphomas of mixed cytological constitution tend to be more rapidly progressive. An early indication of a change in cell differentiation, and so of increasing malignancy, is a notable enlargement of the nucleolus: if this is recognized in part of the tumour in a biopsy speci-men, successive specimens are likely to disclose a progressive change in the character of the cells.

There is seldom any tendency for necrosis to occur in lymphocytic lymphomas unless they have become anaplastic.

When the tumour involves a lymph node affected by chronic lymphadenitis, the fibrotic tissue that has resulted from the inflammatory condition imposes its pattern on the tumour (Fig. 9.232).

Variants

'*T Zone Lymphoma*'.—This uncommon variety of

lymphocytic lymphoma is noted in footnote [||] of Table 9.7 (page 781) (Figs 9.233A and 9.233B).

Diffuse Sclerosing Lymphocytic Lymphoma.—Inter-stitial fibrosis is not a feature of lymphocytic lymphomas, except in the special case of the rare diffuse sclerosing variant ('*fascicular lymphocytic lymphoma*'). This variant occurs oftener in early childhood than at other ages. It has a fine colla-genous stroma: the tumour cells, which usually are well-formed small lymphocytes, are arranged in rows between the fibres, with the consequence that the tumour commonly has a distinctive whorled pattern (Figs 9.234A and 9.234B). Severe anaemia, leucopenia and thrombocytopenia may develop in those cases in which there is extensive involvement of bone marrow.

This 'diffuse' form of sclerosing lymphocytic lymphoma is distinct from the '*nodular sclerotic*

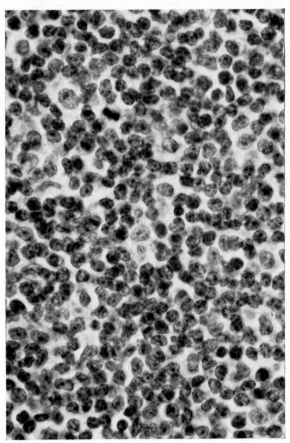

Fig. 9.229. Lymphocytic lymphoma composed of large lymphocytes. The cells are not only larger but also more varied in shape and size than those of the lymphoma of small lymphocytes (see Fig. 9.228). Several mitotic figures are seen. *Haematoxylin–eosin.* × 630.

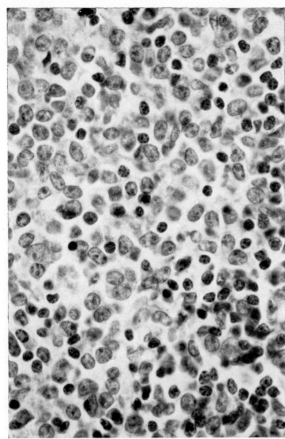

Fig. 9.230. Lymphocytic lymphoma. Most of the tumour in this lymph node consisted of small lymphocytes. In places there were aggregates of substantially larger, paler tumour cells, as in the greater part of this field. The large cells have a more evenly rounded nucleus, with very fine nuclear membrane, pale chromatin and a moderately small nucleolus; multiple nucleoli are rarely present. Compare with Fig. 9.231, in which the larger cells have features that suggest that they are tumour immunoblasts; the large cells in the present picture may be regarded as large lymphocytes that have not undergone transformation into immunoblasts. *Haematoxylin–eosin.* × 630.

lymphosarcoma' defined by Bennett and Millett in 1969.[1459] The nodular sclerotic tumours are characterized by traversal of their substance by bands of collagenous fibres. The tumours that show this pattern include all the histological varieties of lymphomas (Fig. 9.235) except for the well differentiated lymphocytic tumours.[1460] It is said to be a prognostically favourable characteristic.[1461]

Lymphocytic Lymphomas with Protein Deposition in situ.—It seems that any lymphoma that is derived from the 'bursa-equivalent'-dependent system of lymphoid cells (B cells) may produce immuno-

globulins (see Tables 9.6 and 9.7, pages 779 and 780).[1263] This can be confirmed by assay of the amount of immunoglobulin in fresh biopsy material, by histochemical demonstration of diastase-resistant periodic-acid/Schiff-positive inclusions in the tumour cells, by cytochemical demonstration of immunoglobulin on the surface of the tumour cells and by demonstration of protein deposits in their cytoplasm by electron microscopy.[1263] Such studies have shown that these lymphomas may retain the capacity to produce immunoglobulins that is the main function of the normal B cell system. In most instances there is no increase in the amount of immunoglobulin in the blood; when there is an increase, the hyperglobulinaemia is of monoclonal

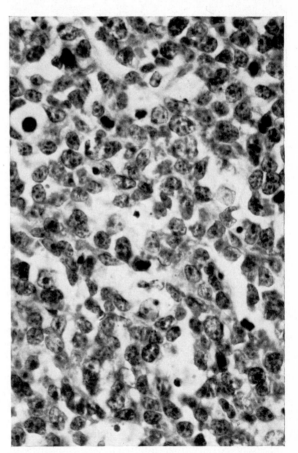

Fig. 9.231. Lymphocytic lymphoma with immunoblastic foci. This field is from a lymph node that was mainly replaced by a lymphoma composed uniformly of small lymphocytes, as in Fig. 9.228. In some parts, such as this, there were aggregates of much larger cells with a pale nucleus. Many of these cells have two or more moderately large, distinct nucleoli. The appearances are those of tumour immunoblasts (compare with Figs 9.262 to 9.265, pages 850 and 851). *Haematoxylin–eosin.* × 630.

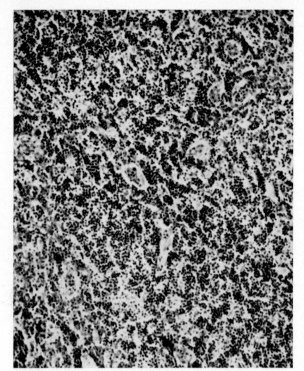

Fig. 9.232. Lymphocytic lymphoma infiltrating a lymph node already the seat of a longstanding chronic non-specific lymphadenitis. The distinct pattern of the tumour in this illustration is probably determined by the increase in the amount of collagenous stroma and the thickening of the walls of the small blood vessels that are consequent on the lymphadenitis. These resistant tissues have kept the infiltrating tumour cells from forming the uniformly cellular mass that is more characteristic of such lymphomas. Compare with Fig. 9.235 (page 826). *Haematoxylin–eosin.* × 110.

type, the protein produced by the tumour cells being of consistent molecular structure and therefore moving with uniform speed on paper electrophoresis to form a tight, concentrated band, and also producing a characteristically 'bowed' anomaly of the arc on immunoelectrophoresis.

In the great majority of immunoglobulin-producing lymphomas there is no clearly evident accumulation of proteinaceous material to be seen in conventional histological preparations. However, in a very small proportion of instances, refractile, intensely eosinophile, homogeneous spherules or coalescent aggregates are seen in the cytoplasm of cells (Fig. 9.236). Some of these cells are macrophages that have ingested the material; others appear to be tumour cells, particularly plasmacytoid cells but occasionally cells that have been interpreted as small lymphocytes, large lymphocytes or immunoblasts. In some cases it has been possible to

show that this eosinophile material contains immunoglobulin, particularly IgM or IgG. It may also give a strong periodic-acid/Schiff reaction; this is not affected by prior incubation with diastase.

Burkitt's Lymphoma[1462]

The condition that has variously been known as the 'lymphoma of childhood in Africa', the 'African lymphoma', Cook's tumour, equatorial arthropod-borne lymphoma and Epstein–Barr lymphoma is

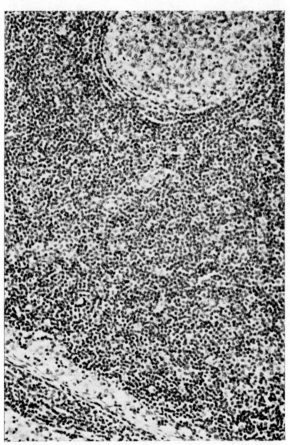

Fig. 9.233A. Lymphocytic lymphoma of the so-called 'T zone' type. This tumour evidently arises from the lymphocytes in the thymus-dependent parts of the lymph nodes—that is, the 'deep cortex' ('paracortical area'), between the follicles. It is thought to be the T lymphocyte equivalent of the lymphomas that arise in the 'bursa-equivalent'-dependent parts, such as the follicle centres. It is a characteristic of the T zone lymphoma that its cells infiltrate the tissues of the affected nodes without destroying the follicles, particularly the germinal centres, which therefore persist, at least for a considerable time. The tumour cells are predominantly well-differentiated lymphocytes. There may be a scattering of solitary larger cells among them, as in the example illustrated. See also Fig. 9.233B. *Haematoxylin–eosin.* × 160.

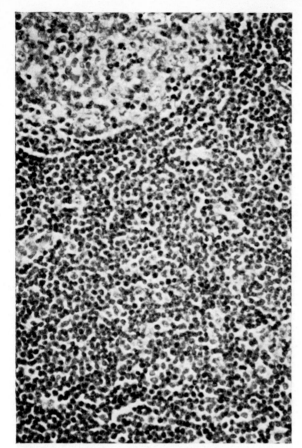

Fig. 9.233B. Higher magnification of field illustrated in Fig. 9.233A. *Haematoxylin–eosin.* × 250.

now most generally and conveniently referred to as Burkitt's lymphoma, or Burkitt's tumour.[1463] It has a long history in Africa,[1464] although the first acceptably detailed description was not recorded until 1904, when Albert Cook observed the disease at the Mengo Hospital in Kampala, Uganda.[1465] Contemporary interest in the condition mainly dates from Burkitt's account, published in 1958[1466] and based on his experiences in Uganda. Previously, series of cases had been included in studies of other forms of cancer in Nigeria,[1467] the Cameroun,[1468] francophone West Africa,[1469] Ghana (then the Gold Coast colony)[1470] and Zaire and Rwanda (then the Belgian Congo and Ruanda-Urundi),[1471] but it was Burkitt who gave the first definitive description of the condition as a tumour entity.[1466] Since then there have been remarkable advances in knowledge of the distribution, aetiology, pathology and treatment of the disease.[1462, 1472, 1473]

Aetiology

Geographical Distribution and the Possibility of an Insect-Borne Agent.—Burkitt's lymphoma occurs both endemically and sporadically. It is endemic in the so-called 'lymphoma belt' of Africa, which stretches right across the continent south of the Sahara and down the east coast of South Africa (it does not include the rest of southern Africa, northern Kenya, Ethiopia and Somalia).[1474] The other endemic area comprises parts of Papua New Guinea.[1475] Sporadic cases[1476–1479]—some of them diagnostically equivocal—have been recognized in Africa outside the lymphoma belt, in southern and south-eastern Asia, in Australia, in Europe and in parts of North and South America (but not in Central America, contrary to a common report, for the supposed occurrence of a case in El Salvador was a misplacement on the map of a case identified in the state of Salvador, in Brazil, where the disease has proved to be frequent enough—for instance, in the state of São Paulo[1480]—to indicate the possibility that there may be an endemic region there).

The geographical distribution of endemic cases within a wide belt of equatorial Africa, and the fall in incidence at altitudes above 1200 m (4000 ft)— practically no cases occur among those who live at

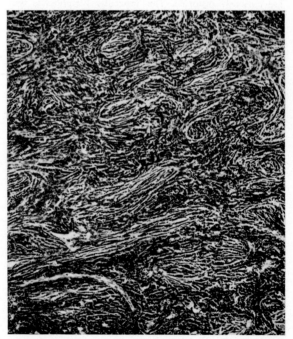

Fig. 9.234A. Lymphocytic lymphoma of the so-called 'fascicular' variety. The whorled pattern of this very uncommon variety is characteristic. See also Fig. 9.234B. *Haematoxylin–eosin.* × 65.

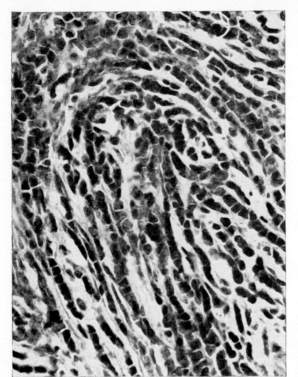

Fig. 9.234B. Same tumour as in Fig. 9.234A. Rows of tumour cells are separated by fine fibrous stroma. Many of the cells are curiously distorted. The 'fascicular lymphocytic lymphoma' is ordinarily seen only in young children. The patient whose biopsy specimen is illustrated here was a man, aged 27. The fascicular pattern was lacking in other parts of the specimen, which showed instead the more typical, diffuse infiltration. This type of tumour is quite distinct from the so-called 'nodular sclerotic lymphosarcoma' (see Fig. 9.235). *Haematoxylin–eosin.* × 330.

above 1500 m (5000 ft)[1481]—led to recognition of the possibility that the disease might be related to climatic conditions, and therefore that it might be borne by arthropods, particularly mosquitoes.[1482] The 'lymphoma belt' coincides with areas in which the annual rainfall is over 50 cm and the mean temperature of the coolest month 16°C.[1482] Further pointers to the likelihood of an infective environmental factor were seen in the age incidence of the disease, with predominant involvement of children (see below). An occasional case is seen among African adults who come from non-endemic areas to live in an endemic region, presumably with no earlier exposure to the causative agent and therefore unimmunized.[1483]

Age.—The disease is said to be unknown before the age of 1 year. It is infrequent in the 2nd and 3rd year of life; its incidence then increases rapidly to its peak

between the 4th and 8th years, thereafter falling sharply.[1484] Few cases are seen after adolescence, apart from those in migrants from other regions (see above). The non-occurrence of the disease in infancy suggests protection by antibodies acquired from the mother. The subsequent rapid rise is typical of arbovirus infection, with exposure to the virus as the child begins to wander abroad independently.

Relation to Malaria.—The endemic distribution of Burkitt's lymphoma in Africa and in Papua New Guinea corresponds to the area of hyperendemic malaria.* The incidence of the tumour has fallen in some regions where malaria has been eradicated.[1485] The geographical occurrence of 'tropical idiopathic splenomegaly' ('big spleen disease'—see page 743),

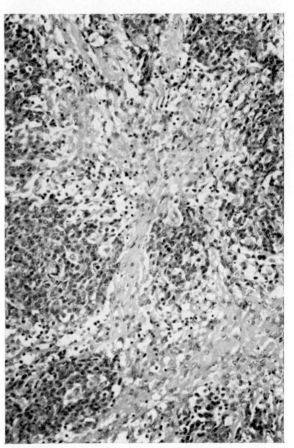

Fig. 9.235. Poorly differentiated lymphocytic lymphoma of the type sometimes described as 'nodular sclerotic', because its substance is broken into distinct cellular foci by the presence of broad strands of collagenous tissue. *Haematoxylin–eosin.* × 160.

* Malaria is said to be hyperendemic when the spleen is palpable in 50 per cent of the children in the area.

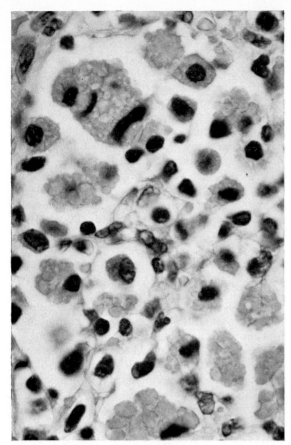

Fig. 9.236.§ Lymphocytic lymphoma with protein elaboration. The cytoplasm of many of the cells in this field of a lymph node biopsy specimen is distended by an accumulation of irregular globules of homogeneous, eosinophile material that is believed to consist largely of immunoglobulin produced by tumour cells. Some of the material has been ingested by phagocytes; some of it is in the cytoplasm of tumour cells. *Haematoxylin–eosin.* × 750.

which is generally believed to be causally associated with chronic malaria, coincides closely with the areas where Burkitt's lymphoma is endemic.[1486] A further observation that possibly links Burkitt's tumour and malaria is the fact that individuals who are heterozygous for haemoglobin A and haemoglobin S (that is, those with haemoglobin AS—the sickle cell trait), and who are known through possession of this trait to have partial protection against infection by *Plasmodium falciparum*, the cause of malignant tertian malaria, have about half the likelihood of developing the tumour that characterizes those with haemoglobin AA.[1487]

Malaria alone cannot be the cause of Burkitt's lymphoma.[1488] It might act with a co-factor—a virus, for instance—to cause the disease,[1486] perhaps by stimulating proliferation of the lymphoid tissues and causing the ordinarily self-limiting lymphocytic proliferation associated with the viral infection to become progressive, or perhaps by interfering with immunological surveillance in such a way that host cells no longer recognize and destroy neoplastic or potentially neoplastic cells.[1488]

Viruses as Possible Aetiological Agents.—Various viruses have come under consideration as potentially a cause of Burkitt's lymphoma. One was the RNA virus (of the so-called togavirus group) that was responsible for an acute epidemic disease (o'nyong-nyong fever) in East Africa in the 1950s and early 1960s:[1489] this virus was carried by the familiar malaria vectors, *Anopheles gambiae* and *Anopheles funestus*, and the distribution of these mosquitoes is similar to that of Burkitt's lymphoma. It is now known that the o'nyong-nyong virus has nothing to do with the occurrence of the tumour. The viruses that have attracted most attention as possible causes of the latter are reoviruses and the herpesvirus that is known as the Epstein–Barr virus.

Reoviruses, predominantly of type 3, were isolated regularly from biopsy specimens in cases of Burkitt's tumour in Uganda[1490] and have been thought to be of indirect aetiological importance (in associaton with other viral or non-viral co-factors).[1491]

The likeliest aetiological agent so far described is the Epstein–Barr virus. This was discovered in 1964[1492] and the information that has since been collected not only points to its causal role in relation to Burkitt's lymphoma but has taken us into a new era of advance in understanding of the pathogenesis of certain types of cancer in man. The importance of the Epstein–Barr virus in relation to Burkitt's lymphoma seems unquestionable, although the nature of the relationship is not yet clear.[1493] The commonest result of infection with this virus is the development of specific antibodies, without any clinical illness; lasting immunity to infectious mononucleosis follows, and the virus may be harboured in the body for life.[1493a] Much less often, infectious mononucleosis results: this is essentially a reversible proliferation of lymphoid cells (see page 647). It is possible that the virus may effect malignant proliferation of lymphoid cells in a very small proportion of infected individuals.[1494] In tropical areas where Burkitt's tumour is endemic, it seems likely that a climate-dependent co-factor operates with the virus to cause the tumour: the co-factor may be some other infection—such as malaria (see above)—that is accompanied by proliferation of the lymphoid tissues.[1486]

Immunological Responses.—Once the possibility that Burkitt's lymphoma might have a viral cause was recognized there was a stimulus to look for evidence of specific immunological responses both to the tumour cells and to the virus or viruses associated with them. Such responses were already known to occur in cases of virus-induced leukaemia and lymphomas in animals, and it seemed probable that they might be found in Burkitt's lymphoma if it also were caused by viral infection. Clinical observations of spontaneous regression[1495] and of the possible importance of the role of the host's reaction to the tumour in determining the success or failure of treatment[1496] indicated the likelihood of specific defensive responses on the part of the host tissues.

Patients with Burkitt's lymphoma and those with nasopharyngeal carcinoma (which also is frequently associated with infection by the Epstein–Barr virus —see page 243, volume 1) regularly have very high titres of circulating antibodies specifically against Epstein–Barr virus.[1497] The titres are much higher than those in most cases of infectious mononucleosis (see page 648); lower titres may be found in the serum of individuals who have a history of infectious mononucleosis in the past and, less frequently, in other people, including a number of healthy people with no history of any illness of a type known to be associated with the presence of this virus.[1498] Antibodies to the Epstein–Barr virus have been found also in a few cases of 'sinus histiocytosis with massive lymphadenopathy' (see page 564).

Cell membrane antigens are found in established cultures of cells that have a considerable load of Epstein–Barr virus and on the cells of Burkitt's lymphoma in biopsy specimens.[1497] These antigens react with antibodies that are present in the serum of the great majority of patients with Burkitt's lymphoma.

Such evidence supports the suggestion that the Epstein–Barr virus is important in the causation of Burkitt's lymphoma, although it does not amount to firm proof.

Practical Aspects of the Host Reaction.[1499]—The lesions of Burkitt's lymphoma are most frequent in organs and tissues that are comparatively poor in lymphoreticular tissue, such as the jaws, ovaries, testes, thyroid, adrenals and breasts. The lymph nodes, with the exception of the abdominal nodes,[1499a] and the spleen and fauciopharyngeal lymphoid tissue are involved relatively rarely. The explanation of this distribution, which is peculiar to Burkitt's lymphoma and quite contrary to the usual predominance of involvement of the lympho-

reticular organs in other types of lymphoma, may relate to the greater chance that the tumour cells may have to survive in an environment lacking the defensive potential of abundant lymphoid tissue.

As in cases of other lymphomas, the prognosis of Burkitt's lymphoma is much influenced by the extent of the disease at the time of starting treatment.[1500] Involvement of the central nervous system, which is by no means rare, and extensive involvement of lymph nodes are prognostically unfavourable, largely through their usual association with increased resistance of the disease to chemotherapy. In other cases, comparatively small amounts of chemotherapy may lead to sustained remissions. Sometimes remission may be unusually delayed, eventually occurring when the disease has seemed wholly resistant to treatment.[1499] Spontaneous remissions have been observed, but are very unusual.[1495] Temporary remissions have been attributed to the administration of serum from patients whose disease had responded to treatment ('convalescent serum'),[1501] but controlled trials have not confirmed such observations.[1502]

The occurrence of remissions, either spontaneously or following treatment with serum from another patient, and the often very marked initial response to chemotherapy support the view that an immunological mechanism may operate. This may be an effect of an unusual degree of antigenicity of the tumour cells. Alternatively, in the majority of cases, it may require the destruction of a large proportion of the tumour cells by cytotoxic drugs before the body can mount an effective immunological defence against the remaining tumour tissue. The latter may possibly undergo changes in antigenic structure as an effect of treatment, with consequent facilitation of the response by normal immunocompetent cells.[1503]

Histopathology[1488, 1504, 1505]

The morbid anatomical and microscopical findings in a series of 557 proven cases of Burkitt's lymphoma seen in Uganda in the period from 1950 to 1965 inclusive have been described by D. H. Wright.[1488, 1504]

Presenting Manifestations.—The commonest presenting manifestation in the Ugandan series was involvement of the jaws (55 per cent), the tumour (Fig. 9.237) being single in about half the cases and multiple in the rest. Radiological examination discloses more instances of multiple tumours than are evident on clinical examination alone. The

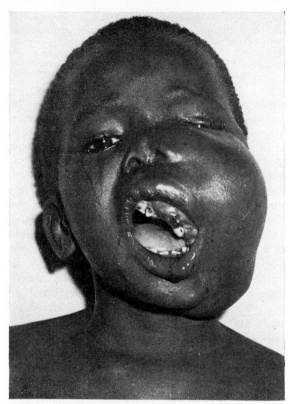

Fig. 9.237.§ This child has Burkitt's lymphoma of the maxilla, with extension into adjacent tissues.

maxillary tumours (Fig. 9.238) tend to spread into the base of the skull and may invade the cranial cavity. Ovarian tumours[1506] were the presenting manifestation in 38 per cent of cases in female patients. Testicular tumours, in contrast, accounted

for only 3·8 per cent of the first symptoms in male patients. Other presenting manifestations are noted in Table 9.13.

Table 9.13. *Main Presenting Clinical Manifestations of Burkitt's Tumour in 557 Cases in Uganda (1950–65)**

Presenting manifestations†	Number of cases	Per cent
Tumour of jaws	306	55
Single tumour of jaws	145	26
Multiple tumours of jaws	161	29
Abdominal swelling	139	25
Ovarian tumours	70	(38% of 183 female patients)
Testicular tumours	14	(3·8% of 372 male patients)
Paraplegia	38	6·8
Tumour of bone other than jaws	37	6·6
Enlargement of superficial lymph nodes	29	5·2
Thyroid tumour	24	4·3
Tumour of a salivary gland	17	3
Mammary tumour‡	9	1·6

* Data from: Wright, D. H., in *Burkitt's Lymphoma*, edited by D. P. Burkitt and D. H. Wright, page 64, table 8.1; Edinburgh and London, 1970.

† More than one organ or structure was the site of a presenting manifestation in a considerable proportion of the cases.

‡ Shepherd, J. J., Wright, D. H., *Brit. J. Surg.*, 1967, **54**, 776.

Necropsy Findings.—The distribution of the tumours at necropsy (Figs 9.239 and 9.240) is shown in Table 9.14. It may be noted that involvement of the central nervous system has been much more frequent

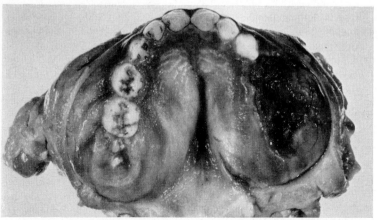

Fig. 9.238.§ Bilateral maxillary involvement by Burkitt's lymphoma, with expansion of the alveolus on each side and encroachment on the hard palate. There is loss of teeth and ulceration on the left side.

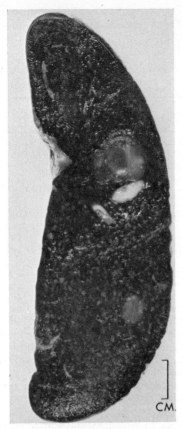

Fig. 9.239. § Spleen of a child who died of Burkitt's lymphoma. Several distinct tumours are present, varying in colour and general appearance. The splenic follicles are prominent and the red pulp is darkened by the presence of malarial pigment. Histological examination showed the lymphomatous tissue to be confined to the obvious masses. The splenic follicles were hyperplastic.

anatomical peculiarities of Burkitt's lymphoma are matched by the distinctiveness of its histological picture.

Histology.—The most striking feature of the histological picture of Burkitt's lymphoma is the so-called 'starry sky'[1508] appearance, which is due to the quite profuse scattering of single, large, pale or vacuolate macrophages among the closely packed, more darkly stained tumour cells (Figs 9.241A and 9.241B). Many of the macrophages contain intensely haematoxyphile round bodies (Flemming's 'stainable bodies'—see page 512 and Fig. 9.4): these are derived from the breakdown of the nuclei of the tumour cells, and it is presumed that the unusual frequency of macrophages in the tumour is a result of a high death rate among its cells.[1509] The 'starry sky' pattern is not pathognomonic, for it may be seen in occasional examples of other lymphomas, although rarely as uniformly widespread and as marked as in Burkitt's lymphoma. Its occurrence in some lymphocytic lymphomas accounts for a proportion of supposed cases of Burkitt's lymphoma

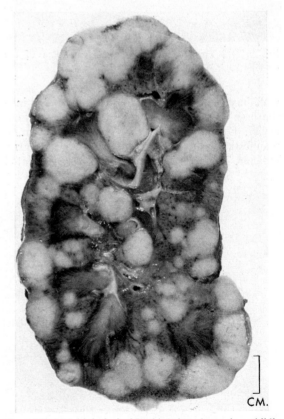

Fig. 9.240. § Multiple foci of Burkitt's lymphoma in a child's kidney.

in some series of post-mortem studies: for instance, there were lesions in the meninges, brain or spinal cord in 81 per cent of cases (21 cases out of 26) in a Nigerian series.[1507] An increase in the frequency of neurological manifestations is attributed to the longer survival of children who, without chemotherapy, would have died earlier in the course of the disease from involvement of other parts of the body.[1504]

The distribution of the lesions—particularly the relative infrequency of involvement of lymphoreticular organs—is another indication of the clear distinction between Burkitt's lymphoma and other lymphomas. Although the series analysed are small, the trend of the differences in distribution of the lesions of Burkitt's lymphoma and those of untreated Hodgkin's disease and of other untreated lymphomas is indicated in Table 9.15. The morbid

Table 9.14. *Distribution of the Tumour at Necropsy in 88 Cases of Burkitt's Lymphoma in Uganda (1953–67)*[*][†]

Organ or tissue	Number of cases	Per cent
Kidneys	64	73
Lymph nodes	60	68
Adrenals	49	56
Jaws	42	48
Pancreas	37	42
Liver	34	39
Thyroid	30	34
Spleen	28	32
Small intestine	24	27
Stomach	20	23
Bones other than the skull	15	17
Brain	15	17
Lungs	13	15
Large intestine	12	14
Spinal cord (compression)	10	11
Breasts	4	5
Ovaries	17	81% of female patients
Testes	7	10% of male patients

[*] Data from: Wright, D. H., in *Burkitt's Lymphoma*, edited by D. P. Burkitt and D. H. Wright, page 65, table 8.2; Edinburgh and London, 1970.

[†] The data tabulated relate to 65 children and 23 adults. There are some significant differences in the distribution of tumours in the two age groups: for instance, tumours were present in the jaws of 57% of the children and in 30% of the adults, in the other bones of 12% of the children and 30% of the adults, and in the breasts in 1·5% of the children and in 13% of the adults.

reported from parts of the world where this disease is not endemic. It is seen also in some non-neoplastic conditions (see, for example, Fig. 9.32, page 555), and it must not be confused with other conditions in which large, pale cells are scattered singly among small lymphoid cells, such as immunoblastic lymphadenopathy (Fig. 9.153, page 704) and some cases of Sézary's syndrome (Fig. 9.276, page 857).

While it is the macrophages that immediately attract attention when sections of Burkitt's lymphoma are examined, their presence is incidental, as has been noted above. The neoplastic cells are those that appear as the dark background against which the macrophages stand out so prominently. They are rounded or somewhat irregular in shape and on average about 12 μm in diameter. Their nucleus is single, round or ovoid, or of irregular outline, and may be notched or cloven. In well-fixed tissue—for instance, at the periphery of a biopsy specimen[1488]—the chromatin is finely or rather coarsely granular, and evenly distributed; in deeper parts of a tumour,

where fixation has been correspondingly somewhat delayed, autolytic changes often make the nucleus appear somewhat vesicular, and the nucleoli, which

Table 9.15. *Distribution of the Tumour at Necropsy in 88 Cases of Burkitt's Lymphoma, 40 Cases of Hodgkin's Disease and 50 Cases of Other Lymphomas*[*]

Organ or tissue	Burkitt's lymphoma (88 cases) %	Hodgkin's disease (40 cases) %	Other lymphomas (50 cases) %
Kidneys	73	10	12
Lymph nodes	68	100	100
Adrenals	56	2·5	6
Jaws	48	0	0
Pancreas	42	7·5	10
Liver	39	57·5	52
Thyroid	34	0	6
Spleen	32	90	92
Small intestine	27	0	4
Stomach	23	2·5	4
Bones other than the skull	17	45	18
Brain	17	0	0
Lungs	15	32·5	16
Large intestine	14	0	2
Spinal cord (lesions causing paraplegia)	11	2·5	2
Breasts	5	0	0
Ovaries	81% of female patients	0 (14 female patients)	5·6% of 18 female patients
Testes	10% of male patients	4·8% of 26 male patients	0

[*] The 88 cases of Burkitt's lymphoma are those to which the data in Table 9.14 relate (Wright, D. H., in *Burkitt's Lymphoma*, edited by D. P. Burkitt and D. H. Wright, page 65, table 8.2; Edinburgh and London, 1970).

The 40 cases of Hodgkin's disease were collected from the records of 11 general teaching hospitals in the United Kingdom and the Republic of Ireland and were selected on the basis of absence of a history of treatment other than with localized X-irradiation and non-specific supportive measures, the availability of a comprehensive post-mortem report and the availability of histological material of a quality adequate to enable an unequivocal histological diagnosis to be made. Most of the cases dated from the 1920s and 1930s; all but two were of the mixed cellularity histological type, the two exceptions being examples of the nodular sclerosis type. The 50 cases of other lymphomas were collected from the same hospitals and were selected on the same basis; 26 were considered to be lymphocytic lymphomas, 15 to be 'immunoblastic lymphomas' and 9 to be pleomorphic or anaplastic undifferentiated lymphomas. Both series were collected over a period of 10 years up to 1960 (Symmers, W. St C., *unpublished series*, including material made available by Professors W. G. Barnard, J. W. S. Blacklock, G. R. Cameron, J. H. Dible, R. A. Q. O'Meara, J. W. Orr, D. S. Russell, R. Scarff, M. J. Stewart and G. Payling Wright).

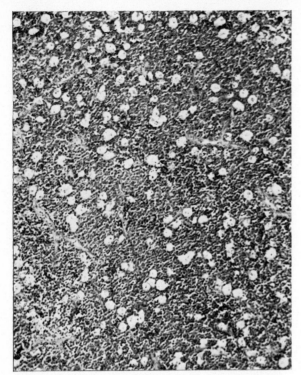

Fig. 9.241A.§ Burkitt's lymphoma. This low magnification shows the characteristic 'starry sky' appearance that results from the contrast between the large, pale macrophages, with their abundant cytoplasm, and the much smaller, closely packed tumour cells, which have little cytoplasm and so form a relatively dense background. It must be remembered that the 'starry sky' picture is not pathognomonic of Burkitt's lymphoma (see Figs 9.244A and 9.276 on pages 834 and 857 respectively). See also Fig. 241B. *Haematoxylin–eosin.* × 75.

are small and haematoxyphile, and from 2 to 5 in number, are the more readily seen.

The cytoplasm of the tumour cells may not be discernible where they are packed closely, as in the deeper parts of a well-fixed specimen. At the cut edge of a specimen, where the cells have tended to become separated although well fixed, it appears as an opaque, sharply defined rim, wider toward one pole, and so staining with eosin and haematoxylin that it has a smoky purplish colour. Its high content of ribonucleic acid, which accounts for the amphiphilia in haematoxylin–eosin preparations, is also shown by its pyroninophilia. Very small, round vacuoles are present in the cytoplasm of many of the cells, although it may be difficult to find them in histological preparations unless fixation has been good and the cells are not pressed together. These vacuoles, which contain neutral fat, are much more readily seen in imprint preparations (Fig. 9.242).

Larger globules of neutral fat are found in the macrophages. Although it is characteristic of Burkitt's lymphoma that lipid is abundant in the tumour, both in the tumour cells and in the macrophages, this is not pathognomonic: some immunoblastic lymphomas, and occasionally other lymphomas, may show the same feature in the cytoplasm of the tumour cells.

There is no increase in the amount of reticulin in the tumours and it is exceptional to see any evidence of collagenous stroma formation, although there may be some thickening of the adventitia of the small blood vessels.

Variants.—Recurrent tumours may show considerable pleomorphism,[1510] with a variable number of binucleate cells, giant cells and maybe cells reminiscent of the Sternberg–Reed cells of Hodgkin's disease (see page 794).[1511] It may be difficult to

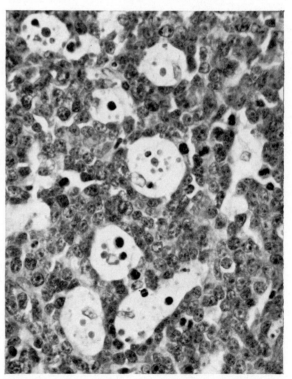

Fig. 9.241B.§ Burkitt's lymphoma. The macrophages are sharply outlined from the surrounding tumour cells. Each has a rather small, pale nucleus; the cytoplasm contains ingested nuclear and other debris (Flemming's 'stainable bodies'—see Fig. 9.4, page 513). The tumour cells have little cytoplasm. Their nucleus contains chromatin that is finely or coarsely distributed; nucleoli are readily seen in many of the cells and are characteristically multiple. Compare with the tumour cells in Fig. 9.244B (page 835). *Haematoxylin–eosin.* × 400.

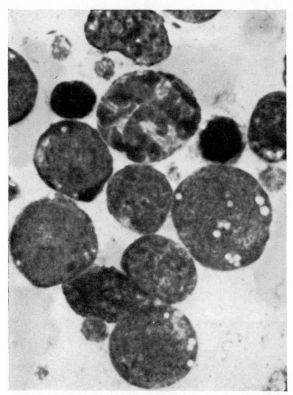

Fig. 9.242.§ 'Imprint' preparation from cut surface of freshly excised tumour tissue in a case of Burkitt's lymphoma. The tumour cells in this field range from 12 to 18 μm in diameter; usually, their range is from 8 to 24 μm and the average cell is from 10 to 12 μm in diameter. The narrow rim of cytoplasm can be seen, darkly stained, in some cells. Cytoplasmic vacuoles are present in most of the cells, varying somewhat in size, and sometimes overlying the nucleus. The vacuoles correspond to the site of lipid material that has been dissolved during fixation of the imprint in alcohol. They are not pathognomonic: identical lipid vacuoles may be found abundantly in the cytoplasm of certain other types of lymphoma, particularly 'histiocytic lymphomas' and possibly other undifferentiated lymphomas, as well as some immunoblastic lymphomas. *May–Grünwald Giemsa.* × 1500.

justify a histological diagnosis of Burkitt's lymphoma in such cases if the previous history is not known and if sections of earlier, typical lesions are not available.[1488]

Position of Burkitt's Lymphoma among the Lymphomas as a Group

The geographical distribution of Burkitt's lymphoma, its relation to the Epstein–Barr virus, its sensitivity to chemotherapy, the distribution of the tumours in the body and the histological picture combine to establish this disease as an entity. Its lymphomatous nature is not in doubt: its cyto-

genesis is far from certain. It has been classed as a 'follicular centre cell lymphoma' of small cells with non-cloven nucleus,[1198] as a 'lymphoblastic lymphoma'[1263] and as an 'undifferentiated lymphoma'.[1512] It is generally considered to be derived from 'bursa-equivalent'-dependent cells (B cells).

Differential Diagnosis

A considerable range of different tumours may simulate the clinical manifestations of Burkitt's lymphoma. Ameloblastomas, fibrous dysplasia and ossifying fibroma, and embryonal sarcomas are among tumours and tumour-like conditions of the jaws that may be mistaken for the lymphoma.[1484] Similarly, the differential diagnosis of tumours in other sites in which Burkitt's lymphoma may present must be carefully considered in each case. There is some tendency to assume that all tumours that might be instances of Burkitt's lymphoma in young African patients, especially in the endemic areas, must be such: this is very far from the case. Nonetheless, Burkitt's lymphoma is the commonest tumour among children in Uganda[1513] and in Ibadan, in Nigeria,[1514] accounting for respectively 50 and 70 per cent of all childhood cancer in these areas.

Histological artefact has been mistaken for the 'starry sky' appearance (Fig. 9.243).

Burkitt's Lymphoma in Britain

A small number of cases clinically and histologically reproducing the picture of Burkitt's lymphoma has been recognized on reviewing the records of children's hospitals in Britain.[1515] In the first edition of this book I mentioned two cases that I had seen here.[1516] One patient was a Jamaican girl, aged 6 years, whose symptoms began shortly before she left the West Indies for the first time: she died in England 8 months later. The histological picture in a biopsy specimen of her maxillary tumour and in tumours in the ovaries, spleen, kidneys, abdominal lymph nodes and heart is identical with that of typical cases of the disease in East Africa. The second patient was a white child who had never been out of Britain: her illness presented with a tumour of the mandible and rapidly increasing enlargement of the cervical and axillary lymph nodes; splenomegaly and a pelvic mass developed; after a transitory response to radiotherapy she died of rapidly progressive heart failure, with radiological evidence of possible tumours protruding from the wall of the right

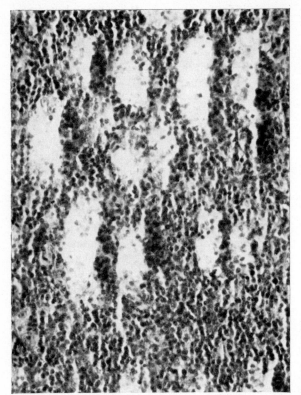

Fig. 9.243.§ This photomicrograph shows the characteristic artefact that results from 'knife chatter' during microtomy. The specimen is a lymph node, and lymphoid tissue is specially prone to this type of artefact, particularly when fixation has been inadequate. The appearances were interpreted by an insufficiently experienced doctor as the 'starry sky' of Burkitt's lymphoma (of which there was no clinical evidence). The report of the findings, illustrated by a photograph similar to this one, was sent to a medical journal for publication as an instance of indigenous Burkitt's lymphoma in Europe: the paper was accepted, and the mistake was recognized only when the proofs were sent in error to a pathologist along with the pulls of some illustrations of his own. *Haematoxylin–eosin.* × 225.

ventricle. There was no necropsy. The histological picture in a well-fixed biopsy specimen from the mandibular tumour and in a cervical lymph node was interpreted as typical of Burkitt's tumour at the time of the original review of the sections (1966): a recent further review does not confirm that diagnosis, for, although the characteristic—but not pathognomonic—'starry sky' appearance is present, the tumour cells themselves appear to be lymphocytes with a compact, uniformly round nucleus, no pyroninophilia of the scanty cytoplasm and no cytoplasmic vacuolation (Figs 9.244A and 9.224B). The tumour could be regarded as an atypical variant

of Burkitt's lymphoma but certainly should not be cited as a classic example.

A more recent case is remarkable because the patient developed Burkitt's lymphoma 2 years after infectious mononucleosis. She is a Scandinavian girl who was found to have infectious mononucleosis at the age of 12 years: the blood picture was characteristic, the Paul–Bunnell reaction was strongly positive and there was a high titre of antibodies against the Epstein–Barr virus. Two years later she was found to have a small tumour in the alveolar process of one maxilla and another in one breast. Both tumours were excised locally: the histological picture was in every respect typical of Burkitt's tumour. Imprint preparations of the mammary tumour were indistinguishable from those in classic cases of the disease (imprints of the maxillary lesion were not available). No virological studies were attempted. The condition has not recurred over a period of almost 4 years since the diagnosis was

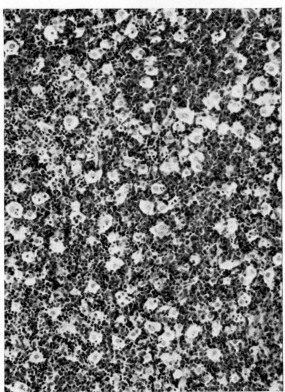

Fig. 9.244A. Well-differentiated lymphocytic lymphoma simulating Burkitt's lymphoma by reason of the profuse scattering of large, solitary macrophages among the tumour cells. Many of the macrophages contain cell debris (Flemming's 'stainable bodies'—see Fig. 9.4, page 513). Compare with Figs 9.241A and 9.241B. See also Fig. 9.244B. *Haematoxylin–eosin.* × 160.

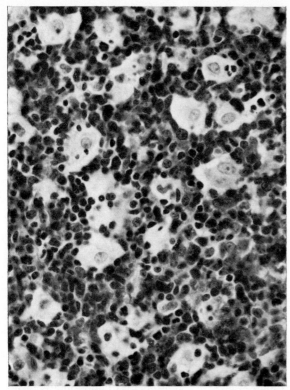

Fig. 9.244B. Higher magnification of part of the field of Fig. 9.244A. Compare the appearance of the tumour cells with that of the tumour cells in Burkitt's lymphoma (Fig. 9.241B). *Haematoxylin–eosin.* × 400.

made; a course of chemotherapy was given as soon as the condition was recognized (about 6 weeks after the surgical treatment). The patient has never travelled outside Scandinavia and the British Isles.[1517]

In common with instances—or supposed instances—of Burkitt's lymphoma occurring in other regions where the disease is not endemic,[1476] all such cases in Britain need to be considered most carefully before acceptance of the diagnosis.

Follicular Lymphoma[1518]

There are differences of opinion about the existence of follicular lymphoma as an entity. In the Rappaport classification of the lymphomas (Table 9.5, page 778)[1262] it is indicated that any cytological type of lymphoma may occur with either a nodular (follicular) pattern or a diffuse (non-follicular) pattern; a follicular lymphoma was not recognized as an entity. In the Lukes–Collins classification (Table 9.6, page 779)[1198] the 'follicular' and 'follicular and diffuse' varieties of lymphomas of follicular centre cells would seem to include tumours that were previously classed by pathologists under the name follicular lymphoma. In the Kiel classification (Table 9.7, page 780)[1264] the follicular lymphomas are included among the lymphomas of germinal centre cells ('centroblastic/centrocytic lymphoma').

For the present it seems still practical to consider follicular lymphoma separately, if only because there are lymphomas of a follicular pattern that have clinical and pathological features in common, and that are sufficiently distinctive to warrant particular consideration.

Synonyms

The first descriptions of follicular lymphoma are usually said to have been by Brill, Baehr and Rosenthal, of the Mount Sinai Hospital in New York, in 1925,[1519] and by Douglas Symmers, of Bellevue Hospital, also in New York, whose independent observations were published in 1927.[1520, 1521] The condition has been known as macrofollicular lymphoma,[1522] follicular lymphoblastoma,[1523] giant follicular lymphadenopathy,[1520] lymphoid follicular reticulosis[1295] and Brill–Symmers disease.[1524] The eponymous term had the double disadvantage of denying the accolade of eponymity to Dr Brill's associates, Baehr and Rosenthal, and of conferring it on Douglas Symmers, who thought this inappropriate,[1525] particularly as his original publication did not clearly distinguish what was to become known as follicular lymphoma from some other forms of follicular lymphadenopathy. Other terms that have been used include Brill's disease[1526] (which is also the name that was used for the mild endemic form of typhus fever that formerly occurred among immigrants in New York—see page 631), giant follicle hyperplasia (which is applied also to a non-neoplastic condition—see page 554), giant follicular hypertrophy[1520] and giant follicular lymphoma.

There are references in the literature well before the 1920s to cases of lymphadenopathy and splenomegaly that in all probability were instances of follicular lymphoma. This admittedly somewhat equivocal term seems as good as any of the others that have been used to describe the disease under discussion, and better than most.

Aetiology

Follicular lymphoma may occur at any age and in both sexes, but it is rather more frequent in women.

Many of the patients are in their 5th or 6th decade at the time of diagnosis. No predisposing causes and no causative factors have been recognized.

Clinical Aspects

Typically, there is a history that enlargement of lymph nodes has been present for many years, or—less often—has come and gone over such a period. Rarely, the first symptoms date from childhood, with a history of recurrent 'glands' that seem to have caused no particular concern to patient, family or doctors. Sometimes there is a history of repeated biopsy of recurrently enlarging nodes, usually in one region. In a proportion of cases the lymphadenopathy is found during a laparotomy, which usually has been undertaken because of some unrelated disease.

The most striking clinical finding is ordinarily the enlargement of the nodes. In the initial stages a single superficial group—most frequently in the groin or in the neck—is affected. Eventually the lymphadenopathy becomes generalized. It is characteristic that nodes tend to be affected that are involved only infrequently by other lymphomas, although they are regularly enlarged in some infections, including the secondary stage of syphilis (see page 613) and rubella (see page 643). These include the retroauricular and occipital nodes, superficial parotid nodes, and supratrochlear and popliteal nodes. Lymphomatous infiltration of the tissue round affected nodes is present in some cases and may be particularly extensive in the mesenteries and retroperitoneal tissue. Enlarged nodes may compress veins, leading to oedema of the limbs and effusion into the serous cavities; the compressed veins may become obliterated by thrombosis.

The fauciopharyngeal lymphoid tissue (particularly the palatine tonsils) may be involved. Infiltration of the skin and subcutaneous tissue and of the conjunctivae and orbits may occur; tumour in the orbital tissue may cause unilateral or bilateral exophthalmos. The liver, lungs, testes and gastric and intestinal mucosa may be conspicuously affected.

Splenomegaly is often present but is seldom of marked degree (see below). Involvement of bone marrow is noted below.

Any of these organs or tissues may be the site of the presenting manifestation. In contrast to other lymphomas, involvement of structures other than lymph nodes and the spleen is usually as well controlled by treatment as the disease in these lymphoreticular organs themselves.

Morbid Anatomy

Lymph Nodes.—Affected lymph nodes generally remain discrete, although in the later stages they may become closely adherent to their neighbours as the tumour becomes invasive and penetrates their capsule. They are smaller than in Hodgkin's disease and less hard than in all but the lymphocytic predominance type of the latter. Their cut surface often has a definite follicular pattern, although this is less evident than in the spleen. The macroscopically visible follicles are up to a millimetre or two in diameter and somewhat whiter and firmer than the surrounding tissue.

Spleen.—The spleen is seldom free from involvement. Its weight is commonly about 350 g and rarely exceeds 500 g, although exceptional specimens weigh several kilograms and considerably surpass the size of the largest spleens from cases of Hodgkin's disease. Splenomegaly of considerable degree may be the presenting manifestation (Figs 9.245A and 9.245B), and in some of these cases no lesions are found elsewhere.[1527] Follicular lymphoma is probably the least rare primary lymphoma of the spleen. Next in frequency is the primary lymphocytic lymphoma, which is sometimes known as the Josselin de Jong lymphoma of the spleen;[1528] this also is a nodular lesion, and it is readily confused with follicular lymphoma macroscopically, although the two tumours are said to be cytologically distinct.[1529]

As in cases of splenomegaly due to other diseases, anaemia, leucopenia and thrombocytopenia may develop as an accompaniment of follicular lymphoma of the spleen (see page 724).

Bone Marrow.—Extensive involvement of the bone marrow is an occasional finding, soft, pinkish tissue taking the place of some proportion of the fatty marrow in the long bones, the appearances macroscopically being those of extended haemopoietic activity or reminiscent of leukaemic marrow (see below).

Histology

The follicle-like structures consist of cells that in most cases are of uniform types, although differing within limits from case to case (see below). The aggregates of cells may be distinct (Fig. 9.246) or

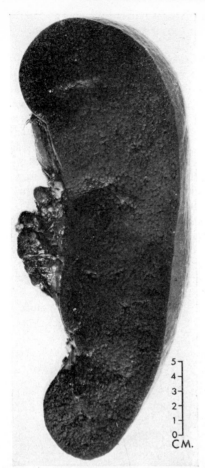

Fig. 9.245A.§ The spleen in a case of follicular lymphoma. Splenomegaly was the presenting manifestation in this case; there was no other clinical abnormality at that time. Splenectomy was performed. Enlargement of abdominal lymph nodes was observed during the operation, and some are seen in the hilum of the spleen in the photograph. The spleen weighed 3500 g. See also Fig. 9.245B, which shows the cut surface of the organ in detail.

means always demonstrable: when present it has some value in drawing attention to the follicular pattern and its probable significance (Figs 9.251 and 9.252).

The follicles are commonly outlined by a fine, capsule-like rim of reticulin fibres. These are probably pre-existing fibres that have been displaced and approximated as the cellular focus has expanded. The contour of the follicles is of limited significance in determining the degree of malignancy. Well-defined follicles are likelier to be a feature of the less malignant examples; coalescent foci, with breaching or loss of the reticulin rim, indicate a more invasive growth, and they are often composed of larger, paler, less differentiated cells. A more important topographical criterion of malignancy is invasion of the tissues round affected nodes (Fig. 9.253).

Tumour Cells.—Most of these tumours consist of small cells with cloven nucleus and a relatively small amount of cytoplasm (Figs 9.254 to 9.256), if cytoplasm is seen at all in the sections. Among the small cells there is a variable proportion of larger cells with a paler, ovoid or round nucleus containing two, and often more, moderately large nucleoli; in addition, there are sometimes occasional macrophages. The small cells are the small follicular centre cells with

ill-defined (Fig. 9.247); they may be round and of uniform size, or—less often—they may vary greatly in shape and in size. They are usually distributed fairly uniformly throughout the affected organ or tissue, replacing the normal lymphoid structure completely (Fig. 9.248); the intervening tissue consists in most cases of cells of the same characteristics as those forming the aggregates, although often compressed between the latter (Fig. 9.249).

Sometimes a narrow, crescentic slit demarcates part of the periphery of the tumour follicles. This appearance is evidently an artefact, occurring during histological processing, particularly when fixation has been inadequate (Fig. 9.250), and it is by no

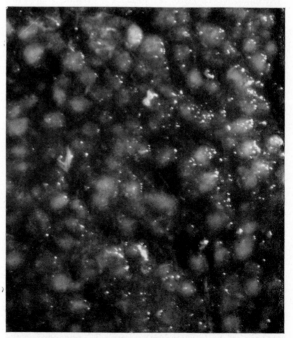

Fig. 9.245B.§ Cut surface of the spleen in Fig. 9.245A, magnified four times to show the tumour follicles.

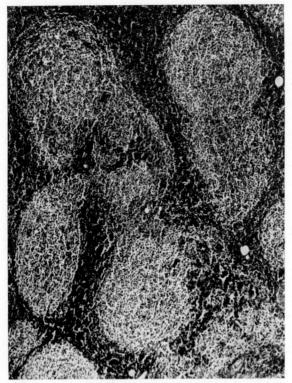

Fig. 9.246. Follicular lymphoma of a lymph node. In this instance the follicle-like collections of tumour cells are clearly seen against the background of small lymphocytes. The uniform cytology of the 'follicles' is evident, even at this magnification. *Haematoxylin–eosin.* × 70.

cloven nucleus of the Lukes–Collins classification of lymphomas (Table 9.6, page 779) and the centro-cytes of the Kiel classification (Table 9.7, page 780); the larger cells (Fig. 9.257) are the large follicular centre cell with cloven nucleus and the centroblast of these classifications respectively. In general, the larger the proportion of the larger, paler cells, the worse the prognosis.

Eventually, anaplastic transformation leads to an overwhelming predominance of the larger cells (see below). This is the finding that is considered to be prognostically of most significance.[1271] The lack of a follicular pattern, which has been considered from the results of some studies to be prognostically grave,[1530] is said by others to be without serious import, provided the cytological composition of the diffuse tumour is characterized by predominance of the small cells, as in the follicular tumours.[1271]

In a series of 540 cases of lymphomas with the cytological constitution referred to above as charac-teristic of follicular lymphoma, 77 per cent were found to have a follicular pattern, 20 per cent a pattern that was partly follicular and partly diffuse, and 3 per cent a wholly diffuse pattern.[1271]

Transitions.—The development of Hodgkin's disease has been reported as a complication of follicluar lymphoma.[1521] This must be a very rare transition, if indeed its occurrence can be confirmed. The few cases that have been shown to me as possible examples have all seemed rather to be cases of the nodular sclerosis type of Hodgkin's disease that, in an earlier biopsy specimen, had shown relatively little fibrosis and cellular pleomorphism, a diagnosis of follicular lymphoma being made through mis-interpretation.

The eventual development of a less differentiated histological picture and the accompanying onset of a rapidly progressive phase of the illness, leading to death, is not so much a transition in the sense of a change in the type of tumour as an anaplastic trans-formation to a more malignant variety of the same tumour. This transformation is manifested histo-

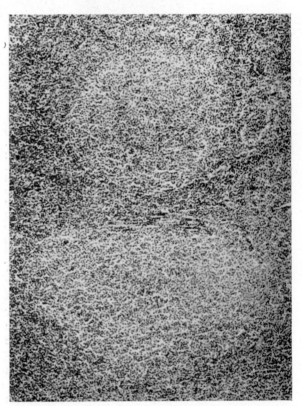

Fig. 9.247. Follicular lymphoma of a lymph node. In this field the two follicle-like aggregates are not very readily distinguished from the background, and the diagnosis could be overlooked. Compare with Fig. 9.246. *Haematoxylin–eosin.* × 75.

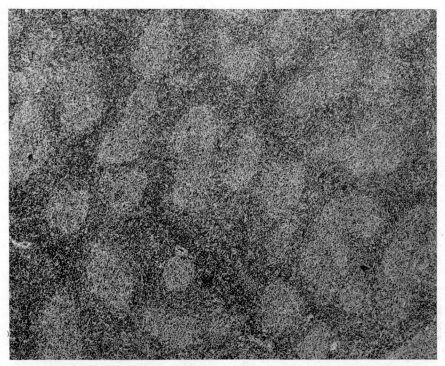

Fig. 9.248.§ Follicular lymphoma of a lymph node. *Haematoxylin–eosin.* × 35.

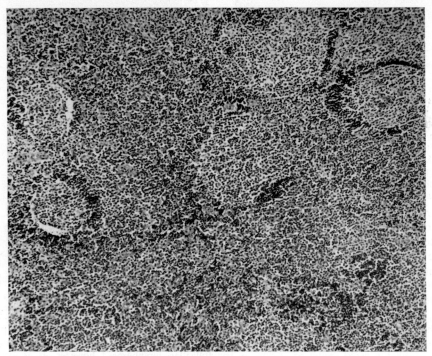

Fig. 9.249. Follicular lymphoma of a lymph node. Some of the tumour follicles are outlined by more darkly stained zones of normal small lymphocytes. Most of the normal structure has been replaced by tumour cells. In places the follicular arrangement of the tumour is no longer evident: the loss of regular follicle-like appearances is usually a feature of the more rapidly progressive tumours, and its observation in a biopsy specimen from a tumour that previously has had a well developed follicle-like structure is likely to indicate an increase in the malignancy of the disease. *Haematoxylin–eosin.* × 85.

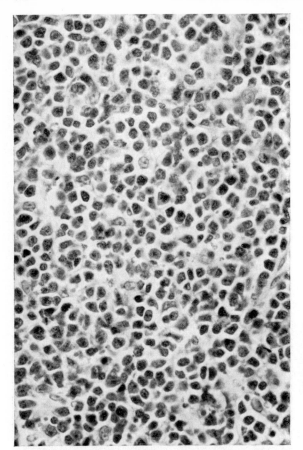

Fig. 9.254. Follicular lymphoma composed of small cells with cloven nucleus. The cells are irregular in shape and contrast notably with the rounded outline of the cells of lymphocytic lymphomas (see Figs 9.228 to 9.230, pages 822 and 823). See also Figs 9.255 to 9.257. *Haematoxylin–eosin.* × 400.

lymphocytic leukaemia and follicular lymphoma accompanied by lymphocytosis, particularly in patients aged under 40 years. But usually the presence of the abnormal cells in blood or marrow films, recognizable by their notched nucleus, readily identifies the condition as the peculiar lymphocytosis of follicular lymphoma.

Nature and Course

Follicular lymphoma, once regarded as a manifestation of hyperplasia or as an unusual inflammatory reaction, is now recognized to be a neoplastic disease of multicentric origin. Once its neoplastic nature was accepted there remained a debate whether it is, at least in a proportion of cases, a benign form of neoplasia, although with an unusually high liability to become malignant, or whether it is

a malignant tumour from its outset. As an unequivocally sarcomatous phase is likely to be the eventual outcome in every case, unless the natural course of the disease can be interrupted successfully by treatment,[1533] it is more of theoretical interest than of practical importance to resolve this question. Until the importance of accurately distinguishing between follicular lymphoma and simple forms of follicular hyperplasia was generally appreciated, the dangers—particularly the high mortality of the untreated disease—were underestimated because of the number of cases of follicular hyperplasia that were misdiagnosed as lymphomatous.

Diagnosis

The diagnosis of follicular lymphoma is exclusively histological. Sometimes it is difficult, and even virtually impossible, to be sure whether a given

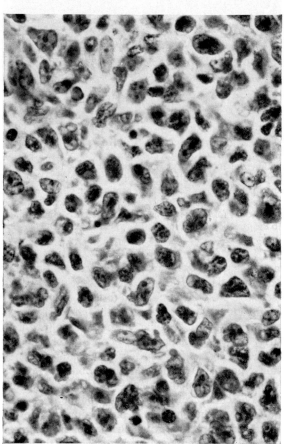

Fig. 9.255. Follicular lymphoma composed of small and large cells with cloven nucleus. The irregularity of the outline of the nucleus and cytoplasm of the cells is evident (see also Fig. 9.254). *Haematoxylin–eosin.* × 630.

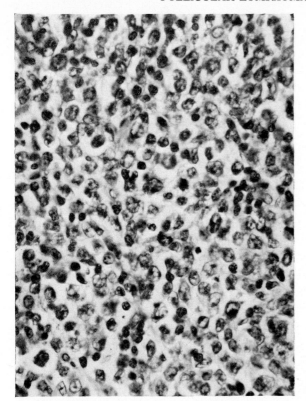

Fig. 9.256. Follicular lymphoma composed of small and large cells with cloven nucleus, but with a substantial proportion of undifferentiated cells with clear, round nucleus. The development of the undifferentiated element was accompanied by rapidly progressive, invasive growth of the tumour, which in earlier biopsy specimens had been composed predominantly of small cells with cloven nucleus (as in Fig. 9.254). *Haematoxylin–eosin.* ×400.

biopsy specimen shows hyperplasia or a follicular lymphoma: this is particularly so if follicles of uniform cytological composition, suggesting the latter diagnosis, are associated with the presence of lymphoid follicles that show the picture of simple follicular hyperplasia ('reactive follicular hyperplasia'—see page 553). The topographical position of the two forms of follicle in a node is not a reliable guide to their identity. Generally, the correct diagnosis can be made without difficulty when all the follicles or follicle-like structures have the same appearance: in particular, the scattering of solitary macrophages that contain Flemming's 'stainable bodies' (see page 512) is a constant characteristic of simple follicular hyperplasia and its presence throughout a uniformly patterned biopsy specimen in a case of follicular lymphadenopathy distinguishes the condition from follicular lymphoma. Similarly, the great size and the bizarre shape of the

follicles of giant follicle hyperplasia (see page 554) should prevent confusion of this infrequent condition with follicular lymphoma, especially as—like simple follicular hyperplasia—it also is characterized by a uniform scattering of macrophages. Diagnostic unanimity in distinguishing between hyperplastic and lymphomatous follicles cannot be expected,[1534] but with care and experience, and clinical consultation, a high degree of accuracy can be achieved.

Other Diagnostic Problems.—Histological appearances that at first sight seem indistinguishable from those typical of follicular lymphoma may be found in apparently localized lesions—for instance, replacing the lymphoid structure of a tonsil, or of a solitary enlarged lymph node, or in a major salivary gland, particularly a parotid gland (see page 966). Each such case must be considered individually. In particular, the appearances of the cells must be

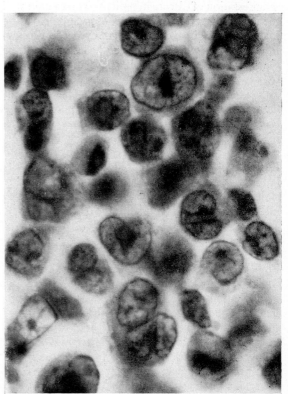

Fig. 9.257. Follicular lymphoma. Large cells with cloven nucleus. The nuclear cleft is much easier to see during microscopy, when the fine focusing adjustment makes it possible to examine each cell in the planes best suited to show this characteristic. However, in this photograph the cleft can be made out, more or less easily, in many of the cells. *Haematoxylin–eosin.* ×1500.

examined in detail: if they lack the characteristics, particularly the nuclear characteristics, that are a feature of follicular lymphomas (see above) and more closely resemble typical small or large lymphocytes, or even immunoblasts (transformed lymphocytes), it is possible that the lesion is an unusual hyperplastic reaction or a neoplasm other than a follicular lymphoma in the narrow sense.

Lymphoid tissue with a follicle-like structure may occur in polypoid form in the rectum or as an infiltrate in the skin, constituting a variety of benign lymphoid polyp of the rectum (see page 1147) or of the lymphomas and pseudolymphomas of the skin (see Chapter 39, Volume 5).

The relation of these strictly local lesions to follicular lymphoma is obscure. The latter may present with any of these manifestations, only later becoming generalized. Sometimes the interval between the development of the localized lesion and ultimate dissemination is many months or even years. In contrast, a localized lesion may be the only manifestation of disease in patients who remain well throughout a period of regular observation covering many years. This seems to be true even of a proportion of cases in which the cells of the lesion are of the type associated with true follicular lymphomas.

Follicle-Like Inflammatory Lesions.—The only inflammatory disease affecting the lymphoid tissues that produces follicle-like lesions that might be mistaken for the lesions of follicular lymphoma is syphilis in the secondary stage (see page 613 and Fig. 9.85).[1535] The epithelioid cell clusters of the latter may have a core of rather small, more darkly staining histiocytes, the picture then being liable to misinterpretation as lymphomatous.

Prognosis

Follicular lymphoma, even when extensive, responds well to radiotherapy and to comparatively low doses of alkylating agents. Its prognosis is much better than that of other lymphomas. The long duration of widespread lymphadenopathy, without other symptoms or signs of illness, and the long remissions that follow successive relapses and further courses of treatment distinguish follicular lymphoma from other lymphomas. Eventually, and often quite suddenly, the disease undergoes a change in character, frank malignancy supervening and leading to death, commonly within about 3 months. The terminal condition is usually an anaplastic sarcomatous transformation or, rather less frequently, the development of an acute leukaemia.[1518] Death

results from effects of the tumours on other structures or from cachexia or infection.

Malabsorption Syndromes and Primary Intestinal Lymphomas

There are three well-defined types of association of a malabsorption syndrome with a malignant intestinal lymphoma. The first, and outside the Middle East the commonest, is represented by the development in the intestine of a solitary lymphoma or of multiple lymphomas as an occasional complication of idiopathic steatorrhoea and similar conditions. The second is the syndrome of the so-called 'Mediterranean lymphoma', which occurs mainly in the Middle East and is characterized by diffuse, widespread lymphomatous change, predominantly in the jejunum: this syndrome may have a peculiarly limited ethnic distribution. The third is the so-called alpha heavy chain disease, in which the occurrence of an immunoglobulin of class A (IgA) that lacks light polypeptide chains is associated with a clinicopathological syndrome that, in the commonest variety of the disease, is identical with the syndrome of the 'Mediterranean lymphoma'.

Solitary and Multiple Intestinal Lymphomas Complicating Idiopathic Steatorrhoea and Similar Malabsorption Syndromes

This type of association of intestinal lymphomas with malabsorption syndromes has no particular geographical distribution. It occurs throughout the world. In the Middle East it is found among Arabs and Jews, and affects the latter irrespective of whether they are of Mediterranean (including North African) stock or of European stock (see 'Mediterranean lymphoma', below).

The association of idiopathic steatorrhoea with an increased liability to the development of a primary intestinal lymphoma has been recognized for many years.[1536] At first the tumour was thought to be the primary condition, causing obstruction of the lymphatic flow,[1536] particularly when there is massive involvement of the mesenteric lymph nodes by the growth.[1537] The present view is that idiopathic steatorrhoea and related diseases (such as gluten-sensitive enteropathy—see page 1084) predispose to the development of the lymphoma.[1538-1540] The tumours develop usually after an interval of several years following the onset of symptoms of malabsorption: in a series of 14 cases the average interval was 21 years,[1539] but in some instances the interval is much less and may be no more than a few months or even weeks.

The tumours arise most frequently in the small intestine and usually,[1539] but not always,[1429] in parts of the bowel affected by the pathological change of which malabsorption is the effect. In a small proportion of cases the tumour arises outside the bowel—for instance, in mesenteric lymph nodes. The intestinal tumours are often multiple; they rarely arise in parts other than the jejunum and the proximal part of the ileum.[1302] In from half to two thirds of the reported cases the tumours have been classified as 'reticulum cell sarcomas', which now would probably be regarded as immunoblastic lymphomas (see page 849). Most of the rest have been described as examples of Hodgkin's disease, with a few instances of 'lymphosarcoma' (lympho-cytic lymphoma) and of pleomorphic lymphomas. It has been pointed out[1541] that the relative propor-tions of the various types of tumour that may develop as a complication of a malabsorption syndrome correspond quite closely to the relative proportions of the types of lymphoma that arise in the ali-mentary tract in the absence of malabsorption:[1542] in particular, the predominance of 'reticulum cell sarcomas' is peculiar to the gastrointestinal tract. It is evident that idiopathic steatorrhoea and related conditions predispose to intestinal lymphomas of the types that arise selectively in the intestine in the absence of these predisposing factors. The frequency of this complication has been recorded as 7 among 70 patients[1543] and 14 among 202 patients,[1539] a range of 7 to 10 per cent.

Pathogenesis.—The pathogenesis of lymphomas that occur as a complication of steatorrhoea is not known. The possibility that the intestinal lesion that results in malabsorption has an autoimmune or other immunological basis—there is commonly a deficiency in the production of immunoglobulins, particularly IgA[1544]—and the long period between the clinical onset of the malabsorption syndrome and the development of the tumour suggest that the occurrence of the latter is related to protracted abnormal stimulation of cells concerned in the immunological responses.

Malabsorption is a common manifestation in patients with the so-called Mediterranean lymphoma (see below).

'Mediterranean Lymphoma'

The condition that has become known, inaccurately, as Mediterranean lymphoma, or Middle Eastern lymphoma, is a form of intestinal lymphoma in which there is diffuse infiltration of the mucous membrane of the jejunum, usually with extension into the duodenum, which may be involved as far upward as the descending part, and into a variable extent of the ileum. The regional lymph nodes are involved also. In contrast to the intestinal lymph-omas referred to opposite and those occurring as a complication of idiopathic steatorrhoea (see above), the so-called Mediterranean lymphoma involves the entire affected length of bowel and there are no interposed areas free from the neoplastic change.

Aetiology.—The disease occurs mainly in young adults and particularly in men. It was first described in 1965, in Israel.[1545] All the patients in the original accounts were Arabs or Jews, and the latter were all of at least second generation Middle Eastern or North African stock; Jews of European origin were unaffected. Later series confirmed this pattern of ethnic predisposition, although very occasionally the disease has been seen in a Jew whose family came to the Middle East from Europe.[1546] Most cases have continued to be observed in the Middle East, but by no means all occur in countries bordering the Mediterranean, and the name 'Mediterranean lymphoma' is for this reason inappropriate. Many of the patients in all countries where the disease has been recognized are from rural areas and belong to economically deprived communities. The disease has been recognized in Iran,[1547] Iraq[1548] and Saudi Arabia,[1549] and possibly in other parts of the world (Pakistan,[1550] Ireland[1551] and South Africa[1552]). It is not certain that all these cases have been identical with the classic cases of the so-called Mediterranean lymphoma; some may well have been instances of alpha heavy chain disease, which differs from 'Mediterranean lymphoma' only in the presence of the abnormal immunoglobulin in the blood and elsewhere (see page 848), and this has not been looked for in every case.

The disease has been seen in Britain in two Jewish siblings who had emigrated from North Africa to Britain in 1966, 6 years before their symptoms developed.[1553] The patients were identical twins, aged 32 years. Another patient whose 'Mediter-ranean lymphoma' was diagnosed in Britain is Maltese and came to this country shortly before his symptoms began.[1553] There was no qualitative abnormality of the plasma proteins in any of these three cases.

'Mediterranean lymphoma' is probably the commonest of all forms of lymphoma in those countries in which it is prevalent, but only among people who belong to the ethnic groups with a liability to the disease (see above).

Clinical Picture.—The clinical onset is often acute, with diarrhoea and abdominal pain. Steatorrhoea and a malabsorption syndrome are constant features; typically, the latter does not include a significant deficiency of vitamin B_{12}, folic acid or iron, and anaemia is not often of notable severity. As the lymphomatous condition extends to the regional lymph nodes, and sometimes farther afield, the patient becomes severely emaciated. Death, usually from cachexia, occurs from 1 to 3 years after the onset of symptoms. Obstruction of the affected part of the bowel and intercurrent infection are occasional causes of death.

Histology.[1554]—It is important to note that the macroscopical appearances of the bowel and of the abdominal lymph nodes may be normal at laparotomy, although in many cases there is evident thickening and induration of the affected small intestine. If the diagnosis is suspected on clinical grounds it may be confirmed by peroral biopsy of the jejunal mucosa.[1547] The jejunal villi are reduced in number and are much shorter and wider than is normal. The surface epithelium is little, if at all, altered. The most characteristic feature is a heavy infiltration of the lamina propria and the adjoining part of the submucosa by plasma cells, with a variable number of lymphocytes and cells that are usually described as 'reticulum cells' (some appear to be histiocytes and others possibly are transformed lymphocytes). Eosinophils and neutrophils may be present. In earlier stages the cellular infiltrate is less abundant and less extensive, and it may be represented by no more than an equivocal increase in the proportion of plasma cells in the lamina propria.

The changes described above merge into those that are considered to indicate that the condition has become frankly lymphomatous, and the distinction between a non-neoplastic stage and the presence of lymphoma is only subjectively determinable in relation to these borderline specimens. The frankly lymphomatous cases are quite easily recognized, the important index being the presence of conspicuously numerous cells that are clearly abnormal. In some instances the predominant tumour cell is plasmacytoid, with an eccentrically placed nucleus and cytoplasm that is amphiphile in haematoxylin–eosin preparations and also pyroninophile. In other cases the majority of the tumour cells are lymphocytes

(Fig. 9.258), which may be small or, usually, large; sometimes the cells have the characteristics of the cells of 'immunoblastic lymphomas' (see page 849) (Fig. 9.259). The proportions of the different types of lymphoma have varied from series to series; the largest number of cases has been variously identified as 'reticulum cell sarcomas' or as 'lymphoblastic lymphosarcomas'.

If laparotomy is performed, or at necropsy, there is often lymphomatous involvement of the mesenteric and other abdominal lymph nodes. In the specimens that I have been shown the tumour in the nodes has been less varied in its cellular composition than the infiltrate in the wall of the bowel, and the appearances have corresponded to those of immunoblastic lymphomas or of plasmacytoid lymphomas

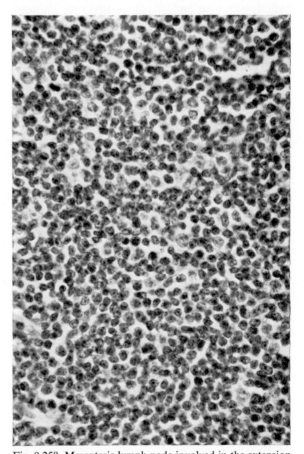

Fig. 9.258. Mesenteric lymph node involved in the extension of the tumour in a case of 'Mediterranean lymphoma'. The tumour in the jejunal mucosa and in the regional lymph nodes was a lymphocytic lymphoma, predominantly composed of well-differentiated lymphocytes of intermediate size, with a proportion of large lymphocytes and of plasmacytoid cells. See also Figs 9.259 and 9.260. *Haematoxylin–eosin.* ×400.

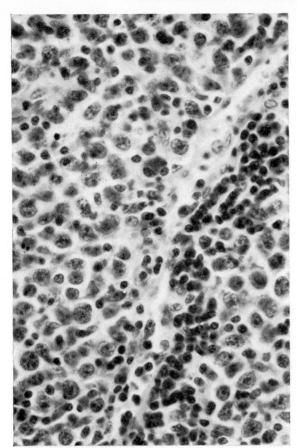

Fig. 9.259. Mesenteric lymph node in another case of 'Mediterranean lymphoma'. The tumour cells in this case are immunoblasts (compare with Fig. 9.258). Some non-neoplastic lymphocytes and plasma cells are included in the field. *Haematoxylin–eosin.* × 400.

according to the Lukes–Collins and Kiel classifications (Tables 9.6 and 9.7, pages 779 and 780).

In some cases multinucleate cells that closely resemble the Warthin–Finkeldey giant cells of measles (see page 641), although on average smaller than these, are present both in the lesions in the bowel and in the affected regional lymph nodes (Fig. 9.260). The significance of this observation is obscure, but inevitably it tends to support the view that there may be an infective—presumptively viral—element in the causation of the disease.

Those mesenteric nodes that are not totally involved by the tumour may show a proliferation of blood vessels and of 'immunoblasts' that is strikingly reminiscent of 'immunoblastic lymphadenopathy' (see page 703). In some cases there are small collections of lipophages in the nodes, mainly in the vicinity of the sinuses: this is a quite frequent finding in mesenteric nodes in cases of any type of malabsorption syndrome.

Relation to Alpha Heavy Chain Disease.—While 'Mediterranean lymphoma' is quite distinct from the syndrome of malabsorption and solitary or multiple discrete intestinal lymphomas (see page 844), its clinicopathological picture merges with that of alpha heavy chain disease (see below). The abnormal immunoglobulin is not present in all the cases of 'Mediterranean lymphoma' in which it is looked for, but it is present frequently enough to suggest that 'Mediterranean lymphoma' and alpha heavy chain disease should not be too dogmatically distinguished as separable entities.

Alpha Heavy Chain Disease (Alpha Chain Disease)

The clinical and histopathological pictures of 'alpha heavy chain disease' are essentially the same

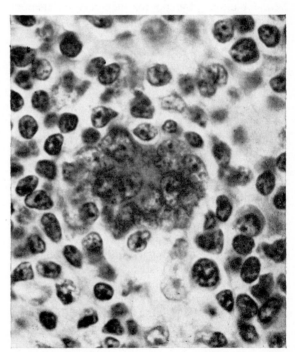

Fig. 9.260. Multinucleate cell in a mesenteric lymph node in a case of 'Mediterranean lymphoma'. The tumour in the jejunum was composed mainly of small and large lymphocytes, with a considerable proportion of plasmacytoid cells. No neoplastic tissue was identified in the regional lymph nodes. Giant cells such as the one in this field were scattered very sparsely both among the tumour cells in the wall of the bowel and in the mesenteric lymph nodes, in which there was also a considerable proportion of plasma cells. The appearances of the giant cells somewhat resemble those of the Warthin–Finkeldey cells in measles (see Figs 9.110A and 9.110B, page 642). *Haematoxylin–eosin.* × 1000.

as those of the non-neoplastic (prelymphomatous) stage of the so-called Mediterranean lymphoma (see above). The patients represent a wider range of ethnic groups than is liable to develop the latter. In addition to people of Mediterranean origin, alpha heavy chain disease has been recognized in patients from Pakistan,[1555] Cambodia,[1556] Argentina,[1557] Colombia,[1557] the United States of America,[1555] Finland,[1555] the Netherlands[1555] and possibly South Africa.[1552] A series of seven cases diagnosed in London comprised patients from as many different parts of the world—Libya, Italy, Greece, Turkey, Iran, Pakistan and Bangladesh.[1558]

Other Aetiological Factors.—Like the so-called Mediterranean lymphoma, alpha heavy chain disease occurs mainly in young adults. There appears to be a preponderance of males, but this may not be as marked as seemed to be the case among some of the earlier published series. The condition is more frequent among the poorer members of affected communities and is relatively rare in those who live in towns.

The Abnormal Protein.—Alpha heavy chain disease was recognized when a Syrian woman with the clinical picture of the 'Mediterranean lymphoma' was found to have an abnormal immunoglobulin of type A in the serum.[1559] The abnormal IgA is devoid of light polypeptide chains and its recognition depends entirely on immunochemical analysis of the serum proteins.[1555] The diagnosis may be beyond the resources of the general laboratory: the heavy chain immunoglobulin is not noticeable in the electrophoretic pattern in about half the cases; in the rest it presents as a broad band in the α_2 and β region. The protein is usually present in urine, but in such small amounts as to be difficult to demonstrate, even in concentrated specimens. Immunoelectrophoretic analysis may give negative results if polyvalent antiserum to normal human serum is used: the analysis must be made with the use of monospecific anti-IgA antiserum. Refined analytical studies are commonly essential if the heavy chain protein is to be demonstrated and identified.[1555]

Histopathology.[1560]—The histological picture of the bowel in alpha heavy chain disease differs from that in cases of 'Mediterranean lymphoma' in the paucity or absence of cells other than plasma cells and small lymphocytes. In particular, the cells described as 'reticulum cells' in the classic accounts of 'Mediterranean lymphoma' (possibly transformed lymphocytes—that is, 'immunoblasts') are very scarce or altogether lacking. Plasma cells account for 70 to 80 per cent of the cells in the lamina propria. They are believed to be the source of the abnormal immunoglobulin.[1557] The cellular infiltrate in the intestine is usually confined to the lamina propria of the mucosa, but—in contrast to 'Mediterranean lymphoma'—the whole length of the small bowel may be involved. Encroachment of the infiltrate into the submucosa is sometimes found. The stomach[1561] and rectum[1562] have been affected in single cases, as have bone marrow and nasopharyngeal lymphoid tissue.[1558] The mesenteric lymph nodes are commonly infiltrated by plasma cells (Fig. 9.261).

The development of a malignant lymphoma has been observed in the case of a patient whose illness was studied over a period of 5 years.[1563] The development of a malignant plasma cell tumour has also been reported.[1564]

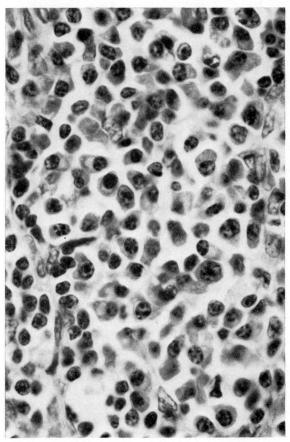

Fig. 9.261. Mesenteric lymph node in a case of alpha heavy chain disease. The node, like the lamina propria of the mucosa of the small intestine, was heavily infiltrated by plasma cells. Some of the cells are binucleate and some are much larger than the majority. *Haematoxylin–eosin.* × 750.

Variant Form.—Very rarely, the presence of alpha heavy chain disease has been accompanied by infiltration of the lungs and enlargement of mediastinal lymph nodes, without evidence of a malabsorption syndrome or of any intestinal involvement.[1565]

Prognosis.—The prognosis of alpha heavy chain disease may be significantly less grave than that of the 'Mediterranean lymphoma'.[1558] However, the discovery that cases of established 'Mediterranean lymphoma' may show the presence of the same abnormal immunoglobulin in the blood is an indication of the association and possible relationship of the two conditions; it also indicates that the prognosis of alpha heavy chain disease may depend on whether it undergoes transition to the lymphomatous state. This transition may be commoner among individuals of the ethnic groups that are predisposed to develop the 'Mediterranean lymphoma' (see page 845).

Complete clinical, immunological and histological recovery has been observed following treatment with prednisone, cyclophosphamide and antibiotics.[1566]

Other Types of 'Heavy Chain Disease'

Gamma Heavy Chain Disease (Gamma Chain Disease).—The first of the heavy chain diseases to be recognized was that in which the immunoglobulin lacking light polypeptide chains is an IgG (Franklin's disease).[1567] The patient had a malignant lymphomatosis. Several more cases of this association have been recognized, but the disease is very rare.[1568] The discovery of alpha heavy chain disease (see above)[1559] and, later, of mu heavy chain disease (see below)[1569] made it expedient that the original variety of this remarkable group of immunoglobulin anomalies be distinguished as gamma heavy chain disease.

Mu Heavy Chain Disease (Mu Chain Disease).— In mu heavy chain disease the immunoglobulin lacking light chains is an IgM. The disease is very rare. It has been associated with myelomatosis[1569] and with chronic lymphocytic leukaemia.[1570]

Immunoblastic Lymphomas (Including Most Tumours Formerly Named 'Reticulum Cell Sarcomas')

Although the reticulum cell is still defined as one of the elements of the reticuloendothelial system (see page 525), the cells that until recently have been regarded as pathological reticulum cells, particularly neoplastic reticulum cells, are now interpreted by various authorities as being in most instances of quite different nature.[1571] The cells that were thought to be neoplastic reticulum cells, and that gave their name to the 'reticulum cell sarcomas' (or reticulosarcomas, according to some*), are now identified as the neoplastic equivalent of transformed lymphocytes ('immunoblasts'—see page 522).[1571, 1572] Most of these tumour immunoblasts are considered to be derived from 'bursa-equivalent'-dependent cells (B cells), a small minority possibly being derived from thymus-dependent cells (T cells).[1198, 1571]

Predisposing Factors.—Although most immunoblastic lymphomas occur without any predisposing factor being apparent, there is a small proportion of cases in which some abnormal immunological state of long standing seems unquestionably to have aetiological significance. Among these disorders are the so-called 'benign lymphoepithelial lesion' of salivary glands (Sjögren's syndrome — see page 952),[1573] alpha heavy chain disease (see page 847)[1563] and 'Mediterranean lymphoma',[1554] immunosuppressive therapy for recipients of organ transplants,[1574] and congenital immunodeficiency states[1201] (see page 770). It is also said that the senescent immunological system may have an increased liability to this type of lymphomatous change.[1198]

Histology.—The main features of these tumours are noted in Table 9.6, footnote [¶] (page 779) and Table 9.7, footnote [***] (page 782). They are illustrated in Figs 9.262 to 9.268.

Necrosis and haemorrhage are less unusual in immunoblastic lymphomas, particularly the less well-differentiated ones (Fig. 9.269), than in other types of lymphoma. The tumours range from comparatively well differentiated growths of more or less uniform cytology (Figs 9.262 to 9.264) to less well-differentiated varieties (Figs 9.265 to 9.267). The cells are often cohesive and this may give them an epithelial appearance: it can be difficult to distinguish between such immunoblastic lymphomas and some anaplastic carcinomas, particularly of squamous origin, including the so-called 'lymphoepitheliomas' of the nasopharynx (see page 241).

* The name reticulosarcoma was proposed by C. Oberling (*Bull. Ass. franç. Cancer*, 1928, **17**, 259) as a generic term for all malignant neoplasms arising in the lymphoreticular organs and tissues. It came to be used in the narrower sense of a sarcoma of reticulum cells.

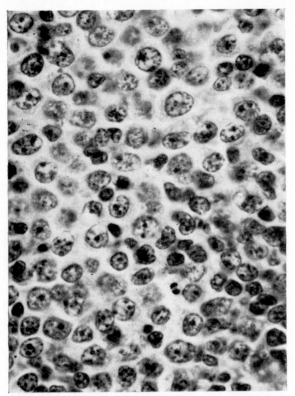

Fig. 9.262. Immunoblastic lymphoma (lymph node biopsy). The nuclei are large, rounded and pale, and contain one to several nucleoli. The cytoplasm of the tumour cells is indistinct, but in general the cells are cohesive. See also Figs 9.263 to 9.268. *Haematoxylin–eosin.* × 750.

Other difficulties in distinguishing between immunoblastic lymphomas and lymphomas of other types are mentioned in the footnotes to Table 9.7 (page 781).

Eosinophils may be present among the tumour cells. In exceptional cases they are very abundant (Fig. 9.268).

Differential Diagnosis.—In a series of 226 cases of lymphadenopathy in which the initial histological diagnosis was 'reticulum cell sarcoma', 165 are considered to have been cases of what now would be called immunoblastic lymphoma, 24 to have been cases of Hodgkin's disease, 8 to have been cases of lymphosarcoma, 23 to have been cases of metastatic tumour (most frequently carcinoma) and 6 to have been non-neoplastic diseases.[1575]

Course.—An immunoblastic lymphoma may arise in any part of the lymphoreticular system or, less frequently, in other organs (see page 820). Some-

times generalization throughout the lymphoreticular organs, particularly lymph nodes, is so rapid that it seems likely that the disease develops more or less simultaneously in multiple foci. In other cases it seems that the tumour spreads by stages from the initial site: in some of these instances it is possible to find seemingly clear evidence of metastasis, such as permeation of the subcapsular sinus of lymph nodes at a distance from the main foci of the disease (Fig. 9.270).

Acute leukaemia occurs as a very rare complication.[1576] It is probably more frequent among children.[1577]

Undifferentiated Lymphomas

By 'undifferentiated lymphoma' is meant a lymphoma composed of cells that cannot with reasonable certainty be identified as the neoplastic equivalent of accepted varieties of normal lymphoreticular cells. Whether a given tumour be regarded as an

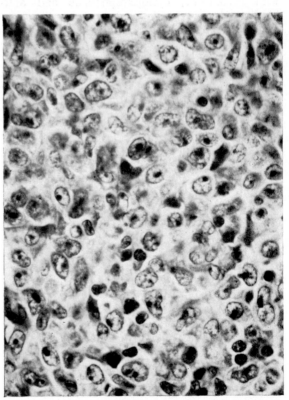

Fig. 9.263. Immunoblastic lymphoma (lymph node biopsy). This tumour is somewhat less well differentiated than that illustrated in Fig. 9.262, but the general features are similar and the cohesiveness of the cells is more evident. *Haematoxylin–eosin.* × 630.

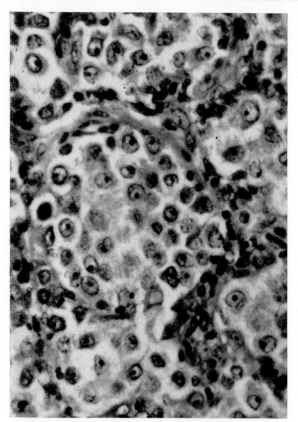

Fig. 9.264. Immunoblastic lymphoma (lymph node biopsy). In this unusual variant the tumour cells tend to be grouped in solid 'alveoli', although this pattern is found only in parts of any given example. The differential diagnosis must include consideration of the possibility that the tumour is a meta-static deposit of a melanoma or of an undifferentiated carcinoma or other tumour. *Haematoxylin–eosin.* × 400.

undifferentiated lymphoma in this sense or be identified with a named cell variety is commonly determined on subjective grounds that reflect the personal experience and inclination of the pathologist.

The category of undifferentiated lymphomas includes the pleomorphic anaplastic lymphomas (Fig. 9.271): among these is the tumour that formerly was often known as 'Hodgkin's sarcoma' (see page 809). The pleomorphic tumours include a wide range of histological pictures. Some of the growths are characterized by the presence of bizarre multi-nucleate giant cells, which may be very numerous or relatively sparse. Others include more or less extensive foci in which there is no division of the cytoplasm, the growth being in the form of a sym-plasma (syncytium), the nuclei scattered through-out a mass of cytoplasm that in some instances can

be followed without evident delimitation through field after field under the high powers of the microscope.

The distinction between the pleomorphic un-differentiated lymphomas and the histiocytic lymphoma (see below) is sometimes arbitrary.

Histiocytic Lymphoma

The histiocytic lymphoma is commonly regarded now as the only true reticulum cell sarcoma. While there continues to be so much other terminological confusion and contradiction in relation to the

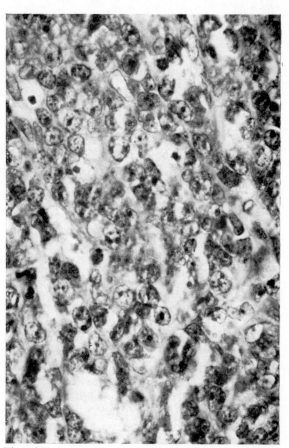

Fig. 9.265. Immunoblastic lymphoma (lymph node biopsy). This tumour is less well differentiated that those already illustrated (Figs 9.262 to 9.264). Although it is difficult to make out detail in the photograph, examination under the microscope showed that many of the tumour nuclei are contained in a continuous mass of cytoplasm (symplasma). Other tumour cells in this field are discrete. An occasional macrophage containing cell debris is present. The practical problem of distinguishing between a lymphoma with this structure and a histiocytic lymphoma is mentioned in the caption of Fig. 9.272 (page 855). *Haematoxylin–eosin.* × 630.

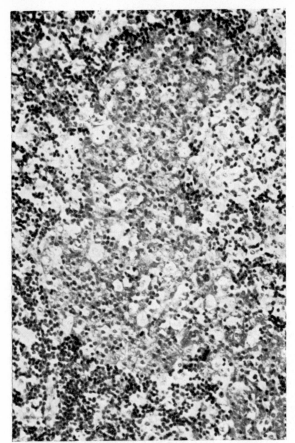

Fig. 9.266. Immunoblastic lymphoma (lymph node biopsy). This field shows a partly symplasmic collection of tumour cells infiltrating the pulp of the node. There is an admixture of lymphocytes and macrophages among the tumour cells. The surrounding lymphoid tissue includes small collections of histiocytes and a scattering of solitary immunoblasts that appear not to be neoplastic. *Haematoxylin–eosin.* × 190.

tumours arising in the lymphoreticular system it is of no particular moment to try to correct the apparent misconception that permits the equation of 'histio-cytic' with 'reticulum cell' as a term descriptive of a particular tumour: maybe it is advantageous to adopt 'histiocytic' in this context rather than per-petuate so compromised a term as 'reticulum cell sarcoma'. The occasionally used name 'histio-sarcoma' has no greater merit than the other terms.

Historical Note.—It was forecast in 1913 by James Ewing that tumours of reticulum cells would be discovered.[1578] The first detailed account of what were supposedly such tumours was given in 1930 by Roulet,[1579] under the name retothelial sarcoma (*Retothelsarkom*). For some 40 years 'reticulum cell sarcomas' were universally recognized as frequent,

readily identifiable, highly malignant tumours aris-ing in the organs of the lymphoreticular system itself or from its cells in other parts of the body. Then, quite suddenly, definition of the immunoblastic lymphoma (see above) led to acceptance of the view that for 40 years we have been wholly wrong in our concept of these tumours: a true 'reticulum cell sarcoma' proves—it seems—to be one of the rarest of all forms of cancer.

Identification.—The identification of reticulum cell tumours (Fig. 9.272) depends on the demonstration of cytochemical and immunological characteristics that are specific to their cells (Table 9.6, footnote [‡‡], page 780). Even when cells with these charac-teristics are found in a tumour they may not be cells of the tumour itself but normal reticulum cells or macrophages that have become incorporated in an immunoblastic or other lymphoma.[1571]

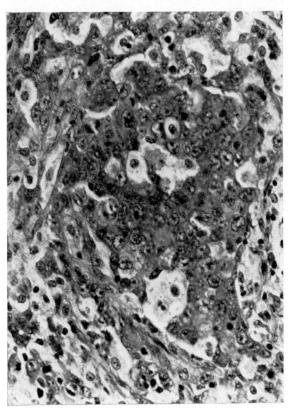

Fig. 9.267. Immunoblastic lymphoma (lymph node biopsy). Symplasmic mass of tumour cells ('syncytial lymphoma'). Mononuclear tumour cells are seen also, and there are some macrophages containing cell debris. Tumours with syncytial features are highly malignant and progress very rapidly. *Haematoxylin–eosin.* × 375.

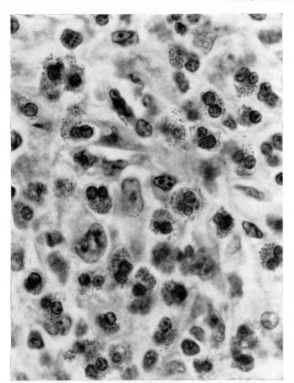

Fig. 9.268. Immunoblastic lymphoma (lymph node biopsy). Eosinophils are very numerous among the tumour cells in this instance. The explanation of this occasional observation is unknown. *Haematoxylin–eosin.* ×950.

Variants and Derivatives.—In exceptional cases, fibrosarcomatous differentiation may develop in parts of the tumour (Fig. 9.273). Monocytic leukaemia is another very rare manifestation (see Fig. 9.274).

Lymphomas of the Skin

Lymphomas may appear in the skin in the course of dissemination or multifocal development of any malignant lymphoma. More rarely, a lymphoma originates in the skin: the primary cutaneous lymphomas may be solitary or, oftener, multifocal lesions, and they may remain confined to the skin or be associated with the appearance of lesions in lymph nodes and elsewhere. The pathology of the cutaneous lesions is considered in Chapter 39. Some general aspects may be mentioned here.

Mycosis Fungoides[1580]

The most familiar lymphomatous disease of the skin is mycosis fungoides, which has been the subject of speculation and controversy since its first descrip-

tion, in 1806[1581] and 1832,[1582] by Jean Louis Alibert, of the Hôpital Saint-Louis, in Paris. Alibert, who saw only one patient with the disease, took the condition for a *pian* (that is, a tumorous or ulcerative state, usually tropical in origin, of which yaws is currently the most generally known example). He named two varieties of pian, ruboid and fungoid, the first being yaws (framboesia) and the second (*pian fungoïde* or *framboesia mycoïdes*) corresponding to

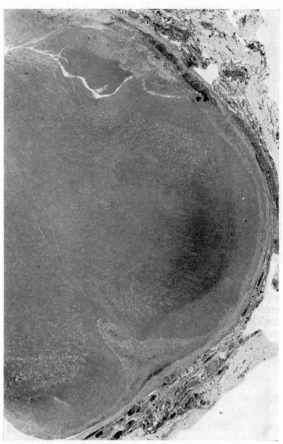

Fig. 9.269. There is almost total necrosis of this lymph node. The patient, a woman of 38 years, had noticed slowly increasing enlargement of cervical, axillary and inguinal lymph nodes for some months when a group in one axilla became suddenly painful and doubled in size within a few days. The biopsy showed the picture illustrated. A much smaller node was adherent to the capsule of the excised necrotic node: the small node was free from necrosis and showed extensive replacement of the normal structure by a well-differentiated immunoblastic lymphoma. The explanation of the massive necrosis was not apparent. However, the patient had been sailing a few days before the acute symptoms began: she had spent some time relaxing in the stern, keeping the tiller steady by bracing it in the armpit in which necrosis of the nodes later developed. See also Fig. 9.28 (page 553). *Haematoxylin–eosin.* ×6.

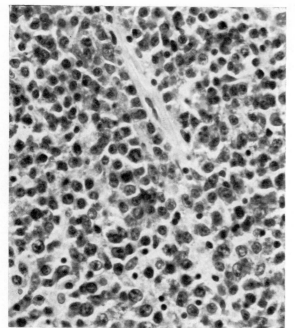

Fig. 9.274. Lymph node biopsy in a case of monocytic leukaemia. The illness presented with painful swelling of the gums, multiple small foci of cutaneous infiltration, and anaemia. There was only slight enlargement of the lymph nodes; this appeared to be of uniform degree throughout the body. The leukaemia was recognized on examination of the blood and bone marrow. The histological picture in the lymph node specimen could not be distinguished from that in cases of diffuse lymphomatous infiltration. *Haematoxylin-eosin.* × 350.

may be used as an adjunct to radiotherapy or electron therapy of the superficial lesions.[1585]

Relation to Other Cutaneous Lymphomas.—Identification of the predominant cell in the lesions of mycosis fungoides as a neoplastic thymus-dependent lymphocyte (T cell) links this condition with at least two other diseases of the skin, Sézary's syndrome and lymphomatoid papulosis, in both of which there is infiltration of the skin by similar cells. The three conditions have been grouped under the term *cutaneous T-cell lymphomas.*[1586]

Lymphomatoid papulosis is the name introduced in 1968[1587] for a condition characterized by the development, over a period of up to many years, of recurrent crops of dermal papules. Clinically and histologically the papules closely resemble the various forms of pityriasis lichenoides except that there is an admixture of atypical cells with a large hyperchromatic nucleus among the predominantly lymphocytic infiltrate in the dermis.[1588] It is ordinarily a benign disease, but generalized malignant

lymphoma developed after 8, 18 and 40 years in three cases among 60 collected from the literature of the period 1956 to 1973.[1589] Sézary's syndrome, in contrast, appears to carry a substantially greater risk of transformation into a frankly lymphomatous or leukaemic state (see below).

Sézary's Syndrome[1590]

Sézary and his colleagues, in 1938, described two cases of generalized erythrodermia in which distinctive large mononuclear cells were present in the blood and in the dermis.[1591, 1592] These cells—the

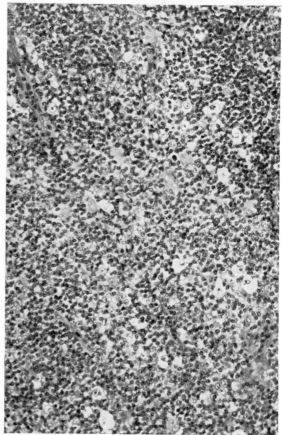

Fig. 9.275A. Lymph node biopsy in a case of mycosis fungoides in the infiltrative (plaque) stage. The node illustrated was in the neck and there were cutaneous lesions of the disease in the area that it drained. Other superficial lymph nodes were also enlarged. The normal structure has been replaced by lymphomatous tissue that consists in part of lymphocytes of intermediate size and in part of rather more pleomorphic tissue, such as that in the photograph, in which atypical reticulum cells are also present. An occasional Sternberg–Reed cell was found (see Fig. 9.275B). *Haematoxylin–eosin.* × 160.

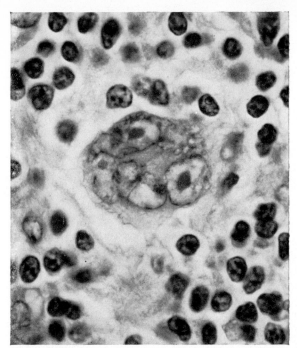

Fig. 9.275B. A Sternberg–Reed cell from the specimen illustrated in Fig. 9.275A. *Haematoxylin–eosin.* × 1000.

so-called Sézary cells, or Lutzner cells[1593]—have now been identified as thymus-dependent cells of a variety peculiar to the syndrome.[1594, 1595] Electron microscopy shows them to have a markedly convoluted nucleus, which has been described as cerebriform.[1593] In histological preparations, under the light microscope, Sézary cells have the appearances of mature lymphocytes, or they may be larger and of somewhat irregular cytoplasmic and nuclear outline. They are associated, both in the cutaneous lesions and in affected lymph nodes and other structures, with a variable proportion of small lymphocytes, plasma cells and histiocytes. In some cases histiocytes are numerous, solitary and rounded, with abundant, opaque, eosinophile cytoplasm (Fig. 9.276).

Nature.—Inconsistencies in defining the syndrome have led to differences of opinion about the nature of the condition. Those who require the association of generalized erythrodermia, lymphadenopathy and the presence of a leukaemic blood picture find the syndrome best regarded as malignant and interpret it as a leukaemic variant of mycosis fungoides.[1264] Those who exclude lymphadenopathy from the essential features of the syndrome find frank malignant change to be comparatively rare, although recognizing that any patient with the

syndrome may eventually develop a lymphoma.[1596] In fact, Sézary's syndrome is considered to account for a considerable proportion of cases of chronic lymphocytic leukaemia of T cell type.[1264]

Lymphadenopathy and Other Internal Lesions.—The changes in affected lymph nodes are mentioned above. Any superficial nodes may be involved, but it is often the inguinal and axillary groups that first attract attention. Early in the disease the changes may be those of a simple non-specific lymphadenitis. More or less well marked features of dermatopathic lymphadenitis soon appear (see page 687), as would

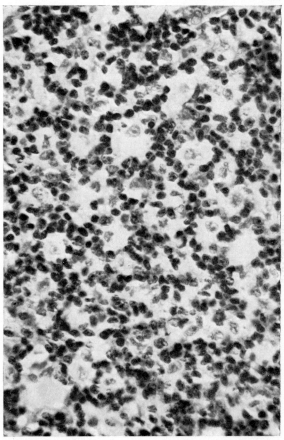

Fig. 9.276.§ Lymph node in a case of Sézary's syndrome in which histiocytes are unusually numerous among the lymphocytes. The peculiar features of the latter cannot be distinguished with the light microscope, although even at this magnification the variability in nuclear size, shape and chromatin content is evident. This photograph is included as much because it shows another example of a condition that may be confused histologically with immunoblastic lymphadenopathy (see Fig. 9.153, page 704), and even with Burkitt's lymphoma (see Figs 9.241A and 9.241B, page 832), as for its intrinsic interest. *Haematoxylin–eosin.* × 400.

be anticipated in view of the severity of the erythro-dermia. Once the characteristic involvement of the blood is established the picture of dermato-pathic lymphadenitis gives place to a total, or almost total, infiltration of the nodes by lymphocytes that include a notable and often predominant proportion of 'Sézary cells' (see above).

The same type of cellular infiltrate may be seen in other organs and tissues.[1597] It is of particular interest, however, that involvement of bone marrow has been found to be no more than slight.[1598]

Kaposi's Sarcoma

Kaposi's sarcoma is not a lymphoma and it is in no way related to the cutaneous lymphomas that have just been discussed. It is mentioned here because it is occasionally complicated by, or accompanied by, some form of malignant lymphoma (see page 713). Also, a peculiar lymphoma-like change has been observed to develop in lymph nodes in some cases: this is noted on page 713. The occurrence of these lymphomas and lymphoma-like conditions may confuse the diagnosis of the underlying condition.

'Malignant Histiocytosis' and Similar Diseases

There is a group of rare fatal diseases of the lympho-reticular system that are characterized by rapidly progressive and widespread proliferation of cells that seem still to be regarded as of reticuloendothelial origin—that is, cells that are believed to be neo-plastic forms of the mononuclear phagocytes. These diseases include Letterer–Siwe disease, 'histiocytic medullary reticulosis', 'hairy cell leukaemia' ('leuk-aemic reticuloendotheliosis') and some even rarer conditions.

Now that some order is appearing in our under-standing of Hodgkin's disease and the other lymph-omas that have been considered in the preceding pages of this chapter, it is to be hoped that the specialists will extend the work that has already started to clarify the still confused subject of the conditions that will be noted briefly here.

Letterer–Siwe Disease[1599, 1600]

This rare condition occurs typically in early child-hood, usually during the first two to three years of life.[1601] Congenital cases have been seen;[1602] exceptionally, it has affected siblings.[1603] A similar condition has been observed very rarely in adults.[1604] Its main features are generalized enlarge-ment of the lymph nodes and enlargement of the spleen and liver, with fever, anaemia (which is usually haemolytic—see page 473), leucopenia, purpuric skin lesions and destructive lesions of the lungs[1605] and, more characteristically, of bones. The pathological change underlying these manifes-tations is a remarkably extensive and cytologically uniform proliferation of cells that conventionally continue to be described as reticulum cells (and may indeed be such). These cells crowd out the normal cells of the lymph nodes (Figs 9.277A, 9.277B and 9.278), spleen and bone marrow and form aggregates in other tissues, such as the dermis. They may be found in the peripheral blood.[1606] The disease usually runs an acute or subacute course; rarely its progress is slower, extending over 4 to 5 years or longer. It was formerly believed to be always fatal, but in exceptional instances recovery has been reported.[1607] However, death may occur within even a few days of the clinical onset.

Adult Form.—A destructive disease of the lungs—sometimes known as Turiaf's disease[1608]—has been described as an adult form of Letterer–Siwe disease. It is one of the rarer causes of the appearances described as 'honeycomb lung' (see page 369, volume 1). Its relation to the disease in children and to the other conditions that are grouped with the latter under the term 'histiocytosis X' (see below) is uncertain.

'Histiocytosis X'

On clinical grounds,[1609] and later on clinical, radio-logical and pathological grounds,[1610, 1611] some authorities suggested that Letterer–Siwe disease could be regarded as the most rapidly progressive member of a triad of related diseases characterized by proliferation of histiocytes. The other members of the triad are Hand–Schüller–Christian disease (see page 763) and eosinophil granuloma of bone (see Chapter 37, Volume 5). The validity of this attempt to group the three diseases together is not universally accepted.[1612] The main grounds for the grouping are two—first, the occasional transition from solitary eosinophil granuloma of bone to the development in several or many bones of lesions that may assume the clinical and radiological charac-teristics usually associated with Hand–Schüller–Christian disease; and second, the similarity of the clinical features of Letterer–Siwe disease to those of the rapidly progressive form of eosinophil granulo-matosis of bone that occurs in young children.

The name 'histiocytosis X' was proposed for this triad[1610] and, being easily assimilable for clinical

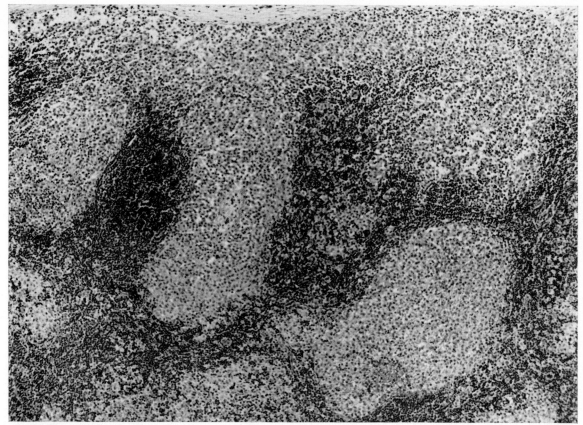

Fig. 9.277A. Lymph node in Letterer–Siwe disease. The subcapsular and trabecular sinuses are filled with pale cells (see Fig. 9.277B). These cells also infiltrate the adjoining pulp, and foci of similar cells have begun to form among the lymphocytes. *Haematoxylin–eosin*. × 90.

use, has persisted. Unfortunately, introduction of the similar term 'lymphogranulomatosis X'[1613] as a synonym for immunoblastic lymphadenopathy (see footnote on page 703) has promoted confusion between these wholly dissimilar, unrelated conditions.

Letterer–Siwe Disease as a Form of 'Malignant Histiocytosis'

Letterer–Siwe disease is sometimes described as a 'non-lipid histiocytosis' (or 'non-lipid reticuloendotheliosis'[1614]). In fact, a few of the proliferating cells may contain a small amount of neutral fat and cholesterol. The proportion of lipid-containing cells is much smaller than in the lesions of Hand–Schüller–Christian disease and in eosinophil granulomas of bone. If the cells that constitute the lesions of Letterer–Siwe disease are histiocytes rather than reticulum cells they show so little evidence of

histiocytic activity (phagocytosis) that the distinction is difficult to recognize.

Letterer–Siwe Disease as a Disease of 'Langerhans Histiocytes'.[1615]

—Studies with the electron microscope have shown that the cells that make up the lesions of Letterer–Siwe disease contain a stable crystal-like structure of constant size and characterized by transverse striation of constant periodicity.[1616] This structure is said to be similar to bodies in the cytoplasm of the Langerhans cells of the epidermis (the cells that are usually still known as melanocytes—see Chapter 39, Volume 5): this finding led to the hypothesis that Letterer–Siwe disease and the other diseases that form the triad of histiocytosis X are a manifestation of proliferation of the Langerhans cells, which some authorities now regard as specialized histiocytes.[1617] The distinctive cytoplasmic body—referred to as the 'X body',[1615] 'Langerhans cell granule',[1618] 'Langerhans organ-

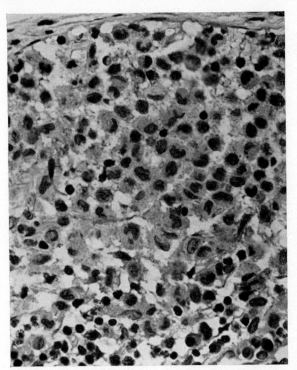

Fig. 9.277B. Higher magnification of part of the subcapsular sinus of the lymph node shown in Fig. 9.277A. 'Reticulum cells' (see text), some showing histiocytic metamorphosis, and eosinophils account for most of the proliferation and infiltration. See also Fig. 9.278. *Haematoxylin–eosin.* × 430.

elle',[1619] 'Langerhans granule'[1620] and 'Birbeck granule'[1621]—has been demonstrated in the cells of the lesions of classic Letterer–Siwe disease[1619] and of a localized eosinophil granuloma[1622] and in the specific pathological cells in the blood stream in a case of generalized histiocytosis,[1620] as well as in the lesions of 'pulmonary histiocytosis X' in an adult[1623] (it was in this last case that the peculiar cytoplasmic body was first observed in the cells of these diseases).

The significance of these findings in relation to the aetiology, pathogenesis and nosological status of Letterer–Siwe disease and the diseases that have been equated with it remains to be confirmed.

'Histiocytic Medullary Reticulosis'*

The condition that is still usually known by the name given it by Robb-Smith, in 1938,[1295] histio-

---

* The topographical designation 'medullary' in this context relates to the presence of the abnormal histiocytes in the pulp (medulla) of the lymph nodes in accordance with the Robb-Smith method of classifying the lymphadenopathies (Robb-Smith, A. H. T., *J. Path. Bact.*, 1938, **47**, 457). It is

cytic medullary reticulosis, is a comparatively rare, rapidly fatal disease that is characterized by fever, considerable splenomegaly, moderate enlargement of lymph nodes, enlargement of the liver and conspicuous haematological disturbances.[1624] Rapidly progressive anaemia, leucopenia and thrombocytopenia result from phagocytosis of blood cells[1625] by abnormal histiocytes that accumulate in large numbers in the lymphoreticular tissues, including the sinuses and pulp of the lymph nodes (Fig. 9.279) and the spleen, liver and bone

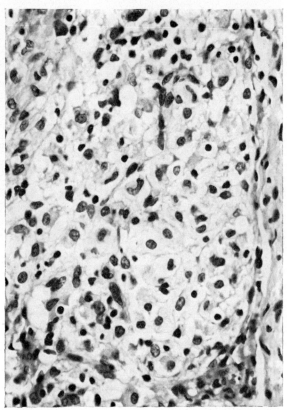

Fig. 9.278. Lymph node in another case of Letterer–Siwe disease. The cells filling the sinus are more histiocytic in appearance than those in Fig. 9.277B and eosinophils are very sparse. The rather distinct outline of the cell margin and the relatively small, centrally placed nucleus give the picture a resemblance to some other forms of histiocytosis. In this instance the child had been inoculated with bacillus Calmette–Guérin (BCG) a few weeks before the onset of the terminal illness: the picture in this biopsy specimen was misinterpreted as 'BCG histiocytosis' (see Fig. 9.78, page 605). *Haematoxylin–eosin.* × 370.

---

not intended to indicate preponderant involvement of the bone marrow (also known as the medulla), contrary to a common misunderstanding that sometimes leads to diagnostic error.

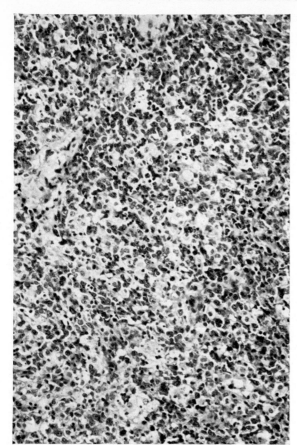

Fig. 9.279. 'Histiocytic medullary reticulosis' (lymph node biopsy). There is a diffuse proliferation of histiocytes, which appear large and pale, and of less mature cells, probably their precursors, which appear smaller and darker, having less cytoplasm and a more compact nucleus. The normal structure of the node has been totally replaced in this field. *Haematoxylin–eosin.* × 160.

marrow. The amount of phagocytosis of erythrocytes, leucocytes and platelets by the pathological histiocytes is seldom approached in other conditions. In contrast, the histiocyte precursors that are said also to be present show no evidence of phagocytosis.

It is necessary to stress that the presence of 'histiocytic medullary reticulosis' should not be suspected merely because proliferation of histiocytes and demonstrable phagocytosis of erythrocytes and other blood cells are observed in a lymphoreticular organ. Some degree of such activity is commonly to be seen, in lymph nodes and elsewhere, in many other conditions, such as the simple lymphadenitis associated with acute inflammation in the drainage area.[1297]

The patient with 'histiocytic medullary reticulosis' is usually acutely ill: diagnostic confusion with benign forms of histiocytosis is not very likely to occur. A point that is said to be of value in distinguishing the histological lesions of malignant histiocytosis, including Letterer–Siwe disease (see above) and 'histiocytic medullary reticulosis', from those of conditions such as 'sinus histiocytosis with massive lymphadenopathy' (see page 564) is the paucity of eosinophils in the latter and their frequently considerable abundance in the malignant conditions.[1626]

'Hairy Cell Leukaemia'[1627]

Nomenclature

It is difficult to conceive how a disease that has become so widely known as 'hairy cell leukaemia' can ever be referred to by any more mundane name. Even the rather odd translations of 'hairy cell' into other languages seem likelier to consolidate the term internationally than cause misunderstanding: neither 'tricholeucocytic leukaemia' nor 'vellutocellular leukaemia' is likely to have preferential currency.* The 'hairy cells' were so named[1628] because their cytoplasm has many fine filamentous projections, well seen under the phase-contrast microscope. This characteristic of the leukaemic cells in the condition that had previously been known as leukaemic reticuloendotheliosis[1629, 1630] encouraged the introduction of the term 'hairy cell leukaemia'.[1631] The term leukaemic reticuloendotheliosis was introduced in 1923 by Ewald, when describing a case of acute leukaemia;[1632] this case was considered by some subsequent writers to have been an example of monocytic leukaemia (Schilling's leukaemia) and for this reason 'leukaemic reticuloendotheliosis' came to be regarded as a synonym of the latter.[1633] Since, 1958, when the disease that was to become known as 'hairy cell leukaemia' was defined in modern terms,[1630] 'leukaemic reticuloendotheliosis' has ceased to be applied to monocytic leukaemia and is now considered by many to be the least unsatisfactory synonym of 'hairy cell leukaemia'.[1634] Nevertheless, while the identity of the neoplastic cell remains uncertain it is difficult to accept a name that has the cytogenetic implications inherent in 'reticuloendotheliosis'. Other proposed

* *Leucémie à cellules chevelues* (or, arguably more appropriate, *velues*) and *Haarzell-Leukämie* (or even *Leukämie mit behaarten Zellen*) compete in print with *leucémie à hairy cells* and *Leukämie mit hairy cells* and *Hairycell-Leukämie*.

names, such as histiocytic leukaemia,[1635] reticulum cell leukaemia,[1636] chronic reticulolymphocytic leukaemia,[1637] lymphoid myelofibrosis[1638] and even 'tricholeucocytic leukaemia'[1639] are no more satisfactory.

Pathology[1627, 1640]

'Hairy cell leukaemia' occurs mainly in men and most frequently after the age of 40 years. Its onset is insidious and its course chronic. Splenomegaly is marked: the pancytopenia that is commonly present may be attributable to 'hypersplenism' (see page 724). A leukaemic blood picture develops during the course of the disease rather than at its onset, and in many cases the white cell count remains below the normal range throughout the illness. There is a relative increase in the number of mononuclear cells in the blood, and most of these appear to be lymphocytes. Careful examination shows that a proportion of the mononuclear cells have the morphological features of 'hairy cells'. These are rather larger than normal large lymphocytes; the characteristic filamentous projections from the cytoplasmic surface may be seen in films stained by Romanowsky methods and examined by the conventional methods of light microscopy.

Attempts to aspirate bone marrow are often unsuccessful. When a sample is obtained, whether by aspiration or excision, or with a biopsy drill, it commonly shows extensive replacement of the normal tissue by the neoplastic cells. In sections there is a fine felt-work of reticulin fibres that only late in the course of the disease gives place to bundles of collagen. The spleen, lymph nodes and liver usually show infiltration by the characteristic cells. The weight of the spleen ranges from 350 g to over 5000 g, the mean being about 1800 g. The leukaemic cells infiltrate the red pulp diffusely and encroach to a limited extent on the white pulp. In the lymph nodes the leukaemic cells occupy mainly the sinuses, particularly the subcapsular sinus; there is also considerable infiltration of the pulp.

In sections the specific cells are large, with abundant, clear or opaque cytoplasm and a nucleus rather larger than that of a mature lymphocyte. The nucleus has a distinct membrane, a fine chromatin pattern and usually one or two rather small, darkly stained nucleoli. Even in histological sections it is possible to make out the fine cytoplasmic processes, which form a delicate system of linkages between adjacent cells (Figs 9.280A and 9.280B). A small number of fibroblasts and small clusters of lymphocytes are interspersed among the 'hairy cells'.

Some Rarer Forms of Generalized 'Histiocytosis'

It is probable that the conditions already referred to in this section—'histiocytosis X' (including Letterer–Siwe disease), 'histiocytic medullary reticulosis' and 'hairy cell leukaemia'—do not account for all the varieties of this pattern of generalized infiltration of the tissues by neoplastic lymphoreticular cells. Among rarer conditions that come within this category are certain examples that have been observed only in particular families. These familial forms of 'histiocytosis' become clinically evident early in infancy and they are rapidly fatal. One, so far identified in only two families,[1641, 1642] is known as *familial haemophagocytic reticulosis (familial histiocytic reticulosis)*. Another, occurring in six sibships of an uncommonly inbred Irish family in the United States of America, has been described as *familial reticuloendotheliosis with eosinophilia.*[1643] The nature and relationship of these genetically determined disorders and their relation to the

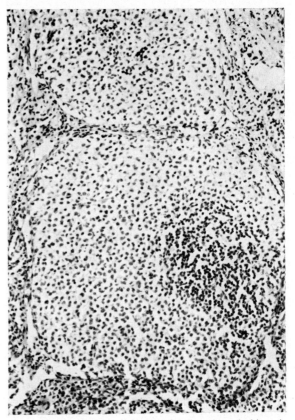

Fig. 9.280A.§ 'Hairy cell leukaemia' (lymph node biopsy). The peripheral sinus is distended by a large accumulation of pale cells that encroach only slightly on the adjoining pulp. See Fig. 9.280B. *Haematoxylin–eosin.* × 130.

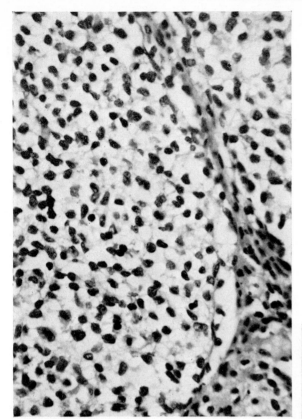

Fig. 9.280B.§ Higher magnification of part of the field illustrated in Fig. 9.280A. The fine cytoplasmic filaments that link adjacent cells are seen. The filaments are much coarser and less numerous in histological preparations than those seen in films under the phase-contrast microscope, but they are equivalent to the latter. The identity of the 'hairy cells' remains uncertain. *Haematoxylin–eosin.* × 400.

various more or less similar, non-familial diseases have not yet been determined.

Other Malignant Diseases Involving the Lymphoreticular System

Although *leukaemia* (particularly lymphocytic leukaemia and monocytic leukaemia) and *myelomas* (both myelomatosis and extraskeletal myelomas) may properly be regarded as neoplastic diseases arising in, or in close histogenetic relation to, the lymphoreticular system, they are dealt with more conveniently in other chapters. Leukaemia is considered mainly in Chapter 8 (pages 478 to 488); for convenience, Sézary's syndrome (page 856) and 'hairy cell leukaemia' (page 861) have been described in this chapter. Myelomatosis is described in Chapter 8 (page 488) and in Chapter 37 (Volume 5);

extraskeletal myelomas are described in Chapter 4 (page 231), Chapter 6 (page 266) and Chapter 7 (page 407).

Metastatic Tumours

The commonest cancerous state of the lymph nodes and spleen is their metastatic involvement by tumours arising in other organs and tissues (see pages 714 and 740 respectively).

The prognostic importance of lymph node involvement in cases of carcinoma is well known. It is not always appreciated how readily secondary deposits in lymph nodes may simulate malignant disease originating in these organs—particularly, of course, when the primary growth remains hidden from clinical observation. Among tumours that are specially liable to be misinterpreted as lymphomas, particularly immunoblastic lymphomas (the former

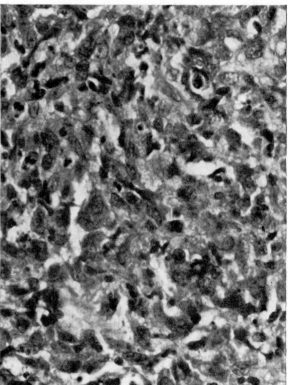

Fig. 9.281. Anaplastic metastatic carcinoma in an inguinal lymph node. The primary growth was in the lower part of the vagina and ranged in structure from unmistakable squamous carcinoma to completely undifferentiated tumour similar to that illustrated. Compare with the undifferentiated lymphoma illustrated in Fig. 9.271 (page 854). *Haematoxylin–eosin.* × 400.

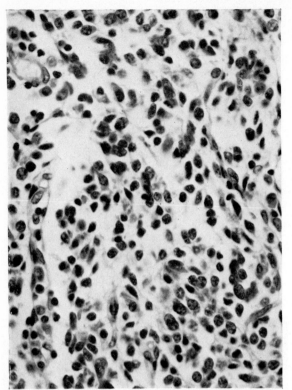

Fig. 9.282. Metastatic neuroblastoma in an inferior deep cervical lymph node of the left side (a 'sentinel' node—see page 715). The primary growth was in the left adrenal gland and had caused no symptoms apart from the enlarging node in the neck. The correct diagnosis was indicated by the presence of rosette-like structures, of which several more or less clearly recognizable examples are included in this field. See also Figs 9.161 (page 714) and 9.283. *Haematoxylin– eosin.* × 400.

'reticulum cell sarcomas'), are metastatic deposits of malignant melanoma (especially when pigment is scanty) and of anaplastic or undifferentiated carcinomas (Fig. 9.281). Rare secondary tumours, such as hepatomas and neuroblastomas (Fig. 9.282), seminoma (Fig. 9.283) and dysgerminoma, are other causes of diagnostic difficulty when lymph node enlargement is the presenting manifestation of the

disease—particularly when the involved nodes are in a part of the body remote from the site of the primary growth. Such problems are mentioned in relation to the accounts of the primary tumours in the corresponding chapters of this book.

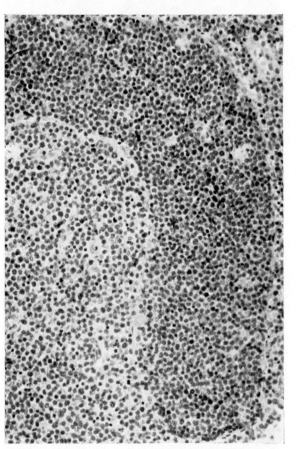

Fig. 9.283. Metastatic seminoma in an axillary lymph node. There were no other symptoms at the time of excision of the node, and the histological picture was interpreted as lymphomatous. The correct diagnosis was made some weeks later when the primary tumour of a testis was found after the patient had asked if he should have treatment for what he thought was a hydrocele. See also Figs 9.161 (page 714) and 9.282. *Haematoxylin–eosin.* × 160.

REFERENCES

INTRODUCTION

1. Yoffey, J. M., Courtice, F. C., *Lymphatics, Lymph and the Lymphomyeloid Complex.* London and New York, 1970.
2. Murphy, J. B., *The Lymphocyte in Resistance to Tissue Grafting, Malignant Disease and Tuberculous Infection.* Rockefeller Institute for Medical Research Monograph No. 21. New York, 1926.

3. Roitt, I. M., Greaves, M. F., Torrigiani, G., Brostoff, J., Playfair, J. H. L., *Lancet,* 1969, **2**, 367.

LYMPHOID SYSTEM

4. Yoffey, J. M., Courtice, F. C., *Lymphatics, Lymph and Lymphoid Tissue,* 2nd edn, page 26. London, 1956.
5. Davies, A. J. S., *Transplant. Rev.,* 1969, **1**, 43.
6. Miller, J. F. A. P., *Brit. med. Bull.,* 1966, **22**, 21.

7. Cooper, M, D., Peterson, R. D. A., South, M. A., *J. exp. Med.*, 1966, **123**, 75.

8. Good, R. A., Papermaster, B. W., *Advanc. Immunol.*, 1964, **4**, 1.

9. Ford, C. E., Micklem, H. S., Evans, E. P., Gray, J. G., Ogden, D. A., *Ann. N.Y. Acad. Sci.*, 1966, **129**, 283.

10. Micklem, H. S., Clarke, C. M., Evans, E. P., Ford, C. E., *Transplantation*, 1968, **6**, 299.

11. Nakamura, K., Metcalf, D., *Brit. J. Cancer*, 1961, **15**, 306.

12. Miller, J. F. A. P., Osoba, D., *Physiol. Rev.*, 1967, **47**, 437.

13. Everett, N. B., Tyler, R. W., *Int. Rev. Cytol.*, 1967, **22**, 205.

14. Metcalf, D., in *The Thymus—Experimental and Clinical Studies*, edited by G. E. W. Wolstenholme and R. Porter. London, 1966.

15. Ernström, U., Larsson, B., *Nature (Lond.)*, 1969, **222**, 279.

16. Burnet, F. M., *The Clonal Selection Theory of Acquired Immunity*. London, 1959.

17. Miller, J. F. A. P., Mitchell, G. F., *Nature (Lond.)*, 1967, **216**, 785.

18. Moore, M. A. S., Owen, J. J. T., *Develop. Biol.*, 1966, **14**, 40.

19. Owen, J. J. T., in *Handbuch der allgemeinen Pathologie*, edited by H.-W. Altmann, F. Büchner, H. Cottier, E. Grundmann, G. Holle, E. Letterer, W. Masshoff, H. Meessen, F. Roulet, G. Seifert and G. Siebert, vol. 7, part 3, page 3. Berlin, Heidelberg and New York, 1970.

20. Archer, O. K., Sutherland, D. E. R., Good, R. A., *Lab. Invest.*, 1964, **13**, 259.

21. Perey, D. Y. E., Frommel, D., Horne, R., Good, R. A., *Lab. Invest.*, 1970, **22**, 212.

22. Gowans, J. L., *Harvey Lect.*, 1968–69, Series 64, 87.

23. Aschoff, L., *Die lymphatischen Organe*. Berlin and Vienna, 1926.

24. Ehrich, W., *Amer. J. Anat.*, 1929, **43**, 347.

25. Kabelitz, H.-J., *Acta haemat. (Basel)*, 1950, **3**, 347.

26. Parrott, D. M. V., de Sousa, M., East, J., *J. exp. Med.*, 1966, **123**, 191.

27. Harris, T. N., Grimm, E., Mertens, E., Ehrich, W. E., *J. exp. Med.*, 1945, **81**, 73.

28. Stutman, O., Yunis, E. J., Good, R. A., *J. exp. Med.*, 1970, **132**, 583.

29. Oort, J., Turk, J. L., *Brit. J. exp. Path.*, 1965, **46**, 147.

30. Gutman, G. A., Weissman, I. L., *Immunology*, 1972, **23**, 465.

31. Sprent, J., Miller, J. F. A. P., *Nature new Biol.*, 1971, **234**, 195.

32. Cunningham, A. J., Smith, J. B., Mercer, E. H., *J. exp. Med.*, 1966, **124**, 701.

33. Hellman, T., in *Handbuch der mikroskopischen Anatomie des Menschen*, edited by W. von Möllendorff, vol. 6, part 4, page 173. Berlin, 1943.

34. Flemming, W., *Arch. mikr. Anat.*, 1885, **24**, 50.

35. Sordat, B., Sordat, M., Hess, M. W., Stoner, R. D., Cottier, H., *J. exp. Med.*, 1970, **131**, 77.

36. Fliedner, T. M., Kesse, M., Cronkite, E. D., Robertson, J. S., *Ann. N.Y. Acad. Sci.*, 1964, **113**, 578.

37. Clawson, C. C., Cooper, M. D., Good, R. A., *Lab. Invest.*, 1967, **16**, 407.

38. Parrott, D. M. V., de Sousa, M. A., *Nature (Lond.)*, 1966, **212**, 1316.

39. Maruyama, K., Masuda, T., *A.R. Inst. Virus Res.*, 1964, **7**, 149.

40. Nossal, G. J. V., Abbot, A., Mitchell, J., Lummus, Z., *J. exp. Med.*, 1968, **127**, 277.

41. Nossal, G. J. V., Ada, G. L., *Antigens, Lymphoid Cells and the Immune Response*. New York, 1971.

42. Ford, W. L., Gowans, J. L., *Proc. roy. Soc. B*, 1967, **168**, 244.

43. Cooper, G. N., Thonard, J. C., Crosby, R. L., Dalbow, M. H., *Aust. J. exp. Biol. med. Sci.*, 1968, **46**, 407.

44. Greaves, M. F., Owen, J. J. T., Raff, M. C., *T and B Lymphocytes: Origins, Properties and Roles in Immune Responses*. Amsterdam and New York, 1974.

45. Henry, K., Goldman, J. M., in *Recent Advances in Pathology*, No. 9, edited by C. V. Harrison and K. Weinbren, page 30. Edinburgh, London and New York, 1975.

46. Medawar, P. B., *Proc. roy. Soc. B*, 1958, **149**, 145.

47. Dutton, R. W., Eady, J. D., *Immunology*, 1964, **7**, 40.

48. Nowell, P. C., *Cancer Res.*, 1960, **21**, 1518.

49. Greaves, M. F., Owen, J. J. T., Raff, M. C., *T and B Lymphocytes: Origins, Properties and Roles in Immune Responses*, chap. 3. Amsterdam and New York, 1974.

50. Bianco, C., Patrick, R., Nussenzweig, V., *J. exp. Med.*, 1970, **132**, 702.

51. Basten, A., Miller, J. F. A. P., Sprent, J., Pye, J., *J. exp. Med.*, 1972, **135**, 610.

52. Eisen, S. A., Wedner, H. J., Parker, C. W., *Immunol. Commun.*, 1972, **1**, 571.

53. Wioland, M., Sabulovic, D., Burg, C., *Nature new Biol.*, 1972, **237**, 275.

54. Lance, E. M., *Clin. exp. Immunol.*, 1970, **6**, 789.

55. Cohen, J. J., Claman, H. N., *J. exp. Med.*, 1971, **133**, 1026.

56. Levine, M. A., Claman, H. N., *Science*, 1970, **167**, 1515.

57. Turk, J. L., Poulter, L. W., *Clin. exp. Immunol.*, 1972, **10**, 285.

58. Bach, J. F., Dardenne, M., *Transplant. Proc.*, 1972, **4**, 345.

59. Bach, J. F., Dardenne, M., *Cell. Immunol.*, 1973, **6**, 394.

60. Uhr, J. W., Scharff, M., *J. exp. Med.*, 1960, **112**, 65.

61. Lukes, R. J., Collins, R. D., in *Malignant Diseases of the Hematopoietic System*, edited by K. Akazaki, page 209. Baltimore and Tokyo, 1973. [*Gann Monogr. Cancer Res.*, No. 15.]

62. Rosenthal, N., *Bull. N.Y. Acad. Med.*, 1954, **30**, 583.

63. Mori, Y., Lennert, K., *Electron Microscopic Atlas of Lymph Node Cytology and Pathology*, page 5. Berlin, Heidelberg and New York, 1969.

64. Zucker-Franklin, D., Davidson, M., Thomas, L., *J. exp. Med.*, 1966, **124**, 533.

65. Furth, R. van, in *Mononuclear Phagocytes*, edited by R. van Furth, page 151. Oxford and Edinburgh, 1970.

66. Osmond, D. G., *Anat. Rec.*, 1969, **165**, 109.

67. Ford, C. E., in *The Thymus: Experimental and Clinical Studies*, edited by G. E. W. Wolstenholme and R. Porter, page 131. London, 1966.

68. Roitt, I. M., Greaves, M. F., Torrigiani, G., Brostoff, J., Playfair, J. H. L., *Lancet*, 1969, **2**, 367.

69. Gowans, J. L., Knight, E. J., *Proc. roy. Soc. B*, 1964, **159**, 257.
70. Ottesen, J., *Acta physiol. scand.*, 1954, **32**, 75.
71. Ford, W. L., *Brit. J. exp. Path.*, 1969, **50**, 257.
72. Buckton, K. E., Court-Brown, W. M., Smith, P. G., *Nature (Lond.)*, 1967, **214**, 470.
73. Nowell, P. C., *Blood*, 1965, **26**, 798.
74. Crowther, D., Fairley, G. H., Sewell, R. L., *J. exp. Med.*, 1969, **129**, 849.
75. Dougherty, T. F., Berliner, M. L., Schneebeli, G. L., Berliner, D. L., *Ann. N.Y. Acad. Sci.*, 1964, **113**, 825.
76. Yoffey, J. M., in *Cell Production and Its Regulation*, edited by G. E. W. Wolstenholme and M. O'Connor, page 1. London, 1960.
77. Carrell, A., *J. exp. Med.*, 1922, **36**, 385.
78. Loutit, J. F., *Lancet*, 1962, **2**, 1106.
79. Burch, P. R. J., Burwell, R. G., *Quart. Rev. Biol.*, 1965, **40**, 252.
80. Thomas, L., in *Cellular and Humoral Aspects of the Hypersensitivity States*, edited by H. S. Lawrence, page 529 (discussion). London, 1959.
81. Warnatz, H., Scheiffart, S. F., *Nature (Lond.)*, 1964, **201**, 408.
82. Hill, W. L., Nissen, B., *J. Immunol.*, 1971, **106**, 421.
83. Byrt, P., Ada, G. L., *Immunology*, 1969, **17**, 503.
84. Greaves, M. F., *Transplant. Rev.*, 1970, **5**, 45.
85. Humphrey, J. H., Roelants, G., Wilcox, N., in *Cell Interaction and Receptor Antibodies in Immune Responses*, edited by O. Makela, A. M. Gross and T. Kosuren, page 123. New York, 1971.
86. Crone, M., Cock, C., Simonsen, M., *Transplant. Rev.*, 1972, **10**, 36.
87. Unanue, E., Cerottini, J., *J. exp. Med.*, 1970, **131**, 711.
88. Huber, H., Fudenberg, H. H., *Int. Arch. Allergy*, 1968, **34**, 18.
89. Kölsch, E., in *Mononuclear Phagocytes*, edited by R. van Furth, page 548. Oxford and Edinburgh, 1970.
90. MacLennon, I. C. M., Hardy, B., Loewi, G., Howard, A., *Brit. J. Cancer*, 1973, **28**, suppl. 1, 7.
91. Fakhri, O., Hobbs, J. R., *Lancet*, 1972, **2**, 403.
92. Roitt, I. M., *Essential Immunology*, 2nd edn, page 233. Oxford, London, Edinburgh and Melbourne, 1974.
93. Alexander, P., Delorme, E., Hamilton, L., Hall, J. G., *Nature (Lond.)*, 1967, **213**, 569.
94. Wilson, D. B., Billingham, R. E., *Advanc. Immunol.*, 1967, **7**, 189.
95. Billingham, R. E., Brent, L., *Transplant. Bull.*, 1957, **4**, 67.
96. Lawrence, H. S., *Advanc. Immunol.*, 1969, **11**, 195.
97. Bloom, B. R., Bennett, B., *Ann. N.Y. Acad. Sci.*, 1970, **169**, 258.
98. Ward, P., Remold, H., David, J., *Cell. Immunol.*, 1970, **1**, 162.
99. Nathan, C., Remold, H., David, J., *J. exp. Med.*, 1971, **133**, 1356.
100. Williams, T. W., Granger, G. A., *J. Immunol.*, 1969, **102**, 911.
101. Mudd, S., *Infectious Agents and Host Reactions*. Philadelphia, London and Toronto, 1970.
102. Mackaness, G. B., in *Mononuclear Phagocytes*, edited by R. van Furth, page 461. Oxford and Edinburgh, 1970.
103. Allison, A., Mallucci, L., *J. exp. Med.*, 1965, **121**, 463.
104. Miller, G., Enders, J., *J. Virol.*, 1968, **2**, 787.
105. Holub, M., *Ann. N.Y. Acad. Sci.*, 1962, **99**, 477.

106. McGregor, D. D., Gowans, J. L., *J. exp. Med.*, 1963, **117**, 303.
107. Miller, J. F. A. P., Mitchell, G. F., *Transplant. Rev.*, 1969, **1**, 3.
108. Claman, H. N., Chaperone, E. A., *Transplant. Rev.*, 1969, **1**, 92.
109. Greaves, M. F., Janossy, G., *Transplant. Rev.*, 1972, **11**, 87.

RETICULOENDOTHELIAL SYSTEM

110. Stuart, A. E., *The Reticulo-Endothelial System*. Edinburgh and London, 1970.
111. *Mononuclear Phagocytes*, edited by R. van Furth. Oxford and Edinburgh, 1970.
112. Metchnikoff, E., *Lectures on the Comparative Pathology of Inflammation* (translated by F. A. Starling and E. H. Starling). London, 1893 [republished: New York, 1968].
113. Ehrlich, P., *Zbl. med. Wiss.*, 1882, **23**, 113.
114. Ehrlich, P., *Dtsch. med. Wschr.*, 1886, **12**, 49.
115. Goldmann, E. E., *Bruns' Beitr. klin. Chir.*, 1909, **64**, 192.
116. Goldmann, E., *Bruns' Beitr. klin. Chir.*, 1912, **78**, 1.
117. Ribbert, H., *Z. allg. Physiol.*, 1904, **4**, 201.
118. Abell, R. G., *Anat. Rec.*, 1940, **78**, 215.
119. Gregersen, M. I., Rawson, R. A., *Amer. J. Physiol.*, 1943, **138**, 698.
120. Cappell, D. F., *J. Path. Bact.*, 1929, **32**, 595, 629, 675.
121. Aschoff, L., Kiyono, K., *Folia haemat. (Frankfurt)*, 1913, **15**, 383.
122. Aschoff, L., *Münch. med. Wschr.*, 1922, **69**, 1352.
123. Aschoff, L., *Ergebn. inn. Med. Kinderheilk.*, 1924, **26**, 1.
124. Cohn, Z. A., in *Mononuclear Phagocytes*, edited by R. van Furth, chap. 8. Oxford and Edinburgh, 1970.
125. Langevoort, H. L., Cohn, Z. A., Hirsch, J. G., Humphrey, J. H., Spector, W. G., Furth, R. van, in *Mononuclear Phagocytes*, edited by R. van Furth, chap. 1. Oxford and Edinburgh, 1970.
126. Kupffer, K. W. von, *Arch. mikr. Anat.*, 1876, **12**, 353.
127. Furth, R. van, *Semin. Hemat.*, 1970, **7**, 125.
128. Furth, R. van, in *Mononuclear Phagocytes*, edited by R. van Furth, chap. 10. Oxford and Edinburgh, 1970.
129. Marshall, A. H. E., *An Outline of the Cytology and Pathology of the Reticular Tissue*, chap. 1. Edinburgh and London, 1956.
130. Maximow, A., in *Handbuch der mikroskopischen Anatomie des Menschen*, edited by W. von Möllendorff, vol. 2, part 1. Berlin, 1927.
131. Thomas, J. A., *Rev. Hémat.*, 1949, **4**, 639.
132. Volterra, M., *Sperimentale*, 1927, **81**, 319.
133. Hirsch, J. G., Fedorko, M. E., in *Mononuclear Phagocytes*, edited by R. van Furth, chap. 2. Oxford and Edinburgh, 1970.
134. Roser, B., in *Mononuclear Phagocytes*, edited by R. van Furth, chap. 11. Oxford and Edinburgh, 1970.
135. Del Río Hortega, P., *Bol. Soc. esp. Biol.*, 1919, **9**, 154.
136. Del Río Hortega, P., Jimenez de Asúa, F., *Arch. Cardiol. Hemat.*, 1921, **2**, 161.
137. Del Río Hortega, P., Jimenez de Asúa, F., *Bol. Soc. esp. Hist. natur.*, 1924, **11**, 7.
138. Maximow, A. A., in *Special Cytology*, edited by E. V. Cowdry, vol. 2, sect. 16. New York, 1932.
139. Stuart, A. E., *The Reticulo-Endothelial System*, page 3. Edinburgh and London, 1970.

140. Biozzi, G., Halpern, B. N., Benacerraf, B., Stiffel, C., in *Physiopathology of the Reticulo-Endothelial System*, edited by B. N. Halpern, page 204. Oxford, 1957.

141. Stuart, A. E., *The Reticulo-Endothelial System*, chap. 3. Edinburgh and London, 1970.

142. Wagner, H. N., Iio, M., *J. clin. Invest.*, 1964, **43**, 1525.

143. Petroff, J. R., *Z. ges. exp. Med.*, 1924, **42**, 242.

144. Murray, I. M., *J. exp. Med.*, 1963, **117**, 139.

145. Heller, J. H., *Endocrinology*, 1955, **56**, 80.

146. Snell, J. F., in *Reticulo-Endothelial Structure and Function*, edited by J. H. Heller, page 321. New York, 1960.

147. Stuart, A. E., *J. Path. Bact.*, 1962, **84**, 193.

148. Kelly, L. S., Brown, B. A., Dobson, E. L., *Proc. Soc. exp. Biol. (N.Y.)*, 1962, **110**, 55.

149. Megirian, R., *J. reticuloendoth. Soc.*, 1965, **2**, 238.

150. Halpern, B. N., Prévot, A.-R., Biozzi, G., Stiffel, C., Mouton, D., Morard, J. C., Bouthillier, Y., Decreusefond, C., *J. reticuloendoth. Soc.*, 1963, **1**, 77.

151. DiCarlo, F. J., Haynes, L. J., Malament, S. G., Phillips, G. E., *Canad. J. Biochem.*, 1963, **41**, 731.

152. Böhme, D., Bouvier, C. A., *Beitr. path. Anat.*, 1960, **122**, 188.

153. Cooper, G. N., Houston, B., *Aust. J. exp. Biol. med. Sci.*, 1964, **42**, 429.

154. Fishman, M., *J. exp. Med.*, 1961, **114**, 837.

155. Unanue, E., Cerottini, J., *J. exp. Med.*, 1970, **131**, 711.

156. Fishman, M., Adler, F. L., *J. exp. Med.*, 1963, **117**, 595.

157. Bessis, M., Breton-Gorius, J., *Blood*, 1962, **19**, 635.

158. Thannhauser, S. J., *Lipidoses—Diseases of the Intracellular Lipid Metabolism*, 3rd edn. New York and London, 1958.

FACTORS THAT AFFECT THE LYMPHORETICULAR TISSUES

159. Yoffey, J. M., Courtice, F. C., *Lymphatics, Lymph and the Lymphomyeloid Complex*, page 804. London and New York, 1970.

160. Warren, S., Bowers, J. Z., *Ann. intern. Med.*, 1950, **32**, 207.

161. Trowell, O. A., *J. Path. Bact.*, 1952, **64**, 687.

162. Martland, H. S., Conlon, P., Knef, J. P., *J. Amer. med. Ass.*, 1925, **85**, 1769.

163. Keuning, F. J., Meer, J. van der, Niewenhuis, P., Oudendijk, P., *Lab. Invest.*, 1963, **12**, 156.

164. Uhr, J. W., Scharff, M., *J. exp. Med.*, 1960, **112**, 65.

165. *Histopathology of Irradiation from External and Internal Sources*, edited by W. Bloom. New York, 1948.

166. Price, C. H. G., *Brit. J. Radiol.*, 1951, **24**, 556.

167. Turk, J. L., Poulter, L. W., *Clin. exp. Immunol.*, 1972, **10**, 285.

168. Miller, J. F. A. P., Mitchell, G. F., *J. exp. Med.*, 1970, **131**, 675.

169. Long, D. H., *Int. Arch. Allergy*, 1957, **10**, 5.

170. Claman, H. N., *New Engl. J. Med.*, 1972, **287**, 388.

171. Hedinger, E., *Frankfurt. Z. Path.*, 1907, **1**, 527.

172. Medlar, E. M., *Amer. J. Path.*, 1927, **3**, 135.

173. Ehrich, W. E., Seifter, J., in *The Effect of ACTH and Cortisone upon Infection and Resistance*, edited by G. Schwartzman, chap. 4. New York, 1953.

174. Axelrod, A. R., Berman, L., *Blood*, 1951, **6**, 434.

175. Ernström, U., Gyllensten, L., *Acta path. microbiol. scand.*, 1959, **47**, 243.

176. Ernström, U., Hedback, A. L., *Acta path. microbiol. scand.*, 1965, **65**, 215.

177. Nicol, T., Zikry, A. A., *Nature (Lond.)*, 1952, **130**, 239.

178. Jackson, C. M., *The Effects of Inanition and Malnutrition upon Growth and Structure*. Philadelphia, 1925.

179. Andreasen, E., *Acta path. microbiol. scand.*, 1943, suppl. 49.

NOMENCLATURE OF DISEASES OF THE LYMPHORETICULAR SYSTEM

180. Hodgkin, T., *Med.-chir. Trans.*, 1832, **17**, 68.

181. Fox, H., *Guy's Hosp. Rep.*, 1936, **86**, 11.

182. Symmers, W. St C., in *Cancer*, edited by R. W. Raven, vol. 2, chap. 24. London, 1958.

183. Dawson, P. J., *Arch. intern. Med.*, 1968, **121**, 288.

184. Carswell, *cited by:* Hodgkin, T. (reference 180, above).

185. New Sydenham Society, *An Atlas of Illustrations of Pathology Compiled (Chiefly from Original Sources) for the New Sydenham Society*, fasc. 12. London, 1898.

186. Craigie, D., *Edinb. med. surg. J.*, 1845, **64**, 400.

187. Bennett, J. H., *Edinb. med. surg. J.*, 1845, **64**, 413.

188. Lautner, *Z. k. k. Ges. Aerzt. Wien*, 1845, 488.

189. Virchow, *Neue Notiz. Geb. Natur- u. Heilk.*, 1845, **36**, 151.

190. Ehrlich, P., *Farbenanalytische Untersuchungen zur Histologie und Klinik*. Berlin, 1891.

191. Cohnheim, J., *Virchows Arch. path. Anat.*, 1865, **33**, 451.

191a. Virchow, *Berl. klin. Wschr.*, 1892, **29**, 288.

191b. Sternberg, C., *Verh. dtsch. path. Ges.*, 1912, **15**, 22.

192. Sternberg, C., in *Handbuch der speziellen pathologischen Anatomie und Histologie*, edited by F. Henke and O. Lubarsch, vol. 1, part 1, page 62. Berlin, 1926.

193. Ewald, O., *Dtsch. Arch. klin. Med.*, 1923, **142**, 222.

194. Letterer, E., *Frankfurt. Z. Path.*, 1924, **30**, 377.

195. Virchow, R., *Die krankhaften Geschwülste*, vol. 2, part 1, page 728. Berlin, 1863.

196. Kundrat, H., *Wien. klin. Wschr.*, 1893, **6**, 211.

197. Ewing, J., *J. med. Res.*, 1913–14, **28**, 1.

198. Oberling, C., *Bull. Ass. franç. Cancer*, 1928, **17**, 259.

199. Roulet, F., *Virchows Arch. path. Anat.*, 1930, **277**, 15.

200. Letterer, E., *Veröff. Gewerbe- u. Konstit. Path.*, 1934, **8**, part 4.

201. Pullinger, B. D., in *Rose Research on Lymphadenoma*, page 115. Bristol and London, 1932.

202. Robb-Smith, A. H. T., *J. Path. Bact.*, 1938, **47**, 457.

203. Robb-Smith, A. H. T., in *Recent Advances in Clinical Pathology*, edited by S. C. Dyke, R. Cruickshank, E. N. Allott, B. L. Della Vida and A. H. T. Robb-Smith, chap. 34. London, 1947.

LYMPH NODES: INTRODUCTION

204. Lennert, K., *Pathologie der Halslymphknoten—Ein Abriss für Pathologen, Kliniker und praktizierende Ärzte*. Berlin, Göttingen and Heidelberg, 1964. [Revised version of: Lennert, K., *Arch. Ohr.-, Nas.-, u. Kehlk.-Heilk.*, 1963, **182**, 1 (Kongressbericht 1963).]

205. Lennert, K., *Lymphknoten—Diagnostik in Schnitt und Ausstrich: A. Cytologie und Lymphadenitis*, in *Handbuch der speziellen pathologischen Anatomie und Histologie*, edited by E. Uehlinger, vol. 1, part 3, book 1. Berlin, Göttingen and Heidelberg, 1961.

206. Yoffey, J. M., Courtice, F. C., *Lymphatics, Lymph and the Lymphomyeloid Complex*, chap. 7. London and New York, 1970.
207. Virchow, R., *Cellular Pathology as Based upon Physiological and Pathological Histology*, translated by F. Chance from the 2nd German edition of *Die Cellularpathologie in ihrer Begründung auf physiologische und pathologische Gewebelehre*, lectures 9 and 10. London, 1860 (republished: New York, 1971).
208. Hellman, T. J., White, G., *Virchows Arch. path. Anat.*, 1930, **278**, 221.

STRUCTURAL ANOMALIES

209. Garret, R., Ada, A. E. W., *Cancer* (*Philad.*), 1957, **10**, 173.
210. Nicholson, G. W. de P., *Studies on Tumour Formation*, page 58. London, 1950.
211. Nicastri, A. D., Foote, F. W., Jr, Frazell, E. L., *J. Amer. med. Ass.*, 1965, **194**, 113.
212. Gricouroff, G., *Bull. Ass. franç. Cancer*, 1962, **49**, 300.
213. Gerard-Marchant, R., *Arch. Path.*, 1964, **77**, 633.
214. Lange, P., *Acta obstet. gynec. scand.*, 1955, **34**, 111.
215. Javert, C. T., *Amer. J. Obstet. Gynec.*, 1951, **62**, 477.
216. Symmers, W. St C., *unpublished observations*.
217. Moloney, G. E., *Brit. med. J.*, 1949, **1**, 435.
218. Koss, L. G., *Cancer* (*Philad.*), 1963, **16**, 1369.
219. McCarthy, S. W., Palmer, A. A., Bale, P. M., Hirst, E., *Pathology*, 1974, **6**, 351.
220. Berg, F. W. T. van den, Kaiserling, E., Lennert, K., *Virchows Arch. Abt. A*, 1976, **371**, 27.
221. Rodriguez, H. A., Ackerman, L. V., *Cancer* (*Philad.*), 1968, **21**, 393.
221a. Albertini, M. von, *Bull. Soc. franç. Derm. Syph.*, 1935, **42**, 1273.
222. Johnson, W. T., Helwig, E. B., *Cancer* (*Philad.*), 1969, **23**, 747.
223. Flendrig, J. A., *Het benigne reuzenlymfoom* (Thesis, Nijmegen). Helmond, The Netherlands, 1969.
224. Anagnostou, D., Harrison, C. V., *J. clin. Path.*, 1972, **25**, 306.
225. Castleman, B., Iverson, L., Pardo Menendez, V., *Cancer* (*Philad.*), 1956, **9**, 822.
226. Tung, K. S. K., McCormack, L. J., *Cancer* (*Philad.*), 1967, **20**, 525.
227. Möbius, G., Schütze, E., *Chirurg*, 1967, **38**, 1.
228. Albrich, W., Schmid, K. O., Friehs, G., Köle, W., Seewann, H. L., *Virchows Arch. Abt. A*, 1973, **358**, 163.
229. Harrison, E. G., Jr, Bernatz, P. E., *Arch. Path.*, 1963, **75**, 284.
230. Holland, P. D. J., *personal communication* (*Dublin*), 1975.
231. Humpherys, S. R., Holley, K. E., Smith, L. H., McIlrath, D. C., *Mayo Clin. Proc.*, 1975, **50**, 317.
232. Denz, F. A., *J. Path. Bact.*, 1947, **59**, 575.
233. Flor, F. S., Pratt, J. H., Dahlin, D. C., *Amer. J. Obstet. Gynec.*, 1957, **73**, 1120.
234. Turner, D. R., *J. Anat.* (*Lond.*), 1969, **104**, 481.
235. Andreasen, E., Gottlieb, O., *Biol. Medd.* (*Kbh.*), 1946, **19**, 1.
236. Haferkamp, O., Rosenau, W., Lennert, K., *Arch. Path.*, 1971, **92**, 81.
237. Dorfman, R. F., Warnke, R., *Hum. Path.*, 1974, **5**, 519.

DEGENERATIVE AND OTHER MISCELLANEOUS CONDITIONS

238. Mackenzie, D. H., *Brit. med. J.*, 1963, **2**, 1449.
239. Symmers, W. St C., *unpublished observations*, 1966, 1972.
240. Sternberg, C., in *Handbuch der speziellen pathologischen Anatomie und Histologie*, edited by F. Henke and O. Lubarsch, vol. 1, part 1, page 265. Berlin, 1926.
241. Sternberg, C., *Verh. dtsch. path. Ges.*, 1905, **9**, 309.
242. Symmers, W. St. C., [Belfast], *unpublished observations*, *circa* 1905–15.
243 Osogoe, B., Courtice, F. C., *Aust. J. exp. Biol. med. Sci.*, 1968, **46**, 515.
244. Davies, J. D., Stansfeld, A. G., *J. clin. Path.*, 1972, **25**, 689.
245. Tanner, N. C., Symmers, W. St C., *unpublished observations*, 1968.
246. Bulloch, W., Schmorl, G., *Beitr. path. Anat.*, 1894, **16**, 247.
247. Sternberg, C., in *Handbuch der speziellen pathologischen Anatomie und Histologie*, edited by F. Henke and O. Lubarsch, vol. 1, part 1, page 308. Berlin, 1926.

LYMPHADENITIS AND OTHER 'REACTIVE' CHANGES IN LYMPH NODES

248. Rutishauser, E., Forouhar, B., *Schweiz. Z. allg. Path.*, 1957, **20**, 98.
249. Chears, W. C., Jr, Hargrove, M. D., Jr, Verner, J. V., Jr, Smith, A. G., Ruffin, J. M., *Amer. J. Med.*, 1961, **30**, 226.
250. Urban, H., *Fortschr. Röntgenstr.*, 1937, **55**, 231.
251. Brunck, H. J., *Frankfurt. Z. Path.*, 1959, **69**, 492.
252. Symmers, W. St C., *unpublished observations*, 1946.
253. Remmele, W., Lennert, K., *Beitr. Klin. Tuberk.*, 1957, **117**, 327.
254. Warner, N. E., Friedman, N. B., *Ann. intern. Med.*, 1956, **45**, 662.
255. Black, M. M., Speer, F. D., *Surg. Gynec. Obstet.*, 1958, **106**, 163.
256. Wartman, W. B., *Brit. J. Cancer*, 1959, **13**, 389.
257. Symmers, W. St C., *Amer. J. Path.*, 1951, **27**, 493.
258. Gorton, G., Linell, F., *Acta radiol.* (*Stockh.*), 1957, **47**, 381.
258a. Lennert, K., in *Handbuch der speziellen pathologischen Anatomie und Histologie*, edited by E. Uehlinger, vol. 1, part 3, book 1, pages 183–187. Berlin, Göttingen and Heidelberg, 1961.
259. Sieracki, J. C., Fisher, E. R., *Amer. J. clin. Path.*, 1973, **59**, 248.
260. Hamazaki, Y., *Virchows Arch. path. Anat.*, 1938, **301**, 490.
261. Wesenberg, W., *Arch. klin. exp. Derm.*, 1966, **227**, 101.
261a. Boyd, J. F., Valentine, J. C., *J. Path.*, 1970, **102**, 58.
262. Bull, T. B., James, K. R., *personal communication*, 1976.
263. Symmers, W. St C., *speculation*, 1949.
264. Rosai, J., Dorfman, R. F., *Cancer* (*Philad.*), 1972, **30**, 1174.
264a. Lampert, F., Lennert, K., *Cancer* (*Philad.*), 1976, **37**, 783.
264b. Destombes, P., *Bull. Soc. Path. exot.*, 1965, **58**, 1169.
264c. Rosai, J., Dorfman, R. F., *Arch. Path.*, 1969, **87**, 63.
265. Robb-Smith, A. H. T., in *Recent Advances in Clinical Pathology*, edited by S. C. Dyke, R. Cruickshank, E. N. Allott, B. L. Della Vida and A. H. T. Robb-Smith, chap. 34 [page 358]. London, 1947.
266. Symmers, W. St C., *unpublished observations*, 1970–76.

267. Sinclair-Smith, C. C., Kahn, L. B., Uys, C. J., *S. Afr. med. J.*, 1974, **48**, 451.
268. Lennert, K., Niedorf, H. R., Blümcke, S., Hardmeier, Th., *Virchows Arch. Abt. B*, 1972, **10**, 14.
269. Lennert, K., in *Handbuch der speziellen pathologischen Anatomie und Histologie*, edited by E. Uehlinger, vol. 1, part 3, book 1, pages 504–509. Berlin, Göttingen and Heidelberg, 1961.
269a. Lober, M., Rawlings, W., Newell, G. R., Reed, R. J., *Cancer (Philad.)*, 1973, **32**, 421.
270. Kinmonth, J. B., *Clin. Sci.*, 1952, **11**, 13.
271. Craig, J. O. M. C., in *A Textbook of Radiology*, 2nd edn, edited by D. Sutton and R. G. Grainger, chap. 32. Edinburgh, London and New York, 1975.
272. Dominok, G. W., *Virchows Arch. path. Anat.*, 1964, **338**, 143.
273. Ravel, R., *Amer. J. clin. Path.*, 1966, **46**, 335.
274. Ahmed, A., Greenwood, N., *J. Path.*, 1973, **111**, 207.
275. Towers, R. P., *J. clin. Path.*, 1957, **10**, 175.
276. Cabanne, F., Michiels, R., Dusserre, P., Bastien, H., Justrabo, E., *Ann. Anat. path.*, 1969, **14**, 419.
277. Cabanne, F., Chapuis, J.-L., Duperrat, B., Putelat, R., *Ann. Anat. path.*, 1966, **11**, 385.
278. Kagan, H. D., *Arch. Otolaryng.*, 1963, **78**, 663.
279. Nosanchuk, J. S., *Arch. Surg.*, 1968, **97**, 583.
280. Symmers, W. St C., *Brit. med. J.*, 1968, **3**, 19.
280a. Christie, A. J., *personal communication (Warren, Michigan)*, 1976.
281. Brock, J., *Dtsch. med. Wschr.*, 1948, **73**, 439.
282. Chevallier, P., Bernard, J., *Les Adénopathies inguinales*. Paris, 1932.
283. Vogels, C., Seeliger, H. P. R., *Med. Mschr.*, 1957, **11**, 648.
284. Bernstein, J. M., Carling, E. Rock, *Brit. med. J.*, 1909, **1**, 319.
285. Howe, C., Miller, W. R., *Ann. intern. Med.*, 1947, **26**, 93.
286. Mollaret, H. H., *Path. et Biol.*, 1971, **19**, 189.
287. Knapp, W., *Ergebn. Mikrobiol.*, 1959, **32**, 196.
288. Donat, R., *Zbl. allg. Path. path. Anat.*, 1952–53, **89**, 347.
289. Akazaki, K., Kozima, M., Hasegawa, H., Murata, J., Uegane, K., Koda, E., *Beitr. path. Anat.*, 1956, **116**, 200.
290. Schmidt, M. B., *Zbl. allg. Path. path. Anat.*, 1907, **18**, 593.
291. Story, P., Hanbury, W. J., *J. Path. Bact.*, 1957, **73**, 443.
292. Symmers, W. St C., *unpublished observations*, 1946–48.
293. Bojsen-Møller, J., *Acta path. microbiol. scand. B*, 1972, suppl. 229.
294. Seeliger, H. P. R., Meyer, V. F., Eyer, H., *Listeriosis*. New York, 1961.
295. Seeliger, H. P. R., Emmerling, P., Emmerling, H., *Dtsch. med. Wschr.*, 1968, **93**, 2037.
296. Murray, E. G. D., Webb, R. A., Swann, M. B. R., *J. Path. Bact.*, 1926, **29**, 407.
297. Gray, M. L., Killinger, A. H., *Bact. Rev.*, 1966, **30**, 309.
298. Hyslop, N. St. G., Osborne, A. D., *Vet. Rec.*, 1959, **71**, 1082.
299. Louria, D. B., Hensle, T., Armstrong, D., Collins, H. S., Blevins, A., Krugman, D., Buse, M., *Ann. intern. Med.*, 1967, **67**, 261.
300. Simpson, J. F., *J. Neurol. Neurosurg. Psychiat.*, 1971, **34**, 657.
301. Hood, M., *Pediatrics*, 1961, **27**, 390.

302. Reiss, H. J., Potel, J., Krebs, A., *Z. ges. inn. Med.*, 1951, **6**, 451.
303. Nyfeldt, A., *C.R. Soc. Biol. (Paris)*, 1929, **101**, 590.
304. Knott, F. A., Wright, G. Payling, Symmers, W. St C., *unpublished observations*, 1945–50.
305. Nyfeldt, A., *Zbl. Vet.-Med.*, 1958, Beiheft 1, 86.
306. Stanley, N. F., *Aust. J. exp. Biol. med. Sci.*, 1949, **27**, 133.
307. Taylor, L., Carslaw, R. W., *Lancet*, 1967, **1**, 1214.
308. Sternberg, C., in *Handbuch der speziellen pathologischen Anatomie und Histologie*, edited by F. Henke and O. Lubarsch, vol. 1, part 1, page 308. Berlin, 1926.
308a. Dutz, W., Kohout, E., in *Pathology Annual*, vol. 6, edited by S. C. Sommers, page 209. New York and London, 1971.
309. Klein, F., Walker, J. S., Fitzpatrick, D. F., Lincoln, R. E., Mahlandt, B. G., Jones, W. I., Dobbs, J. P., Hendrix, K. J., *J. infect. Dis.*, 1966, **116**, 123.
310. Symmers, W. St C., *unpublished observation*.
311. Smith, H., Stoner, H. B., *Fed. Proc.*, 1967, **26**, 1554.
312. Dalldorf, F. G., Beall, F. A., *Arch. Path.*, 1967, **83**, 154.
313. Wätjen, J., Reimann, W., *Beitr. path. Anat.*, 1937, **99**, 115.
314. Kettler, L.-H., *Virchows Arch. path. Anat.*, 1947, **314**, 358.
315. Günther, G. W., *Frankfurt. Z. Path.*, 1940, **54**, 550.
316. Dürck, H., *Beitr. path. Anat.*, 1904, **36**, suppl. 6, 1.
317. Masshoff, W., *Dtsch. med. Wschr.*, 1953, **78**, 532.
318. Vortel, V., Jindrák, K., Výmola, F., *Virchows Arch. path. Anat.*, 1958, **331**, 631.
319. Lennert, K., in *Handbuch der speziellen pathologischen Anatomie und Histologie*, edited by E. Uehlinger, vol. 1, part 3, book 1, page 217. Berlin, Göttingen and Heidelberg, 1961.
320. Hecker, W. C., *Arch. Kinderheilk.*, 1957, **156**, 151.
321. Symmers, W. St C., *unpublished observation*, 1967.
322. Elliot Smith, A., *personal communication (Oxford)*, 1969.
323. McCoy, G. W., *Publ. Hlth Bull. (Wash.)*, 1911, No. 43, 53.
324. McCoy, G. W., Chapin, C. W., *J. infect. Dis.*, 1912, **10**, 61.
325. Burroughs, A. L., Holdenried, R., Longanecker, D. S., Meyer, K. F., *J. infect. Dis.*, 1945, **76**, 115.
326. Wherry, W. B., Lamb, B. H., *J. infect. Dis.*, 1914, **15**, 331.
327. Jusatz, H. J., *Z. Hyg. Infekt.-Kr.*, 1961, **148**, 69.
328. Schulten, H., *Ergebn. inn. Med. Kinderheilk.*, 1945, **64**, 1160.
329. Brewis, E. G., Drennan, A. M., Mackie, T. J., Symmers, W. St C., *unpublished observations (Edinburgh)*, 1942–43.
330. Houston, T., Kane, F. F., M'Caw, I. H., *unpublished case (Belfast)*, 1941.
331. Peeney, A. L. P., Smallwood, H. M., Symmers, W. St C., *unpublished case (Birmingham)*, 1952.
332. Baker, W. H. J., Christie, D. R., Valteris, K., *personal communication (Hereford)*, 1976.
333. Ringertz, O., Dahlstrand, S., *Acta path. microbiol. scand.*, 1968, **72**, 464.
334. Overholt, E. L., Tigertt, W. D., Kadull, P. J., Ward, M. K., *Amer. J. Med.*, 1961, **30**, 785.
335. Collett, R., *Forh. Vidensk.-Selsk. (Kristiania)*, 1895, **3**, 1.
336. Thjøtta, T., *Bull. Hyg. (Lond.)*, 1931, **5**, 490.
337. Olin, G., *Bull. Off. int. Hyg. publ.*, 1938, **30**, 2804.

338. Ohara, H., *Zbl. Bakt., I. Abt. Orig.*, 1930, **117**, 440.
339. Dahlstrand, S., Ringertz, O., Zetterberg, B., *Scand. J. infect. Dis.*, 1971, **3**, 7.
340. Schuermann, H., Reich, H., *Arch. Derm. Syph. (Berl.)*, 1950, **190**, 579.
341. Meyer, M., *Z. Laryng. Rhinol.*, 1953, **32**, 525.
342. Randerath, E., *Virchows Arch. path. Anat.*, 1944, **312**, 165.
343. Francis, E., Callender, G. R., *Arch. Path. (Chic.)*, 1927, **3**, 577.
344. Starck, H. J., *Zbl. allg. Path. path. Anat.*, 1952–53, **89**, 233.
345. Albertini, A. von, Lieberherr, W., *Frankfurt. Z. Path.*, 1937, **51**, 69.
346. Janbon, M., Bertrand, L., *Rev. Prat. (Paris)*, 1955, **5**, 233.
347. Hendricks, S. L., *Amer. J. publ. Hlth*, 1955, **45**, 1282.
348. Bevan, L. E. W., *Trans. roy. Soc. trop. Med. Hyg.*, 1921–22, **15**, 215.
349. Bang, B., *Z. Thiermed.*, 1897, **1**, 241.
350. Bruce, D., *Practitioner*, 1887, **39**, 161
351. Zammit, T., in *Reports of the Commission Appointed by the Admiralty, the War Office, and the Civil Government of Malta, for the Investigation of Mediterranean Fever, under the Supervision of an Advisory Committee of the Royal Society*, part 3, page 83; part 4, page 96. London, 1905–07.
352. Galbraith, N. S., Ross, M. S., de Mowbray, R. R., Payne, D. J. H., *Brit. med. J.*, 1969, **1**, 612.
352a. Scottish Brucellosis Symposium, *Scot. med. J.*, 1976, **21**, 123.
353. Forbus, W. D., *Reaction to Injury—Pathology for Students of Disease Based on the Functional and Morphological Responses of Tissues to Injurious Agents*, [vol. 1] pages 641–649. Baltimore, 1943.
354. Parsons, P. B., Poston, M. A., *Sth. med. J. (Bgham, Ala.)*, 1939, **32**, 7.
355. Rabson, S. M., *Amer. J. clin. Path.*, 1939, **9**, 604.
356. Lennert, K., in *Handbuch der speziellen pathologischen Anatomie und Histologie*, edited by E. Uehlinger, vol. 1, part 3, book 1, page 296. Berlin, Göttingen and Heidelberg, 1961.
357. Michel-Béchet, R., Puig, R., Charvet, P., *Localisations viscérales et aspects chirurgicaux des brucelloses*. Paris, 1939.
358. Kerr, W. R., Coghlan, J. D., Payne, D. J. H., Robertson, L., *Lancet*, 1966, **2**, 1181.
358a. Leading Article, *Brit. med. J.*, 1977, **1**, 466.
359. Public Health Laboratory Service Working Party, *Lancet*, 1972, **1**, 676.
360. Murdock, C. R., Symmers, W. St C., *unpublished observations (Belfast)*, 1940–42.
360a. Donovan, C., *Indian med. Gaz.*, 1905, **40**, 411.
360b. Goldberg, J., *Brit. J. vener. Dis.*, 1959, **35**, 266.
360c. Rajam, R. V., Rangiah, P. N., *Donovanosis (Granuloma Inguinale, Granuloma Venereum)*. Geneva, 1954. [*Wld Hlth Org. Monogr. Ser.*, 1954, No. 24.]
360d. *Manual of Histologic Staining Methods of the Armed Forces Institute of Pathology*, 3rd edn, edited by L. G. Luna, chap. 9. New York, Toronto, London and Sydney, 1968.
361. Carter, G. R., *Advanc. vet. Sci.*, 1967, **11**, 321.
362. Hubbert, W. T., Rosen, M. N., *Amer. J. publ. Hlth*, 1970, **60**, 1103, 1109.
363. André, R., Dreyfus, B., *Bull. Soc. méd. Hôp. Paris*, 1952, **68**, 157.

364. Corry, D. C., Naftalin, J. M., Vollum, R. L., *unpublished case (Oxford)*, 1947.
365. Robins, G. D., *Stud. roy. Victoria Hosp., Montreal*, 1906, **2**, 1.
366. M'Fadyean, J., *J. comp. Path.*, 1904, **17**, 295.
367. Piggott, J. A., Hochholzer, L., *Arch. Path.*, 1970, **90**, 101.
368. Thin, R. N. T., Brown, M., Stewart, J. B., Garrett, C. J., *Quart. J. Med.*, 1970, N.S. **39**, 115.
369. Ranke, E., *Münch. med. Wschr.*, 1917, **64**, 305.
370. Parrot, J., *C.R. Soc. Biol. (Paris)*, 1876, sér. 6, **3**, 308.
371. Koch, R., *Dtsch. med. Wschr.*, 1891, **17**, 101, 1189.
372. Iles, P. B., Emerson, P. A., *Brit. med. J.*, 1974, **1**, 143.
373. Public Health Laboratory Service Report, *Brit. med. J.*, 1976, **1**, 658.
374. Calmette, A., *L'Infection bacillaire et la tuberculose chez l'homme et chez les animaux*. Paris, 1920.
375. Wolff, E., *Berl. klin. Wschr.*, 1912, **58**, 1531.
376. Tamura, M., Ogawa, G., Sagawa, I., Amano, S., *Amer. Rev. Tuberc.*, 1955, **71**, 465.
377. Ngu, V. A., in *Companion to Surgery in Africa*, edited by W. W. Davey. Edinburgh and London, 1968.
378. Hoda, S., Rab, S. M., *Brit. med. J.*, 1974, **3**, 786.
379. Brailey, M., *Bull. Johns Hopk. Hosp.*, 1937, **61**, 258.
380. Die Säuglingstuberkulose in Lübeck, *Arb. Reichsgesund.-Amte*, 1935, **69**, 1–406.
381. Rennke, H., Lennert, K., *Virchows Arch. Abt. A*, 1973, **358**, 241.
382. Trautmann, F. O. P., Trautmann, M., *Samml. selt. klin. Fälle*, 1955, **10**, 7.
383. Sachsse, B., *Folia haemat. (Lpz.)*, 1958, n.F. **2**, 212.
384. Koch, O., *Tuberk.-Arzt*, 1952, **6**, 67.
385. Landolt, R., *Statistische Betrachtungen über die Tuberkulosebefunde im Sektionsgut des Schweizerischen Forschungsinstitutes für Tuberkulose in Davos*. Inaug.-Diss., Zürich, 1955.
386. Beitzke, H., *Ergebn. ges. Tuberk.- u. Lung.-Forsch.*, 1953, **11**, 177.
387. Symmers, W. St C., *unpublished observation*, 1974.
388. Koch, R., *Dtsch. med. Wschr.*, 1897, **23**, 209.
389. Weiss, D. W., Wells, A. Q., *Amer. Rev. resp. Dis.*, 1960, **81**, 518.
390. Dubos, R., *Amer. Rev. resp. Dis.*, 1964, **90**, 505.
391. Webb, G. B., Williams, W. W., *J. Amer. med. Ass.*, 1911, **57**, 1431.
392. Medical Research Council Report, *Bull. Wld Hlth Org.*, 1972, **46**, 371.
393. Calmette, A., Guérin, C., *C.R. Acad. Sci. (Paris)*, 1909, **149**, 716.
394. Weill-Hallé, B., Turpin, R., *Bull. Soc. méd. Hôp. Paris*, 1925, **49**, 1589.
395. Hart, P. D'Arcy, *Brit. med. J.*, 1967, **1**, 587.
396. Calmette, A., Guérin, C., Boquet, A., Nègre, L., *La Vaccination préventive contre la tuberculose par le BCG*. Paris, 1927.
397. Wallgren, A., *J. Amer. med. Ass.*, 1928, **91**, 1876.
398. Kaplan, I., *Lancet*, 1966, **2**, 393.
399. Hsing, C. T., *Bull. Wld Hlth Org.*, 1954, **11**, 1023.
400. Stoppelman, M. R. H., Drion, E. F., *Ned. T. Geneesk.*, 1956, **100**, 2584.
401. Mande, R., Fillastre, C., Herrault, A., *Rev. Tuberc. (Paris)*, 1958, **22**, 165.
402. Holm, J., *Publ. Hlth Rep. (Wash.)*, 1946, **61**, 1298.
403. Carlgren, L. E., Hansson, C. G., Henricsson, L., Wåhlén, P., *Acta paediat. (Uppsala)*, 1966, **55**, 636.

404. Symmers, W. St C., in *Drug-Induced Diseases—Second Symposium Organized by the Boerhaave Courses for Post-Graduate Medical Education, State University of Leyden, October 1964*, edited by L. Meyler and H. M. Peck, page 108 [Case 2]. Amsterdam, New York, London, Milan, Tokyo and Buenos Aires, 1965.

405. Kaiserling, E., Lennert, K., Nitsch, K., Drescher, J., *Virchows Arch. Abt. A*, 1972, **355**, 333.

406. Desikan, K. V., Job, C. K., *Int. J. Leprosy*, 1966, **34**, 147.

407. Miller, J., *J. Path. Bact.*, 1905, **10**, i.

408. Keay, A. J., *Tubercle (Edinb.)*, 1969, **50**, suppl., 85.

409. Runyon, E. H., *Med. Clin. N. Amer.*, 1959, **43**, 273.

410. Cruickshank, R., *personal communication (Edinburgh)*, 1973.

411. Tacquet, A., Devulder, B., Tison, F., *Maroc méd.*, 1966, **45**, 501.

412. Nnochiri, E., *personal communication (London)*, 1972.

413. Seldam, R. E. J. ten, *personal communication (Perth, Western Australia)*, 1969.

414. Marks, J., *Tubercle (Edinb.)*, 1969, **50**, suppl., 78.

415. Morris, C. A., Grant, G. H., Everall, P. H., Myres, A. T. M., *J. clin. Path.*, 1973, **26**, 422.

416. Büngeler, W., *Virchows Arch. path. Anat.*, 1943, **310**, 566.

417. Virchow, R., *Die krankhaften Geschwülste*. Berlin, 1863. [Translation of part relating to leprosy: Fite, G. L., *Int. J. Leprosy*, 1954, **22**, 71, 205 (Virchow's account of the characteristic cells is on pages 207–209).]

417a. Herxheimer, G., *Virchows Arch. path. Anat.*, 1923, **245**, 403.

418. Neisser, A., *Breslau. aerztl. Z.*, 1879, **1**, 200.

419. Cowdry, E. V., *Amer. J. Path.*, 1940, **16**, 103.

420. Furniss, A. L., *Indian J. med. Sci.*, 1953, **7**, 475.

421. Hamazaki, Y., *Acta path. jap.*, 1950, **1**, 1.

422. Kirsch, E., *Virchows Arch. path. Anat.*, 1950, **317**, 602.

423. Ridley, D. S., Jopling, W. H., *Int. J. Leprosy*, 1966, **34**, 255.

424. Symmers, W. St C., *Brit. med. J.*, 1970, **4**, 763 [Cases 3–5].

425. Purchase, H. S., *J. comp. Path.*, 1944, **54**, 238.

426. Magnusson, H., *Vet. Rec.*, 1938, **50**, 1459.

427. Bull, L. B., Dickinson, C. G., *Aust. vet. J.*, 1935, **11**, 126.

428. Blackwell, J. B., Smith, F. H., Joyce, P. R., *Pathology*, 1974, **6**, 243.

429. Symmers, W. St C., *unpublished observations*, 1975–76.

430. Leading Article, *Brit. med. J.*, 1970, **4**, 67.

431. Hartsock, R. J., Halling, L. W., King, F. M., *Amer. J. clin. Path.*, 1970, **53**, 304.

432. Turner, D. R., Wright, D. J. M., *J. Path.*, 1973, **110**, 305.

433. Wassermann, A., Neisser, A., Bruck, C., *Dtsch. med. Wschr.*, 1906, **32**, 745.

434. Cummer, C. L., *Amer. J. Syph.*, 1928, **12**, 13.

435. Gaedeke, R., *Arch. Derm. Syph. (Berl.)*, 1948, **186**, 612.

436. Schneider, P., *Verh. dtsch. Ges. Path.*, 1928, **23**, 177.

437. Symmers, W. St C., in *Systemic Mycoses—A Ciba Foundation Symposium: In Commemoration of William Balfour Baikie*, edited by G. E. W. Wolstenholme and R. Porter, page 26. London, 1968.

438. Symmers, W. St C., in *Anatomic and Clinical Pathology—Proceedings of the VIII World Congress of Anatomic and Clinical Pathology: Munich, 12–16 September 1972*, edited by M. Nordmann, R. Merten and H. Lommel, page 255. Amsterdam and New York, 1973.

439. Symmers, W. St C., in *Opportunistic Fungal Infections—Proceedings of the Second International Conference*, edited by E. W. Chick, A. Balows and M. L. Furcolow, chap. 23. Springfield, Illinois, 1975.

440. Fetter, B. F., *Arch. Path.*, 1961, **71**, 416.

441. Grocott, R. G., *Amer. J. clin. Path.*, 1955, **25**, 975.

442. Symmers, W. St C., *Curiosa—A Miscellany of Clinical and Pathological Experiences*, chapters 1–4. London, 1974.

443. Flamm, H., Jonas, R., *Wien. klin. Wschr.*, 1956, **68**, 671.

444. Shrewsbury, J. F. D., *personal communication (Birmingham)*, 1948.

445. Symmers, W. St C., *Amer. J. clin. Path.*, 1966, **46**, 514 [Cases 31 and 32].

446. Symmers, W. St C., *Amer. J. clin. Path.*, 1966, **46**, 514 [Case 14].

447. Symmers, W. St C., in *Drug-Induced Diseases—Second Symposium Organized by the Boerhaave Courses for Post-Graduate Medical Education, State University of Leyden, October 1964*, edited by L. Meyler and H. M. Peck, page 108 [page 113, para. (b)]. Amsterdam, New York, London, Milan, Tokyo and Buenos Aires, 1965.

448. Symmers, W. St C., *Curiosa—A Miscellany of Clinical and Pathological Experiences*, chap. 23. London, 1974.

449. Majocchi, D., *Boll. real. Accad. med. Roma*, 1883, **9**, 220.

450. Mikhail, G. R., *Int. J. Derm.*, 1970, **9**, 41.

451. Okudaira, M., *Acta path. jap.*, 1956, **6**, 207 [Case 8].

452. Bénard, P., Drouhet, E., Nadal, C., René-Corail, L., *Sem. thér.*, 1961, **37**, 133.

453. Marton, K., Cherid, A., *Int. J. Derm.*, 1973, **12**, 295.

454. Symmers, W. St C., *personal observations*, 1954–74.

454a. Tolentino, P., Borrone, C., *Scand. J. infect. Dis.*, 1976, **8**, 61.

455. MacGillivray, J. B., *J. clin. Path.*, 1966, **19**, 424.

455a. Talerman, A., Bradley, J. M., Woodland, B., *J. med. Microbiol.*, 1970, **3**, 633.

456. Dangerfield, L. F., Gear, J., *S. Afr. med. J.*, 1941, **15**, 128.

457. Helm, M. A. F., Berman, C., in *Sporotrichosis Infection on Mines of the Witwatersrand—A Symposium*, page 59. Johannesburg, 1947.

458. Du Toit, C. J., *Proc. Mine med. Offrs' Ass.*, 1942, **22**, 111.

459. Tsai, C. Y., Lu, C., Wang, L. T., Hsu, T. L., Sung, J. L., *Amer. J. clin. Path.*, 1966, **46**, 99.

460. Ajello, A., in *Histoplasmosis—Proceedings of the Second National Conference Held at the Center for Disease Control, Atlanta, Georgia*, edited by L. Ajello, E. W. Chick, M. L. Furcolow and A. Balows, chap. 15. Springfield, Illinois, 1971.

461. Straub, M., Schwarz, J., *Amer. J. clin. Path.*, 1955, **25**, 727.

462. Dovenbarger, W. V., Tsubura, E., Schwarz, J., Baum, G. L., *J. thorac. cardiovasc. Surg.*, 1961, **42**, 193.

463. Tesh, R. B., Schneidau, J. D., Jr, *New Engl. J. Med.*, 1966, **275**, 597.

464. Zung-Pah Woo, Reimann, H. A., *J. Amer. med. Ass.*, 1957, **164**, 1092.
465. Cockshott, W. P., Lucas, A. O., *Quart. J. Med.*, 1964, N.S. **33**, 223.
466. Drouhet, E., *Ann. Soc. belge Méd. trop.*, 1972, **52**, 391.
467. Fiese, M. J., *Coccidioidomycosis*, pages 111 and 141. Springfield, Illinois, 1958.
468. Wilson, J. W., Smith, C. E., Plunkett, O. A., *Calif. Med.*, 1953, **79**, 233.
469. Vaněk, J., Schwarz, J., Hakim, S., *Amer. J. clin. Path.*, 1970, **54**, 384.
470. Wilson, J. W., Cawley, E. P., Weidman, F. D., Gilmer, W. S., *A.M.A. Arch. Derm.*, 1955, **71**, 39.
471. Yarzábal, L. A., in *Paracoccidioidomycosis—Proceedings of the First Pan American Symposium, 25–27 October 1971, Medellín, Colombia*, page 261. Washington, D.C., 1972.
472. Salfelder, K., Doehnert, G., Doehnert, H.-R., *Virchows Arch. Abt. A*, 1969, **348**, 51.
473. Lutz, A., *Brazil-med.*, 1908, **22**, 121, 141.
474. Costa, P. D. da, Oliveira, N. C. de, Picanço, M., Guedes e Silva, J. B., *Hospital (Rio de J.)*, 1970, **77**, 805.
475. Bettarello, A., Magaldi, C., Amato Netto, V., *Rev. Hosp. Clín. Fac. Med. S. Paulo*, 1972, **27**, 245.
476. Lôbo, J., *Rev. méd. Pernambuco*, 1931, **1**, 763.
477. Wiersema, J. P., in *Human Infection with Fungi, Actinomycetes and Algae*, edited by R. D. Baker, page 577. New York, Heidelberg and Berlin, 1971.
478. Destombes, P., Ravisse, P., *Bull. Soc. Path. exot.*, 1964, **57**, 1018.
479. Caldwell, D. K., Caldwell, M. C., Woodard, J. C., Ajello, L., Kaplan, W., McClure, H. M., *Amer. J. trop. Med. Hyg.*, 1975, **24**, 105.
480. Symmers, W. St C., *unpublished observation*, 1976.
481. Symmers, W. St C., *Amer. J. clin. Path.*, 1966, **46**, 514 [Case 9].
482. Lie Kian Joe, Njo-Injo Tjoei Eng, Pohan, A., Meulen, H. van der, Emmons, C. W., *A.M.A. Arch. Derm.*, 1956, **74**, 378.
483. Symmers, W. St C., *Proc. roy. Soc. Med.*, 1964, **57**, 405 [Fig. 1].
484. Symmers, W. St C., *Ann. Soc. belge Méd. trop.*, 1972, **52**, 365 [Fig. 16].
485. Symmers, W. St C., *Ann. Soc. belge Méd. trop.*, 1972, **52**, 365 [Fig. 32].
486. Symmers, W. St C., in *Drug-Induced Diseases—Second Symposium Organized by the Boerhaave Courses for Post-Graduate Medical Education, State University of Leyden, October 1964*, edited by L. Meyler and H. M. Peck, page 108 [Case 6]. Amsterdam, New York, London, Milan, Tokyo and Buenos Aires, 1965.
487. Brandsberg, J. W., Tosh, T. E., Furcolow, M. L., *New Engl. J. Med.*, 1964, **270**, 874.
488. Symmers, W. St C., *unpublished observations*, 1967, 1972.
489. Lacaz, C. da S., Ferri, R. G., Raphael, A., Fava Netto, C., Minami, P. S., Castro, R. M., Dillon, N. L., *Hospital (Rio de J.)*, 1967, **71**, 7.
490. Angulo O., A., Carbonell, L., *Mycopathologia (Den Haag)*, 1961, **15**, 61.
491. Winn, W. A., *personal communication (Springville, California)*, 1965.
492. Henderson, D. W., Humeniuk, V., Meadows, R., Forbes, I. J., *Pathology*, 1974, **6**, 235.

493. Fetter, B. F., Klintworth, G. K., Nielsen, H. S., Jr, in *Human Infection with Fungi, Actinomycetes and Algae*, edited by R. D. Baker, page 1081. New York, Heidelberg and Berlin, 1971.
494. Sudman, M. S., *Amer. J. clin. Path.*, 1974, **61**, 10.
494a. Davies, R. R., Wilkinson, J. L., *Ann. trop. Med. Parasit.*, 1967, **61**, 112.
494b. Symmers, W. St C., in *Anatomic and Clinical Pathology—Proceedings of the VIII World Congress of Anatomic and Clinical Pathology: Munich, 12–16 September 1972*, edited by M. Nordmann, R. Merten and H. Lommel, page 255 [Fig. 6]. Amsterdam and New York, 1973.
495. Brill, N. E., *Amer. J. med. Sci.*, 1910, **139**, 484.
496. Zinsser, H., *Amer. J. Hyg.*, 1934, **20**, 513.
497. Traub, R., Wisseman, C. L., *Bull. Wld Hlth. Org.*, 1968, **39**, 209.
498. Lackman, D. B., *Clin. Pediat. (Philad.)*, 1963, **2**, 296.
499. Ash, J. E., *Amer. J. trop. Med.*, 1947, **27**, 483.
500. Eshchar, J., Waron, M., Alkan, W. J., *J. Amer. med. Ass.*, 1966, **195**, 390.
501. Whittick, J. W., *Brit. med. J.*, 1950, **1**, 979.
502. Page, L. A., *Int. J. system. Bact.*, 1966, **16**, 223.
503. Jones, H., Rake, G., Stearns, B., *J. infect. Dis.*, 1945, **76**, 55.
504. Meyer, K. F., *Ann. N.Y. Acad. Sci.*, 1953, **56**, 545.
505. Durand, Nicolas, J., Favre, *Bull. Soc. méd. Hôp. Paris*, 1913, 3. sér., **35**, 274.
506. Frei, W. S., *Klin. Wschr.*, 1925, **4**, 2148.
507. Smith, E. B., Custer, R. P., *J. Urol. (Baltimore)*, 1950, **63**, 546.
508. Favre, M., *Ann. Derm. Syph. (Paris)*, 1949, 8. sér., **9**, 249.
509. Stewart, D. B., in *Lymphogranuloma Venereum—Epidemiological, Clinical, Surgical and Therapeutic Aspects Based on a Study in the Caribbean*, edited by M. M. Sigel, chap. 6. Coral Gables, Florida, 1962.
510. Jørgensen, L., *Acta path. microbiol. scand.*, 1959, **47**, 113.
511. Hellerström, S., *Acta derm.-venereol. (Stockh.)*, 1929, suppl. 1.
512. Hamperl, H., *personal communication (Bonn)*, 1974.
513. Miyagawa, Y., Mitamura, T., Yaoi, H., Ishii, N., Okanishi, J., *Jap. J. exp. Med.*, 1935, **13**, 1.
514. Gamna, C., *Presse méd.*, 1924, **32**, 404.
515. Favre, M., *Presse méd.*, 1924, **32**, 651.
516. Debré, R., Job, J.-C., *Acta paediat. (Uppsala)*, 1954, **43**, suppl. 96.
517. Gsell, O., Gsell-Busse, M., *Ergebn. inn. Med. Kinderheilk.*, 1957, n.F. **9**, 76.
518. Gräff, S., *Mschr. Kinderheilk.*, 1954, **102**, 232.
519. Mollaret, P., Reilly, J., Bastin, R., Tournier, P., *Bull. Soc. méd. Hôp. Paris*, 1950, **66**, 424.
520. Wegman, T., Usteri, C., Hedinger, C., *Schweiz. med. Wschr.*, 1951, **81**, 853.
521. Daniels, W. B., MacMurray, F. G., *Ann. intern. Med.*, 1952, **37**, 697.
522. Floros, A., *Wien. klin. Wschr.*, 1952, **64**, 963.
523. Debré, R., Lamy, M., Jammet, M.-L., Costil, L., Mozziconacci, P., *Bull. Soc. méd. Hôp. Paris*, 1950, **66**, 76.
524. Foshay, L., *Lancet*, 1952, **1**, 673.
525. Daniels, W. B., MacMurray, F. G., *J. Amer. med. Ass.*, 1954, **154**, 1247.
526. Lennert, K., in *Handbuch der speziellen pathologischen*

Anatomie und Histologie, edited by E. Uehlinger, vol. 1, part 3, book 1, page 234. Berlin, Göttingen and Heidelberg, 1961.

527. Symmers, W. St C., *unpublished observations*, 1946–75.

528. Usteri, C., Wegmann, T., Hedinger, C., *Schweiz. med. Wschr.*, 1952, **82**, 1287.

529. Peeney, A. L. P., Shrewsbury, J. F. D., Symmers, W. St C., Thomson, A. P. D., *unpublished observations*, 1950.

530. Mollaret, P., Reilly, J., Bastin, R., Tournier, P., *Presse méd.*, 1951, **59**, 701.

531. Petzetakis, M., *Zbl. Bakt.*, *I. Abt. Orig.*, 1937, **139**, 397.

532. Guttmann, P. H., *Calif. Med.*, 1955, **82**, 25.

533. Boyd, G. L., Craig, G., *J. Pediat.*, 1961, **59**, 313.

534. Epstein, M. A., Achong, B. G., in *Burkitt's Lymphoma*, edited by D. P. Burkitt and D. H. Wright, chap. 22. Edinburgh and London, 1970.

535. Henle, G., Henle, W., Diehl, V., *Proc. nat. Acad. Sci. (Wash.)*, 1968, **59**, 94.

536. Warthin, A. S., *Arch. Path. (Chic.)*, 1931, **11**, 864.

536a. Finkeldey, W., *Virchows Arch. path. Anat.*, 1931, **281**, 323.

537. Ciaccio, C., *Virchows Arch. path. Anat.*, 1910, **199**, 378.

538. Alagna, G., *Arch. Laryng. Rhin. (Berl.)*, 1911, **25**, 527.

538a. Eck, H., *Frankfurt. Z. Path.*, 1944, **58**, 147.

539. Symmers, W. St C., *Curiosa—A Miscellany of Clinical and Pathological Experiences*, chap. 5. London, 1974.

539a. Dorfman, R. F., Herweg, J. C., *J. Amer. med. Ass.*, 1966, **198**, 230.

540. Lennert, K., in *Handbuch der speziellen pathologischen Anatomie und Histologie*, edited by E. Uehlinger, vol. 1, part 3, book 1, page 336. Berlin, Göttingen and Heidelberg, 1961.

541. Sommers, S. C., Wilson, J. C., Hartman, F. W., *J. exp. Med.*, 1951, **93**, 505.

542. Joklik, W. K., *Ann. Rev. Microbiol.*, 1968, **22**, 305.

543. Evans, W. E. D., *unpublished observations (Charing Cross Hospital Medical School, London)*, 1960.

544. Lukes, R. J., Collins, R. D., *Brit. J. Cancer*, 1975, **31**, suppl. 2, 1.

545. Hartsock, R. J., *Cancer (Philad.)*, 1968, **21**, 632.

546. Symmers, W. St C., *unpublished observations*, 1966–75.

547. Bartley, E. O., Biggart, J. H., Blair, E. M. McV., Graham, N. C., Hickey, E. M., Houston, T., McCoy, J. H., Reilly, L. V., Smyth, J. A., Symmers, W. St C., Wilson, W. J., *unpublished observation (Belfast)*, 1940.

548. Verlinde, J. D., *T. Diergeneesk.*, 1951, **76**, 334.

549. Büttner, D., Giese, H., Müller, G., Peters, D., *Arch. ges. Virusforsch.*, 1964, **14**, 657.

550. Symmers, W. St C., Webster, J. M., *unpublished observation (Birmingham)*, 1950.

551. Tomlinson, T. H., Jr, *Amer. J. Path.*, 1939, **15**, 523.

552. Fruhling, L., Sacrez, R., Le Gal, Y., Porte, P., Dorner, M., *Ann. Anat. path.*, 1959, N.S. **4**, 574.

553. Seifert, G., Oehme, J., *Pathologie und Klinik der Cytomegalie*, page 32. Leipzig, 1957.

554. Klemola, E., *Ann. intern. Med.*, 1973, **79**, 267.

555. Jordan, M. C., Rousseau, W. E., Stewart, J. A., Noble, G. R., Chin, T. D. Y., *Ann. intern. Med.*, 1973, **79**, 153.

556. Kantor, G. L., Goldberg, L. S., *Semin. Hemat.*, 1971, **8**, 261.

557. Pfeiffer, E., *Jb. Kinderheilk.*, 1889, **29**, 257.

558. Filatov, N. F., [*Lectures on Acute Infectious Diseases of Children*—in Russian], vol. 1, page 13. Moscow, 1885. [German translation: *Vorlesungen über acute Infectionskrankheiten im Kindesalter—autorisierte, vom Verfasser ergänzte deutsche Ausgabe*, translated from the 2nd Russian edition by L. Polonsky; Vienna and Leipzig, 1897.]

559. Türk, W., *Wien. med. Wschr.*, 1907, **20**, 157.

559a. Sprunt, T. P., Evans, F. A., *Bull. Johns Hopk. Hosp.*, 1920, **31**, 410.

560. Paul, J. R., Bunnell, W. W., *Amer. J. med. Sci.*, 1932, **183**, 90.

561. Davidsohn, I., *Amer. J. Dis. Child.*, 1935, **49**, 1222.

562. Niederman, J. C., McCollum, R. W., Henle, G., Henle, W., *J. Amer. med. Ass.*, 1968, **203**, 205.

563. Hubler, W. L., Bailey, A. A., Campbell, D. C., Mathieson, D. R., *Proc. Mayo Clin.*, 1951, **26**, 313.

564. Reske-Nielsen, E., Mogensen, E. F., *Acta haemat. (Basel)*, 1955, **13**, 387.

565. Finch, S. C., in *Infectious Mononucleosis*, edited by R. L. Carter and H. G. Penman, chap. 2. Oxford and Edinburgh, 1969.

566. Marshall, S., Millingen, K. S., *Brit. med. J.*, 1952, **1**, 1325.

567. Worlledge, S. M., Dacie, J. V., in *Infectious Mononucleosis*, edited by R. L. Carter and H. G. Penman, chap. 5. Oxford and Edinburgh, 1969.

568. Damashek, W., in *Infectious Mononucleosis*, edited by R. L. Carter and H. G. Penman, chap. 13. Oxford and Edinburgh, 1969.

569. Greaves, M. F., Owen, J. J. T., Raff, M. C., *T and B Lymphocytes: Origins, Properties and Roles in Immune Responses*, page 74. Amsterdam and New York, 1974.

570. Shisido, A., Honjo, S., Suganuma, M., Ohtaki, S., Hikita, M., Fijuwara, T., Takasaka, M., *Jap. J. med. Sci. Biol.*, 1965, **18**, 73.

571. Grient, A. J. van der, in *Side Effects of Drugs—A Survey of Unwanted Effects of Drugs Reported in 1965–1967*, vol. 6, edited by L. Meyler and A. Herxheimer, page 242. Amsterdam, 1968.

572. Citron, K. M., in *Side Effects of Drugs—A Survey of Unwanted Effects of Drugs Reported in 1968–1971*, vol. 7, edited by L. Meyler and A. Herxheimer, page 429. Amsterdam, 1972.

573. Hoagland, R. J., *Infectious Mononucleosis*. New York and London, 1967.

574. Wood, T. A., Frenkel, E. P., *Amer. J. Med.*, 1967, **43**, 923.

575. Wulff, H. R., *Scand. J. Haemat.*, 1965, **2**, 179.

576. Sharp, A. A., in *Infectious Mononucleosis*, edited by R. L. Carter and H. G. Penman, chap. 6. Oxford, 1969.

577. Baron, D. N., Bell, J. L., Dunnet, W. N., *J. clin. Path.*, 1965, **18**, 209.

578. Kilpatrick, Z. M., *Arch. intern. Med.*, 1966, **117**, 47.

579. Webster, S. G. P., *Brit. med. J.*, 1968, **2**, 411.

580. Lennert, K., in *Handbuch der speziellen pathologischen Anatomie und Histologie*, edited by E. Uehlinger, vol. 1, part 3, book 1, page 326. Berlin, Göttingen and Heidelberg, 1961.

580a. Gowing, N. F. C., in *Pathology Annual*, vol. 10, edited by S. C. Sommers, page 1. New York, 1975.

581. Gall, E. A., Stout, H. A., *Amer. J. Path.*, 1940, **16**, 433.

582. Lennert, K., *Verh. dtsch. Ges. Path.*, 1959, **42**, 203.

583. Symmers, W. St C., *unpublished observations*, 1975–76.

584. Symmers, W. St C., in *Systemic Pathology*, 1st edn, edited by G. Payling Wright and W. St C. Symmers, vol. 1, page 228. London, 1966.

585. Marinesco, G., *La Lymphocytose infectieuse aigue*. Paris, 1965.

586. Smith, C. H., *Amer. J. Dis. Child.*, 1941, **62**, 231.

587. Dunn, H. G., *Brit. med. J.*, 1952, **1**, 78.

588. Meyer, J. M., *Amer. J. clin. Path.*, 1946, **16**, 244.

589. Olson, L. C., Miller, G., Hanshaw, J. B., *Lancet*, 1964, **1**, 200.

590. Areán, V. M., Echevarría, R., in *Pathology of Protozoal and Helminthic Diseases with Clinical Correlation*, edited by R. A. Marcial-Rojas and E. Moreno, chap. 12. Baltimore, 1971.

591. Frenkel, J. K., in *Pathology of Protozoal and Helminthic Diseases with Clinical Correlation*, edited by R. A. Marcial-Rojas and E. Moreno, chap. 13. Baltimore, 1971.

592. Frenkel, J. K., in *The Coccidia*—Eimeria, Isospora, Toxoplasma, *and Related Genera*, edited by D. M. Hammond and P. L. Long, chap. 9. Baltimore and London, 1973.

593. Nicolle, C., Manceaux, L., *C.R. Acad. Sci. (Paris)*, 1908, **147**, 763.

594. Splendore, A., *Rev. Soc. Sci. S. Paulo*, 1908, **3**, 109.

595. Janků, J., *Čas. Lék. čes.*, 1923, **62**, 1021.

596. Wolf, A., Cowen, D., *Bull. neurol. Inst. N.Y.*, 1937, **6**, 306.

597. Siim, J. C., *J. Amer. med. Ass.*, 1951, **147**, 1641.

598. Siim, J. C., *Ann. N.Y. Acad. Sci.*, 1956, **64**, 185.

599. Beattie, C. P., in *Recent Advances in Medical Microbiology*, edited by A. P. Waterson, chap. 9. London, 1967.

600. Desmonts, G., Couvreur, J., Ben-Rachid, M. S., *Arch. franç. Pédiat.*, 1965, **22**, 1183.

601. Desmonts, G., in *Toxoplasmosis*, edited by D. Hentsch, page 137. Bern, 1971.

602. Frenkel, J. K., in *Pathology of the Nervous System*, edited by J. Minckler, vol. 3, page 2521. New York, 1972.

603. Feldman, H. A., *Amer. J. Dis. Child.*, 1953, **86**, 487.

604. Sabin, A. B., Eichenwald, H., Feldman, H. A., Jacobs, L., *J. Amer. med. Ass.*, 1952, **150**, 1063.

605. Alexander, C. M., Callister, J. W., *A.M.A. Arch. Path.*, 1955, **60**, 563.

606. Garcia, A. G. P., *Arch. Dis. Childh.*, 1968, **43**, 705.

607. Sever, J. L., Berendes, H., Weiss, W., Drage, J. S., Hardy, J., Gilkeson, M. R., Roberts, J. M., in *Prevention of Mental Retardation through Control of Infectious Disease*, edited by H. Eichenwald, page 37. Washington, D.C., 1966.

608. Frenkel, J. K., in *Comparative Aspects of Reproductive Failure*, edited by K. Benirschke, page 279. Berlin, Heidelberg and New York, 1967.

609. Durge, N. G., Baqai, M. U., Ward, R., *Lancet*, 1967, **2**, 155.

610. Chandar, K., Mair, H. J., Mair, N. S., *Brit. med. J.*, 1968, **1**, 158.

611. Hooper, A. D., *A.M.A. Arch. Path.*, 1957, **64**, 1.

612. Vischer, T. L., Bernheim, C., Engelbrecht, E., *Lancet*, 1967, **2**, 919.

613. Kalderon, A. E., Kikkawa, Y., Bernstein, J., *Arch. intern. Med.*, 1964, **114**, 95.

614. Bobowski, S. J., Reed, W. G., *A.M.A. Arch. Path.*, 1958, **65**, 460.

615. Zimmerman, L. E., *Surv. Ophthal.*, 1961, **6**, 832.

616. Couvreur, J., Desmonts, G., *Develop. Med. Child Neurol.*, 1962, **4**, 519.

616a. Longmore, H. J. A., *Brit. med. J.*, 1977, **1**, 490.

617. Bernard, J., Boiron, M., Levy, J. P., Ripault, J., Desmonts, G., *Nouv. Rev. franç. Hémat.*, 1962, **2**, 910.

618. Cheever, A. W., Valsamis, M. P., Rabson, A. S., *New Engl. J. Med.*, 1965, **272**, 26.

619. Symmers, W. St C., *Curiosa—A Miscellany of Clinical and Pathological Experiences*, chap. 25. London, 1974.

620. Reynolds, E. S., Walls, K. W., Pfeiffer, R. I., *Arch. intern. Med.*, 1966, **118**, 401.

621. Robb-Smith, A. H. T., in *Recent Advances in Clinical Pathology*, edited by S. C. Dyke, R. Cruickshank, E. N. Allott, B. L. Della Vida and A. H. T. Robb-Smith, chap. 34. London, 1947.

622. Piringer-Kuchinka, A., *Verh. dtsch. Ges. Path.*, 1953, **36**, 352.

623. Bamler, H., Schulthess, G. von, *Schweiz. med. Wschr.*, 1955, **85**, 1070.

624. Lennert, K., in *Handbuch der speziellen pathologischen Anatomie und Histologie*, edited by E. Uehlinger, vol. 1, part 3, book 1, page 343. Berlin, Göttingen and Heidelberg, 1961.

625. Piringer-Kuchinka, A., Martin, I., Thalhammer, O., *Virchows Arch. path. Anat.*, 1958, **331**, 522.

626. Roth, F., Piekarski, G., *Virchows Arch. path. Anat.*, 1959, **332**, 181.

626a. Beverley, J. K. A., Fleck, D. G., Kwantes, W., Ludlam, G. B., *J. Hyg. (Lond.)*, 1976, **76**, 215.

627. Stansfeld, A. G., *J. clin. Path.*, 1961, **14**, 565.

628. Sabin, A. B., Feldman, H. A., *Science*, 1948, **108**, 660.

629. Desmonts, G., Couvreur, J., Alison, F., Baudelot, J., Gerbeaux, J., Lelong, M., *Rev. franç. Étud. clin. biol.*, 1965, **10**, 952.

630. Kean, B. H., Kimball, A. C., Christenson, W. N., *J. Amer. med. Ass.*, 1969, **208**, 1002.

631. Jacobs, L., *Advanc. Parasit.*, 1967, **5**, 1.

632. Jacobs, L., *Ann. Rev. Microbiol.*, 1963, **17**, 429.

633. Hutchison, W. M., Dunachie, J. F., Work, K., *Acta path. microbiol. scand.*, 1968, **74**, 462.

634. Frenkel, J. K., Dubey, J. P., Miller, N. L., *Science*, 1970, **167**, 893.

635. Sabin, A. B., *Advanc. Pediat.*, 1942, **1**, 1.

636. Frenkel, J. K., Weber, R. W., Lunde, M. N., *J. Amer. med. Ass.*, 1960, **173**, 1471.

637. Neu, H. C., *J. Amer. med. Ass.*, 1967, **202**, 844.

638. Siegel, S. E., Lunde, M. N., Gelderman, A. H., Halterman, R. H., Brown, J. A., Levine, A. S., Graw, R. G., *Blood*, 1971, **37**, 388.

639. Levi, G. C., Hyakutake, S., Amato, V., Correa, M. O. A., *Rev. Soc. bras. Med. trop.*, 1968, **2**, 275.

640. Rommel, M., Breuning, J., *Berl. Münch. tierärztl. Wschr.*, 1967, **80**, 365.

641. Minter, D. M., in *Manson's Tropical Diseases*, 17th edn, edited by C. Wilcocks and P. E. C. Manson-Bahr, page 1072. London, 1972.

642. Adler, S., Foner, A., Montiglio, B., *Trans. roy. Soc. trop. Med. Hyg.*, 1966, **60**, 380.

643. Lacaz, C. da S., Baruzzi, R. G., Siqueira, W., Jr, *Introdução à Geografia médica do Brasil*, page 274. São Paulo, 1972.

644. Manson-Bahr, P. E. C., *Trans. roy. Soc. trop. Med. Hyg.*, 1959, **53**, 123, 136.

645. Bhattacharyya, M. N., *Indian J. med. Sci.*, 1955, **10**, 602.
646. Moškovskij, S. D., Duhanina, N. N., *Bull. Wld Hlth Org.*, 1971, **44**, 529.
647. Chung, H. L., *Chin. med. J.*, 1953, **71**, 421.
648. Das Gupta, N. N., Guha, A., De, N., *Exp. Cell Res.*, 1954, **6**, 353.
649. Sen Gupta, P. C., Mukherjee, A. M., *J. Indian med. Ass.*, 1968, **50**, 1.
650. Angevine, D. M., Hamilton, T. R., Wallace, F. G., Hazard, J. B., *Amer. J. med. Sci.*, 1945, **210**, 33.
651. Fenech, F. F., Xuereb, G. P., *personal communication (Malta)*, 1970.
652. Cachia, E. A., Fenech, F. F., *Trans. roy. Soc. trop. Med. Hyg.*, 1964, **58**, 234.
653. Bassett-Smith, P. W., *Brit. med. J.*, 1914, **2**, 1058.
654. Lipscomb, F. E., Gibson, M. O. J., *Brit. med. J.*, 1944, **1**, 492.
655. Bell, D. W., Carmichael, J. A. G., Williams, R. S., Holman, R. L., Stewart, P. D., *Brit. med. J.*, 1958, **2**, 740.
656. Cole, A. C. E., *Trans. roy. Soc. trop. Med. Hyg.*, 1943–44, **37**, 409.
657. Symmers, W. St C., *unpublished observation*, 1975.
658. Montenegro, D., *Amer. J. trop. Med.*, 1924, **4**, 331.
659. Wilcocks, C., Manson-Bahr, P. E. C., *Manson's Tropical Diseases*, 17th edn, pages 119, 131. London, 1972.
660. Knight, R., Woodruff, A. W., Pettit, J. E., *Trans. roy. Soc. trop. Med. Hyg.*, 1967, **61**, 701.
661. Paola, D. de, Silva, J. R. da, *Ergebn. allg. Path. path. Anat.*, 1960, **39**, 1.
662. Symmers, W. St C., *Lancet*, 1960, **1**, 127.
663. Selberg, W., *Verh. dtsch. Ges. Path.*, 1950, **32**, 90.
664. Pessôa, S. B., *Arch. Hig. (S. Paulo)*, 1961, **26**, 41.
665. Convit, J., Kerdel Vegas, F. T., *Arch. Derm.*, 1965, **91**, 439.
666. Manson-Bahr, P. E. C., Winslow, D. J., in *Pathology of Protozoal and Helminthic Diseases with Clinical Correlation*, edited by R. A. Marcial-Rojas and E. Moreno, chap. 4. Baltimore, 1971.
667. Destombes, P., *Bull. Soc. Path. exot.*, 1960, **53**, 299.
668. Price, E. W., Fitzherbert, M., *Ethiop. med. J.*, 1965, **3**, 57.
669. Hutt, M. S. R., Wilks, N. E., in *Pathology of Protozoal and Helminthic Diseases with Clinical Correlation*, edited by R. A. Marcial-Rojas and E. Moreno, chap. 1. Baltimore, 1971.
670. Wilcocks, C., Manson-Bahr, P. E. C., *Manson's Tropical Diseases*, 17th edn, page 953. London, 1972.
671. Minter, D. M., in *Manson's Tropical Diseases*, 17th edn, edited by C. Wilcocks and P. E. C. Manson-Bahr, page 1106. London, 1972.
672. Winterbottom, T., *An Account of the Native Africans in the Neighbourhood of Sierra Leone; to Which Is Added an Account of the Present State of Medicine among Them*, vol. 2, page 29. London, 1803.
673. Harding, R. D., Hawking, F., *Lancet*, 1944, **2**, 835.
674. Symmers, W. St C., *unpublished studies of biopsy specimens (5 cases) referred by H. D. Ross (Salisbury, Rhodesia)*, 1961–63.
675. Lumb, G., *Tumours of Lymphoid Tissue*, page 166. Edinburgh and London, 1954.
676. Lanham, S. M., *Nature (Lond.)*, 1968, **218**, 1273.

676a. Godfrey, D. G., Lanham, S. M., *Trans. roy. Soc. trop. Med. Hyg.*, 1971, **65**, 248.
676b. Spencer, H. C., Jr, Gibson, J. J., Jr, Brodsky, R. E., Schultz, M. G., *Ann. intern. Med.*, 1975, **82**, 633.
676c. Symmers, W. St C., *unpublished observations*, 1972, 1975.
677. Andrade, Z. A., Andrade, S. G., in *Pathology of Protozoal and Helminthic Diseases with Clinical Correlation*, edited by R. A. Marcial-Rojas and E. Moreno, chap. 2. Baltimore, 1971.
678. Chagas, C., *Mem. Inst. Osw. Cruz*, 1909, **1**, 158.
679. Romaña, C., *Mem. Inst. Osw. Cruz*, 1943, **39**, 253.
680. Laranja, F. S., Dias, E., Nobrega, G., Miranda, A., *Circulation*, 1956, **14**, 1035.
681. Hutt, M. S. R., Köberle, F., Salfelder, K., in *Spezielle pathologische Anatomie—Ein Lehr- und Nachschlagewerk*, edited by W. Doerr, G. Seifert and E. Uehlinger, vol. 8 (*Tropical Pathology*, by H. Spencer, A. D. Dayan, J. B. Gibson, R. G. Huntsman, M. S. R. Hutt, G. C. Jenkins, F. Köberle, B. G. Maegraith and K. Salfelder), chap. 12 [page 381]. Berlin, Heidelberg and New York, 1973.
682. World Health Organization, *Wld Hlth Org. techn. Rep. Ser.*, 1960, No. 202 [page 4].
683. Sherman, I. W., Mudd, J. B., Trager, W., *Nature (Lond.)*, 1965, **208**, 691.
684. Winslow, D. J., Connor, D. H., Sprinz, H., in *Pathology of Protozoal and Helminthic Diseases with Clinical Correlation*, edited by R. A. Marcial-Rojas and E. Moreno, chap. 10 [page 213]. Baltimore, 1971.
685. Škrabalo, Z., in *Pathology of Protozoal and Helminthic Diseases with Clinical Correlation*, edited by R. A. Marcial-Rojas and E. Moreno, chap. 11 (and addendum, page 232).
686. Editorial, *Lancet*, 1976, **1**, 1001.
687. Škrabalo, Z., Deanović, Z., *Docum. Med. geogr. trop. (Amst.)*, 1957, **9**, 11.
688. Garnham, P. C. C., Donnelly, J., Hoogstraal, H., Kennedy, C. C., Walton, G. A., *Brit. med. J.*, 1969, **4**, 768.
689. Scholtens, R. G., Braff, E. H., Healy, G. R., Gleason, N., *Amer. J. trop. Med. Hyg.*, 1968, **17**, 810.
690. Anderson, A. E., Cassaday, P. B., Healy, G. R., *Amer. J. clin. Path.*, 1974, **62**, 612.
691. Tanaka, H., Hall, W. T., Sheffield, J. B., Moore, D. H., *J. Bact.*, 1965, **90**, 1735.
692. Weinman, D., *Trans. Amer. phil. Soc.*, 1944, **33**, part 3, 243.
693. Pinkerton, H., Weinman, D. J., *Proc. Soc. exp. Biol. (N.Y.)*, 1937, **37**, 587.
694. Walle, W. van der, *Docum. Med. geogr. trop. (Amst.)*, 1957, **9**, 149.
695. Stoll, N. R., *J. Parasit.*, 1947, **33**, 1.
696. Tokumo, S., *Hiroshima J. med. Sci.*, 1956, **5**, 21.
697. Marcial-Rojas, R. A., in *Pathology of Protozoal and Helminthic Diseases with Clinical Correlation*, edited by R. A. Marcial-Rojas and E. Moreno, chap. 37. Baltimore, 1971.
698. Winter, H., *Z. klin. Med.*, 1955, **153**, 407.
699. Ribas-Mujal, D., in *Pathology of Protozoal and Helminthic Diseases with Clinical Correlation*, edited by R. A. Marcial-Rojas and E. Moreno, chap. 36. Baltimore, 1971.
700. *Trichinosis in Man and Animals*, edited by S. E. Gould. Springfield, Illinois, 1970.
701. Virchow, R., *Virchows Arch. path. Anat.*, 1860, **18**, 330.

702. Baar, H. S., Dyke, S. C., Symmers, W. St C., *unpublished observation*, 1948.
703. Kirsten, K., *cited by:* Lennert, K., in *Handbuch der speziellen pathologischen Anatomie und Histologie*, edited by E. Uehlinger, vol. 1, part 3, book 1, pages 440–441 (Figs 279 and 280). Berlin, Göttingen and Heidelberg, 1961.
704. Deeds, D. D., *Amer. J. Obstet. Gynec.*, 1947, **54**, 890.
705. Kastranek, F., *Wien. klin. Wschr.*, 1948, **60**, 51.
706. Symmers, W. St C., *Arch. Path. (Chic.)*, 1950, **50**, 475 [page 497].
707. Lake, N. C., Symmers, W. St C., *unpublished observation*, 1955.
708. O'Connor, F. W., Hulse, C. R., *Trans. roy. Soc. trop. Med. Hyg.*, 1931–32, **25**, 445.
709. Bras, G., Lie Kian Joe, *Docum. neerl. indones. Morb. trop.*, 1951, **3**, 289.
710. Meyers, F. M., Kouwenaar, W., *Geneesk. T. Ned.-Ind.*, 1939, **79**, 853.
711. Lie Kian Joe, *Amer. J. trop. Med. Hyg.*, 1962, **11**, 646.
712. Turner, L. H., *Trans. roy. Soc. trop. Med. Hyg.*, 1959, **53**, 154.
713. Spencer, H., in *Spezielle pathologische Anatomie—Ein Lehr- und Nachschlagewerk*, edited by W. Doerr, G. Seifert and E. Uehlinger, vol. 8 (*Tropical Pathology*, by H. Spencer, A. D. Dayan, J. B. Gibson, R. G. Huntsman, M. S. R. Hutt, G. C. Jenkins, F. Köberle, B. G. Maegraith and K. Salfelder), chap. 16 [pages 543–544]. Berlin, Heidelberg and New York, 1973.
714. Connor, D. H., *Hum. Path.*, 1970, **1**, 553.
715. Price, D. L., Hopps, H. C., in *Pathology of Protozoal and Helminthic Diseases with Clinical Correlation*, edited by R. A. Marcial-Rojas and E. Moreno, chap. 52. Baltimore, 1971.
716. Beaver, P. C., Orihel, T. C., *Amer. J. trop. Med. Hyg.*, 1965, **14**, 1010.
717. Abadie, S. H., Swartzwelder, J. C., Holman, R. L., *Amer. J. trop. Med. Hyg.*, 1965, **14**, 117.
718. Orihel, T. C., Beaver, P. C., *Amer. J. trop. Med. Hyg.*, 1965, **14**, 1030.
719. Rosenblatt, P., Beaver, P. C., Orihel, T. C., *Amer. J. trop. Med. Hyg.*, 1962, **11**, 641.
720. Muller, R., *Advanc. Parasit.*, 1971, **9**, 73.
721. Riou, M., *Bull. Soc. Path. exot.*, 1934, **27**, 86.
722. Faust, E. C., Russell, P. F., Jung, R. C., *Craig and Faust's Clinical Parasitology*, 8th edn, page 535. Philadelphia, 1970.
723. Symmers, W. St C., *unpublished observations*, 1958, 1972, 1973.
723a. Virchow, R., *Verh. phys.-med. Ges. Würzb.*, 1855, **6**, 84.
724. Tansurat, P., in *Pathology of Protozoal and Helminthic Diseases with Clinical Correlation*, edited by R. A. Marcial-Rojas and E. Moreno, chap. 29. Baltimore, 1971.
725. Buckley, J. J. C., Crook, E. A., Symmers, W. St C., *unpublished observation*, 1966.
726. Sadun, E. H., Sung Shen Lin, Williams, J. E., *Amer. J. trop. Med. Hyg.*, 1958, **7**, 494.
727. Symmers, W. St C., *unpublished observations (Egypt)*, 1941.
728. Chai Hong Chung, in *Pathology of Protozoal and Helminthic Diseases with Clinical Correlation*, edited by R. A. Marcial-Rojas and E. Moreno, chap. 24. Baltimore, 1971.
729. Donges, J., *Z. Tropenmed. Parasit.*, 1966, **17**, 252.
730. Hunter, D., *The Diseases of Occupations*, 5th edn, page 399. London, 1975.
731. Dutra, F. R., *Amer. J. Path.*, 1948, **24**, 1137.
732. Hardy, H. L., *Amer. Rev. Tuberc.*, 1956, **74**, 885.
733. Dobson, R. L., Weaver, J. C., Lewis, L., *Ann. intern. Med.*, 1953, **38**, 312.
734. Dutra, F. R., *Arch. Derm. Syph. (Chic.)*, 1949, **60**, 1140.
735. Lennert, K., in *Handbuch der speziellen pathologischen Anatomie und Histologie*, edited by E. Uehlinger, vol. 1, part 3, book 1, page 316. Berlin, Göttingen and Heidelberg, 1961.
736. Scadding, J. G., *Sarcoidosis*, chap. 22. London, 1967.
737. Dutra, F. R., Cholak, J., Hubbard, D. M., *Amer. J. clin. Path.*, 1949, **19**, 229.
738. Patter, W. N. van, Bargen, J. A., Dockerty, M. B., Feldman, W. H., Mayo, C. W., Waugh, J. M., *Gastroenterology*, 1954, **26**, 347.
739. Lennert, K., in *Handbuch der speziellen pathologischen Anatomie und Histologie*, edited by E. Uehlinger, vol. 1, part 3, book 1, page 426. Berlin, Göttingen and Heidelberg, 1961.
740. Wuketich, S., *Frankfurt. Z. Path.*, 1959, **70**, 187.
741. Symmers, W. St C., *unpublished observations*, 1958–69.
742. Saunders, J., *Brit. med. J.*, 1976, **1**, 437.
743. Lennert, K., in *Handbuch der speziellen pathologischen Anatomie und Histologie*, edited by E. Uehlinger, vol. 1, part 3, book 1, page 310, table 27. Berlin, Göttingen and Heidelberg, 1961.
743a. Stengel, A., *Trans. Ass. Amer. Phycns*, 1904, **19**, 174.
743b. Wolbach, S. B., *J. med. Res.*, 1911, **24**, 243.
743c. Robb-Smith, A. H. T., *J. Path. Bact.*, 1938, **47**, 457.
744. Pautrier, L. M., Woringer, F., *Bull. Soc. franç. Derm. Syph.*, 1932, **39**, 947.
745. Pautrier, L. M., Woringer, F., *Ann. Derm. Syph. (Paris)*, 1937, sér. 8, **7**, 258.
746. Laymon, C. W., Jackson, R., *A.M.A. Arch. Derm. Syph.*, 1955, **71**, 303.
747. Lennert, K., Elschner, H., *Frankfurt. Z. Path.*, 1954, **65**, 559.
748. Laipply, T. C., White, C. J., *A.M.A. Arch. Derm. Syph.*, 1951, **63**, 611.
749. Jarrett, A., Kellett, H. S., *Brit. J. Derm.*, 1951, **63**, 343.
750. Churg, J., Strauss, L., *Amer. J. Path.*, 1951, **27**, 277.
751. Braunstein, H., Gall, E. A., *cited by:* Lennert, K., in *Handbuch der speziellen pathologischen Anatomie und Histologie*, edited by E. Uehlinger, vol. 1, part 3, book 1, page 383. Berlin, Göttingen and Heidelberg, 1961.
752. Lennert, K., in *Handbuch der speziellen pathologischen Anatomie und Histologie*, edited by E. Uehlinger, vol. 1, part 3, book 1, page 385. Berlin, Göttingen and Heidelberg, 1961.
753. Symmers, W. St C., *unpublished observations*, 1960–75.
754. Gardner, D. L., *Pathology of the Connective Tissue Diseases*. London, 1965.
755. Motulsky, A. G., Weinberg, S., Saphir, O., Rosenberg, E., *A.M.A. Arch. intern. Med.*, 1952, **90**, 660.
756. Felty, A. R., *Bull. Johns Hopk. Hosp.*, 1924, **35**, 16.
757. Chauffard, A., Ramon, F., *Rev. Méd. (Paris)*, 1896, **16**, 345.
758. Still, G. F., *Med.-chir. Trans.*, 1896–97, **80**, 47.
759. Cruickshank, B., *Scot. med. J.*, 1958, **3**, 110.
760. Missen, G. A. K., Taylor, J. D., *J. Path. Bact.*, 1956, **71**, 179.

761. Ennevaara, K., Oka, M., *Ann. rheum. Dis.*, 1964, **23**, 131.

762. Dubois, E. L., in *Lupus Erythematosus—A Review of the Current Status of Discoid and Systemic Lupus Erythematosus and Their Variants*, edited by E. L. Dubois, chap. 9. New York, Toronto, Sydney and London, 1966.

763. Moore, R. D., Weisberger, A. S., Bowerfind, E. S., Jr, *A.M.A. Arch. Path.*, 1956, **62**, 472.

764. Klemperer, P., Gueft, B., Lee, S. L., Leuchtenberger, C., Pollister, A. W., *Arch. Path. (Chic.)*, 1950, **49**, 503.

765. Vazquez, J. J., Dixon, F. J., *Lab. Invest.*, 1957, **6**, 205.

766. Symmers, W. St C., in *Eight Colloquia on Clinical Pathology*, edited by M. Welsch, P. Dustin and J. Dagnelie, page 749. Brussels, 1958.

767. Weiss, R. S., Swift, S., *A.M.A. Arch. Derm.*, 1955, **72**, 103.

768. Ball, J., Davson, J., *J. Path. Bact.*, 1949, **61**, 569.

769. Graciansky, P. de, *Sem. Hôp. Paris*, 1953, **29**, 1621.

770. Symmers, W. St C., *unpublished observations*, 1966.

771. Symmers, W. St C., *Lancet*, 1956, **1**, 592 [Case 1].

772. Wegener, F., *Verh. dtsch. path. Ges.*, 1936, **29**, 202.

773. Wegener, F., *Beitr. path. Anat.*, 1939, **102**, 36.

774. Taylor, L. R. S., Plummer, N. S., Symmers, W. St C., *unpublished observations*, 1960–62.

775. Symmers, W. St C., *J. clin. Path.*, 1960, **13**, 1.

IATROGENIC LYMPHADENOPATHY

776. Ben-Ishay, D., *Lancet*, 1961, **1**, 476.

777. Theodoropoulos, G., Makkous, A., Constantoulakis, M., *J. clin. Path.*, 1968, **21**, 492.

778. Reynolds, J. S., *Ann. Allergy*, 1966, **24**, 337.

779. Rich, A. R., in *Sensitivity Reactions to Drugs—A Symposium Organized by the Council for International Organizations of Medical Sciences*, edited by M. L. Rosenheim, R. Moulton, S. Moeschlin and W. St C. Symmers, page 196. Oxford, 1958.

780. Jaffiol, C., Mary, P., Pastorello, R., *Méd. intern.*, 1966, **1**, 167.

781. Queries and Answers, *Brit. med. J.*, 1933, **1**, 903.

782. Merritt, H. H., Putnam, T. J., *J. Amer. med. Ass.*, 1938, **111**, 1068.

783. Butler, T. C., *J. Pharmacol. exp. Ther.*, 1953, **109**, 340.

784. Saltzstein, S. L., Ackerman, L. V., *Cancer (Philad.)*, 1959, **12**, 164.

785. Krasznai, G., Györy [*sic*] [Győry], Gy., *J. Path. Bact.*, 1968, **95**, 314.

786. Krasznai, G., Szegedi, Gy., *Acta morph. Acad. Sci. hung.*, 1969, **17**, 175.

787. Gams, R. A., Neal, J. A., Conrad, F. G., *Ann. intern. Med.*, 1968, **69**, 557.

788. Lukes, R. J., Tindle, B. H., *New Engl. J. Med.*, 1975, **292**, 1.

789. Hyman, G. A., Sommers, S. C., *Blood*, 1966, **28**, 416.

790. Cloake, P. C., Symmers, D., Symmers, W. St C., *unpublished observations (Birmingham, England; New York)*, 1949–50.

791. Elliott, F. A., *personal communication (London)*, 1959.

792. Langlands, A. O., Maclean, N., Pearson, J. G., Williamson, E. R. D., *Brit. med. J.*, 1967, **1**, 215.

793. Symmers, W. St C., *unpublished observations*, 1970–75.

794. Woodbury, D. M., Fingl, E., in *The Pharmacological Basis of Therapeutics*, 5th edn, edited by L. S. Goodman, A. Gilman, A. G. Gilman and G. B. Koelle, chap. 13. New York, Toronto and London, 1975.

795. Krasznai, G., Szegedi, Gy., *Frankfurt. Z. Path.*, 1967, **77**, 313.

OTHER DISEASES AFFECTING LYMPH NODES

796. Germann, H.-J., Westerhausen, M., Maas, D., *Verh. dtsch. Ges. inn. Med.*, 1972, **78**, 908.

797. Westerhausen, M., Oehlert, W., *Dtsch. med. Wschr.*, 1972, **97**, 1407.

798. Frizzera, G., Moran, E. M., Rappaport, H., *Lancet*, 1974, **1**, 1070.

799. Radaszkiewicz, T., Lennert, K., *Dtsch. med. Wschr.*, 1975, **100**, 1157.

800. Moore, S. B., Harrison, E. G., Jr, Weiland, L. H., *Mayo Clin. Proc.*, 1976, **51**, 273.

800a. Toth, J., Garam, T., *Lancet*, 1977, **1**, 102.

801. Waldenström, J., *Acta med. scand.*, 1944, **117**, 216.

801a. Harrison, C. V., *J. clin. Path.*, 1972, **25**, 12.

802. Dutcher, T. F., Fahey, J. L., *J. nat. Cancer Inst.*, 1959, **22**, 887.

803. Lennert, K., *Pathologie der Halslymphknoten—Ein Abriss für Pathologen, Kliniker und praktizierende Ärzte*, page 83. Berlin, Göttingen and Heidelberg, 1964. [Revised version of: Lennert, K., *Arch. Ohr.-, Nas.-, u. Kehlk.-Heilk.*, 1963, **182**, 1 (Kongressbericht 1963) (page 83).]

804. Forget, B. G., Squires, J. W., Sheldon, H., *Arch. intern. Med.*, 1966, **118**, 363.

805. Moore, D. F., Migliore, P. J., Shullenberger, C. C., Alexanian, R., *Ann. intern. Med.*, 1970, **72**, 43.

806. Lennart, P., Wallenius, G., Werner, I., *Acta med. scand.*, 1960, **168**, 431.

807. Symmers, W. St C., *unpublished observations*, 1966–75.

808. Ritzmann, S. E., Thurm, R. H., Truax, W. E., Levin, W. C., *Arch. intern. Med.*, 1960, **105**, 939.

809. Nathan, D. G., Baehner, R. L., *Progr. Hemat.*, 1971, **7**, 235.

810. Quie, P. G., *Curr. Probl. Pediat.*, 1971–72, **11**, 1.

811. Berendes, H., Bridges, R. A., Good, R. A., *Minn. Med.*, 1957, **40**, 309.

812. Landing, B. H., Shirkey, H. S., *Pediatrics*, 1957, **20**, 431.

813. Holmes, B., Quie, P. G., Windhorst, D. B., Good, R. A., *Lancet*, 1966, **1**, 1225.

814. Azimi, P., Bodenbender, J. G., Hintz, R. L., Kontras, S. B., *Lancet*, 1968, **1**, 208.

815. Macfarlane, P. S., Speirs, A. L., Sommerville, R. G., *Lancet*, 1967, **1**, 408.

816. Windhorst, D. B., Holmes, B., Good, R. A., *Lancet*, 1967, **1**, 737.

817. Andersen, V., Koch, C., Vejlsgaard, R., Wilken-Jensen, K., *Acta paediat. (Uppsala)*, 1968, **57**, 110.

818. Quie, P. G., White, J. G., Holmes, B., Good, R. A., *J. clin. Invest.*, 1967, **46**, 668.

819. Carson, M. J., Chadwick, D. L., Brubaker, C. A., Cleland, R. S., Landing, B. H., *Pediatrics*, 1965, **35**, 405.

820. Symchych, P. S., Wanstrup, J., Andersen, V., *Acta path. microbiol. scand.*, 1968, **74**, 179.

821. Bannatyne, R. M., Skowron, P. N., Weber, J. L., *J. Pediat.*, 1969, **75**, 236.

822. Davis, S. D., Schaller, J., Wedgewood, R. J., *Lancet*, 1966, **1**, 1013.

823. Miller, M. E., Oski, F. A., Harris, M. B., *Lancet*, 1971, **1**, 665.

824. Bartman, J., van de Velde, R., Friedman, F., *Pediatrics*, 1967, **40**, 1000.

824a. *Symposium on Kaposi's Sarcoma*, edited by L. V. Ackerman and J. F. Murray. Basel and New York, 1963. [Reprinted from: *Acta Un. int. Cancer*, 1962, **18**, No. 3.]

824b. Bhana, D., Templeton, A. C., Master, S. P., Kyalwazi, S. K., *Brit. J. Cancer*, 1970, **24**, 464.

824c. Davies, J. N. P., Lothe, F., in *Symposium on Kaposi's Sarcoma*, edited by L. V. Ackerman and J. F. Murray, page 81. Basel and New York, 1963. [Reprinted from: *Acta Un. int. Cancer*, 1962, **18**, 394.]

824d. Slavin, G., Cameron, H. MacD., Singh, H., *Brit. J. Cancer*, 1969, **13**, 349.

824e. Templeton, A. C., *Cancer (Philad.)*, 1972, **30**, 854.

824f. Murray, J. F., Lothe, F., in *Symposium on Kaposi's Sarcoma*, edited by L. V. Ackerman and J. F. Murray, page 100. Basel and New York, 1963. [Reprinted from: *Acta Un. int. Cancer*, 1962, **18**, 413.]

824g. Oettlé, A. G., in *Symposium on Kaposi's Sarcoma*, edited by L. V. Ackerman and J. F. Murray, page 17. Basel and New York, 1963. [Reprinted from: *Acta Un. int. Cancer*, 1962, **18**, 330.]

824h. Lubin, J., Rywlin, A. M., *Arch. Path.*, 1971, **92**, 338.

824i. Mazzaferri, E. L., Penn, G. M., *Arch. intern. Med.*, 1968, **122**, 521.

824j. Symmers, W. St C., *unpublished observation*, 1976.

824k. Wigley, J. E. M., Rees, D. L., Symmers, W. St C., *Proc. roy. Soc. Med.*, 1955, **48**, 449.

824m. Warner, T. F. C. S., O'Loughlin, S., *Lancet*, 1975, **2**, 687.

824n. Zak, F. G., Solomon, A., Fellner, M. J., *J. Path. Bact.*, 1966, **92**, 594.

824p. Burkitt, D. P., *Brit. med. J.*, 1970, **4**, 424.

824q. Giraldo, G., Beth, E., Coeur, P., Vogel, C. L., Dhru, D. S., *J. nat. Cancer Inst.*, 1972, **49**, 1495.

825. Viacava, E. P., Pack, G. T., *Arch. Surg.*, 1944, **48**, 109.

826. Virchow, R., *Med. Reform*, 1848–49, **1–2**, 248.

827. Troisier, *Bull. Soc. méd. Hôp. Paris*, 1886, 3. sér., **3**, 394.

828. Troisier, *Arch. gén. Méd.*, 1889, **1**, 129, 297.

LYMPH NODE BIOPSY

829. Dorfman, R. F., Warnke, R., *Hum. Path.*, 1974, **5**, 519.

830. Kirk, C. J. C., Peel, R. N., James, K. R., Kershaw, Y., *Basic Medical Laboratory Technology*, chap. 24. Tunbridge Wells, Kent, 1975.

831. Lennert, K., *Lymphknoten—Diagnostik in Schnitt und Ausstrich: A. Cytologie und Lymphadenitis*, in *Handbuch der speziellen pathologischen Anatomie und Histologie*, edited by E. Uehlinger, vol. 1, part 3, book 1. Berlin, Göttingen and Heidelberg, 1961.

832. Roitt, I. M., *Essential Immunology*, 2nd edn, page 55. Oxford, London, Edinburgh and Melbourne, 1974.

833. Henry, K., *Brit. J. Cancer*, 1975, **31**, suppl. 2, 73.

834. Cottier, H., Turk, J., Sobin, L., *Bull. Wld Hlth Org.*, 1972, **47**, 375, 409.

THE SPLEEN

835. *Die Milz—Struktur, Funktion, Pathologie, Klinik, Therapie: The Spleen—Structure, Function, Pathology, Clinical Aspects, Therapy*, edited by K. Lennert and D. Harms. Berlin, Heidelberg and New York, 1970.

836. Boyd, E., *Arch. Path. (Chic.)*, 1933, **16**, 350.

837. Weiss, L., *Semin. Hemat.*, 1965, **2**, 205.

838. King, J. T., Puchter, H., Sweat, F., *Arch. Path.*, 1968, **85**, 237.

839. Wennberg, E., Weiss, L., *Ann. Rev. Med.*, 1969, **20**, 29.

840. Rappaport, H., in *Die Milz: The Spleen*, edited by K. Lennert and D. Harms, page 24. Berlin, Heidelberg and New York, 1970.

841. Wolf, R., Fischer, J., in *Die Milz: The Spleen*, edited by K. Lennert and D. Harms, page 113. Berlin, Heidelberg and New York, 1970.

842. Pettit, J. E., Williams, E. D., Glass, H. I., Lewis, S. M., Szur, L., Wicks, C. J., *Brit. J. Haemat.*, 1971, **20**, 575.

843. Barcroft, J., Barcroft, H., *J. Physiol. (Lond.)*, 1923–24, **58**, 138.

844. Berendes, M., *Blood*, 1959, **14**, 558.

845. Jandl, J. H., *J. Lab. clin. Med.*, 1960, **55**, 663.

846. Murphy, J. R., *J. Lab. clin. Med.*, 1962, **60**, 32.

847. Prankerd, T. A. J., *Quart. J. Med.*, 1960, N.S. **29**, 199.

848. Jordan, H. E., *Physiol. Rev.*, 1942, **22**, 375.

849. Wiland, E. K., Smith, E. B., *Amer. J. clin. Path.*, 1956, **26**, 619.

850. Perry, S., Irvin, G. L., Whang, J., *Blood*, 1967, **29**, 22.

851. Raff, M. C., Wortis, H. H., *Immunology*, 1970, **18**, 931.

852. Osmond, D. G., *Anat. Rec.*, 1969, **165**, 109.

853. Penny, R., Rozenberg, M. C., Firkin, B. G., *Blood*, 1966, **27**, 1.

854. Ljungqvist, U., *Acta chir. scand.*, 1970, suppl. 411, 1.

855. Hirsch, J., McBride, J. A., Dacie, J. V., *Aust. Ann. Med.*, 1966, **15**, 122.

856. McMillan, R., Scott, J. L., *Blood*, 1968, **32**, 738.

857. Scott, J. L., McMillan, R., Davidson, J. G., Marino, J. V., *Blood*, 1971, **38**, 162.

858. McBride, J. A., Dacie, J. V., Shapley, R., *Brit. J. Haemat.*, 1968, **14**, 225.

859. Ek, J. I., Rayner, S., *Acta med. scand.*, 1950, **137**, 417.

860. Krumbhaar, E. B., *Amer. J. med. Sci.*, 1932, **184**, 215.

861. Doan, C. A., *Bull. N.Y. Acad. Med.*, 1949, **25**, 625.

862. Singer, K., Weisz, L., *Amer. J. med. Sci.*, 1945, **210**, 301.

863. Harker, L. A., *J. Lab. clin. Med.*, 1971, **77**, 247.

864. Aster, R. H., *Blood*, 1969, **34**, 117.

865. Teir, H., Wikström, S., in *Die Milz: The Spleen*, edited by K. Lennert and D. Harms, page 317. Berlin, Heidelberg and New York, 1970.

866. Noyes, W. D., Bothwell, T. H., Finch, C. A., *Brit. J. Haemat.*, 1960, **6**, 43.

867. Rizza, C. R., Eipe, J., *Brit. J. Haemat.*, 1971, **20**, 629.

868. Harms, D., in *Die Milz: The Spleen*, edited by K. Lennert and D. Harms, page 306. Berlin, Heidelberg and New York, 1970.

869. Askonas, B. A., Humphrey, J. H., *Biochem. J.*, 1958, **68**, 252.

870. Rowley, D. A., *J. Immunol.*, 1950, **65**, 515.

871. Selawry, H. S., Starr, J. L., *J. Immunol.*, 1971, **106**, 349, 358.

872. Claret, I., Morales, L., Montaner, A., *J. pediat. Surg.*, 1975, **10**, 59.

873. Ramsay, L. E., Bouskill, K. C., *J. roy. nav. med. Serv.*, 1973, **59**, 102.

874. Leading Article, *Lancet*, 1976, **1**, 1167.

875. Erickson, W. D., Burgert, E. O., Jr, Lynn, H. B., *Amer. J. Dis. Child.*, 1968, **116**, 1.

876. King, H., Shumacker, H. B., Jr, *Ann. Surg.*, 1952, **136**, 239.

877. Horan, M., Colebatch, J. H., *Arch. Dis. Childh.*, 1962, **37**, 398.

878. Robinson, T. W., Sturgeon, P., *Pediatrics*, 1960, **25**, 941.

879. Lozzio, B. B., Wargon, L. B., *Immunology*, 1974, **27**, 167.

880. Thurman, W. G., *Amer. J. Dis. Child.*, 1963, **105**, 138.

881. Lawkowicz, W., Krzeminska-Lawkowiczowa, I., Kraj, M., Rostkowska, J., Ciesluk, S., *Arch. Immunol. Ther. exp. (Warsz.)*, 1974, **22**, 711.

882. Schumacher, M. J., *Arch. Dis. Childh.*, 1970, **45**, 114.

883. Crosby, W. H., *Ann. Rev. Med.*, 1963, **14**, 349.

884. Howell, W. H., *J. Morph.*, 1890-91, **4**, 57.

885. Jolly, J. M. J., *Traité technique d'hématologie—morphologie, histogenèse, histophysiologie, histopathologie.* Paris, 1923.

886. Wiedermann, B., Wondrak, E., *Z. ges. inn. Med.*, 1962, **17**, 20.

887. Löffler, H., in *Die Milz: The Spleen*, edited by K. Lennert and D. Harms, page 196. Berlin, Heidelberg and New York, 1970.

888. Hutchison, H. E., Ferguson-Smith, M. A., *J. clin. Path.*, 1959, **12**, 451.

889. Doniach, I., Grüneberg, H., Pearson, J. E. G., *J. Path. Bact.*, 1943, **55**, 23.

890. Heinz, R., *Virchows Arch. path. Anat.*, 1890, **122**, 112.

891. Allen, D. W., Jandl, J. H., *J. clin. Invest.*, 1961, **40**, 454.

892. Beutler, E., Dern, R. J., Alving, A. S., *J. Lab. clin. Med.*, 1955, **45**, 40.

893. Selwyn, J. G., *Brit. J. Haemat.*, 1955, **1**, 173.

894. Lipson, R. L., Bayrd, E. D., Watkins, C. H., *Amer. J. clin. Path.*, 1959, **32**, 526.

895. Hirsh, J., Dacie, J. V., *Brit. J. Haemat.*, 1966, **12**, 44.

896. Dameshek, W., *Leukopenia and Agranulocytosis.* New York, 1944.

897. Dameshek, W., Estren, I., *The Spleen and Hypersplenism.* New York and London, 1947.

898. Dameshek, W., *Bull. N.Y. Acad. Med.*, 1955, **31**, 113.

899. Hayhoe, F. G. J., Whitby, L., *Quart. J. Med.*, 1955, N.S. **24**, 365.

900. Heinle, R. W., Holden, W. D., *Surg. Gynec. Obstet.*, 1949, **89**, 79.

901. Wiseman, B. K., Doan, C. A., *Ann. intern. Med.*, 1942, **16**, 1097.

902. Aster, R. H., *J. clin. Invest.*, 1966, **45**, 645.

903. Crosby, W. H., Ruiz, F., *Blood*, 1962, **20**, 793.

904. Ruhenstroth-Bauer, G., *Semin. Hemat.*, 1965, **2**, 229.

905. Dacie, J. V., Brain, M. C., Harrison, C. V., Lewis, S. M., Worlledge, S. M., *Brit. J. Haemat.*, 1969, **17**, 317.

906. Jandl, J. H., Jacob, H. S., Daland, G. A., *New Engl. J. Med.*, 1961, **264**, 1063.

907. Engelbreth-Holm, J., *Amer. J. med. Sci.*, 1938, **195**, 32.

908. Symmers, W. St C., *unpublished observations*, 1972–76.

909. Meyer, A., *Dtsch. med. Wschr.*, 1931, **57**, 226.

910. Cartwright, G. E., Chung, H.-L., Chang, A., *Blood*, 1948, **3**, 249.

911. Marcial-Rojas, R. A., in *Pathology of Protozoal and Helminthic Diseases with Clinical Correlation*, edited by R. A. Marcial-Rojas and E. Moreno, pages 397–398. Baltimore, 1971.

912. Bertino, J., Myerson, R. M., *Arch. intern. Med.*, 1960, **106**, 213.

913. De Gruchy, G. C., Langley, G. R., *Aust. Ann. Med.*, 1961, **10**, 292.

914. Richmond, J., Donaldson, G. W. K., Williams, R., Hamilton, P. J. S., Hutt, M. S. R., *Brit. J. Haemat.*, 1967, **13**, 348.

915. Stathers, G. M., Ma, M. H., Blackburn, C. R. B., *Aust. Ann. Med.*, 1968, **17**, 12.

916. Girsh, L. S., Myerson, R. M., *Amer. J. clin. Path.*, 1957, **27**, 328.

917. Medoff, A. S., Bayrd, E. D., *Ann. intern. Med.*, 1954, **40**, 481.

918. Florentin, P., Chalnot, P., Michon, P., *Rev. belge Path.*, 1955, **24**, 501.

919. Schrijver, H., Verdonk, G. J., *Acta med. scand.*, 1957, **158**, 235.

920. Schultz, J. C., Denny, W. F., Ross, S. W., *Amer. J. med. Sci.*, 1964, **247**, 30.

921. Putschar, W. G. J., Manion, W. C., *Amer. J. clin. Path.*, 1956, **26**, 429.

922. Lyons, W. S., Hanlon, D. G., Helmholz, H. F., Dushane, J. W., Edwards, J. E., *Proc. Mayo Clin.*, 1957, **32**, 277.

923. Kevy, S. V., Tefft, M., Vawter, G. F., Rosen, F. S., *Pediatrics*, 1968, **42**, 752.

924. Greenberg, S. D., *A.M.A. Arch. Path.*, 1957, **63**, 333.

925. Halpert, B., Gyorkey, F., *A.M.A. Arch. Path.*, 1957, **64**, 266.

926. Edington, G. M., *Trans. roy. Soc. trop. Med. Hyg.*, 1955, **49**, 253.

927. Edington, G. M., *J. clin. Path.*, 1957, **10**, 182.

928. Diggs, L. W., *J. Amer. med. Ass.*, 1935, **104**, 538.

929. Pearson, H. A., Spencer, R. P., Cornelius, E. A., *New Engl. J. Med.*, 1969, **281**, 923.

930. Marsh, G. W., Stewart, J. S., *Brit. J. Haemat.*, 1970, **19**, 445.

931. Crome, P., Mollison, P. L., *Brit. J. Haemat.*, 1964, **10**, 137.

932. Martin, J. B., Bell, H. E., *Canad. med. Ass. J.*, 1965, **92**, 875.

933. Weatherall, D. J., Bradley, J., in *Blood and Its Disorders*, edited by R. M. Hardisty and D. J. Weatherall, chap. 30 [page 1443]. Oxford, London, Edinburgh and Melbourne, 1974.

934. Hardisty, R. M., Wolff, H. H., *Brit. J. Haemat.*, 1955, **1**, 390.

935. Wagner von Jauregg, J., *Jb. Psychiat.*, 1887, **7**, 94.

936. Wagner von Jauregg, J., *Psychiat.-neurol. Wschr.*, 1918–19, **20**, 132, 251.

937. Garamella, J. J., Hay, L. J., *Ann. Surg.*, 1954, **140**, 107.

938. Schlüter, E., Scholz, I. von, Stutte, H. J., *Virchows Arch. Abt. A*, 1975, **368**, 205.

939. Bhagwandeen, S. B., *The Clinico-Pathological Manifestations of Schistosomiasis in the African and the Indian in Durban*, page 133. Pietermaritzburg, 1968.

939a. Gandy, C., *Bull. Soc. anat. Paris*, 1905, **80**, 872.

939b. Gamna, C., *Haematologica*, 1923, **4**, 129.

940. Round Table Discussion, in *Die Milz: The Spleen*, edited by K. Lennert and D. Harms, page 419. Berlin, Heidelberg and New York, 1970.

941. Rotter, R., Luttgens, W. F., Peterson, W. L., Stock, A. E., Motulsky, A. G., *Ann. intern. Med.*, 1956, **44**, 257.

942. Feitis, H., *Beitr. path. Anat.*, 1921, **68**, 297.

943. Magnus, H. A., *J. Path. Bact.*, 1937, **44**, 103.

944. Ball, J., Davson, J., *J. Path. Bact.*, 1949, **61**, 569.

945. Teilum, G., *Amer. J. Path.*, 1948, **24**, 389.

946. Kaiser, I. H., *Bull. Johns Hopk. Hosp.*, 1942, **71**, 31.
947. Denko, C. W., Zumpft, C. W., *Arthr. and Rheum.*, 1962, **5**, 478.
948. Hunt, A. C., Bothwell, P. W., *J. clin. Path.*, 1967, **20**, 267.
949. Symmers, W. St C., *unpublished observations.*
950. Straub, M., Schwarz, J., *Amer. Rev. resp. Dis.*, 1960, **82**, 528.
951. Salfelder, K., Schwarz, J., *Dtsch. med. Wschr.*, 1967, **92**, 1468.
952. Okudaira, M., Straub, M., Schwarz, J., *Amer. J. Path.*, 1961, **39**, 599.
953. Yow, E. M., Brennan, J. C., Nathan, M. H., Israel, L., *Ann. intern. Med.*, 1961, **55**, 307.
954. Schwarz, J., in *Human Infection with Fungi, Actinomycetes and Algae*, edited by R. D. Baker, page 92. New York, Heidelberg and Berlin, 1971.
955. Smith, E. B., Custer, R. P., *Blood*, 1946, **1**, 317.
956. Hutt, M. S. R., Wilks, N. E., in *Pathology of Protozoal and Helminthic Diseases with Clinical Correlation*, edited by R. A. Marcial-Rojas and E. Moreno, chap. 1. Baltimore, 1971.
956a. Dhayagude, R. G., Amin, B. M., *Amer. J. Path.*, 1942, **18**, 351.
957. Piyaratn, P., Pradatsundarasar, A., *Amer. J. trop. Med. Hyg.*, 1961, **10**, 839.
958. Sar, A. van der, Hartz, H., *Amer. J. trop. Med.*, 1945, **25**, 83.
959. Symmers, W. St C., *unpublished observations*, 1967, 1969.
960. Poole, J. B., Marcial-Rojas, R. A., in *Pathology of Protozoal and Helminthic Diseases with Clinical Correlation*, edited by R. A. Marcial-Rojas and E. Moreno, chap. 33. Baltimore, 1971.
961. Raper, A. B., *J. Path. Bact.*, 1959, **78**, 1.
962. Parker, E. F., Brown, A. G., *Surgery*, 1948, **24**, 708.
963. Elliot Smith, A., Other, A. N., Symmers, W. St C., Tanner, N. C., *unpublished observation*, 1956–66.
964. Bostick, W. L., *Amer. J. Path.*, 1945, **21**, 1143.
965. Berge, Th., *Acta path. microbiol. scand.*, 1965, **63**, 333.
966. Tasker, R. G., *J. clin. Path.*, 1958, **11**, 142.
967. Willis, R. A., *The Borderline of Embryology and Pathology*, chap. 9. London, 1962.
968. Symmers, W. St C., *unpublished observation*, 1946.
969. Schuster, N. H., *J. Path. Bact.*, 1937, **44**, 29.
970. Wright, M., *Arch. Path. (Chic.)*, 1949, **47**, 180.
971. Willis, R. A., *The Spread of Tumours in the Human Body*, 2nd edn, page 206. London, 1952.
972. Berge, Th., *Acta path. microbiol. scand.*, 1967, suppl. 188.
973. Harman, J. W., Dacorso, P., *Arch. Path. (Chic.)*, 1948, **45**, 179.
974. Rappaport, H., Crosby, W. H., *Amer. J. Path.*, 1957, **33**, 429.
974a. Cruickshank, B., *personal communication*, 1972.
975. Dollberg, L., Casper, J., Djaldetti, M., Klibansky, C., DeVries, A., *Amer. J. clin. Path.*, 1965, **43**, 16.
976. Quinton, S. W., Wurzel, H., Czernobilsky, B., *Amer. J. clin. Path.*, 1967, **47**, 484.
977. Sen Gupta, P. C., Chatterjea, J. B., Mukherjee, A. M., Chatterji, A., *Blood*, 1960, **16**, 1039.
978. Hill, J. M., Speer, R. J., Gedikoglu, H., *Amer. J. clin. Path.*, 1963, **39**, 607.
979. Wetherley-Mein, G., in *Blood and Its Disorders*, edited by R. M. Hardisty and D. J. Weatherall, page 1181. Oxford, London, Edinburgh and Melbourne, 1974.

980. Wilcocks, C., Manson-Bahr, P. E. C., *Manson's Tropical Diseases*, 17th edn, page 128. London, 1972.
981. Marsden, P. D., Hutt, M. S. R., Wilks, N. E., Voller, A., Blackman, V., Shah, K. K., Connor, D. H., Hamilton, P. J. S., Banwell, J. G., Lunn, H. F., *Brit. med. J.*, 1965, **1**, 89.
982. Marsden, P. D., Hamilton, P. J. S., *Brit. med. J.*, 1969, **1**, 99.
983. Cattoir, E., Marill, F. G., *Cah. méd. Un. franç.*, 1950, **5**, 585.
984. Fawdrey, A. L., *Trans. roy. Soc. trop. Med. Hyg.*, 1955, **49**, 387.
985. Chaudhuri, R. N., Saha, T. K., Basu, S. P., Mukherjee, A. M., *Indian J. med. Res.*, 1956, **44**, 305.
986. Pitney, W. R., *Trans. roy. Soc. trop. Med. Hyg.*, 1968, **62**, 717.
987. Cook, J., McFadzean, A. J. S., Todd, D., *Brit. med. J.*, 1963, **2**, 337.
988. Williams, R., Parsonson, A., Somers, K., Hamilton, P. J. S., *Lancet*, 1966, **1**, 329.
989. Anand, S. V., Davey, W. W., *Brit. J. Surg.*, 1965, **52**, 335.
990. Watson-Williams, E. J., Allan, N. C., Fleming, A. F., *Brit. med. J.*, 1967, **4**, 416.
991. Boyer, J. L., Sen Gupta, K. P., Biswas, S. K., Pal, N. C., Basu Mallick, K. C., Iber, F. L., Basu, A. K., *Ann. intern. Med.*, 1967, **66**, 41.
992. Hamilton, P. J. S., Hutt, M. S. R., Wilks, N. E., Olweny, C., Ndawula, R. L., Mwanje, L., *E. Afr. med. J.*, 1965, **42**, 191.
993. Pitney, W. R., Pryor, D. S., Tait Smith, A., *J. Path. Bact.*, 1968, **95**, 417.
994. Hermann, R. E., DeHaven, K. E., Hawk, W. A., *Ann. Surg.*, 1968, **168**, 896.

SARCOIDOSIS
995. Scadding, J. G., *Sarcoidosis*. London, 1967.
996. *Fifth International Conference on Sarcoidosis*, edited by L. Levinský and F. Macholda. Praha, 1971.
997. Leitner, S. J., *Der Morbus Besnier-Boeck-Schaumann —Chronische epitheloidzellige Reticuloendotheliose oder Granulomatose*, 2nd edn. Basel, 1949.
998. Longcope, W. T., Freiman, D. G., *A Study of Sarcoidosis*. Baltimore, 1952. [Reprinted from: *Medicine (Baltimore)*, 1952, **31**, 1.]
999. Besnier, E., *Ann. Derm. Syph. (Paris)*, 1889, 2 sér., **10**, 333.
1000. Tenneson, M., *Ann. Derm. Syph. (Paris)*, 1892, 3 sér., **3**, 1142.
1001. Hutchinson, J., *Arch. Surg. (Lond.)*, 1897–98, **9**, 307.
1002. Boeck, C., *Norsk Mag. Lægevidensk.*, 1899, 4 r., **14**, 1321 [English translation in: *J. cutan. gen.-urin. Dis.*, 1899, **17**, 543].
1003. Boeck, C., *Arch. Derm. Syph. (Wien u. Lpz.)*, 1905, **73**, 71, 301.
1004. Boeck, C., *Arch. Derm. Syph. (Wien u. Lpz.)*, 1916, **121**, 707.
1005. Kuznitzky, E., Bittorf, A., *Münch. med. Wschr.*, 1915, **62**, 1349.
1006. Schaumann, J., *'Sur le lupus pernio'—Mémoire présenté en novembre 1914 à la Société française de dermatologie et de syphiligraphie pour le Prix Zambaco*. Stockholm, 1934.
1007. Kreibich, K., *Arch. Derm. Syph. (Wien u. Lpz.)*, 1904, **71**, 3.

1008. Rieder, H., *Fortschr. Röntgenstr.*, 1910, **15**, 125.
1009. Jüngling, O., *Fortschr. Röntgenstr.*, 1919–21, **27**, 375.
1010. Jüngling, O., *Bruns' Beitr. klin. Chir.*, 1928, **143**, 401.
1011. Bruins Slot, W. J., *Ned. T. Geneesk.*, 1936, **80**, 2859.
1012. Pautrier, L. M., *Bull. Soc. méd. Hôp. Paris*, 1937, **53**, 1608.
1013. Heerfordt, C. F., *Albrecht v. Graefes Arch. Ophthal.*, 1909, **70**, 254.
1014. Darier, J., Roussy, G., *Arch. Méd. exp.*, 1906, **18**, 1.
1015. Löfgren, S., *Acta med. scand.*, 1946, suppl. 174.
1016. Löfgren, S., *Acta med. scand.*, 1953, **145**, 424, 465.
1017. Scadding, J. G., *Sarcoidosis*, page 46, table 4.1. London, 1967.
1018. James, I., Wilson, A. J., *Brit. J. Surg.*, 1945–46, **33**, 280.
1019. Schaumann, J., *Acta med. scand.*, 1941, **106**, 239.
1020. Mohri, N., *Virchows Arch. Abt. A*, 1974, **362**, 259.
1021. Williams, W. Jones, *J. Path. Bact.*, 1960, **79**, 193.
1022. Doniach, I., Wright, E. A., *J. Path. Bact.*, 1951, **63**, 69.
1023. Cunningham, J. A., *Amer. J. Path.*, 1951, **27**, 761.
1024. Lombardo, C., *Sperimentale*, 1914, **68**, 329.
1025. Winkler, M., *Arch. Derm. Syph. (Wien u. Lpz.)*, 1905, **77**, 1.
1026. Wolbach, S. B., *J. med. Res.*, 1911, **24**, 243.
1027. Splendore, A., *Rev. Soc. cient. S. Paulo*, 1908, **3**, 62.
1027a. Hoeppli, R., *Chin. med. J.*, 1932, **46**, 1179.
1028. Weiss, J. A., *Laryngoscope (St Louis)*, 1960, **70**, 1351.
1029. Gravesen, P. B., *Lymphogranulomatosis benigna.* Odense, 1942.
1030. Larsson, L. G., *Acta radiol. (Stockh.)*, 1951, **36**, 361.
1031. Lindsay, J. R., Perlman, H. B., *Ann. Otol. (St Louis)*, 1951, **60**, 549.
1032. Trible, W. H., *A.M.A. Arch. Otolaryng.*, 1958, **68**, 382.
1033. Schiessle, W., Könn, G., Wurm, K., Reindell, H., *J. franç. Méd. Chir. thor.*, 1963, **17**, 465.
1034. Scadding, J. G., *Sarcoidosis*, page 435. London, 1967.
1035. Kovnat, P. J., Donohue, R. F., *Ann. intern. Med.*, 1965, **62**, 120.
1036. Löfgren, S., Wahlgren, F., *Acta derm.-venereol. (Stockh.)*, 1949, **29**, 1.
1037. James, D. G., *Brit. med. J.*, 1961, **1**, 853.
1038. Wallace, S. L., Lattes, R., Malia, J. P., Ragan, C., *Ann. intern. Med.*, 1958, **48**, 497.
1039. Powell, L. W., Jr, *Amer. J. clin. Path.*, 1953, **23**, 881.
1040. Gardner-Thorpe, C., *Neurology (Minneap.)*, 1972, **22**, 971.
1041. James, D. G., *Quart. J. Med.*, 1959, N.S. **28**, 109.
1042. Gilg, I., *Kliniske undersøgelser over Boecks sarcoid (sarcoidose)—behandling og forløb*, page 139 [English summary: page 178]. København, 1955.
1043. Nou, E., *Acta tuberc. scand.*, 1965, **46**, 147.
1044. Jordon, J. W., Osborne, E. D., *Arch. Derm. Syph. (Chic.)*, 1937, **35**, 663.
1045. Goobar, J. E., Gilmer, W. S., Jr, Carroll, D. S., Clark, G. M., *J. Amer. med. Ass.*, 1961, **178**, 1162.
1046. Gormsen, H., *Acta med. scand.*, 1948, suppl. 213, 154.
1047. Sokoloff, L., Bunim, J. J., *New Engl. J. Med.*, 1959, **260**, 841.
1048. Moreau, R., *Bull. Acad. nat. Méd. (Paris)*, 1949, **133**, 89.
1049. Martenstein, H., *Arch. Derm. Syph. (Berl.)*, 1924, **147**, 70.
1050. Perkins, E. S., *Trans. ophthal. Soc. U.K.*, 1958, **78**, 511.
1051. Scadding, J. G., *Sarcoidosis*, chap. 8. London, 1967.
1052. Crick, R., Hoyle, C., Smellie, H., *Brit. J. Ophthal.*, 1961, **45**, 461.
1053. Zimmerman, L. E., Maumenee, A. E., *Amer. Rev. resp. Dis.*, 1961, **84**, No. 5, part 2, 42.
1054. Bornstein, J. S., Frank, M. I., Radner, D. B., *New Engl. J. Med.*, 1962, **267**, 60.
1055. Ricker, W., Clark, M., *Amer. J. clin. Path.*, 1949, **19**, 725.
1056. Meyer, J. S., Foley, J. M., Campagna-Pinto, D., *A.M.A. Arch. Neurol. Psychiat.*, 1953, **69**, 587.
1057. Walker, A. G., *Postgrad. med. J.*, 1961, **37**, 431.
1058. Jefferson, M., *Brain*, 1957, **80**, 540.
1059. Wood, E. H., Bream, C. A., *Radiology*, 1959, **73**, 226.
1060. Longcope, W. T., Freiman, D. G., *A Study of Sarcoidosis* [case 15]. Baltimore, 1952. [Reprinted from: *Medicine (Baltimore)*, 1952, **31**, 1.]
1061. Jefferson, M., *Brain*, 1957, **80**, 540 [case 5].
1062. Skealy, C. N., Kahama, L., Engel, F. L., McPherson, H. T., *Amer. J. Med.*, 1961, **30**, 46.
1063. Ricker, W., Clark, M., *Amer. J. clin. Path.*, 1949, **19**, 725 [Cases 10 and 11].
1064. Pinkerton, H., Iverson, L., *A.M.A. Arch. intern. Med.*, 1952, **90**, 456.
1065. Taylor, A. B., *J. Obstet. Gynaec. Brit. Emp.*, 1960, **67**, 32.
1066. Cowdell, R. H., *Quart. J. Med.*, 1954, N.S. **23**, 29.
1067. Symmers, W. St C., *unpublished observations*, 1975.
1068. Reisner, D., *Amer. Rev. Tuberc.*, 1944, **39**, 437.
1069. Löfgren, S., Snellman, B., Lindgren, A. G. H., *Acta med. scand.*, 1957, **159**, 295.
1070. Scholz, D. A., Keating, F. R., Jr, *Amer. J. Med.*, 1956, **21**, 75.
1071. Jackson, W. P. U., Dancaster, C., *J. clin. Endocr.*, 1959, **19**, 658.
1072. Rhodes, J., Reynolds, E. H., Fitzgerald, J. D., Fourman, P., *Lancet*, 1963, **2**, 598.
1073. Polachek, A. A., Matre, W. J., *Amer. J. dig. Dis.*, 1964, **9**, 429.
1074. Palmer, E. D., *J. Lab. clin. Med.*, 1958, **52**, 231.
1075. Pearce, J., Ehrlich, A., *Ann. Surg.*, 1955, **141**, 115.
1076. Allen, E. H., Batten, J. C., Jefferson, K., *Brit. J. Radiol.*, 1956, **29**, 56.
1077. Macleod, I. B., Jenkins, A. M., Gill, W., *J. roy. Coll. Surg. Edinb.*, 1965, **10**, 319.
1078. Phear, D. N., *Lancet*, 1958, **2**, 1250.
1079. Becker, W. F., Coleman, W. D., *Ann. Surg.*, 1961, **153**, 987.
1080. Mather, G., Dawson, J., Hoyle, C., *Quart. J. Med.*, 1955, N.S. **24**, 331.
1081. Porter, G. H., *Arch. intern. Med.*, 1961, **108**, 483.
1082. Porter, G. H., *New Engl. J. Med.*, 1960, **263**, 1350.
1083. Moyer, J. H., Ackerman, A. J., *Amer. Rev. Tuberc.*, 1950, **61**, 299 [case 9].
1084. Israel, H. L., Sones, M., *Arch. intern. Med.*, 1964, **113**, 255.
1085. Kveim, A., *Nord. Med.*, 1941, **9**, 169.
1086. Williams, R. H., Nickerson, D. A., *Proc. Soc. exp. Biol. (N.Y.)*, 1935, **33**, 403.
1087. Appel, B., *Arch. Derm. Syph. (Chic.)*, 1941, **43**, 172.
1088. Siltzbach, L. E., Ehrlich, J. C., *Amer. J. Med.*, 1954, **16**, 790.
1089. Siltzbach, L. E., *J. Amer. med. Ass.*, 1961, **178**, 476.
1090. Siltzbach, L. E., *Amer. Rev. resp. Dis.*, 1961, **84**, No. 5, part 2, 89.
1091. Sones, M., Israel, H. L., Krain, R., Beerman, H., *J. invest. Derm.*, 1955, **24**, 353.
1092. Hart, P. D'Arcy, Mitchell, D. N., Sutherland, I., *Brit. med. J.*, 1964, **1**, 795.

1093. Daniel, T. M., Schneider, G. W., *Amer. Rev. resp. Dis.*, 1962, **86**, 98.
1094. Refvem, O., *Acta med. scand.*, 1954, suppl. 294.
1095. Zettergren, L., *Acta Soc. Med. upsalien.*, suppl. 5.
1096. Pinner, M., *Amer. Rev. Tuberc.*, 1938, **37**, 690.
1097. Nethercott, S. E., Strawbridge, W. G., *Lancet*, 1956, **2**, 1132.
1098. Cummings, M. M., Hudgins, P. C., *Amer. J. med. Sci.*, 1958, **236**, 311.
1099. Cummings, M. M., Dunner, E., Schmidt, R. H., Jr, Barnwell, J. B., *Postgrad. Med.*, 1956, **19**, 437.
1100. Proceedings of International Conference on Sarcoidosis, 1960, *Amer. Rev. resp. Dis.*, 1961, **84**, No. 5, part 2.
1101. Plummer, N. S., Symmers, W. St C., Winner, H. I., *Brit. med. J.*, 1957, **2**, 599.
1102. Harris, T. R., Blumenfeld, H. B., Cruthirds, T. P., McCall, C. B., *Arch. intern. Med.*, 1965, **115**, 637.
1103. Furcolow, M. L., *personal communication*, 1972.
1104. Huntington, R. W., Jr, *personal communication*, 1965.
1105. Scadding, J. G., *Sarcoidosis*, chap. 23. London, 1967.
1106. Hopkins, A., *J. Neurol. Neurosurg. Psychiat.*, 1974, **37**, 644.
1107. Salvesen, H. A., *Acta med. scand.*, 1935, **86**, 127 [case 4].
1108. Taylor, A. J., *Brit. J. Tuberc.*, 1958, **52**, 70 [case 1].
1109. Scadding, J. G., *Sarcoidosis*, chap. 25. London, 1967.
1110. Michael, M., Jr, Cole, R. M., Beeson, P. B., Olson, B. J., *Amer. Rev. Tuberc.*, 1950, **62**, 403.
1111. Fletcher, G. H., *Cent. Afr. J. Med.*, 1966, **12**, 29.
1112. Wade, H. H., *Int. J. Leprosy*, 1962, **30**, 342.
1113. Shattock, S. G., *Proc. roy. Soc. Med.*, 1916–17, **10**, Sect. Path., 6.
1114. Löfgren, S., Snellman, B., Nordenstam, H., *Acta chir. scand.*, 1955, **108**, 405.
1115. Symmers, W. St C., *Brit. med. J.*, 1956, **2**, 786.

LIPIDOSES AND OTHER STORAGE DISEASES
1116. Hug, G., in *The Liver*, edited by E. A. Gall and F. K. Mostofi, page 48. Baltimore, 1973.
1117. Thannhauser, S. J., *Lipidoses—Diseases of the Intracellular Lipid Metabolism*, 3rd edn. New York and London, 1958.
1118. Zöllner, N., Wolfram, G., in *Biochemical Disorders in Human Disease*, 3rd edn, edited by R. H. S. Thompson and I. D. P. Wootton, chap. 17. London, 1970.
1119. Neufeld, E. F., Fratantoni, J. G., *Science*, 1970, **169**, 141.
1120. Hunter, C., *Proc. roy. Soc. Med.*, 1916–17, **10**, Sect. Dis. Child., 104.
1121. Hurler, G., *Z. Kinderheilk.*, 1919, **24**, 220.
1122. Pfaundler, M., *Jb. Kinderheilk.*, 1920, **92**, 421.
1123. Rywlin, A. M., Lopez-Gomez, A., Tachmes, P., Pardo, V., *Amer. J. clin. Path.*, 1971, **56**, 572.
1124. Howell, R. R., in *The Metabolic Basis of Inherited Disease*, edited by J. B. Stanbury, J. B. Wyngaarden and D. S. Fredrickson, 3rd edn, page 149. New York and London, 1972.
1125. Ryman, B. E., *J. clin. Path.*, 1974, **27**, suppl. (Roy. Coll. Path.) 8, 106.
1126. Andersen, D. H., *Lab. Invest.*, 1956, **5**, 11.
1127. Bürger, M., Grütz, O., *Arch. Derm. Syph. (Berl.)*, 1932, **166**, 542.
1128. Booth, D. A., Goodwin, H., Cumings, J. N., *J. Lipid Res.*, 1966, **7**, 337.
1129. Meyer, K., Grumbach, M. M., Linker, A., Hoffmann, P., *Proc. Soc. exp. Biol. (N.Y.)*, 1958, **97**, 273.
1130. Fabry, J., *Arch. Derm. Syph. (Wien. u. Lpz.)*, 1898, **43**, 187.
1131. Anderson, W., *Brit. J. Derm.*, 1898, **10**, 113.
1132. Sweeley, C. C., Klionsky, B., in *The Metabolic Basis of Inherited Disease*, edited by J. B. Stanbury, J. B. Wyngaarden and D. S. Fredrickson, 2nd edn, page 618. New York and London, 1966.
1133. Krabbe, K., *Brain*, 1916, **39**, 74.
1134. Peiffer, J., *Arch. Psychiat. Nervenkr.*, 1957, **195**, 446.
1135. Hager, H., Oehlert, W., *Méd. et Hyg. (Genève)*, 1958, **16**, 84.
1136. Norman, R. M., Urich, H., Lloyd, O. C., *J. Path. Bact.*, 1956, **72**, 121.
1137. Maloney, A. F. J., Cumings, J. N., *J. Neurol. Neurosurg. Psychiat.*, 1960, **23**, 207.
1138. Groen, J. J., *Arch. intern. Med.*, 1964, **113**, 543.
1139. Gaucher, P. C., *De l'Épithélioma primitif de la rate; hypertrophie idiopathique de la rate sans leucémie.* Thesis, Paris, 1882.
1139a. Schlagenhaufer, F., *Virchows Arch. path. Anat.*, 1907, **187**, 125.
1140. Marchand, F., *Münch. med. Wschr.*, 1907, **54**, 1102.
1141. Epstein, E., *Biochem. Z.*, 1924, **145**, 398.
1142. Lieb, H., *Hoppe-Seylers Z. physiol. Chem.*, 1924, **140**, 305.
1143. Thannhauser, S. J., *Ass. Res. nerv. Dis. Proc.*, 1953, **32**, 238.
1144. Fisher, E. R., Reidbord, H., *Amer. J. Path.*, 1962, **41**, 679.
1145. Czitober, H., Gründig, E., Schobel, B., *Klin. Wschr.*, 1964, **42**, 1179.
1146. Gründig, E., Czitober, H., Schobel, B., *Clin. chim. Acta*, 1965, **12**, 157.
1147. Hillborg, P. O., Estborn, B., *Acta paediat. (Uppsala)*, 1964, **53**, 558.
1148. Svennerholm, E., Svennerholm, L., *Nature (Lond.)*, 1963, **198**, 688.
1149. Gerken, H., Wiedemann, H. R., *Ann. paediat. (Basel)*, 1964, **203**, 328.
1150. Symmers, W. St C., *unpublished observations*, 1966–68.
1151. Brady, R. O., *Clin. Chem.*, 1967, **13**, 565.
1152. Niemann, A., *Jb. Kinderheilk.*, 1914, **79**, 1.
1153. Pick, L., *Ergebn. inn. Med. Kinderheilk.*, 1926, **29**, 519.
1154. Crocker, A. C., Farber, S., *Medicine (Baltimore)*, 1958, **37**, 1.
1155. Terry, R. D., Sperry, W. M., Brodoff, B., *Amer. J. Path.*, 1954, **30**, 263.
1156. Fredrickson, D. S., in *The Metabolic Basis of Inherited Disease*, edited by J. B. Stanbury, J. B. Wyngaarden and D. S. Fredrickson, 2nd edn, page 580. New York and London, 1966.
1157. Schiff, F., *Jb. Kinderheilk.*, 1926, **112**, 1.
1158. O'Brien, J. S., Stern, M. D., Landing, B. H., O'Brien, J. K., Donnell, G. N., *Amer. J. Dis. Child.*, 1965, **109**, 338.
1159. Cumings, J. N., *personal communication*, 1967.
1160. *Cerebral Lipidoses*, edited by L. van Bogaert, J. N. Cumings and A. Lowenthal. Oxford, 1957.
1161. Hand, A., *Proc. path. Soc. Philad.*, 1893, **16**, 282.
1162. Hand, A., *Arch. Pediat.*, 1893, **10**, 673.
1163. Hand, A., *Amer. J. med. Sci.*, 1920, **162**, 509.
1164. Schüller, A., *Fortschr. Röntgenstr.*, 1915–16, **23**, 12.
1165. Christian, H. A., in *Contributions to Medical and Biological Research, Dedicated to Sir William Osler,*

Bart., M.D., F.R.S., in Honour of His Seventieth Birthday, July 12, 1919, by His Pupils and Coworkers, vol. 1, page 390. New York, 1919.

1166. Christian, H. A., *Med. Clin. N. Amer.*, 1920, **3**, 849.

1167. Henschen, F., *Acta paediat. (Uppsala)*, 1931, **12**, suppl. 6.

1168. Oswald, N., Parkinson, T., *Quart. J. Med.*, 1949, N.S. **18**, 1.

1169. Engelbreth-Holm, J., Teilum, G., Christensen, E., *Acta med. scand.*, 1944, **118**, 292.

1170. *Manual of Histologic Staining Methods of the Armed Forces Institute of Pathology*, 3rd edn, edited by L. G. Luna, chap. 9. New York, Toronto, London and Sydney, 1968.

1171. Jaffe, H. L., Lichtenstein, L., *Arch. Path. (Chic.)*, 1944, **37**, 99.

1172. Farber, S., *Amer. J. Path.*, 1941, **17**, 625.

1173. Thannhauser, S. J., *J. Mt Sinai Hosp.*, 1950, **17**, 90.

1174. Lichtenstein, L., *A.M.A. Arch. Path.*, 1953, **56**, 84.

1175. Nash, F. W., Cavanagh, J. B., *Arch. Dis. Childh.*, 1952, **27**, 391.

1176. Hirschhorn, K., Wilkinson, F. C., *Amer. J. Med.*, 1959, **26**, 60.

1177. Thannhauser, S. J., Magendantz, H., *Ann. intern. Med.*, 1938, **11**, 1662.

1178. Holt, L. E., Jr, Aylward, F. X., Timbres, H. G., *Johns Hopk. Hosp. Bull.*, 1939, **64**, 279.

1179. Elliot Smith, A., *personal communication (Oxford)*, circa 1956.

1180. Zöllner, N., *Dtsch. med. Wschr.*, 1959, **84**, 386.

1181. Chapman, F. D., Kinney, T. D., *Amer. J. Dis. Child.*, 1941, **62**, 1014.

1182. Nevin, N. C., Cumings, J. N., McKeown, F., *Brain*, 1967, **90**, 419.

1183. Refsum, S., *Nord. Med.*, 1945, **28**, 2682.

1184. Refsum, S., *Acta psychiat. scand.*, 1946, suppl. 38.

1185. Pearse, A. G. E., *Histochemistry—Theoretical and Applied*, 3rd edn, vol. 2, page 1083. Edinburgh and London, 1972.

1186. Einarson, L., Telford, I. A., *Anat. Skr.*, 1960, **3**, 5.

1186a. Oppenheimer, E. H., Andrews, E. C., Jr, *Pediatrics*, 1959, **23**, 1091.

1186b. Silverstein, M. N., Ellefson, R. D., Ahern, E. J., *New Engl. J. Med.*, 1970, **282**, 1.

1186c. Silverstein, M. N., Ellefson, R. D., *Semin. Hemat.*, 1972, **9**, 299.

LYMPHOMAS

1187. *The Registrar General's Statistical Review of England and Wales for the Year 1973*, Part 1(A). London, 1975.

1188. Symmers, W. St C., in *Systemic Pathology*, 1st edn, edited by G. Payling Wright and W. St C. Symmers, chap. 5 [page 247]. London, 1966.

1189. Lee, Y.-T. N., Spratt, J. S., Jr, *Malignant Lymphoma: Nodal and Extranodal Diseases*, chap. 8 [page 273]. New York and London, 1974.

1190. Ultmann, J. E., Hyman, G. A., Calder, B., *Blood*, 1963, **21**, 282.

1191. Woolner, L. B., McConahey, W. M., Beahrs, O. H., *J. clin. Endocr.*, 1959, **19**, 53.

1192. Azzopardi, J. G., Evans, D. J., *J. clin. Path.*, 1971, **24**, 744.

1193. Sataline, L. R., Mobley, E. M., Kirkham, W., *Gastroenterology*, 1963, **44**, 342.

1194. Cammarata, R. J., Rodnan, G. P., Jensen, W. N., *Arch. intern. Med.*, 1963, **111**, 330.

1195. Howqua, J., Mackay, I. R., *Blood*, 1963, **22**, 191.

1196. Harvey, A. McG., Shulman, L. E., Tumulty, P. A., Conley, C. L., Schoenrich, E. H., *Medicine (Baltimore)*, 1954, **33**, 291 [page 347].

1197. Fudenberg, H. H., *Arthr. and Rheum.*, 1966, **9**, 464.

1198. Lukes, R. J., Collins, R. D., *Brit. J. Cancer*, 1975, **31**, suppl. 2, 1.

1199. Page, A. R., Hansen, A. E., Good, R. A., *Blood*, 1963, **21**, 197.

1200. Green, I., Litwin, S., Adlersberg, R., Rubin, I., *Arch. intern. Med.*, 1966, **118**, 592.

1201. Dent, P. B., Peterson, R. D. A., Good, R. A., in *Immunologic Deficiency Disease in Man*, edited by D. Bergsma and R. A. Good, page 443. New York, 1968.

1202. Penn, I., *Recent Results Cancer Res.*, 1970, **35**, 1.

1203. Schwartz, R. S., André-Schwartz, J., *Ann. Rev. Med.*, 1968, **19**, 269.

1204. Burnet, F. M., *Lancet*, 1967, **1**, 1171.

1205. Walford, R. L., Hildemann, W. H., *Amer. J. Path.*, 1965, **46**, 713.

1206. Wilson, W. E. C., Kirkpatrick, C. H., in *Experience in Renal Transplantation*, edited by T. E. Starzl, page 239. Philadelphia and London, 1964.

1207. Schwartz, R. S., André-Schwartz, J., Armstrong, M. Y. K., Beldotti, C., *Ann. N.Y. Acad. Sci.*, 1966, **129**, 804.

1208. Smithers, D. W., Peckham, M. J., in *Hodgkin's Disease*, edited by D. Smithers, G. Hamilton Fairley, T. J. McElwain and M. J. Peckham, chap. 25. Edinburgh and London, 1973.

1209. Peckham, M. J., Guay, J-P., Hamlin, I. M. E., Lukes, R. J., *Brit. J. Cancer*, 1975, **31**, suppl. 2, 413.

1210. Richmond, J., Sherman, R. S., Diamond, H. D., Craver, L. F., *Amer. J. Med.*, 1962, **32**, 184.

1211. Whitcomb, M. E., Schwarz, M. I., Keller, A. R., Flannery, E. P., Blom, J., *Amer. Rev. resp. Dis.*, 1972, **106**, 79.

1212. Currie, S., Henson, R. A., Morgan, H. G., Poole, A. J., *Brain*, 1970, **93**, 629.

1213. Aström, K. E., Mancall, E. L., Richardson, E. P., Jr, *Brain*, 1958, **81**, 93.

1214. Wilkinson, M., Croft, P. B., Urich, H., *Proc. roy. Soc. Med.*, 1967, **60**, 683.

1215. Ultmann, J. E., Cunningham, J. K., Gellhorn, A., *Cancer Res.*, 1966, **26**, 1047.

1216. Westling, P., *Acta radiol. (Stockh.)*, 1965, suppl. 245, 5.

1217. Azzopardi, J. G., Lehner, T., *J. clin. Path.*, 1966, **19**, 539.

1218. Gazet, J.-C., in *Hodgkin's Disease*, edited by D. Smithers, G. Hamilton Fairley, T. J. McElwain and M. J. Peckham, chap. 20. Edinburgh and London, 1973.

1219. Prager, D., Sembrot, J., Southard, M., *Cancer (Philad.)*, 1972, **29**, 458.

1220. Kritzler, R. A., *Amer. J. Med.*, 1958, **25**, 532.

1221. Kagan, A. R., Morton, D. L., Hafermann, M. D., Johnson, R. E., *Radiology*, 1969, **92**, 632.

1222. Carbone, P. P., Kaplan, H. S., Musshoff, K., Smithers, D. W., Tubiana, M., *Cancer Res.*, 1971, **31**, 1860.

1223. Rosenberg, S. A., *Cancer Res.*, 1966, **26**, 1310.

1224. Lukes, R. J., Craver, L. F., Hall, T. C., Rappaport, H., Ruben, P., *Cancer Res.*, 1966, **26**, 1311.

1225. Moran, E. M., Ultmann, J. E., Ferguson, D. J.,

Hoffer, P. B., Ranniger, K., Rappaport, H., *Brit. J. Cancer*, 1975, **31**, suppl. 2, 228.

1226. *Hodgkin's Disease*, edited by D. Smithers, G. Hamilton Fairley, T. J. McElwain and M. J. Peckham, appendix 2, page 250. Edinburgh and London, 1973.

1227. Macdonald, J. S., Peckham, M. J., in *Hodgkin's Disease*, edited by D. Smithers, G. Hamilton Fairley, T. J. McElwain and M. J. Peckham, chap. 18. Edinburgh and London, 1973.

1228. McCready, V. R., in *Hodgkin's Disease*, edited by D. Smithers, G. Hamilton Fairley, T. J. McElwain and M. J. Peckham, chap. 19. Edinburgh and London, 1973.

1229. Gilbert, R., *Amer. J. Roentgenol.*, 1939, **41**, 198.

1230. Pusey, W. A., *J. Amer. med. Ass.*, 1902, **38**, 166.

1231. Gowing, N. F. C., in *Hodgkin's Disease*, edited by D. Smithers, G. Hamilton Fairley, T. J. McElwain and M. J. Peckham, chap. 4. Edinburgh and London, 1973.

1232. Littman, M. L., Walter, J. E., *Amer. J. Med.*, 1968, **45**, 922.

1233. Scadding, J. G., *Sarcoidosis*, page 448. London, 1967.

1234. Symmers, W. St C., *unpublished series*.

1235. Partridge, B. M., Winner, H. I., *Lancet*, 1966, **2**, 1251.

1236. Symmers, W. St C., *Lancet*, 1967, **1**, 159.

1237. Brincker, H., *Acta path. microbiol. scand. A*, 1970, **78**, 19.

1238. Chase, M. W., *Cancer Res.*, 1966, **26**, 1097.

1239. Haynes, W. F., Jr, Begg, C. F., *Cancer (Philad.)*, 1957, **10**, 1221.

1240. Schein, P. S., Vickers, H. R., *Arch. Derm.*, 1972, **105**, 244.

1241. Skinsnes, O. K., *Ann. N.Y. Acad. Sci.*, 1968, **154**, 19.

1242. Moore, R. D., *Ohio St. med. J.*, 1953, **49**, 512.

1243. Casazza, A. R., Duvall, C. P., Carbone, P. P., *Cancer Res.*, 1966, **26**, 1290.

1244. Sinkovics, J. G., Smith, J. P., *Cancer (Philad.)*, 1969, **24**, 631.

1245. Symmers, W. St C., *Proc. roy. Soc. Med.*, 1965, **58**, 341 [Case 3]; and in *Drug-Induced Diseases— Second Symposium Organized by the Boerhaave Courses for Post-Graduate Medical Education, State University of Leyden, October 1964*, edited by L. Meyler and H. M. Peck, page 108 [Case 16, page 145]—Amsterdam, New York, London, Milan, Tokyo and Buenos Aires, 1965.

1246. Louria, D. B., Hensle, T., Armstrong, D., Collins, H. S., Blevins, A., Krugman, D., Buse, M., *Ann. intern. Med.*, 1967, **67**, 261.

1247. Buchner, L. H., Schneierson, S. S., *Amer. J. Med.*, 1968, **45**, 904.

1248. Symmers, W. St C., *J. clin. Path.*, 1960, **13**, 1 [Case 3].

1249. Wong, T.-W., Warner, N. E., *Arch. Path.*, 1962, **74**, 403.

1250. Lynfield, Y. L., Farhangi, M., Runnels, J. L., *J. Amer. med. Ass.*, 1969, **207**, 944.

1251. Sokal, J. E., Firat, D., *Amer. J. Med.*, 1965, **39**, 452.

1252. Paradinas, F. J., Wiltshaw, E., *J. clin. Path.*, 1972, **25**, 233.

1253. Vogel, C. L., Cohen, M. H., Powell, R. D., De Vita, V. T., *Ann. intern. Med.*, 1968, **68**, 97.

1254. Humphries, K. R., Ngan, H., James, K., *Thorax*, 1968, **23**, 100.

1255. Vietzke, W. M., Gelderman, A. H., Grimley, P. M., Valsamis, M. P., *Cancer (Philad.)*, 1968, **21**, 816.

1256. Barlotta, F. M., Ochoa, M., Jr, Neu, H. C., Ultmann, J. E., *Ann. intern. Med.*, 1969, **70**, 517.

1257. Symmers, W. St C., *Proc. roy. Soc. Med.*, 1965, **58**, 341 [Case 4]; and in *Drug-Induced Diseases— Second Symposium Organized by the Boerhaave Courses for Post-Graduate Medical Education, State University of Leyden, October 1964*, edited by L. Meyler and H. M. Peck, page 108 [Case 17, page 146]—Amsterdam, New York, London, Milan, Tokyo and Buenos Aires, 1965.

1258. Schier, W. W., Roth, A., Ostroff, G., Schrift, M. H., *Amer. J. Med.*, 1956, **20**, 94.

1259. Aisenberg, A. C., *Cancer Res.*, 1966, **26**, 1152.

1259a. Fairley, G. Hamilton, Scott, R. Bodley, *Brit. med. J.*, 1961, **2**, 920.

1260. Symmers, W. St C., in *Drug-Induced Diseases— Second Symposium Organized by the Boerhaave Courses for Post-Graduate Medical Education, State University of Leyden, October 1964*, edited by L. Meyler and H. M. Peck, page 108 [Case 6, page 122]. Amsterdam, New York, London, Milan, Tokyo and Buenos Aires, 1965.

1261. Rappaport, H., Winter, W. J., Hicks, E. B., *Cancer (Philad.)*, 1956, **9**, 792.

1262. Rappaport, H., *Tumors of the Hematopoietic System* (Atlas of Tumor Pathology, sect. 3, fasc. 8), page F8–97. Washington, D.C., 1966.

1263. Lennert, K., Stein, H., Kaiserling, E., *Brit. J. Cancer*, 1975, **31**, suppl. 2, 29.

1264. Lennert, K., Mohri, N., Stein, H., Kaiserling, E., Müller-Hermelink, H. K., *Malignant Lymphomas Other than Hodgkin's Disease*. Berlin, Heidelberg and New York, 1977 [in press].

1265. Gerard-Marchant [Gérard-Marchant], R., Hamlin, I., Lennert, K., Rilke, F., Stansfeld, A. G., Unnik, J. A. M. van, *Lancet*, 1974, **2**, 406.

1266. Dorfman, R. F., *Lancet*, 1974, **1**, 1295.

1267. Bennett, M. H., Farrer-Brown, G., Henry, K., Jelliffe, A. M., *Lancet*, 1974, **2**, 405.

1268. Diebold, J., *Nouv. Presse méd.*, 1974, **3**, 1818.

1269. Kay, H. E. M., *Lancet*, 1974, **2**, 586.

1270. Bradfield, J. W. B., *Lancet*, 1974, **2**, 652.

1271. Lennert, K., Mohri, N., Stein, H., Kaiserling, E., *Brit. J. Haemat.*, 1975, **31**, suppl., 193.

1272. Smith, H. A., *Amer. J. clin. Path.*, 1962, **38**, 75.

1273. Holzworth, J., *J. Amer. vet. med. Ass.*, 1960, **136**, 47.

1274. Sandersleben, J., *Arch. exp. Vet.-Med.*, 1961, **15**, 620.

1275. Smith, H. A., *Path. vet.*, 1965, **2**, 68.

1276. Squire, R. A., *Cornell Vet.*, 1964, **54**, 97.

1277. Forbus, W. D., Davis, C. L., *Amer. J. Path.*, 1946, **22**, 35.

1278. *Hodgkin's Disease*, edited by D. Smithers, G. Hamilton Fairley, T. J. McElwain and M. J. Peckham. Edinburgh and London, 1973.

1279. Hodgkin, T., *Med.-chir. Trans.*, 1832, **17**, 68.

1280. Malpighi, M., *De viscerum structura exercitatio anatomica*, page 125. Bononiae [Bologna], 1666. [English translation: *Ann. med. Hist.*, 1925, **7**, 245.]

1281. Wilks, S., *Guy's Hosp. Rep.*, 1865, **11**, 56.

1282. Fox, H., *Guy's Hosp. Rep.*, 1936, **86**, 11.

1282a. Ober, W. B., *N.Y. St. J. Med.*, 1977, **77**, 126.

1283. Lukes, R. J., *Amer. J. Roentgenol.*, 1963, **90**, 944.

1284. Jackson, H., Jr, Parker, F., Jr, *Hodgkin's Disease and Allied Disorders*, chap. 1, sect. 2. New York, 1947.

1285. Edington, G. M., Osunkoya, B. O., Hendrickse, M., *J. nat. Cancer Inst.*, 1973, **50**, 1633.

1286. Lukes, R. J., Butler, J. J., Hicks, E. B., *Cancer* (*Philad.*), 1966, **19**, 317.

1287. Cross, R. M., *J. clin. Path.*, 1969, **22**, 165.

1288. Bonfils, É. A., *Quelques réflexions sur un cas d'hypertrophie ganglionnaire générale—avec fistules lymphatiques et avec cachexie, sans leucémie.* Clermont, 1857.

1289. Wunderlich, C. A., *Arch. physiol. Heilk.*, 1858, **2**, 123.

1290. Billroth, T., *Wien. med. Wschr.*, 1871, **21**, 1065.

1291. Benda, C., *Verh. dtsch. path. Ges.*, 1904, **7**, 123.

1292. Grosz, S., *Beitr. path. Anat.*, 1906, **39**, 405.

1293. Mallory, F. B., *The Principles of Pathologic Histology*, page 326. Philadelphia and London, 1914.

1294. Fraenkel, E., in *Handbuch der speziellen pathologischen Anatomie und Histologie*, vol. 1, part 1, edited by F. Henke and O. Lubarsch, page 349. Berlin, 1926.

1295. Robb-Smith, A. H. T., *J. Path. Bact.*, 1938, **47**, 457.

1296. Jackson, H., Jr, *Surg. Gynec. Obstet.*, 1937, **64**, 465.

1297. Robb-Smith, A. H. T., in *Recent Advances in Clinical Pathology*, edited by S. C. Dyke, R. Cruickshank, E. N. Allott, B. L. Della Vida and A. H. T. Robb-Smith, chap. 34. London, 1947.

1298. Harrison, C. V., *J. Path. Bact.*, 1952, **64**, 513.

1299. Lumb, G., *Tumours of Lymphoid Tissue*, chap. 7. Edinburgh and London, 1954.

1300. Symmers, W. St C., in *Cancer*, edited by R. W. Raven, vol. 2, part 2, chap. 24. London, 1958.

1301. Ben-Asher, H., *Amer. J. Gastroent.*, 1971, **56**, 446.

1302. Cornes, J. S., *Proc. roy. Soc. Med.*, 1967, **60**, 732.

1303. Perry, P. M., Cross, R. M., Morson, B. C., *Proc. roy. Soc. Med.*, 1972, **65**, 72.

1304. Kern, W. H., Crepeau, A. G., Jones, J. C., *Cancer* (*Philad.*), 1961, **14**, 1151.

1305. Marshall, G., Roessmann, U., Noort, S. van den, *Cancer* (*Philad.*), 1968, **22**, 621.

1306. McGregor, J. K., *Amer. J. Surg.*, 1960, **99**, 348.

1307. Jackson, F. C., Ney, E. C., Fisher, E. R., *Ann. Surg.*, 1959, **150**, 1000.

1308. Rappaport, H., Berard, C. W., Butler, J. J., Dorfman, R. F., Lukes, R. J., Thomas, L. B., *Cancer Res.*, 1971, **31**, 1864.

1309. Smithers, D. W., in *Hodgkin's Disease*, edited by D. Smithers, G. Hamilton Fairley, T. J. McElwain and M. J. Peckham, chap. 3. Edinburgh and London, 1973.

1310. Symmers, W. St. C. [Belfast, 1919], Biggart, J. H. [Belfast, 1944], *unpublished observation communicated by J. H. Biggart to the Pathological Society of Great Britain and Ireland*, 1951.

1311. Strum, S. B., Rappaport, H., *Amer. J. Med.*, 1971, **51**, 222.

1312. Murchison, C., *Trans. path. Soc. Lond.*, 1870, **21**, 372.

1313. Pel, P. K., *Berl. klin. Wschr.*, 1885, **22**, 3.

1314. Ebstein, W., *Berl. klin. Wschr.*, 1887, **24**, 565.

1315. Hutchinson, E. C., Leonard, B. J., Maudsley, C., Yates, P. O., *Brain*, 1958, **81**, 75.

1316. Croft, P. B., Urich, H., Wilkinson, M., *Brain*, 1967, **90**, 31.

1317. Brain, Wilkinson, M., *Brain*, 1965, **88**, 465.

1318. Bluefarb, S. M., *Cutaneous Manifestations of the Malignant Lymphomas.* Springfield, Illinois, 1959.

1319. Wasserman, L. R., Stats, D., Schwartz, L., Fudenberg, H., *Amer. J. Med.*, 1955, **18**, 961.

1320. Bowdler, A. J., Prankerd, T. A. J., *Brit. med. J.*, 1962, **1**, 1169.

1321. Yonet, H. M., Vigliano, E. M., Horowitz, H. I., *Amer. J. med. Sci.*, 1967, **254**, 48.

1322. Bowdler, A. J., Glick, I. W., *Ann. intern. Med.*, 1966, **65**, 761.

1323. Goguel, A., Helpt-Eppinger, M., Teillet, F., Weil, M., Jacquillat, C., Bernard, J., *Nouv. Rev. franç. Hémat.*, 1969, **9**, 581.

1324. Peckham, M. J., McElwain, T. J., in *Hodgkin's Disease*, edited by D. Smithers, G. Hamilton Fairley, T. J. McElwain and M. J. Peckham, chap. 24. Edinburgh and London, 1973.

1325. Jelliffe, A. M., Millett, Y. L., Marston, J. A. P., Bennett, M. H., Farrer-Brown, G., Kendall, B., Keeling, D. H., *Clin. Radiol.*, 1970, **21**, 439.

1326. Delarue, J., Diebold, J., *Virchows Arch. Abt. A*, 1971, **353**, 27.

1327. Farrer-Brown, G., Bennett, M. H., Harrison, C. V., Millett, Y., Jelliffe, A. M., *J. clin. Path.*, 1972, **25**, 294.

1328. Greenfield, W. S., *Trans. path. Soc. Lond.*, 1878, **29**, 272.

1329. Sutton, *Trans. path. Soc. Lond.*, 1878, **29**, 342.

1330. Coupland, S., *Trans. path. Soc. Lond.*, 1878, **29**, 363.

1331. Sternberg, C., *Z. Heilk.*, 1898, **19**, 21.

1332. Reed, D. M., *Johns Hopk. Hosp. Rep.*, 1902, **10**, 133.

1333. Andrewes, F. W., *Trans. path. Soc. Lond.*, 1902, **53**, 305.

1334. Tindle, B. H., Parker, J. W., Lukes, R. J., *Amer. J. clin. Path.*, 1972, **58**, 607.

1335. Doyle, A. P., Hellström, H. R., *Ann. intern. Med.*, 1963, **59**, 363.

1336. Schnitzer, B., *Lancet*, 1970, **1**, 1399.

1337. Strum, S. B., Park, J. K., Rappaport, H., *Cancer* (*Philad.*), 1970, **26**, 176.

1338. Rappaport, H., *Tumors of the Hematopoietic System* (Atlas of Tumor Pathology, sect. 3, fasc. 8), page F8–156. Washington, D.C., 1966.

1339. Brincker, H., *Acta path. microbiol. scand. A*, 1970, **78**, 19.

1340. Kadin, M. E., Donaldson, S. S., Dorfman, R. F., *New Engl. J. Med.*, 1970, **283**, 859.

1341. Strum, S. B., Rappaport, H., *Arch. Path.*, 1971, **91**, 127.

1342. Lennert, K., Mestdagh, J., *Virchows Arch. Abt. A*, 1968, **344**, 1.

1343. Leading Article, *Lancet*, 1976, **2**, 507.

1344. Lennert, K., *Frankfurt. Z. Path.*, 1953, **64**, 343.

1345. Robb-Smith, A. H. T., *Lancet*, 1976, **2**, 970.

1346. Sahakian, G. J., Al-Mondhiry, H., Lacher, M. J., Connolly, C. E., *Cancer* (*Philad.*), 1974, **33**, 1369.

1347. Ezdinli, E. Z., Sokal, J. E., Aungst, C. W., Kim, U., Sandberg, A. A., *Ann. intern. Med.*, 1969, **71**, 1097.

1348. Wrigley, P. F. M., Fairley, G. Hamilton, Matthias, J. Q., in *Hodgkin's Disease*, edited by D. Smithers, G. Hamilton Fairley, T. J. McElwain and M. J. Peckham, chap. 16. Edinburgh and London, 1973.

1349. Han, J., *Cancer* (*Philad.*), 1971, **28**, 300.

1350. Burns, C. P., Stuernholm, R. L., Kellermeyer, R. U., *Cancer* (*Philad.*), 1971, **27**, 806.

1351. Swain, W. R., Windschitl, H. E., Doccherhohnen, A., Bankole, R. O., Bates, H. A., *Cancer* (*Philad.*), 1971, **27**, 569.

1352. Yamasaki, M., *Z. Heilk.*, 1904, **25**, 269.

1353. McFadden, G. D. F., Thomson, W. W. D., *unpublished observation* (*Belfast*), 1939.

1354. Symmers, D., *Arch. intern. Med.*, 1944, **74**, 163.

1355. Loehry, C. A., *Brit. med. J.*, 1964, **2**, 1594.

1356. Pack, G. T., Molander, D. W., *Cancer Res.*, 1966, **26**, 1254.

1357. Thomson, A. D., *Brit. J. Cancer*, 1955, **9**, 37.

1358. Marshall, A. H. E., Wood, C., *J. Path. Bact.*, 1957, **73**, 163.

1359. Gowing, N. F. C., in *Hodgkin's Disease*, edited by D. Smithers, G. Hamilton Fairley, T. J. McElwain and M. J. Peckham, chap. 17. Edinburgh and London, 1973.

1360. Smithers, D. W., in *Hodgkin's Disease*, edited by D. Smithers, G. Hamilton Fairley, T. J. McElwain and M. J. Peckham, chap. 11. Edinburgh and London, 1973.

1361. Sutcliffe, S. B. J., Wrigley, P. F. M., Smyth, J. F., Webb, J. A. W., Tucker, A. K., Beard, M. E. J., Irving, M., Stansfeld, A. G., Malpas, J. S., Crowther, D., Whitehouse, J. M. A., *Brit. med. J.*, 1976, **4**, 1343.

1362. Lukes, R. J., Collins, R. D., *Cancer (Philad.)*, 1974, **34**, 1488.

1363. Smithers, D. W., in *Hodgkin's Disease*, edited by D. Smithers, G. Hamilton Fairley, T. J. McElwain and M. J. Peckham, chap. 1. Edinburgh and London, 1973.

1364. Schwartz, R. S., Beldotti, L., *Science*, 1965, **149**, 1511.

1365. Vianna, N. J., Greenwald, P., Davies, J. N. P., *Lancet*, 1971, **1**, 1209.

1366. Vianna, N. J., Greenwald, P., Brady, J., Polan, A. K., Dwork, A., Mauro, J., Davies, J. N. P., *Ann. intern. Med.*, 1972, **77**, 169.

1367. Vianna, N. J., Polan, A. K., *New Engl. J. Med.*, 1973, **289**, 499.

1368. Wagener, D. J. Th., Haanen, C., *Lancet*, 1975, **2**, 747.

1369. Alderson, M. R., Nayak, R., *Brit. J. prev. soc. Med.*, 1971, **25**, 168.

1370. Milham, S., *New Engl. J. Med.*, 1974, **290**, 1329.

1371. Hoover, R., *New Engl. J. Med.*, 1974, **291**, 473.

1372. Vianna, N. J., Polan, A. K., Keogh, M. D., Greenwald, P., *Lancet*, 1974, **2**, 131.

1373. Smith, P. G., Kinlen, L. J., Doll, R., *Lancet*, 1974, **2**, 525.

1374. Razis, D. V., Diamond, H. D., Craver, L. F., *Ann. intern. Med.*, 1959, **51**, 933.

1375. Smithers, D. W., *Brit. med. J.*, 1967, **2**, 263, 337.

1376. Berliner, A. D., Distenfeld, A., *J. Amer. med. Ass.*, 1972, **221**, 703.

1377. Priesel, A., Winkelbauer, A., *Virchows Arch. path. Anat.*, 1926, **262**, 749.

1378. Cridland, M. D., *Brit. med. J.*, 1965, **2**, 820.

1379. Becker, G., *Strahlentherapie*, 1971, **141**, 156.

1380. Falkson, H. C., *Brit. med. J.*, 1965, **2**, 171.

1381. Fraumeni, J. F., Li, F. P., *J. nat. Cancer Inst.*, 1969, **42**, 681.

1382. Levine, P. H., Ablashi, D. V., Berard, C. W., Carbone, P. P., Waggoner, D. E., Malan, L., *Cancer (Philad.)*, 1971, **27**, 416.

1383. Johansson, B., Klein, G., Henle, W., Henle, G., *Int. J. Cancer*, 1970, **6**, 450.

1384. Goldman, J. M., Aisenberg, A. C., *Cancer (Philad.)*, 1970, **26**, 327.

1385. Rosdahl, N., Olesen Larsen, S., Clemmesen, J., *Brit. med. J.*, 1974, **2**, 253.

1386. Hyams, L., Wydner, E. L., *J. chron. Dis.*, 1968, **21**, 391.

1387. Vianna, N. J., Greenwald, P., Davies, J. N. P., *Lancet*, 1971, **1**, 431.

1388. Vianna, N. J., Greenwald, P., Davies, J. N. P., *Lancet*, 1971, **1**, 733.

1389. Vianna, N. J., *Cancer Res.*, 1974, **34**, 1149.

1390. Wolman, I. J., *Quart. Rev. Pediat.*, 1956, **2**, 109.

1391. MacMahon, B., *Cancer Res.*, 1966, **26**, 1189.

1392. Miller, R. W., *J. Amer. med. Ass.*, 1966, **198**, 1216.

1393. Leading Article, *Brit. med. J.*, 1975, **1**, 351.

1394. Aisenberg, A. C., *J. clin. Invest.*, 1962, **41**, 1964.

1395. Morgenfeld, M. D., Bomchil, G., *New Engl. J. Med.*, 1968, **278**, 565.

1396. Goffinet, D. R., Glatstein, E. J., Merigan, T. O., *Ann. intern. Med.*, 1972, **76**, 235.

1397. Brown, R. S., Haynes, H. A., Foley, H. T., Godwin, H. A., Berard, C. W., Carbone, P. P., *Ann. intern. Med.*, 1967, **67**, 291.

1398. Hoffbrand, B. I., *Brit. med. J.*, 1964, **1**, 1156.

1399. Miller, D. G., *Ann. intern. Med.*, 1962, **57**, 703.

1400. Goldman, J. M., Hobbs, J. R., *Immunology*, 1967, **13**, 421.

1401. Schier, W. W., Roth, A., Ostroff, G., Schrift, M. H., *Amer. J. Med.*, 1956, **20**, 94.

1402. Libansky, J., *Blood*, 1965, **25**, 169.

1403. Aisenberg, A. C., Leskowitz, S., *New Engl. J. Med.*, 1963, **268**, 1269.

1404. Hancock, B. W., Bruce, L., Ward, A. M., Richmond, J., *Brit. med. J.*, 1976, **1**, 313.

1405. Casazza, A. R., Duvall, C. P., Carbone, P. P., *Cancer Res.*, 1966, **26**, 1290.

1406. Canellos, G. P., DeVita, V. T., Arseneau, J. C., Whang-Peng, J., Johnson, R. E. C., *Lancet*, 1975, **1**, 947.

1407. Falk, J., Osoba, D., *Lancet*, 1971, **2**, 1118.

1408. Li, F. P., Fraumeni, J. F., Mantel, N., Miller, R. W., *J. nat. Cancer Inst.*, 1969, **43**, 1159.

1409. Olin, R., *Lancet*, 1976, **2**, 916.

1410. Symmers, W. St C., *J. clin. Path.*, 1968, **21**, 650.

1411. Coppleson, L. W., Factor, R. M., Strum, S. B., Graff, P. W., Rappaport, H., *J. nat. Cancer Inst.*, 1970, **45**, 731.

1412. Crum, E. D., Ng, A. B. P., Tsoa, L.-l., Kellermeyer, R. W., *Amer. J. clin. Path.*, 1974, **61**, 403.

1413. Krasznai, G., Keresztury, S., Szücs, L., *J. clin. Path.*, 1967, **20**, 841.

1414. Gordon, M. H., *Brit. med. J.*, 1933, **1**, 641.

1414a. Turner, J. C., Jackson, H., Jr, Parker, F., Jr, *Amer. J. med. Sci.*, 1938, **195**, 27.

1415. Symposium on Non-Hodgkin's Lymphomata, *Brit. J. Cancer*, 1975, **31**, suppl. 2.

1416. Brown, T. C., Peters, M. V., Bergsagel, D. E., Reid, J., *Brit. J. Cancer*, 1975, **31**, suppl. 2, 174.

1417. Unnik, J. A. M. van, Breur, K., Burgers, J. M. V., Cleton, F., Hart, A. A. M., Stenfert Kroese, W. F., Somers, R., Turnhout, J. M. M. P. M. van, *Brit. J. Cancer*, 1975, **31**, suppl. 2, 201.

1418. Butler, J. J., Stryker, J. A., Shullenberger, C. C., *Brit. J. Cancer*, 1975, **31**, suppl. 2, 208.

1419. Musshoff, K., Schmidt-Vollmer, H., *Brit. J. Cancer*, 1975, **31**, suppl. 2, 425.

1420. Skarin, A. T., Davey, F. R., Moloney, W. C., *Arch. intern. Med.*, 1971, **127**, 259.

1421. Rosenberg, S. A., Diamond, H. D., Jaslowitz, B., Craver, L. F., *Medicine (Baltimore)*, 1961, **40**, 31.

1422. Al-Saleem, T., Harwick, R., Robbins, R., Blady, J. V., *Cancer (Philad.)*, 1970, **26**, 1383.

1423. Banfi, A., Bonadonna, G., Ricci, S. B., Milani, F.,

Molinari, R., Monfardini, S., Zucali, R., *Brit. med. J.*, 1972, **3**, 140.

1424. Banfi, A., Bonadonna, G., Carnevali, G., Molinari, R., Monfardini, S., Salvini, E., *Cancer (Philad.)*, 1970, **26**, 341.

1425. Saltzstein, S. L., in *Pathology Annual*, edited by S. C. Sommers, vol. 4, page 159. New York and London, 1969.

1426. Jenkins, B. A. Gwynne, Salm, R., *Brit. J. Dis. Chest*, 1971, **65**, 225.

1427. Rubin, M., *J. thorac. cardiovasc. Surg.*, 1968, **56**, 293.

1428. Heerden, J. A. van, Harrison, E. G., Jr, Bernatz, P. E., Kiely, J. M., *Dis. Chest*, 1970, **57**, 518.

1429. Naqvi, M. S., Burrows, L., Kark, A. E., *Ann. Surg.*, 1969, **170**, 221.

1430. Cathcart, R. S., Sutton, J. P., Gregorie, H. B., Jr, *Ann. Surg.*, 1971, **173**, 398.

1431. Dawson, I. M. P., Cornes, J. S., Morson, B. C., *Brit. J. Surg.*, 1961–62, **49**, 80.

1432. Cornes, J. S., Wallace, M. H., Morson, B. C., *J. Path. Bact.*, 1961, **82**, 371.

1433. Al-Khateeb, A. K., *Int. Surg.*, 1970, **54**, 295.

1434. Torres, A., Bollozos, G. D., *Cancer (Philad.)*, 1971, **27**, 1492.

1435. Molander, D. W., Pack, G. T., *Amer. J. Roentgenol.*, 1965, **93**, 154.

1436. Shoji, H., Miller, T. R., *Cancer (Philad.)*, 1971, **28**, 1234.

1437. Molander, D. W., Pack, G. T., *Rev. Surg.*, 1963, **20**, 3.

1438. Schaumburg, H. H., Plank, C. R., Adams, R. D., *Neurology (Minneap.)*, 1972, **22**, 396.

1439. Troland, C. E., Sahyoun, P. F., Mandeville, F. B., *J. Neuropath. exp. Neurol.*, 1950, **9**, 332.

1440. Plafker, J., Martinez, A. J., Rosenblum, W. I., *Sth. med. J. (Bgham, Ala.)*, 1972, **65**, 385.

1441. Schneck, S. A., Penn, I., *Lancet*, 1971, **1**, 983.

1442. Griffin, J. W., Thompson, R. W., Mitchinson, M. J., Kiewiet, J. C. de, Welland, F. H., *Amer. J. Med.*, 1971, **51**, 200.

1443. Morgan, G., *J. clin. Path.*, 1971, **24**, 585.

1444. Reese, A. B., *Tumors of the Eye and Adnexa* (Atlas of Tumor Pathology, sect. 10, fasc. 38), page F38–177. Washington, D.C., 1956.

1445. Lawler, M. R., Jr, Richie, R. E., *Cancer (Philad.)*, 1967, **20**, 1438.

1446. Hamlin, J. A., Kagan, A. R., Friedman, N. B., *Cancer (Philad.)*, 1972, **29**, 1352.

1447. Nelson, G. A., Dockerty, M. B., Pratt, J. H., ReMine, W. H., *Amer. J. Obstet. Gynec.*, 1958, **76**, 861.

1448. Mahran, M., Iskander, S. G., *Int. J. Gynaec. Obstet.*, 1972, **10**, 81.

1449. Wright, C. J. E., *Amer. J. Obstet. Gynec.*, 1973, **117**, 114.

1450. Woolner, L. B., McConahey, W. M., Beahrs, O. H., Black, R. M., *Amer. J. Surg.*, 1966, **111**, 502.

1451. Sparagana, M., *J. Amer. Geriat. Soc.*, 1970, **18**, 550.

1452. Walt, A. J., Woolner, L. B., Black, B. M., *Cancer (Philad.)*, 1957, **10**, 663.

1453. Javier, B. V., Yount, W. J., Crosby, D. J., Hall, T. C., *Dis. Chest*, 1967, **52**, 481.

1454. Roberts, W. C., Glancy, D. L., DeVita, V. T., Jr, *Amer. J. Cardiol.*, 1968, **22**, 85.

1455. Pierce, J. C., Madge, G. E., Lee, H. M., Hume, D. M., *J. Amer. med. Ass.*, 1972, **219**, 1593.

1456. Virchow, R., *Die krankhaften Geschwülste*, vol. 2, part 1, page 728. Berlin, 1863.

1457. Dreschfeld, J., *Dtsch. med. Wschr.*, 1891, **17**, 1175.

1458. Kundrat, H., *Wien. klin. Wschr.*, 1893, **6**, 211.

1459. Bennett, M. H., Millett, Y. L., *Clin. Radiol.*, 1969, **20**, 339.

1460. Bennett, M. H., *Brit. J. Cancer*, 1975, **31**, suppl. 2, 44.

1461. Millett, Y. L., Bennett, M. H., Jelliffe, A. M., Farrer-Brown, G., *Brit. J. Cancer*, 1969, **23**, 683.

1462. *Burkitt's Lymphoma*, edited by D. P. Burkitt and D. H. Wright. Edinburgh and London, 1970.

1463. Roulet, F. C., in *The Lymphoreticular Tumours in Africa: Les Tumeurs lymphoréticulaires en Afrique— A Symposium Organized by the International Union Against Cancer—Paris 1963*, edited by F. C. Roulet, pages vii, ix. Basel and New York, 1964.

1464. Hutt, M. S. R., in *Burkitt's Lymphoma*, edited by D. P. Burkitt and D. H. Wright, chap. 1. Edinburgh and London, 1970.

1465. Cook, A., *cited by:* Davies, J. N. P., Elmes, S., Hutt, M. S. R., Timavalye, L. A. R., Owor, R., Shaper, L., *Brit. med. J.*, 1964, **1**, 259, 336.

1466. Burkitt, D., *Brit. J. Surg.*, 1958–59, **46**, 218.

1467. Elmes, B. G. T., Baldwin, R. B. T., *Ann. trop. Med. Parasit.*, 1947, **41**, 321.

1468. Capponi, M., *Bull. Soc. Path. exot.*, 1953, **46**, 605.

1469. Camain, R., *Bull. Soc. Path. exot.*, 1954, **47**, 614.

1470. Edington, G. M., *Brit. J. Cancer*, 1956, **10**, 595.

1471. Thijs, S., *Ann. Soc. belge Méd. trop.*, 1957, **37**, 483.

1472. *The Lymphoreticular Tumours in Africa: Les Tumeurs lymphoréticulaires en Afrique—A Symposium Organized by the International Union Against Cancer— Paris 1963*, edited by F. C. Roulet. Basel and New York, 1964.

1473. *Treatment of Burkitt's Tumour—Proceedings of a Conference Organized by the Chemotherapy Panel of the International Union Against Cancer*, edited by J. H. Burchenal and D. P. Burkitt. Berlin, Heidelberg and New York, 1967.

1474. Burkitt, D. P., in *Burkitt's Lymphoma*, edited by D. P. Burkitt and D. H. Wright, chap. 17. Edinburgh and London, 1970.

1475. Booth, K., Burkitt, D., Bassett, D. J., Cooke, R. A., Biddulph, J., *Brit. J. Cancer*, 1967, **21**, 657.

1476. Case Reports of Burkitt's Lymphoma outside Africa, *Int. J. Cancer*, 1967, **2**, 581–611.

1477. Burkitt, D., *Int. J. Cancer*, 1967, **2**, 562.

1478. Hoogstraten, J., *Int. J. Cancer*, 1967, **2**, 566.

1479. Shanmugaratnam, K., Tan, K. K., Lee, K. W., *Int. J. Cancer*, 1967, **2**, 576.

1480. Dalldorf, G., Carvalho, R. P. S., Jamra, M., Frost, P., Erlich, D., Marigo, C., *J. Amer. med. Ass.*, 1969, **208**, 1365.

1481. Burkitt, D. P., *Brit. J. Cancer*, 1962, **16**, 379.

1482. Haddow, A. J., in *Burkitt's Lymphoma*, edited by D. P. Burkitt and D. H. Wright, chap. 18. Edinburgh and London, 1970.

1483. Burkitt, D., Wright, D., *Brit. med. J.*, 1966, **1**, 569.

1484. Burkitt, D. P., in *Burkitt's Lymphoma*, edited by D. P. Burkitt and D. H. Wright, chap. 2. Edinburgh and London, 1970.

1485. Chapman D. S., Jenkins, T., *Med. Proc.*, 1963, **9**, 320.

1486. Burkitt, D. P., in *Burkitt's Lymphoma*, edited by D. P. Burkitt and D. H. Wright, chap. 19. Edinburgh and London, 1970.

1487. Pike, M. C., Morrow, R. H., Kisuule, A., Mafigiri, J., *Brit. J. prev. soc. Med.*, 1970, **24**, 39.

1488. Wright, D. H., in *Pathology Annual*, edited by S. C.

Sommers, vol. 6, page 337. New York and London, 1971.

1489. Williams, M. C., Woodall, J. P., Corbet, P. S., Gillett, J. D., *Trans. roy. Soc. trop. Med. Hyg.*, 1965, **59**, 300.

1490. Bell, T. M., Massie, A., Ross, M. G. R., Simpson, D. I. H., Griffin, E., *Brit. med. J.*, 1966, **1**, 1514.

1491. Bell, T. M., in *Burkitt's Lymphoma*, edited by D. P. Burkitt and D. H. Wright, chap. 21. Edinburgh and London, 1970.

1492. Epstein, M. A., Achong, B. G., Barr, Y. M., *Lancet*, 1964, **1**, 702.

1493. Epstein, M. A., Achong, B. G., in *Burkitt's Lymphoma*, edited by D. P. Burkitt and D. H. Wright, chap. 22. Edinburgh and London, 1970.

1493a. Epstein, M. A., Achong, B. G., *Lancet*, 1973, **2**, 836.

1494. Allison, A. C., *Lancet*, 1968, **1**, 1141.

1495. Burkitt, D. P., Kyalwazi, S. K., *Brit. J. Cancer*, 1967, **21**, 14.

1496. Burkitt, D., in *Treatment of Burkitt's Tumour— Proceedings of a Conference Organized by the Chemotherapy Panel of the International Union Against Cancer*, edited by J. H. Burchenal and D. P. Burkitt, page 197. Berlin, Heidelberg and New York, 1967.

1497. Klein, G., in *Burkitt's Lymphoma*, edited by D. P. Burkitt and D. H. Wright, chap. 16. Edinburgh and London, 1970.

1498. Goldman, M., Reisher, J. I., Bushar, H. F., *Lancet*, 1968, **1**, 1156.

1499. Ngu, V. A., Burkitt, D. P., Osunkoya, B. O., in *Burkitt's Lymphoma*, edited by D. P. Burkitt and D. H. Wright, chap. 14. Edinburgh and London, 1970.

1499a. Wright, D. H., *Brit. J. Surg.*, 1964, **51**, 245.

1500. Clifford, P., Singh, S., Stjernswärd, J., Klein, G., *Cancer Res.*, 1967, **27**, 2578.

1501. Ngu, V. A., *Brit. med. J.*, 1966, **1**, 345.

1502. Fass, L., Herberman, R. B., Ziegler, J., Morrow, R. H., Jr, *J. nat. Cancer Inst.*, 1970, **44**, 145.

1503. Stjernswärd, J., Clifford, P., Svedmyr, E., in *Burkitt's Lymphoma*, edited by D. P. Burkitt and D. H. Wright, chap. 15. Edinburgh and London, 1970.

1504. Wright, D. H., in *Burkitt's Lymphoma*, edited by D. P. Burkitt and D. H. Wright, chaps 8 and 9. Edinburgh and London, 1970.

1505. Histopathological Definition of Burkitt's Tumour, *Bull. Wld Hlth Org.*, 1969, **40**, 601 [memorandum drafted by C. Berard, G. T. O'Conor, L. B. Thomas and H. Torloni and signed by 14 other pathologists].

1506. Brew, D. St. J., Jackson, J. G., *Brit. J. Cancer*, 1960, **14**, 621.

1507. Janota, I., *Brit. J. Cancer*, 1966, **20**, 47.

1508. O'Conor, G. T., *Cancer (Philad.)*, 1961, **14**, 270.

1509. Cooper, E. H., Frank, G. L., Wright, D. H., *Europ. J. Cancer*, 1966, **2**, 377.

1510. Osunkoya, B. O., Ngu, V. A., Mottram, F. C., *Cancer (Philad.)*, 1970, **25**, 505.

1511. Wright, D. H., *Lancet*, 1970, **1**, 1052.

1512. Rappaport, H., *Tumors of the Hematopoietic System* (Atlas of Tumor Pathology, sect. 3, fasc. 8), page F8–99. Washington, D.C., 1966.

1513. Clift, R. A., Wright, D. H., Clifford, P., *Blood*, 1963, **22**, 243.

1514. Edington, G. M., Maclean, C. M. U., *Brit. J. Cancer*, 1965, **19**, 471.

1515. Wright, D. H., *personal communication*, 1964.

1516. Symmers, W. St C., in *Systemic Pathology*, 1st edn, edited by G. Payling Wright and W. St C. Symmers, chap. 5 [page 268]. London, 1966.

1517. Symmers, W. St C., *unpublished observation*, 1973.

1518. Spiro, S., Galton, D. A. G., Wiltshaw, E., Lohmann, R. C., *Brit. J. Cancer*, 1975, **31**, suppl. 2, 60.

1519. Brill, N. E., Baehr, G., Rosenthal, N., *J. Amer. med. Ass.*, 1925, **84**, 668.

1520. Symmers, D., *Arch. Path. (Chic.)*, 1927, **3**, 816.

1521. Symmers, D., *Arch. Path. (Chic.)*, 1938, **26**, 603.

1522. Wright, C. J. E., *Amer. J. Path.*, 1956, **32**, 201.

1523. Baehr, G., *Trans. Ass. Amer. Phycns*, 1932, **47**, 330.

1524. Craver, L. F., *Med. Clin. N. Amer.*, 1934, **18**, 703.

1525. Symmers, D., *personal communication*, 1950.

1526. Nicol, J. E., *Canad. med. Ass. J.*, 1940, **43**, 151.

1527. Hickling, R. A., *Brit. med. J.*, 1960, **1**, 1464.

1528. Josselin de Jong, R. de, *Beitr. path. Anat.*, 1921, **69**, 185.

1529. Delarue, J., Diebold, J., *Ann. Anat. path.*, 1969, **14**, 25.

1530. Dorfman, R. F., *Lancet*, 1974, **2**, 961.

1531. Anday, G. J., Schmitz, H. L., *A.M.A. Arch. intern. Med.*, 1952, **89**, 621.

1532. Rosenthal, N., Dreskin, O. H., Vural, I. C., Zak, F. G., *Acta haemat. (Basel)*, 1952, **8**, 368.

1533. Blumenberg, R. M., Olson, K. B., Stein, A. A., Hawkins, T. L., *Amer. J. Med.*, 1963, **35**, 832.

1534. Sandnes, K., Iversen, O. H., *Beitr. Path.*, 1971, **144**, 158.

1535. Evans, N., *Arch. Path. (Chic.)*, 1944, **37**, 175.

1536. Fairley, N. Hamilton, Mackie, F. P., *Brit. med. J.*, 1937, **1**, 375.

1537. Kent, T. H., *Arch. Path.*, 1964, **78**, 97.

1538. Gough, K. R., Read, A. E., Naish, J. M., *Gut*, 1962, **3**, 232.

1539. Harris, O. D., Cooke, W. T., Thompson, H., Waterhouse, J. A. H., *Amer. J. Med.*, 1967, **42**, 899.

1540. Whitehead, R., *Gut*, 1968, **9**, 569.

1541. Harrison, C. V., in *Recent Advances in Pathology*, No. 9, edited by C. V. Harrison and K. Weinbren, page 84. Edinburgh, London and New York, 1975.

1542. Azzopardi, J. G., Menzies, T., *Brit. J. Surg.*, 1959–60, **47**, 358.

1543. Austad, W. I., Cornes, J. S., Gough, K. R., McCarthy, C. F., Read, A. E., *Amer. J. dig. Dis.*, 1967, **12**, 475.

1544. Beale, A. J., Parish, W. E., Douglas, A. P., Hobbs, J. R., *Lancet*, 1971, **1**, 1198.

1545. Ramot, B., Shahin, N., Bubis, J. J., *Israel J. med. Sci.*, 1965, **1**, 221.

1546. Ramot, B., *Ann. Rev. Med.*, 1971, **22**, 19.

1547. Haghighi, P., Nasr, K., in *Pathology Annual*, edited by S. C. Sommers, vol. 8, page 231. New York, 1973.

1548. Al-Saleem, T., al-Bahrani, Z., *Cancer (Philad.)*, 1973, **31**, 291.

1549. Chowdhary, A. H., *personal communication (Riyadh)*, 1975.

1550. Farooki, M. A., *personal communication (Riyadh)*, 1975.

1551. Hourihane, D. O'B., Weir, D. G., *Gastroenterology*, 1970, **59**, 130.

1552. Novis, B. H., Bank, S., Marks, I. N., Selzer, G., Kahn, L., Sealy, R., *Quart. J. Med.*, 1971, N.S. **40**, 521.

1553. Symmers, W. St C., *unpublished observations*, 1972.

1554. Rappaport, H., Ramot, B., Hulu, N., Park, J. K., *Cancer (Philad.)*, 1972, **29**, 1502.

1555. Seligmann, M., *Brit. J. Cancer*, 1975, **31**, suppl. 2, 356.

1556. Rambaud, J.-C., Matuchansky, C., Bognel, J.-C., Bognel, C., Bernier, J.-J., Scotto, J., Perol, C., Ferrier, J.-P., Mihaesco, E., Hurez, D., Seligmann, M., *Ann. Méd. intern.*, 1970, **121**, 135.

1557. Seligmann, M., Mihaesco, E., Frangione, B., *Ann. N.Y. Acad. Sci.*, 1971, **190**, 487.

1558. Doe, W. F., *Brit. J. Cancer*, 1975, **31**, suppl. 2, 350.

1559. Rambaud, J.-C., Bognel, C., Prost, A., Bernier, J.-J., Le Quintrec, Y., Lambling, A., Danon, F., Hurez, D., Seligmann, M., *Digestion*, 1968, **1**, 321.

1560. Doe, W. F., Henry, K., Hobbs, J. R., Jones, F. Avery, Dent, C. E., Booth, C. C., *Gut*, 1972, **13**, 947.

1561. Berenguer, J., Garrido, G., Sanchez-Cuenca, J. M., Tamarit, L., Sala, T., Rodrigo, M., Calabuig, J. R., Baguena, J., *Arch. Mal. Appar. dig.*, 1972, **61**, 95c.

1562. Laroche, C., Seligmann, M., Merillon, H., Turpin, G., Marche, C., Cerf, M., Lemaigre, G., Forest, M., Hurez, D., *Presse méd.*, 1970, **78**, 55.

1563. Bognel, J.-C., Rambaud, J.-C., Modigliani, R., Matuchansky, C., Bognel, C., Bernier, J.-J., Scotto, J., Hautefeuille, P., Mihaesco, E., Hurez, D., Preud'Homme, J. L., Seligmann, M., *Rev. europ. Étud. clin. biol.*, 1972, **17**, 362.

1564. Doe, W. F., Henry, K., *unpublished observation* (cited in reference 1558, above).

1565. Florin-Christensen, A., Doniach, D., Newcomb, P. B., *Brit. med. J.*, 1974, **2**, 413.

1566. Manousos, O. N., Economidou, J. C., Georgiadou, D. E., Pratsika-Ougourloglou, K. G., Hadziyannis, S. J., Merikas, G. E., Henry, K., Doe, W. F., *Brit. med. J.*, 1974, **2**, 409.

1567. Franklin, E. C., Lowenstein, J., Bigelow, B., Meltzer, M., *Amer. J. Med.*, 1964, **37**, 332.

1568. Seligmann, M., *Europ. J. clin. biol. Res.*, 1972, **17**, 349.

1569. Takahashi, M., Yagi, Y., Moore, G. E., Pressman, D., *J. Immunol.*, 1969, **102**, 1274.

1570. Frangione, B., Franklin, E. C., *Semin. Hemat.*, 1973, **10**, 53.

1571. Stein, H., Kaiserling, E., Lennert, K., *Virchows Arch. Abt. A*, 1974, **364**, 51.

1572. Lukes, R. J., Collins, R. D., in *Malignant Diseases of the Hematopoietic System*, edited by K. Akazaki, page 209. Baltimore and Tokyo, 1973. [*Gann Monogr. Cancer Res.*, No. 15.]

1573. Talal, N., Sokoloff, L., Barth, W. F., *Amer. J. Med.*, 1967, **43**, 50.

1574. Penn, I., Halgrimson, C. G., Starzel, T. E., *Transplant. Proc.*, 1971, **3**, 773.

1575. Symmers, W. St C., *J. clin. Path.*, 1968, **21**, 654.

1576. Mathé, G., Belpomme, D., Dantchev, D., Pouillart, P., Jasmin, C., Misset, J. L., Musset, M., Amiel, J. L., Schlumberger, J. R., Schwarzenberg, L., Hayat, M., Vassel, F. de, Lafleur, M., *Biomedicine*, 1974, **20**, 333.

1577. Borella, L., *Cancer (Philad.)*, 1964, **17**, 26.

1578. Ewing, J., *J. med. Res.*, 1913–14, **28**, 1.

1579. Roulet, F., *Virchows Arch. path. Anat.*, 1930, **277**, 15.

1580. Brehmer-Andersson, E., *Acta derm.-venereol. (Stockh.)*, 1976, **56**, suppl. 75.

1581. Alibert, J. L., *Description des maladies de la peau observées à l'hôpital Saint-Louis, et exposition des meilleures méthodes suivies pour leur traitement*, page 157 (plate 36). Paris, 1806.

1582. Alibert, J. L., *Monographie des dermatoses ou précis théorique et pratique des maladies de la peau*. Paris, 1832.

1583. Rappaport, H., Edgcomb, J., Thomas, L., *Amer. J. clin. Path.*, 1968, **50**, 625.

1584. Epstein, E. H., Jr, Levin, D. L., Croft, J. D., Jr, Lutzner, M. A., *Medicine (Baltimore)*, 1972, **15**, 61.

1585. Griem, M. L., Moran, E. M., Ferguson, D. J., Mettler, F. A., Griem, S. F., *Brit. J. Cancer*, 1975, **31**, suppl. 2, 362.

1586. Lutzner, M., Edelson, R., Schein, P., Green, I., Kirkpatrick, C., Ahmed, A., *Ann. intern. Med.*, 1975, **83**, 534.

1587. Macaulay, W. L., *Arch. Derm.*, 1968, **97**, 23.

1588. Black, M. M., Wilson Jones, E., *Brit. J. Derm.*, 1972. **86**, 329.

1589. Brehmer-Andersson, E., *Acta derm.-venereol. (Stockh.)*, 1976, **56**, suppl. 75 [page 117].

1590. Winkelmann, R. K., Linman, J. W., *Amer. J. Med.*, 1973, **55**, 192.

1591. Sézary, A., Bouvrain, Y., *Bull. Soc. franç. Derm. Syph.*, 1938, **45**, 254.

1592. Sézary, A., Horowitz, A., Maschas, H., *Bull. Soc. franç. Derm. Syph.*, 1938, **45**, 395.

1593. Lutzner, M. A., Jordan, H. W., *Blood*, 1968, **31**, 719.

1594. Brouet, J.-C., Flandrin, G., Seligmann, M., *New Engl. J. Med.*, 1973, **289**, 341.

1595. Symposium on the Sezary [*sic*] Cell, *Mayo Clin. Proc.*, 1974, **49**, 513.

1596. Winkelmann, R. K., in *Proceedings of the 14th International Congress of Dermatology, Padua and Venice, 1972*, edited by F. Flarer, F. Serri and D. W. K. Cotton, page 14. Amsterdam and New York, 1974.

1597. Paradinas, F. J., Harrison, K. M., *Cancer (Philad.)*, 1974, **33**, 1068.

1598. Edelson, R. L., Lutzner, M. A., Kirkpatrick, C. H., Shevach, E. M., Green, I., *Mayo Clin. Proc.*, 1974, **49**, 558.

1599. Letterer, E., *Frankfurt. Z. Path.*, 1924, **30**, 377.

1600. Siwe, S. A., *Zbl. Kinderheilk.*, 1933, **55**, 212.

1601. Siwe, S., *Advanc. Pediat.*, 1949, **4**, 117.

1602. Nezelof, C., *Rev. franç. Étud. clin. biol.*, 1966, **11**, 22.

1603. Juberg, R. C., Kloepfer, H. W., Oberman, H. A., *Pediatrics*, 1970, **45**, 753.

1604. Pruzanski, W., Altman, R., *Arch. intern. Med.*, 1964, **113**, 261.

1605. McKeown, F., *J. Path. Bact.*, 1954, **68**, 147.

1606. Orchard, N. P., *Arch. Dis. Childh.*, 1950, **25**, 151.

1607. Doede, K. G., Rappaport, H., *Cancer (Philad.)*, 1967, **20**, 1782.

1608. Turiaf, J., *Poumon*, 1969, **35**, 725.

1609. Wallgren, A., *Amer. J. Dis. Child.*, 1940, **60**, 471.

1610. Lichtenstein, L., *A.M.A. Arch. Path.*, 1953, **56**, 84.

1611. Lichtenstein, L., *J. Bone Jt Surg.*, 1964, **41A**, 76.

1612. Lieberman, P. H., Jones, C. R., Dargeon, H. W. K., Begg, C. F., *Medicine (Baltimore)*, 1969, **48**, 375.

1613. Radaszkiewicz, T., Lennert, K., *Dtsch. med. Wschr.*, 1975, **100**, 1157.

1614. Schafer, E. L., *Amer. J. Path.*, 1949, **25**, 49.

1615. Nezelof, C., Basset, F., Rousseau, M. F., *Biomedicine*, 1973, **18**, 365.

1616. Tusques, J., Pradal, G., *J. Microsc. (Paris)*, 1968, **8**, 113.

1617. Breathnach, A. S., *Arch. Biochim. Cosmét.*, 1968, **11**, 11.

1618. Wolff, K., *J. Cell Biol.*, 1967, **35**, 468.

1619. Niebauer, G., Krawezyk, W. S., Wilgram, G. F., *Arch. klin. exp. Derm.*, 1970, **239**, 125.

1620. Inamura, M., Sakamoto, S., Hanazono, H., *Cancer (Philad.)*, 1971, **28**, 467.

1621. Hoshino, T., Kukita, A., Sato, S., *J. Electron Microsc.*, 1970, **19**, 271.

1622. Morales, A. R., Fine, G., Horn, R. C., Watson, J. H. L., *Lab. Invest.*, 1969, **20**, 412.

1623. Basset, F., Turiaf, J., *C.R. Acad. Sci. (Paris)*, 1965, **261**, 3701.

1624. Scott, R. Bodley, Robb-Smith, A. H. T., *Lancet*, 1939, **2**, 194.

1625. Natelson, E. A., Lynch, E. C., Hettig, R. A., Alfrey, C. P., Jr, *Arch. intern. Med.*, 1968, **122**, 223.

1626. Rosai, J., Dorfman, R. F., *Cancer (Philad.)*, 1972, **30**, 1174.

1627. Burke, J. S., Byrne, G. E., Jr, Rappaport, H., *Cancer (Philad.)*, 1974, **33**, 1399.

1628. Schrek, R., Donnelly, W. J., *Blood*, 1966, **27**, 199.

1629. Gosselin, G. R., Hanlon, D. G., Pease, G. L., *Canad. med. Ass. J.*, 1956, **74**, 886.

1630. Bouroncle, B. A., Wiseman, B. K., Doan, C. A., *Blood*, 1958, **13**, 609.

1631. Plenderleith, I. H., *Canad. med. Ass. J.*, 1970, **102**, 1056.

1632. Ewald, O., *Dtsch. Arch. klin. Med.*, 1923, **142**, 222.

1633. Foord, A. G., Parson, L., Butt, E. M., *J. Amer. med. Ass.*, 1933, **101**, 1859.

1634. Katayama, I., Finkel, H. E., *Amer. J. Med.*, 1974, **57**, 115.

1635. Beachey, E. H., Hashimoto, K., Burkett, L. L., *Clin. Res.*, 1969, **17**, 530.

1636. Lee, S. L., Rosner, F., Rosenthal, N., Rosenthal, R. L., *N.Y. St. J. Med.*, 1969, **69**, 422.

1637. Rubin, A. D., Douglas, S. D., Chessin, L. N., Glade, P. R., Dameshek, W., *Amer. J. Med.*, 1969, **47**, 149.

1638. Duhamel, G., *Acta haemat. (Basel)*, 1971, **45**, 89.

1639. Daniel, M. T., Flandrin, G., *Lab. Invest.*, 1974, **30**, 1.

1640. Vykoupil, K. F., Thiele, J., Georgii, A., *Virchows Arch. Abt. A*, 1976, **370**, 273.

1641. Farquhar, J. W., MacGregor, A. R., Richmond, J., *Brit. med. J.*, 1958, **2**, 1561.

1642. Marrian, V. J., Sanerkin, N. G., *J. clin. Path.*, 1963, **16**, 65.

1643. Omenn, G. S., *New Engl. J. Med.*, 1965, **273**, 427.

ACKNOWLEDGEMENTS FOR ILLUSTRATIONS

The photomicrographs that have been added to this chapter for the second edition of the book were prepared with the collaboration of Mr R. S. Barnett, Department of Histopathology, Charing Cross Hospital Medical School, London.

Fig. 9.10. Reproduced by permission of the author and publishers, Messrs Oliver and Boyd (Longman Group Ltd), from: Marshall, A. H. E., *An Outline of the Cytology and Pathology of the Reticular Tissue*; Edinburgh and London, 1956 (Fig. 9).

Fig. 9.14. Histological preparation provided by Dr R. H. Cowdell, Radcliffe Infirmary, Oxford.

Fig. 9.16. Histological preparation provided by Dr S. W. McCarthy, Kanematsu Institute, Sydney Hospital, Sydney, New South Wales, Australia.

Fig. 9.19. Histological preparation provided by Dr F. J. Paradinas, Charing Cross Hospital Medical School, London; illustrated by permission of Professor N. F. C. Gowing, Dr A. L. Levene and Mr R. W. Raven, Royal Marsden Hospital, London.

Figs 9.24, 62. Histological preparations provided by Dr K. Valteris, County Hospital, Hereford.

Fig. 9.26. Specimen provided by Dr P. Kidd and Dr F. Kurrein, Worcester Royal Infirmary, Worcester.

Figs 9.32, 186, 187, 189, 194, 195, 210, 245A, 245B, 248. Reproduced by permission of the editor and publishers, Messrs Butterworth & Company (Publishers) Ltd, from: Symmers, W. St C., in *Cancer*, edited by R. W. Raven, vol. 2, chap. 24; London, 1958 (Figs 269a, 270–274, 277 and 278).

Fig. 9.44B (lower magnification picture). Photomicrograph provided by Mr K. R. James and Mr R. S. Barnett, Department of Histopathology, Charing Cross Hospital Medical School, London.

Fig. 9.49. Histological preparation provided by Professor F. Cabanne, Faculty of Medicine and Pharmacy, Dijon, France.

Fig. 9.58. Histological preparation provided by Dr J. Grant, London School of Hygiene and Tropical Medicine (University of London), London.

Figs 9.71, 164, 171, 191, 194, 195. Pathology Museum, Charing Cross Hospital Medical School, London; reproduced by permission of the Curator, Dr F. J. Paradinas; photographs by Miss P. M. Turnbull, Charing Cross Hospital Medical School.

Fig. 9.81. Reproduced by permission of the editor from: Symmers, W. St C., *Brit. med. J.*, 1970, **4**, 763 (Fig. 3).

Fig. 9.98. Reproduced by permission of the editor and publishers, The University of Arizona Press, from: Symmers, W. St C., in *Coccidioidomycosis*, edited by L. Ajello, page 301; Tucson, Arizona, 1967 (Fig. 3).

Fig. 9.99. Reproduced by permission of the Director of the Prins Leopold Instituut voor Tropische Geneeskunde, Antwerp, Belgium, from: Symmers, W. St C., in *International Colloquium on Medical Mycology 6-XII-1963–8-XII-1963*, page 281; Antwerp, 1963 (Fig. 9) [and by permission of the editor from: Symmers, W. St C., *Ann. Soc. belge Méd. trop.*, 1964, **44**, 869 (Fig. 9)]. Specimen provided by the late Dr W. E. D. Evans, Charing Cross Hospital Medical School, London.

Fig. 9.101. Histological preparation provided by Dr R. Meadows, The Queen Elizabeth Hospital, Woodville, South Australia.

Fig. 9.128. Histological preparation lent for photography by Professor K. Lennert, Pathological Institute of the University of Kiel, Germany. Photographed by permission of W. H. Kirsten, MD, University of Chicago, Chicago, Illinois, United States of America, who originally provided the preparation for the use of Professor Lennert (Lennert, K., in *Handbuch der speziellen pathologischen Anatomie und Histologie*, edited by E. Uehlinger, vol. 1, part 3, book 1, Figs 279 and 280, page 440; Berlin, Göttingen and Heidelberg, 1961).

Fig. 9.129. Histological preparation lent for photography by Professor K. Lennert, Pathological Institute of the University of Kiel, Germany.

Fig. 9.131. Specimen provided by the late Dr W. E. D. Evans, Charing Cross Hospital Medical School, London.

Fig. 9.132. Histological preparation provided by Associate Professor K. Prathap, University of Malaya, Kuala Lumpur, Malaysia.

Fig. 9.162. Specimen presented to Charing Cross Hospital Medical School, London, by Dr G. W. Storey, National Temperance Hospital, London, and York District Hospital, York.

Fig. 9.163. Histological preparation provided by Dr S. B. Bhagwandeen, Monash University, Clayton, Victoria, Australia, formerly of the University of Zambia School of Medicine, Lusaka, Zambia.

Fig. 9.170. Specimen provided by the late Dr W. E. D. Evans, Charing Cross Hospital Medical School, London; photograph by Miss P. M. Turnbull, Charing Cross Hospital Medical School.

Fig. 9.172. Histological preparation provided by Dr Tatsuo Yoneyama, University of Kentucky College of Medicine, Lexington, Kentucky, United States of America.

Figs 9.190A, 190B. Histological preparations provided by Dr G. A. C. Summers, County Hospital, York, and York District Hospital.

Figs 9.193A, 193B. Gordon Museum, Guy's Hospital, London; reproduced by permission of the Curator, Mr J. D. Maynard; photographs by Miss P. M. Turnbull, Charing Cross Hospital Medical School, London.

Fig. 9.211. Reproduced by permission of the editors and publishers, Excerpta Medica Foundation, from: Symmers, W. St C., in *Drug-Induced Diseases—Second Symposium Organized by the Boerhaave Courses for Post-Graduate Medical Education, State University of Leyden, October 1964*, edited by L. Meyler and H. M. Peck, page 108; Amsterdam, New York, London, Milan, Tokyo and Buenos Aires, 1965 (Fig. 7).

Figs 9.236, 280A, 280B. Histological preparations provided by Dr F. J. Paradinas, Charing Cross Hospital Medical School, London.

Fig. 9.237. Photograph provided by Professor D. H. Wright, The University of Southampton Faculty of Medicine, formerly of Makerere College Medical School, Kampala, Uganda, and reproduced by permission of Mr D. P. Burkitt, External Scientific Staff of the Medical Research Council (United Kingdom), formerly of Mulago Hospital, Kampala.

Fig. 9.238. Reproduced by permission of the author, editor and publishers from: Wright, D. H., *Brit. J. Surg.*, 1964, **51**, 245.

Figs 9.239, 240, 241A. Photographs provided in 1965 by Professor D. H. Wright, The University of Southampton Faculty of Medicine, formerly of Makerere College, Kampala, Uganda.

Fig. 9.241B. Specimen provided by Professor D. H. Wright, The University of Southampton Faculty of Medicine, Southampton.

Fig. 9.242. Preparation lent for photography by Professor D. H. Wright, The University of Southampton Faculty of Medicine, Southampton.

Fig. 9.243. Histological preparation provided by the author of the paper mentioned in the caption, who suggested that the history be noted in this chapter.

Fig. 9.276. Histological preparation provided by Dr F. J. Paradinas, Charing Cross Hospital Medical School, London, and Dr Kathleen M. Harrison, Royal East Sussex Hospital, Hastings.

10: *The Thymus Gland*

by Kristin Henry

CONTENTS

10: *The Thymus Gland*

by Kristin Henry

INTRODUCTION

Development

The thymus is a highly specialized organ that in most mammals—including man—is situated in the anterior mediastinum. It arises as a paired structure from the endoderm of the third and, possibly, fourth branchial pouches of each side of the neck during the sixth intrauterine week: it thus shares a common origin with the inferior parathyroid glands. Probably there is also a contribution from the ectoderm of the cervical sinus.[1] By a process of downward migration most of the left and right lobes come to lie in the anterior mediastinum in front of the great vessels at the base of the heart and the pericardium. Only the upper pole of each lobe remains in the neck, where it is closely applied to the trachea. In view of the migration of the developing thymus it is not surprising that there may be partial or complete failure of descent into the mediastinum, resulting in ectopic thymic tissue in the neck; aberrant descent may result in the misplacement of thymic tissue in the mediastinum itself. In some series aberrant nodules of thymic tissue have been found in as many as 20 per cent of individuals.[2]

The epithelial nature of the thymus is clearly evident by the end of the second intrauterine month. Soon after that there is a process of cortication (or lobulation). Lymphocytes are seen within the cortical areas toward the ninth week of intrauterine life; this is in contrast to lymph nodes and spleen, in which they do not make their appearance until the twelfth week.[3] In the past there has been controversy about the origin of the thymic lymphocytes (thymocytes): there is now convincing evidence that they are derived from immigrant bone marrow cells[4] that differentiate within the environment of the thymic epithelium. They do not, as was formerly suggested, develop from the epithelial cells themselves. For some time after birth the thymus is the most active lymphopoietic tissue in the body, with a mitotic rate far exceeding that of the peripheral lymphoid tissue.[5] The intense lymphopoiesis is independent of any extrinsic mechanism; it is related to the thymic epithelial cells.[6] For reasons that are as yet poorly understood, the vast majority of thymic lymphocytes are short-lived and die *in situ*;[7] but it appears that—at least in fetal and early postnatal life—some thymic lymphocytes are seeded to peripheral lymphoid tissue and have a long life.[8]

The thymus grows rapidly *in utero* and reaches its greatest weight in proportion to body weight at birth (mean weight 22 g). Its weight is greatest at puberty (mean weight 34 g). There is a wide variation in weight at any age.[9] Following puberty there is a gradual reduction in the thymic parenchyma and replacement with fatty tissue, but it is important to realize that the thymus never disappears completely. This normal process is referred to as physiological (or age) involution and must not be confused with the very marked and rapid decrease in size—stress (or accidental) involution—that is seen in a variety of illnesses, such as neoplasia and infection, and following treatment with X-rays and cytotoxic drugs and the administration of metabolically active steroids. Stress involution also occurs during pregnancy and lactation. The mechanism of thymic involution entails a massive depletion of cortical lymphocytes and is mediated through the pituitary-adrenal axis.[10] It was failure to appreciate the effects of stress and hormonal influences, together with the wide variation in thymic weight at different ages, that led in the past to normal thymus glands being described as enlarged or persistent, and to the concept of status thymicolymphaticus. Status thymicolymphaticus was the term used in instances of sudden death, from trivial causes, in which the thymus was thought to be enlarged. A committee was set up to investigate this condition:[9] it found no evidence for the existence of status thymicolymphaticus, taking into account the known wide variation in thymic weight at any given age, and the fact that it is precisely in patients dying suddenly that there would be no time for stress involution to occur. However, some pathologists continued to

---

References to Other Chapters: A list of the chapters in each of the five volumes is on page v at the front of this volume.

believe in the entity,[11] or in a very rare association between a liability to sudden death and a large thymus with hyperplasia of other lymphoid tissues.[12]

Structure

The two lobes of the thymus are invested in loose connective tissue that is fused anteriorly to form a continuous sheet. The two lobes, although in close apposition, are not fused (Fig. 10.1). Each lobe has a capsule and is divided into many lobules by connective tissue septa (Fig. 10.2). In the normal thymus (Fig. 10.3) argyrophile reticulin fibres are confined to blood vessels, septa and the capsule. They are absent from the parenchyma of the gland, and in particular at the corticomedullary junction. In certain diseases, as mentioned later, the amount of reticulin is increased and its arrangement is altered.

The basic structural unit of the thymus is the lobule. Each lobule comprises the peripheral, darkly staining, lymphocytic cortex and the inner, paler medulla (Fig. 10.4). Although appearing different in stained sections, the structure of cortex and medulla is essentially the same in that both are composed of a mixture of lymphocytes and epithelial cells, the lymphocytes lying within a meshwork composed of the cytoplasmic processes of epithelial cells. Lymphocytes are very numerous and closely packed in the cortex and it is for this reason that the attenuated epithelial cells of this

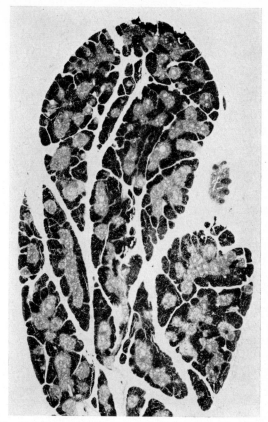

Fig. 10.2.§ Normal thymus at age of nine years. The lobular structure and distinct differentiation of the darkly staining cortex and palely staining medulla are well seen. *Haematoxylin–eosin.* × 8.

part, which are found mainly beneath the capsule and along the septa and round blood vessels, tend to be obscured. In contrast, lymphocytes are fewer in number in the medulla, where they are scattered among the numerous thymic epithelial cells. It will be noted that these are referred to here as epithelial cells rather than as 'epithelial reticular cells', since the latter term—still commonly applied to them—misleadingly suggests that they have a mesenchymal derivation. Electron microscopy has confirmed their epithelial nature (Fig. 10.5): they contain numerous tonofilaments and show desmosomal attachments, and a basement membrane is seen wherever they abut on connective tissue.

Also found within the medulla are the distinctive structures known as Hassall's corpuscles (Fig. 10.6). These are complex tubular structures derived from aggregates of thymic epithelial cells, as has been confirmed by ultrastructural studies (Fig. 10.7). They show varying degrees of keratinization and

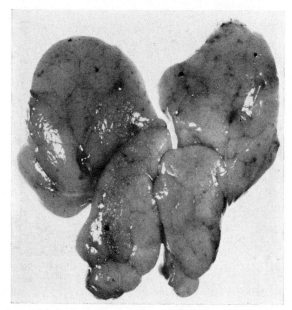

Fig. 10.1.§ Normal fetal thymus at 32 weeks. The left and right lobes are separate. Twice natural size.

§ See *Acknowledgements*, page 924.

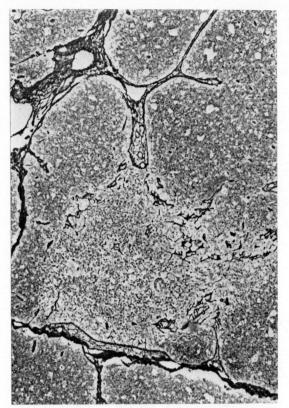

Fig. 10.3. Distribution of argyrophile reticulin fibres in the normal thymus of a child. These fibres are present only round blood vessels and in the capsule and septa. *Gordon and Sweet method for reticulin.* × 50.

central cystic change and it is a common finding to see degenerate cells, particularly lymphocytes and eosinophils, within cystic Hassall's corpuscles. Far from being effete structures, Hassall's corpuscles (in common with the solitary epithelial cells in the medulla) secrete a sulphated acid mucopolysaccharide (Fig. 10.6B).[13, 14]

Other cells in the thymus include eosinophils, a few macrophages, the so-called periodic-acid/Schiff-positive ('PAS-positive') cells, and the myoid or striated muscle cells. The PAS-positive cells[15] are found mainly at the corticomedullary junction and are particularly prominent in the involuting thymus: it is not yet known whether they are specialized macrophages or altered epithelial cells. Myoid cells are of particular interest because of their possible relation to myasthenia gravis.[16] These cells have been known since the latter half of the last century:[17] they were called myoid cells by Hammar because —although he believed them to be hypertrophied reticular cells (that is, epithelial cells)—he wanted to stress their similarity to striated muscle. It is

surprising that their existence was virtually ignored until 1966, when attention was again drawn to them.[13, 18] Not only do these cells share certain light microscopical and ultrastructural features with striated muscle (Figs 10.8 and 10.9), they are also antigenically similar, as is shown by their cross-reactivity with sera containing anti-striated-muscle antibody ('myoid antibody'). In certain species, particularly among reptiles and birds, they are numerous. In the human thymus they are few in number: they are most plentiful at birth (Fig. 10.8A) but can be found at all ages if carefully searched for (Fig. 10.8B). The reason myoid cells are difficult to detect is that the thick myosin and thin actin myofilaments are not always organized into sarcomeres;[19] when present, sarcomeres are often arranged in a haphazard fashion (Fig. 10.9).

In most accounts of thymic structure it is stated that lymphoid follicles with germinal centres are not seen in the normal gland. This is incorrect,

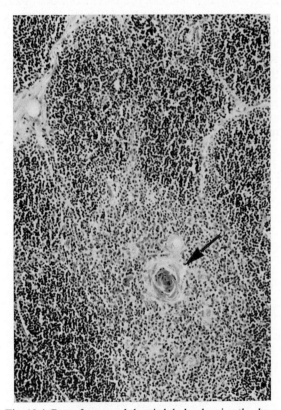

Fig. 10.4. Part of a normal thymic lobule, showing the dense aggregation of lymphocytes in the cortex and the comparative pallor of the medulla, where lymphocytes are fewer and the epithelial component more conspicuous. The field includes a large Hassall's corpuscle (arrow) that has undergone cystic change centrally. *Haematoxylin–eosin.* × 120.

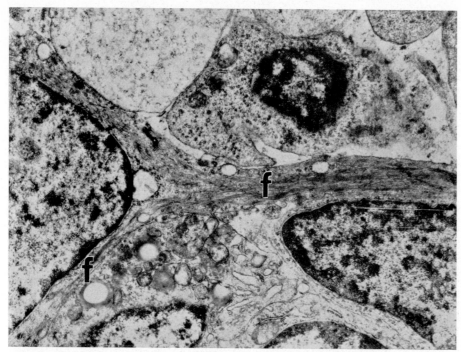

Fig. 10.5. Electron micrograph of part of an epithelial cell of the thymic cortex. A long extension of its cytoplasm between the lymphocytes contains numerous tonofilaments (f, f). × 12 000.

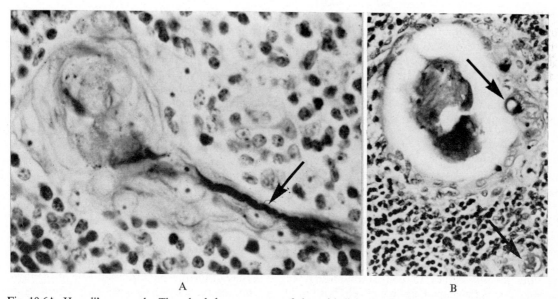

A   B

Fig. 10.6A. Hassall's corpuscle. The whorled arrangement of the epithelial cells forming the corpuscle is seen. The arrow points to a skein of tonofibrils (the electron microscope shows these to be bundles of tonofilaments). *Phospho-tungstic acid haematoxylin.* × 640.

Fig. 10.6B. Hassall's corpuscles. The arrows point to intracellular mucin. *Alcian blue; periodic-acid/Schiff.* × 300.

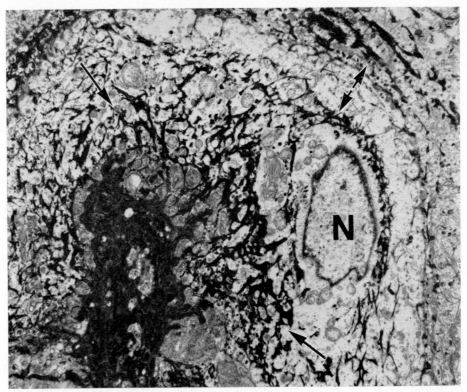

Fig. 10.7. Electron micrograph of part of a Hassall's corpuscle. The arrows point to parts of the abundant, dense, fibrillary material (keratin) in the cytoplasm of an epithelial cell. The nucleus of an epithelial cell is also seen (N). ×4800.

for it is not uncommon to find them occasionally in the otherwise normal thymus, particularly in children (Fig. 10.10), adolescents and young adults.[20] Their frequency as recorded by different observers has varied, these variations doubtless reflecting differing sources of material and the care with which they have been sought.[21]

Involution

With increasing age there is a gradual loss of thymic parenchyma, which is replaced by adipose tissue (Fig. 10.11). This process of age involution[22] is most marked in the cortical areas, due to a decrease in the number of lymphocytes, which normally are most numerous there. At first the general architectural pattern is well preserved but with advancing age the thymus comes to consist of strands of shrunken, spindle-shaped, epithelial cells with only a sprinkling of lymphocytes (Fig. 10.12). In stress or accidental involution[10] also there is a marked loss of lymphocytes from cortical areas: if the stimulus is continued the weight of the thymus is greatly reduced and the histological picture is characterized by irregular lobules consisting of spindle-shaped epithelial cells with only occasional lymphocytes; there is complete loss of differentiation between cortex and medulla (Fig. 10.13). Hassall's corpuscles may show conspicuous cystic change and appear to be increased in number: they are not really more numerous but simply seem so because of the loss of other elements. Another common feature of the involuted thymus is the presence of elongated cystic spaces lined by squamous epithelium: these are derived from Hassall's corpuscles (Fig. 10.14).[20]

Functional Aspects

Study of the growth curve of the thymus indicates that it is functionally at its most active around the time of birth. The important role of the thymus in immunity was recognized only comparatively recently. Although thymic abnormalities were known to occur in some human diseases (for instance, acromegaly[23] and thyrotoxicosis[24]), and had also been related to the development of certain naturally occurring, virus-induced leukaemias in

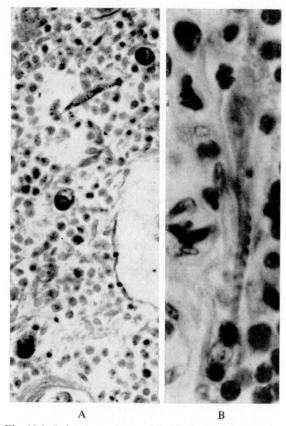

A   B

Fig. 10.8. Striated muscle (myoid) cells in thymus. *Phosphotungstic acid haematoxylin.*

A. Thymus of a stillborn baby (38 weeks' gestation). Only the elongated cell, cut lengthwise in the upper part of the field, shows cross striation. × 350.

B. Thymus of an adult. Myoid cell of tadpole-like appearance, with distinct cross-striation, in the corticomedullary junctional zone. × 1400.

animals,[25] it was only in 1954 that the first real clue linking the thymus with immune function was discovered: this was the observation of a patient with a thymoma accompanied by hypogamma-globulinaemia and other immune defects.[26] In 1960 Miller[27] performed his classic experiments of thymectomy in newborn mice and showed conclusively that the thymus was essential for the development of normal cell-mediated immunity and for certain humoral immune responses. He then demonstrated that similar immune defects could be produced in adult mice if thymectomy was preceded by sublethal irradiation.[28] In both situations—neonatally thymectomized mice and thymectomized irradiated adult mice—the immune defects could be corrected by thymus grafting, by infusion of lymphocytes and by injecting thymic

extracts. It was later shown that lasting restoration of normal immunological activity was dependent not on thymic lymphocytes but on thymic epithelial cells, which secrete hormonal ('humoral') substances.[29] There is also experimental evidence of functional collaboration between bone marrow lymphocytes and thymic and thoracic duct lymphocytes.[30]

It is now generally accepted that the thymus, like the bursa of Fabricius in birds, is a primary or central lymphoid organ. It is responsible for the production, differentiation and direction of a population of antigen-reactive small lymphocytes (which are concerned primarily with cell-mediated immunity) and of a population of 'memory cells' primed by previous contact with antigen. Thymus-dependent lymphocytes are currently known as T lymphocytes[31] and distinguished from the bone-marrow dependent ('bursa dependent') B lymphocytes. The majority of T lymphocytes are long-lived and recirculate between lymph and

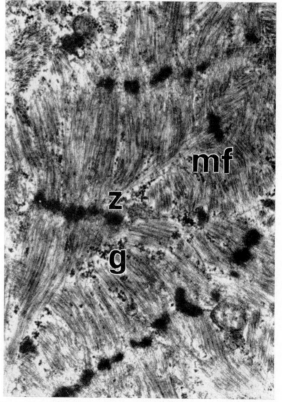

Fig. 10.9. Electron micrograph of cytoplasm of a myoid cell. The sarcomeres are arranged in a disorderly manner. Z lines (Z), myofilaments (mf) and glycogen granules (g) are indicated. × 48 000.

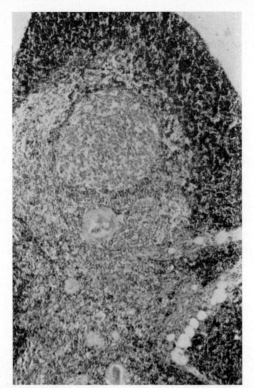

Fig. 10.10. There is a lymphoid follicle with a large germinal centre in the medullary part of this field. Normal thymus of a child of nine years. *Haematoxylin–eosin.* × 120.

vascular compartments by way of the specialized postcapillary venules (see page 519).[32] In the peripheral lymphoreticular tissues they are identified with particular areas:[33] in lymph nodes the thymus-dependent areas are the deep or paracortical zones[34] and in the spleen they are the perifollicular arterial lymphoid sheaths.[35]

THYMIC APLASIA AND HYPOPLASIA

Immune Deficiency States

Hypoplasia of the thymus is associated with various immune deficiency states (Fig. 10.15). Although rare, this association supports the concept that the development of the immune system in man is similar to that in animals. Only the commoner syndromes in which the defect is linked with thymic abnormality will be described.

Reticular Dysgenesis

The severest of the immune deficiency syndromes is reticular dysgenesis.[36, 37] In this condition there is failure of development of bone marrow precursor cells, with consequent severe leucopenia affecting both the lymphoid and the myeloid series of cells. The thymus is vestigial and contains neither lympho-cytes nor Hassall's corpuscles. The disease is fatal, resulting in still birth or in death within a few weeks of birth.

Swiss Type of Hypogammaglobulinaemia (Glanzmann–Riniker Disease)

Hypogammaglobulinaemia ('agammaglobulin-aemia') of the Swiss type is usually familial and its incidence is consistent with an autosomal recessive mode of inheritance. It was first described in Switzerland.[38] Affected infants are subject to many types of infection—bacterial, fungal, protozoal and viral—within the first few months of life: they usually die before the age of two years. There is an extreme degree of thymic hypoplasia; this is usually associated with failure of the thymus to

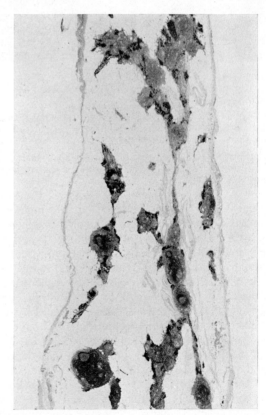

Fig. 10.11. Thymus of a woman, aged 44. Adipose tissue replacing thymic parenchyma—normal age involution. *Haematoxylin–eosin.* × 8.

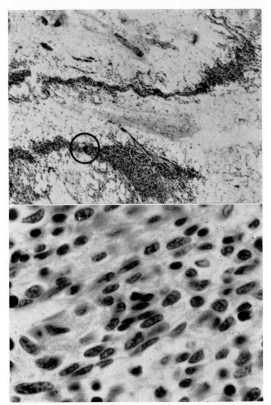

Fig. 10.12. Marked normal, involutional replacement of the thymic parenchyma by adipose tissue: a manifestation of ageing. The parenchyma is reduced to attenuated, irregular strands of tissue. The encircled area in the upper photograph includes the field illustrated in the lower photograph which shows spindle cell metamorphosis of the epithelial cells. *Haematoxylin–eosin.* Upper: ×30. Lower: ×350.

descend from the neck into the mediastinum. The gland weighs about 3 g (the normal weight of the thymus at birth is about 22 g). Microscopy shows a total absence of lymphocytes and Hassall's corpuscles and no distinction between cortex and medulla (Fig. 10.16). The peripheral lymphoid tissues are also underdeveloped, being deficient both in the T lymphocyte (thymus-dependent) paracortical areas and in the B lymphocyte ('bursa-equivalent'-dependent) follicles with their germinal centres and plasma cells. The basic fault is in the lymphoid stem cell, which normally interacts with the thymus and the bursa-equivalent.[39] There is consequent failure of both cell-mediated and humoral immunity.

Thymic Alymphoplasia[39]

The clinical picture of this condition is similar to that of the Swiss type of hypogammaglobulinaemia

except that progress of the disease is less rapid and there is longer survival. In contrast to Swiss hypogammaglobulinaemia the condition occurs only in boys and is probably linked to the X chromosome.

Thymic Dysplasia[40]

Thymic dysplasia is distinguished from the Swiss type of hypogammaglobulinaemia and from thymic alymphoplasia by the fact that, although the thymus is rudimentary and epithelial, the immune defect predominantly involves cellular immunity, with only a partial disorder of immunoglobulin production.

DiGeorge Syndrome[41, 41a]

This condition results from arrested development of the third and possibly of the fourth branchial arches. In addition to a vestigial thymus, there is

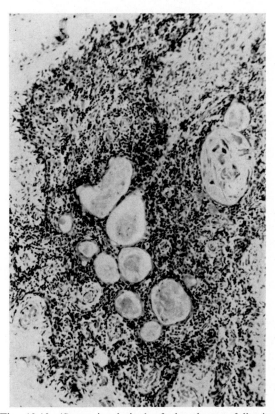

Fig. 10.13. 'Stress involution' of the thymus following corticosteroid therapy. The patient was a baby, aged nine months. The thymic architecture is much distorted. There is loss of lymphocytes from the cortex and the epithelial cells show spindle-shape metamorphosis. Hassall's corpuscles are notably cystic and crowded together. *Haematoxylin–eosin.* ×100.

Q

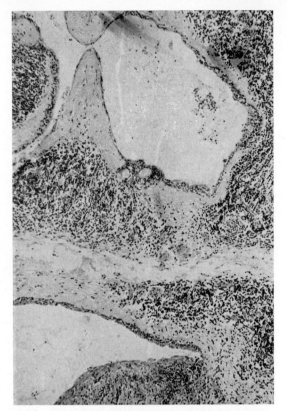

Fig. 10.14. Marked cystic change in an involuted thymus. The patient was a man, aged 42, with rheumatic heart disease. The cysts are lined by squamous epithelium. *Haematoxylin–eosin.* × 80.

absence or hypoplasia of the parathyroids; anomalies of the heart and great vessels are usually also present. If the baby survives the hypoparathyroidism in the neonatal period, it is likely to die during the following months from the infections that it lacks the capacity to combat successfully. The immune deficiency has been successfully treated by transplantation of fetal thymic tissue.[42]

Nezelof's Syndrome[43]

The thymic abnormality in Nezelof's syndrome is similar to that of the DiGeorge syndrome except that there is no hypoparathyroidism. The failure of development involves only that part of the branchial entoderm that should differentiate into thymic epithelium.

Ataxia-Telangiectasia[44]

Ataxia-telangiectasia (ataxia telangiectatica; Louis-Bar's syndrome[45]) is a hereditary autosomal reces-

sive disease that involves several body systems. The principal manifestations are cerebellar ataxia, oculocutaneous telangiectasia, mental deterioration and immune deficiency. The major immune defect is in cell-mediated immunity and results in susceptibility to sinusitis and recurrent bronchopulmonary infection. It is associated with hypoplasia or aplasia of the thymus. Death usually occurs in the second or third decade from chronic respiratory infection or lymphoma. The condition probably results from a failure of development of mesenchymal cells.

Wiskott–Aldrich Syndrome[46, 47]

The Wiskott–Aldrich syndrome is a hereditary disease transmitted as a sex-linked recessive trait. It is characterized by a very severe immune deficiency, with recurrent infection, eczematous dermatitis and thrombocytopenia. Infection is the usual cause of death; malignant lymphoma develops in some cases. The immune defect is principally in cell-mediated immunity; a curious feature of the disease is that the defect becomes severer as the child grows older. The thymus is small but of normal structure, apart from showing stress involution as an accompaniment of the terminal infection. In contrast, the peripheral lymphoid tissue shows progressive depletion of T-lymphocyte-dependent areas and there is lymphocytopenia. It is thought that the essential fault is an inability of the T lymphocytes to recognize antigen.[48]

Bruton Type of Hypogammaglobulinaemia[49]

This X-chromosome-linked condition may be mentioned as an example of an immune deficiency state predominantly affecting humoral immunity. The thymus is normal—apart from stress involution —and the T lymphocytes are present in normal numbers and so the thymus-dependent areas in the peripheral lymphoid tissue are not depleted; in contrast, there is a total absence of lymphoid follicles with germinal centres, and of plasma cells, reflecting a deficiency of B lymphocytes (see page 519).

Acquired Hypogammaglobulinaemia

The clinical manifestations accompanying acquired hypogammaglobulinaemia vary.[50, 51] It is of interest and practical importance that patients with this condition are unusually liable to develop thymoma, lymphoma and various autoimmune diseases,

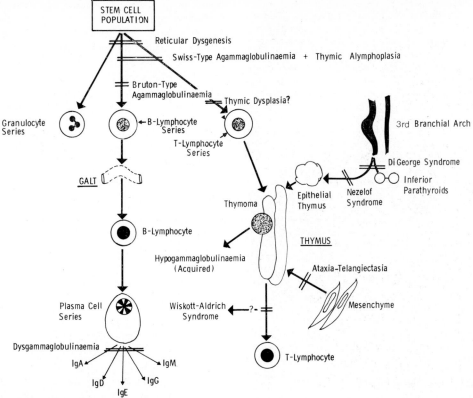

Fig. 10.15.§ Diagrammatic representation of immune deficiency states. The double lines across the pathways of normal development indicate the site at which the block occurs in the deficiency states named. GALT: gut-associated lymphoid tissue.

including haemolytic anaemia and gastric mucosal atrophy leading to pernicious anaemia.

THYMIC HYPERPLASIA

True hyperplasia of the thymus is rare and seems to be linked with endocrine abnormalities. For instance, it has been recognized for many years that there is enlargement of the thymus in cases of thyrotoxicosis.[52] This enlargement is due to a true hyperplasia involving the cortex and medulla: the weight of the the thymus is well above the normal range. Hyperplasia of the thymus in thyrotoxicosis is associated with generalized hyperplasia of the lymphoreticular tissue throughout the body and is thought to be related to the raised level of circulating thyroxine.[53] Other conditions in which thymic hyperplasia occurs include chronic adrenal cortical insufficiency (Addison's disease), acromegaly,[54] congenital absence of the pituitary gland and anencephaly. In some of these conditions the

hyperplasia of the thymus is due to lack of corticotrophin.[55]

The debatable application of the term thymic hyperplasia to the changes in the thymus in cases of myasthenia gravis without thymoma is mentioned below.

THE THYMUS AND MYASTHENIA GRAVIS

The occurrence of abnormalities of the thymus in association with myasthenia gravis has been known since 1901, when a case of this disease was reported in which there was a mediastinal tumour involving the thymus.[56] Following this observation there were numerous accounts of thymic abnormalities found at necropsy in cases of myasthenia gravis. These conditions ranged from thymomas to 'hyperplasia', 'persistence' and subinvolution of the gland. Further evidence of the association of thymic abnormalities and myasthenia gravis was the demonstration that some patients with the latter, particularly young

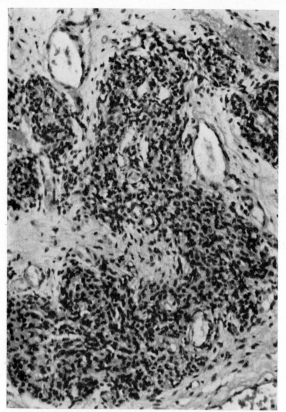

Fig. 10.16.§ Thymus in a case of the Swiss type of hypo-gammaglobulinaemia. The patient was a boy, aged eight months. The lobules are irregular and lack corticomedullary demarcation. The cells are mostly spindle-shaped epithelial cells. There are no Hassall's corpuscles. *Haematoxylin–eosin.* × 200.

women without tumours, benefit from thymec-tomy.[57]

The relation between myasthenia gravis and thymoma ('thymomatous myasthenia gravis') is considered on page 920.

The Thymus in Cases of Myasthenia Gravis without Thymoma ('Non-Thymomatous Myasthenia Gravis')

It was not until 1943 that the remarkable changes in the thymus in cases of myasthenia gravis without thymoma ('non-thymomatous myasthenia gravis') were recognized.[58] They are characterized by the presence within the medulla of numerous lymphoid follicles with active germinal centres, often resulting in appreciable expansion of this part of the gland (Fig. 10.17). There is no significant increase in the weight of the thymus, since the cortex usually

shows some degree of involution, with lymphocyte depletion appropriate to the age of the patient. The lymphoid follicles in the thymic medulla are similar to those in lymph nodes and other lymphoreticular tissue (Fig. 10.18). Sometimes the increase in the number of the follicles is relatively small, particularly in older patients. There does not appear to be any correlation between the number of follicles and the severity of the myasthenia.[59]

Other microscopical abnormalities in the thymus in these cases include an overall increase in the number of lymphocytes and plasma cells and of their immediate precursors in the medulla. There is also a great increase in the reticulin fibre content, particularly round lymphoid follicles and at the corticomedullary junction (Fig. 10.19): taken with the other abnormalities this is indicative of a chronic inflammatory process. Ultrastructural studies confirm and extend this view (Fig. 10.20). There is no constant abnormality at the level of light micro-

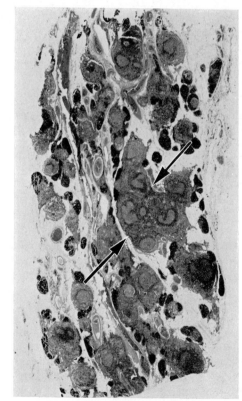

Fig. 10.17.§ Thymus of a woman, aged 33, who had myasthenia gravis without a thymoma. The medulla is notably expanded in some areas (for instance, between the arrows): it contains numerous lymphoid follicles, with germinal centres and often irregular in outline. *Haematoxylin–eosin.* × 8.

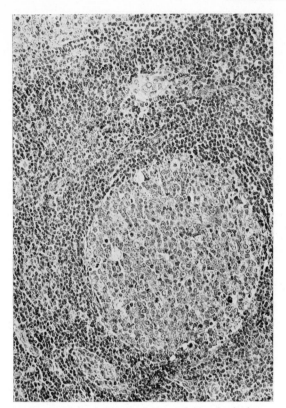

Fig. 10.18.§ Thymus of a woman, aged 30, who had myasthenia gravis without a thymoma. The field includes parts of adjacent medullary lymphoid follicles with active germinal centres. Epithelial cells and Hassall's corpuscles are seen in the intervening zone. See also Fig. 10.19. *Haematoxylin–eosin.* × 120.

particularly easy to identify in the thymus in cases of myasthenia gravis and are more numerous than in normal individuals of similar age.[62] In view of the increase in the number of the myoid cells it is possible that they provide an antigen that provokes an autoimmune state and consequent local inflammatory response. However, it should be pointed out that only 30 per cent of patients with non-thymomatous myasthenia gravis possess an auto-antibody to striated muscle ('myoid antibody'):[63] in contrast, this antibody is present in 95 per cent of patients with thymomatous myasthenia gravis.

Thymitis has been proposed as a term more appropriate for these changes than thymic hyperplasia,[64] since the chronic inflammatory process appears similar to that occurring in the thyroid gland in Hashimoto's thyroiditis. Indeed, it was this similarity that led to the suggestion that myasthenia gravis itself might be an autoimmune disease.[65]

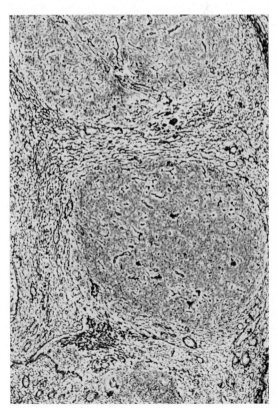

Fig. 10.19. Same thymus as in Fig. 10.18. Reticulin fibres are numerous in the tissue round the germinal centres of the lymphoid follicles. Compare with the normal thymus illustrated in Fig. 10.3, in which reticulin fibres are characteristically sparse. *Gordon and Sweet method for reticulin.* × 120.

scopy in the epithelial network, but Hassall's corpuscles are sometimes increased in number and may show cystic change and, occasionally, increased secretory activity.[60]

About 80 per cent of patients with myasthenia gravis and no thymoma show these microscopical abnormalities in the thymus. In contrast to thymomatous myasthenia gravis, which tends to occur in older patients (see page 920), the non-thymomatous disease is seen most frequently in women between 15 and 35 years.

Thymic hyperplasia is the term that has been used most commonly to describe the changes in the gland in cases of myasthenia unassociated with thymoma. The hyperplastic changes are confined to the medullary lymphoid tissue and have been interpreted as a reaction to an unknown stimulus affecting the thymus primarily, since there is no generalized lymphoid hyperplasia.[61] In this context it is interesting that myoid cells (Fig. 10.8) are

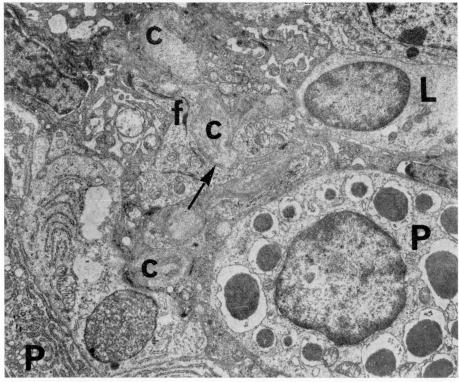

Fig. 10.20. Electron micrograph of the thymic medulla in a case of myasthenia gravis. The main features are the presence of plasma cells (P, P) and increased amounts of connective tissue (c, c, c) between the processes of epithelial cells. The cisternae of the rough endoplasm of the plasma cell to the right of the field, below, are distended and contain electron-dense secretory products. Other features illustrated are a lymphocyte (L), tonofilaments (f) and basement membrane (arrow). × 6000.

It must be emphasized that the formation of lymphoid follicles within the thymus is not specific to myasthenia gravis. They are found in the thymus of some healthy people. They are also found in the thymus of patients with various diseases, including Addison's disease, autoimmune thyroiditis, rheumatoid arthritis, rheumatic heart disease and systemic lupus erythematosus. However, the lymphoid follicles in the thymus in these conditions are never as numerous or as prominent as in myasthenia gravis. It is of interest in the context of thyroid disease that some patients with myasthenia gravis show evidence of thyroid dysfunction.[66]

The Relation between Pathological Changes in the Thymus and Myasthenia Gravis

While there is no doubt that a relation exists between abnormalities of the thymus and myasthenia gravis, the nature of this association is not wholly understood. Its existence is indicated by the fact that after thymectomy there is a notable increase in the occurrence of remissions, and often complete cure of the myasthenic condition, particularly in non-thymomatous myasthenia gravis and when the duration of the disease has been short;[67] older patients are less likely to benefit from thymectomy —when they do so the results are less complete. Interestingly, there are well-documented reports of the onset of myasthenia gravis years after the excision of a symptomless thymoma.

That the muscle autoantibody (myoid antibody) is not the cause of the myasthenic symptoms is indicated by the following observations:[68] (1) myoid antibody is present in patients with a thymoma that is not associated with myasthenia gravis; (2) the myoid antibody is not directed at the motor endplate, which is the site of the lesion in myasthenia gravis; (3) there is no correlation between the presence or absence of myoid antibody and the severity of the myasthenia; and (4) in transient neonatal myasthenia gravis there is no correlation with myoid antibody. These considerations led to the suggestion that the abnormal thymus is the site of elaboration of a neuromuscular blocking agent, and that patients with thymoma and myoid antibodies but no evidence of myasthenia gravis have an effective means of successfully inactivating these substances.[69] The changes in the thymus in cases of myasthenia gravis in the absence of a thymoma were interpreted as a pre-neoplastic transformation, and the presence of the auto-antibody as merely an indicator of the disease. The induction of autoimmune thymitis in guinea-pigs, and the demonstration of a neuromuscular block that is prevented by thymectomy prior to immunization is further evidence for the production of a neuromuscular blocking agent, which has been named thymin.[70] It is postulated that the presence of a thymoma represents a distinct condition and that it is the tumour that is the cause of an auto-immune thymitis.

An alternative hypothesis is that the neuro-muscular lesion in myasthenia gravis is the result of a cell-mediated autoimmune mechanism.[71] This suggestion is based on a histological review of thymectomy specimens from patients with the disease: the findings indicate that the length of the interval between thymectomy and the sub-sequent remission of symptoms is proportional to the number of active germinal centres in the thymus. It thus appears that the essential patho-logical process is the generation within these active germinal centres of immunocompetent lymphocytes capable of inducing and sustaining cell-mediated autoimmune neuromuscular injury. This hypothesis can be applied also to thymo-matous myasthenia gravis, since similar patho-logical changes are commonly found in the thymic tissue apart from the tumour.

It remains to be shown which aetiological mechanism—neuromuscular blockade or cell-mediated immunity—is responsible. In either case, the explanation of the underlying 'inflammatory' follicular hyperplasia of the lymphoid tissue in the medulla of the thymus has yet to be found. The possibility of viral or bacterial infection has not been excluded. The relation of the thymic myoid cells to myasthenia gravis has not been established.

INFECTION AND THE THYMUS

Usually, the only thymic manifestation of infective disease is the occurrence of non-specific involutional changes (see page 894). Acute specific thymitis may occur in certain infections, such as influenza,[72] measles and miliary tuberculosis. The histological appearances are those characteristic of the infections as they are seen in the tissues of the lymphoreticular system (see, for instance, page 641). Similarly, thymitis may develop in the course of brucellosis and infectious mononucleosis.

True abscesses of the thymus are very rare: they are usually a result of septicaemia caused by pyo-genic organisms. The condition that sometimes is still referred to as Dubois's abscess is not an abscess at all but the outcome of leakage of the contents of a thymic cyst, resulting in the develop-ment of a surrounding granuloma (see page 919).

TUMOURS OF THE THYMUS

The tumours that arise in the thymus are peculiarly interesting, in particular because some 30 per cent are associated with systemic disorders. Myasthenia gravis is the commonest of the latter: a thymoma is present in about 15 per cent of patients with this disease.[73] Conditions more rarely associated with thymic tumours include hypogammaglobulinaemia, hypoplastic anaemia, myositis, systemic lupus erythematosus and Cushing's syndrome (see below).

It has become clear that tumours of the thymus, whether accompanied by systemic disease or not, are less rare than was previously supposed.[74] They are seldom seen in patients below 20 years of age; the mean age at which they are recognized is about 48 years.[75]

It is important to note that the term thymoma is applied to any neoplasm arising in the thymus. It does not denote a special histological type of tumour or indicate whether a tumour is benign or malig-nant.

Classification

Many classifications of thymic tumours have been proposed: none is entirely satisfactory. They range from the simple, such as one that divides thymic tumours into two groups according to whether or not they are associated with myasthenia gravis,[76] to the exceedingly complex, such as the embryo-logical classification of Lowenhaupt.[77] Most classi-fications are based on histological appearances. In 1957, Thomson and Thackray, from a study of 67 examples, proposed a division of thymic tumours into three main groups—epithelial, lymphoid and teratomatous.[78] They subdivided the epithelial group into five main categories—(a) differentiated or epidermoid tumours, (b) oval cell and spindle cell tumours, (c) thymic lymphoepitheliomas, (d) granulomatous thymomas and (e) undifferentiated epithelial tumours: the epithelial subgroups accounted for 54 of their 67 tumours. In contrast, Castleman, in a monograph published in 1955, did not attempt to classify the tumours but simply described a number of histological patterns observed in a series of these tumours.[79] Lattes, in 1962, published a study of 107 primary neoplasms of the thymus:[80] he recognized four main types—predominantly lymphoid, predominantly epithelial, predominantly spindle-celled and predominantly rosette-forming tumours. Another classification is that of Friedman, based on a study of 55 thymic tumours:[81] he defined them as (a) lymphoepithelial tumours, (b) teratoid tumours, (c) lymphomas and (d) myoid tumours—a previously undefined category.

The difficulty of classification is mainly due to the very wide range of histological appearances. While most thymic tumours are composed of two cell types, the epithelial cell and the lymphocyte, there is considerable variation in the appearance and arrangement of the epithelial cells and in the arrangement of the lymphocytes in relation to the epithelial component. In addition, the proportion of lymphocytes to epithelial cells may vary in different areas of any tumour, and even in adjacent lobules. Thus, not only do thymic tumours differ one from another but there may be substantial differences in appearance in different areas of the same tumour. Growing knowledge of thymic structure and function and the work of reference centres where thymic tumours can be collected and studied specially should lead to an acceptable classification.

It is proposed to discuss thymic tumours here under four headings: (1) mixed lymphocytic and epithelial thymoma (including the so-called 'granulomatous' thymoma); (2) teratomatous and teratoid tumours; (3) other essentially thymic tumours (pure epithelial thymoma; thymolipoma; tumours of myoid origin); and (4) a miscellaneous group of conditions that are not peculiar to the thymus (lymphomas, leukaemia, secondary tumours).

Mixed Lymphocytic and Epithelial Thymoma

The majority of thymic tumours are composed of a mixture of thymic epithelial cells and lymphocytes and fall into this group. Typically, these tumours are well encapsulated and confined to one lobe (Fig. 10.21). Involvement of both lobes is a late occurrence except in the case of some more rapidly growing tumours. The capsule may be very thick

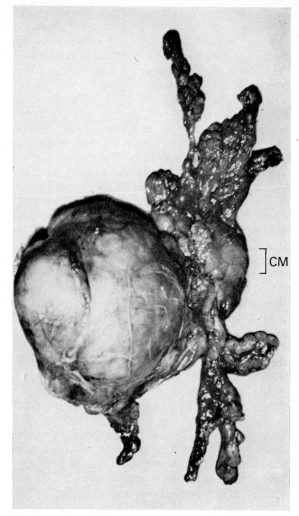

Fig. 10.21. Resected thymus of a man, aged 42, with myasthenia gravis. A thymoma occupies most of one lobe. The other lobe is not involved.

and contain calcific plaques, suggesting that the tumour has been present for a considerable time.

The cut surface usually shows a lobular pattern; the lobules vary in size and are separated by bands of connective tissue that sometimes are very broad and dense. Cystic change is not uncommon (Fig. 10.22) and may be so extensive that there is little solid tumour. About a quarter of these growths invade neighbouring structures such as the pericardium and pleura (Fig. 10.23) or compress the great vessels, leading to the syndrome of mediastinal obstruction. Even in these cases the lobular structure of the tumour is still evident.

The weight of thymomas associated with myasthenia gravis ranges from 10 to 150 g, the average

to the epithelial cells: these are the tumours that are usually designated *lymphoepitheliomas*.

The epithelial cells in a given thymoma tend to be of uniform size. Frequently they are large and plump, and have an oval, vesicular nucleus and indistinctly outlined, eosinophile cytoplasm (Fig. 10.29): this type of epithelial cell is commonly seen in thymomas associated with myasthenia gravis and has sometimes been regarded as characteristic of that disease, although in fact it may occur in other thymomas. Oval and spindle-shaped epithelial cells are commonly present. Tumours in which there is a preponderance of the latter are often described as *spindle cell thymomas* (Fig. 10.30). The presence of these cells may give the tissue an appearance that closely resembles some connective tissue tumours, especially when the cells are arranged in whorls: however, the frequent transition between the spindle-shaped cells and recognizably

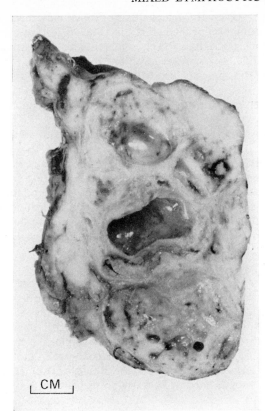

Fig. 10.22. Resected thymoma in a case of myasthenia gravis. The patient was a woman, aged 38. The cut surface discloses the marked cystic degeneration that is not uncommon in mixed lymphocytic and epithelial thymomas.

being 70 g;[79] in cases without myasthenia the weight may be as much as 300 g and more.[79]

Histology

Microscopy reveals a great range of appearances, largely dependent on the relative proportion of the lymphocytic and epithelial components and the variation in appearance and arrangement of the epithelial cells. Some tumours are predominantly epithelial (Figs 10.24 and 10.25); others are predominantly lymphocytic (Figs 10.26 and 10.27), the epithelial component sometimes being so obscured that the appearances may be incorrectly interpreted as lymphomatous. There is also variation in the proportion of one cell type to another within different areas of the same tumour and even within adjacent lobules (Fig. 10.28). Some tumours show a fairly even and consistent admixture of epithelial cells and lymphocytes (Fig. 10.29), although there may be considerable variation in the arrangement of the lymphocytes in relation

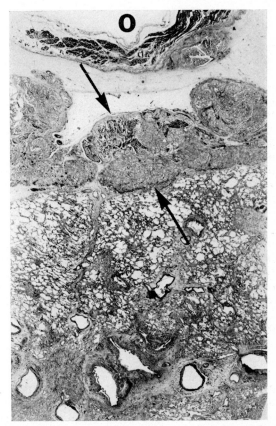

Fig. 10.23. Invasion of the pleura (arrows) by a mixed lymphocytic and epithelial thymoma. The patient did not have myasthenia gravis. There is no extension into the substance of the lung (below). The oesophagus is at the top of the field (O). *Haematoxylin–eosin.* × 5.

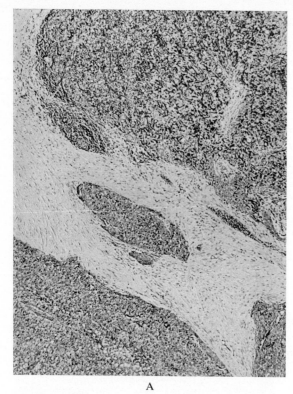

A

Fig. 10.24.§ Mixed lymphocytic and epithelial thymoma. The patient was a man, aged 55, with myasthenia gravis. See also Fig. 10.38 (page 918). *Haematoxylin–eosin.*

A.§ Solid masses of tumour cells are separated by dense fibrous tissue. × 65.

B.§ The predominantly epithelial nature of this specimen is seen well at the higher magnification. Many of the cells are vacuolate. Those abutting on the connective tissue tend to be arranged in a polarized manner (arrow). × 160.

epithelial cells establishes their identity. The epithelial nature of the spindle cell thymomas is also supported by the frequent occurrence of spindle-shaped epithelial cells in involuted thymus glands (see page 898) and by the ultrastructural characteristics of the cells. Purely or predominantly spindle-celled thymomas are not associated with myasthenia gravis (unless the histological appearances are a result of preoperative radiation, which leads to loss of the lymphocytic component and spindle-cell metamorphosis of the epithelial component of mixed lymphocytic and epithelial thymomas). They are associated with other systemic disorders, notably systemic lupus erythematosus, hypoplastic anaemia and hypogamma-globulinaemia.

The epithelial component of some tumours may show a more differentiated or epidermoid appear-ance (Figs 10.24 and 10.25). Sometimes there is vacuolation of the cytoplasm (Fig. 10.24B) or even mucin secretion. Rarely, differentiated cells are so distinctly squamous in nature that they may form keratin 'pearls' (Fig. 10.31): such structures are to be distinguished from neoplastic Hassall's corpuscles, formed in thymomas (an uncommon occurrence), and from pre-existing Hassall's corpuscles that have been enveloped by a tumour in the course of its growth. In contrast to such differentiated tumours there are those that consist of very undifferentiated epithelium, ranging from anaplastic growths with numerous mitotic figures (Fig. 10.32) to those in which the epithelium is multinucleate or syncytial, at least in part, and shows much variation in nuclear structure and size (Fig. 10.33).

Patterns.—The wide range of appearance of the epithelial cells of these tumours is matched by the variation in their arrangement; several distinctive histological patterns result. Spindle cell change, with consequent resemblance to connective tissue tumours, has been mentioned above. Another pattern is characterized by the presence of numerous microcysts lined by flattened epithelial cells, a sieve-

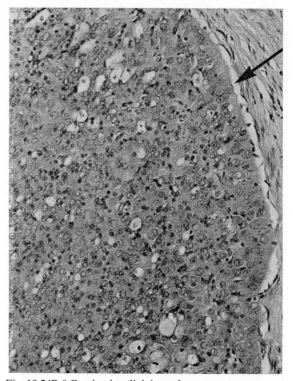

Fig. 10.24B.§ Caption in adjoining column.

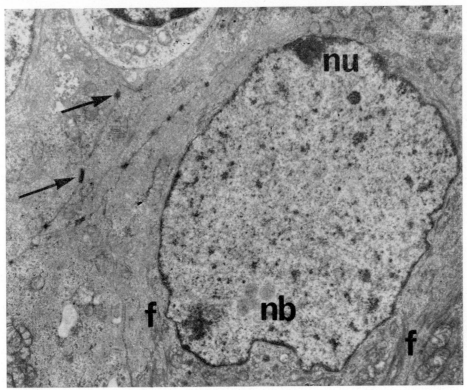

Fig. 10.25.§ Electron micrograph of the thymoma illustrated in Fig. 10.24. The cytoplasm of the epithelial tumour cells contains tonofilaments (f, f) and the cells are connected through many desmosomes (arrows). The nucleus has an open structure; there is margination of chromatin, a nucleolus (nu) and collections of nuclear bodies (nb). ×9000.

like appearance resulting (Fig. 10.34). The cysts may contain proteinaceous material. This cystic structure may be of relatively limited extent; in other instances, cysts are numerous and widespread and give the growth a superficial resemblance to a lymphangioma. It is very unusual for the whole of a tumour to show such a pattern: if sufficient material is sectioned the essentially thymic nature is revealed.

Another pattern is composed of small, scattered cyst-like spaces against a background of epithelial cells (Fig. 10.35). These spaces may appear empty or may contain lymphocytes. They are not true cysts but originate by widening of the circum-vascular spaces (Fig. 10.35B). The importance of this appearance is that it has been described as the histological pattern most characteristic of the thymomas that are associated with myasthenia gravis: in fact, however, the same pattern may be seen in the absence of myasthenia gravis (Fig. 10.35).

Where the epithelial cells of thymomas abut on connective tissue they commonly show orientation in a palisade-like arrangement (Figs 10.24B and 10.36). Other arrangements that may be seen in the epithelial component are glandular and adenomatoid patterns and rosette formation. Whatever the histological pattern, there is usually a striking lobulation of the tumour by fibrous bands that traverse it.

The So-called Granulomatous Thymoma

The name granulomatous thymoma was introduced to categorize a group of epithelial thymic tumours typified by areas of necrosis and by fibrosis and the presence of eosinophils.[82] Often these tumours include very large cells with conspicuous, hyperchromatic nuclei that resemble the 'Sternberg–Reed' cells of Hodgkin's disease. Many of the tumours that may be included under this term are examples of mediastinal involvement in nodular sclerotic Hodgkin's disease (see page 805);[83] others are mediastinal tumours such as teratomas and

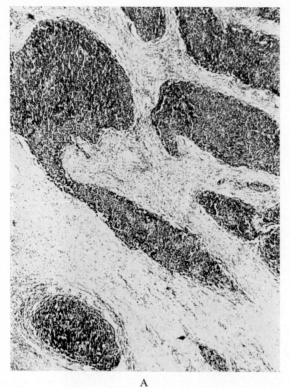

A

Fig. 10.26.§ Mixed lymphocytic and epithelial thymoma composed predominantly of lymphocytes. The patient was a woman, aged 42, with myasthenia gravis. *Haematoxylin–eosin.*

A.§ The low magnification shows the lobular pattern clearly, with intersecting bands of fibrous tissue separating the cellular masses. ×65.

B. Higher magnification, showing relatively few epithelial cells (arrows) among the lymphocytes. ×160.

seminomas in which there is a marked granulomatous response (see page 914).

In a small proportion of cases the granulomatous thymoma is a distinct variant of the mixed lymphocytic and epithelial thymoma (see page 908). This variant has a lobular pattern reminiscent of thymic lobulation (Fig. 10.37A). There are often areas of necrosis. The pleomorphic cellular content of the tumour includes lymphocytes, neutrophils and eosinophils, epithelial tumour cells and large, atypical mononuclear cells. It is possible to recognize transition between the atypical cells and the epithelial cells (Fig. 10.37B). The distinction from Hodgkin's disease depends to some extent on the absence of typical 'Sternberg–Reed' cells. This variety of granulomatous thymoma may occur in association with myasthenia gravis.

Lymphocytes in Mixed Lymphocytic and Epithelial Thymomas

While a lymphocytic component is present in every variant of the mixed lymphocytic and epithelial thymoma, it may be very sparse or show variation from one area to another (Figs 10.24, 26, 28, 33 and 35). The arrangement of the lymphocytes in relation to the epithelial cells also varies: they may be distributed in strands or festoons between the epithelial cells (Fig. 10.29) and, because of their circumvascular arrangement, they may appear in parallel lines (Fig. 10.38) when the vessels are cut lengthwise. They also accumulate in the small pseudocysts (that is, widened circumvascular spaces) that are referred to above (Fig. 10.35).

There are no morphological features that distinguish the lymphocytes of these tumours from normal thymic lymphocytes or from the small lymphocytes in other parts of the body (Figs 10.26 and 27). There is one immunological difference between thymoma lymphocytes and normal thymic lymphocytes: the tumour cells (like the small lymphocytes of normal blood and lymph) are transformed into pyroninophile blast cells by lymphocyte transformation agents such as the plant mitogen, phytohaemagglutinin (see page 522).[84]

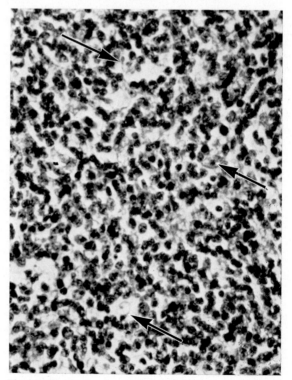

Fig. 10.26B. Caption in adjoining column.

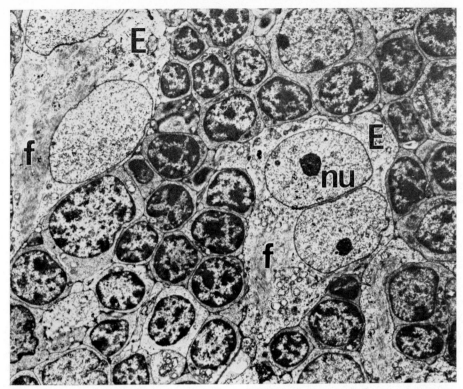

Fig. 10.27. Electron micrograph of the thymoma illustrated in Fig. 10.26. Two binucleate epithelial cells (E, E) are present among the many small lymphocytes. Tonofilaments (f, f) and a nucleolus (nu) are indicated. × 2800.

This suggests that the lymphocytes of thymomas are immunologically competent lymphocytes rather than neoplastic derivatives of the non-competent thymic lymphocytes. The lymphocytes in thymomas may therefore be present as an immune response to thymic epithelial tumour cell antigen, a manifestation comparable to similar findings in epithelial tumours arising in other parts of the body.

Malignancy of Thymomas

Judged by the criterion of local invasiveness, some 25 per cent of thymomas are malignant. In these cases there is direct invasion of mediastinal structures, including the pericardium, great vessels and pleura. The pleura, including that of the interlobar fissures, may be so extensively involved that the lungs are encased (Fig. 10.23): it is not surprising that some thymomas with pleural or pericardial involvement have been mistaken for mesotheliomas (see page 407). Although the lungs may be greatly compressed by a thymoma it is unusual for their parenchyma to be invaded.

The tumour may spread into the neck, downward to involve the diaphragm, and forward through the intercostal spaces or even through the sternum into the subcutaneous tissue of the chest wall, where it may fungate through the skin. In exceptional cases, nodules of tumour not connected with the main mass are present in the pericardium or pleura. There are few acceptable reports of metastasis to more distant sites.[85] It seems probable that in some recorded instances of supposed metastasis the diagnosis of thymoma was incorrect or the findings were the result of direct extension—for example, through the diaphragm into the liver.

Most thymomas grow slowly and are long confined to one lobe of the gland. Apart from their extension into adjoining tissues, the invasive tumours are not distinguished by any special histological features from those that remain encapsulated. Mitotic activity is not particularly helpful in prognostication since mitotic figures are infrequent in most thymomas of mixed lymphocytic and epithelial structure, whatever the histological subtype. The proportion of cells in mitosis is notably increased only in very rapidly growing

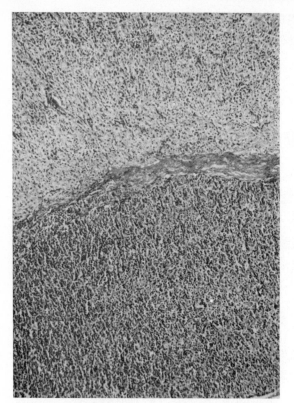

Fig. 10.28. Mixed lymphocytic and epithelial thymoma. The patient was a man, aged 72; he did not have myasthenia gravis. This field shows that one lobule (upper) is predominantly epithelial and another predominantly lymphocytic. *Haematoxylin–eosin.* × 60.

thymomas: in these the epithelial component is usually so undifferentiated that the malignancy of the growth is not in doubt (Fig. 10.32). The most important prognostic criteria are size and encapsulation. The tumours that present early, and therefore while they are still comparatively small, carry the best prognosis: indeed, there is no evidence that such tumours, if adequately excised, ever recur. Diagnosis at this most favourable stage is usually attributable to the presence of systemic symptoms, such as myasthenia.

Ectopic thymic tissue is not uncommon: it may be found anywhere from the neck to the diaphragm (see page 894). Occasionally, a thymoma originates in ectopic tissue (Fig. 10.39): like other thymomas it may be associated with systemic disorders. Failure to appreciate that ectopic thymomas occur has led to such tumours being misinterpreted as metastatic growths originating in other parts of the body.

Teratomatous and Teratoid Tumours of the Thymus

Most mediastinal tumours that may be placed under this heading fall into one of two groups—teratomas and so-called seminomas. Embryonal carcinoma and choriocarcinoma have also been described.

Teratoma.—Most of the teratomas that develop in the anterior mediastinum are benign dermoid cysts. Thymic tissue can usually be identified in the wall of these cysts, and this has led to the suggestion that all anterior mediastinal teratomas result from faults in the development of the thymus.[86] However, it should be borne in mind that any large tumour or cyst in the anterior mediastinum is likely to be in contact with the thymus and so may incorporate thymic tissue.

'Seminoma'.—The so-called mediastinal seminoma occurs in young males. There is good evidence that

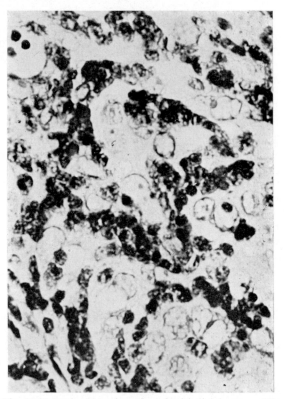

Fig. 10.29.§ Mixed lymphocytic and epithelial thymoma. The patient was a woman, aged 30, with myasthenia gravis. The epithelial cells have an indistinct outline and watery-looking cytoplasm, and a large, vesicular nucleus with prominent nucleolus. The lymphocytes are distributed in festoons between the epithelial cells. *Haematoxylin–eosin.* × 750.

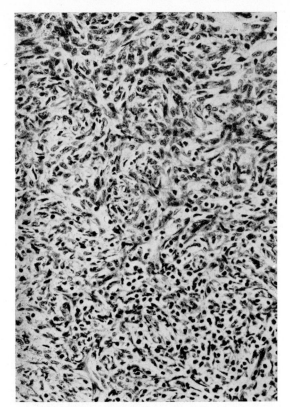

Fig. 10.30.§ Mixed epithelial and lymphocytic thymoma of spindle-celled type ('spindle cell thymoma'). The patient was a man, aged 63; he did not have myasthenia gravis. There is a scattering of lymphocytes among the epithelial cells. See also Fig. 10.34. *Haematoxylin–eosin.* × 200.

it originates in the thymus, although its cytogenesis is unknown. Histologically (Fig. 10.40B), it is identical with seminoma of the testis (see Chapter 26) and dysgerminoma of the ovary (see Chapter 27). As in these gonadal tumours, it is often possible to identify teratoid elements in the thymic 'seminoma' (Fig. 10.40A)[87] and a relation to teratomas is likely. The prognosis is similar to that of the testicular seminoma. It is important to remember than an intrathoracic secondary deposit of a primary gonadal tumour can be mistaken for this mediastinal tumour.

Other Essentially Thymic Tumours

Pure Epithelial Thymoma ('Carcinoid-Like Tumour of the Thymus')

This rare tumour, which—confusingly—has also been referred to as thymic adenoma, small cell carcinoma and carcinoid tumour of the thymus, is associated with Cushing's syndrome. It resembles none of the other varieties of thymoma but consists entirely of nests and masses of uniform epithelial cells. The cells have a moderate amount of eosinophile cytoplasm and a centrally located, round to oval nucleus. Only an occasional mitotic figure is seen. There is only a scanty stroma, in the form of thin septa. Lymphocytes are absent. A relation between these tumours, bronchial carcinoids and 'oat cell' carcinomas of lung with Cushing's syndrome (see page 403) has been suggested.[88]

Carcinoid tumours (argentaffinomas) not associated with Cushing's syndrome also occur, rarely, in the thymus (Fig. 10.41).[89]

Thymolipoma

The thymolipoma is a rare hamartoma that grossly appears to be composed of adipose tissue. On microscopy, however, there is an intimate relation between the fatty tissue and thymic tissue.[90] Some

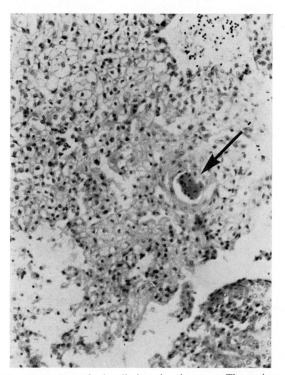

Fig. 10.31. Part of a locally invasive thymoma. The patient was a man, aged 53; he did not have myasthenia. The tumour is a mixed lymphocytic and epithelial thymoma, with a well-differentiated epithelial component and the formation of keratin 'pearls' (arrow). A microcyst is seen in the upper right corner: some lymphocytes are present in its lumen. *Haematoxylin–eosin.* × 120.

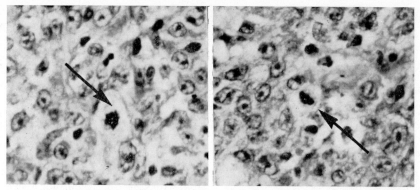

Fig. 10.32. Two fields showing the structure of a locally invasive thymoma. The patient was a woman, aged 28; she did not have myasthenia. The tumour is a mixed lymphocytic and epithelial thymoma that is composed predominantly of undifferentiated epithelial cells. Mitotic figures are conspicuous (arrows). *Haematoxylin–eosin.* × 350.

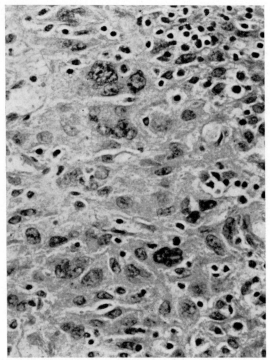

Fig. 10.33. Locally invasive thymoma. The patient was a woman, aged 82; she did not have myasthenia. The epithelial cells include some with a much enlarged nucleus, multinucleate forms, and the development of a syncytial arrangement. *Haematoxylin–eosin.* × 550.

of these tumours have attained a very large size—up to 6000 g.[91] An association with myasthenia gravis has not been reported. In one case the tumour was accompanied by hypoplastic anaemia[92] and in another by thyrotoxicosis.[93]

Myoid Cell Tumours

Myosarcoma arising in the thymus[81] and a less malignant variant showing differentiation toward

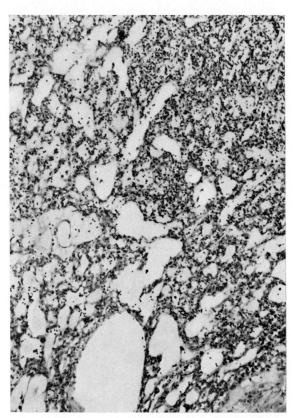

Fig. 10.34. Another field from the mixed lymphocytic and epithelial thymoma illustrated in Fig. 10.30. Here the presence of many thin-walled spaces gives the picture a resemblance to that of a lymphangioma. *Haematoxylin–eosin.* × 100.

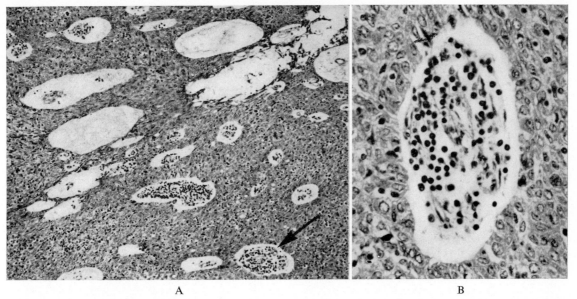

A   B

Fig. 10.35.§ Mixed lymphocytic and epithelial thymoma. The patient was a man, aged 43; he did not have myasthenia. *Haematoxylin–eosin.*

A. In this field many cyst-like spaces are seen, some of them empty and others containing lymphocytes. × 100.

B. Higher magnification of the cyst-like space indicated by the arrow in Fig. 10.35A: it is now clear that this appearance is due to widening of the circumvascular space and that there is no true cyst. × 200.

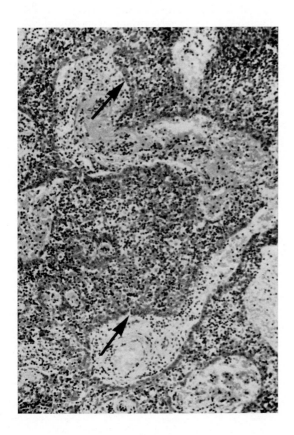

both epithelial cell and myoid cell formation[94] have been recorded. Thymic tumours of myoid cell origin or with a conspicuous myoid cell component are probably not as rare as has been supposed.

Miscellaneous Neoplastic Conditions

Lymphomas and Leukaemia

All types of lymphoma and leukaemia may involve the thymus.[95] Occasionally, enlargement of the gland caused by lymphomatous or leukaemic infiltration may be the first evidence of disease.[96] In cases of leukaemia the diagnosis is usually evident. It may be more difficult to distinguish lymphomas from true thymomas, particularly if the disease is confined to the mediastinum at the time of diagnosis. The histological types of thymoma likeliest to be confused with lymphoma are the predominantly lymphocytic thymomas (which closely resemble lymphocytic lymphomas), thymomas in which the epithelial component is undifferentiated

Fig. 10.36. Mixed lymphocytic and epithelial thymoma. The patient was a man, aged 45; he did not have myasthenia. This tumour shows well-marked palisading of the epithelial component where it abuts on the connective tissue (arrows). *Haematoxylin–eosin.* × 120.

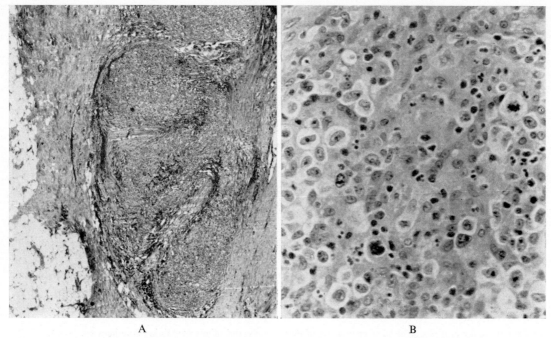

A   B

Fig. 10.37.§ The so-called granulomatous thymoma. The patient was a woman, aged 33. *Haematoxylin–eosin.*

A. At low magnification the lobular pattern of the tumour is evident, and reminiscent of the lobulation of the normal thymus. × 40.

B. In this pleomorphic cellular area the transition from large, atypical, mononuclear cells at the periphery of the field to the recognizably epithelial cells at the centre is seen. Many neutrophils and some lymphocytes are present also. × 300.

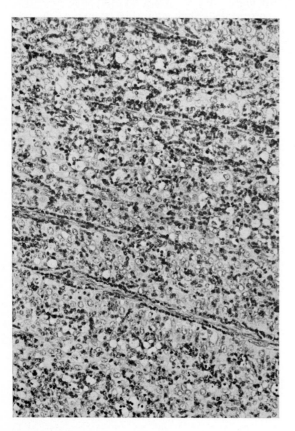

(which may resemble 'reticulum cell' sarcomas) and granulomatous thymomas (which resemble nodular sclerotic Hodgkin's disease). Provided that a sufficiently thorough further microscopical study is made of mediastinal tumours that are histologically equivocal on initial examination, thymomas can usually be distinguished from lymphomas because histological criteria typical of the former will be disclosed in some part of the specimen. The distinction is important since the two classes of tumour require different treatment.

Secondary Tumours

The thymus may be directly invaded by tumours in adjacent parts, such as a primary bronchial carcinoma or a metastatic growth in mediastinal lymph nodes. It is rare for the thymus to be involved by haematogenous or lymphatic spread from other sites.[95] Microscopical examination usually provides the correct diagnosis in such

Fig. 10.38.§ Mixed lymphocytic and epithelial thymoma (same specimen as in Fig. 10.24). This field illustrates the conspicuous lymphocytic 'cuffing' of the longitudinally cut blood vessels. *Haematoxylin–eosin.* × 160.

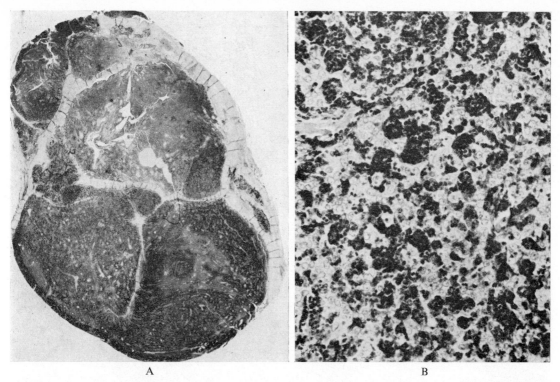

Fig. 10.39.§ Mixed lymphocytic and epithelial thymoma arising in ectopic thymic tissue in the neck. The patient was a woman, aged 38, with myasthenia gravis. A mediastinal thymoma was also present, in the normal site of the thymus. *Haematoxylin–eosin.* A:§ ×5. B: ×120.

cases, but there are some instances in which it is difficult to distinguish with certainty between secondary carcinoma and thymoma.

Angiofollicular Lymph Node Hyperplasia[97]

This condition, sometimes referred to as the 'giant mediastinal lymph node' or 'mediastinal lymph node hyperplasia',[98] is described on page 544. Although it is a disease of lymph nodes, not of the thymus, it is important in relation to the latter because it may be mistaken for a thymoma. Two factors contribute to this confusion: the large size of the mass, and the possibility of misinterpreting the hyalinized vascular structures in the germinal centres as Hassall's corpuscles.

THYMIC CYSTS

Cystic change is fairly common in the involuted thymus and results from degeneration of Hassall's corpuscles (see page 895). Multiple small cysts of this type are found particularly often in the thymus of infants with congenital syphilis.

Larger cysts also occur in the thymus. Their origin is uncertain. Many authors indeed restrict the term thymic cyst to non-neoplastic cysts that are large enough to be visible to the naked eye and that have a capsule in which thymic tissue is present.[99] These simple cysts are lined by epithelium that may be columnar, flattened, squamous (Fig. 10.42) or ciliate. While some of them may be derived from remnants of the parts of the branchial endoderm (or of the ectoderm of the cervical sinus) from which the thymus develops (see page 894), the evidence available points to origin of the majority in degenerating Hassall's corpuscles[100] and so to their acquired nature.

Other cysts involving the thymus or occurring in its vicinity include lymphatic cysts, bronchiogenic cysts, dermoid cysts (see above) and cystic degeneration in thymomas.[101] Cystic degeneration is not infrequent in thymomas (Fig. 10.22): if extensive it may obscure the thymic origin of the tumour.

Leakage of the contents of any variety of thymic cyst results in an accumulation of macrophages and foreign body giant cells in relation to the escaped fatty matter, often accompanied by the development

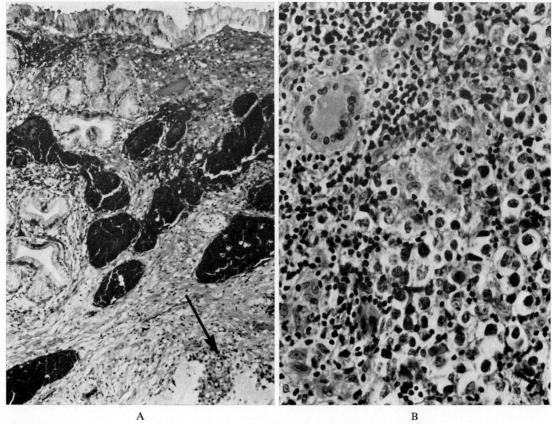

A   B

Fig. 10.40. Parts of a large seminoma that arose in a mediastinal teratoma of thymic origin. The patient was a boy, aged 11 years. *Haematoxylin–eosin.*

A. The arrow points to a seminomatous focus adjoining teratomatous neuroglial tissue. The rest of the field consists largely of teratomatous glandular elements. The very dark areas are blood-filled spaces. × 100.

B. At higher magnification the characteristic features of the seminoma are evident. Histiocytes are present among the typical seminoma cells and there is a multinucleate cell. The lymphocytic element is conspicuous. × 300.

of a granulomatous response in the wall of the cyst itself (Fig. 10.42). The occurrence of such inflammatory changes in association with the small cysts that often characterize the thymus of infants with congenital syphilis (see above) accounts for the non-suppurative inflammatory lesion that formerly was known as a Dubois abscess (see page 907).[102]

THYMOMAS AND SYSTEMIC DISORDERS

Many systemic disorders are known to occur in association with primary tumours of the thymus gland. While some associations may be coincidental, there is no doubt that there is a direct relation between certain diseases and the presence of a thymoma. The occurrence of these conditions as an accompaniment of the tumours provides important indications of the functions of the thymus.

Myasthenia Gravis

The occurrence of a thymoma as an accompaniment of myasthenia gravis has been recognized for many years. Some 10 to 15 per cent of patients with myasthenia gravis have a thymoma; correspondingly, about 30 per cent of thymomas are associated with myasthenia gravis. Myasthenia gravis in association with thymoma occurs at a later age and tends to be severer and more refractory to treatment than when there is no tumour (see page 904). In some series there has been a preponderance of men aged from 40 to 60 years:[103] in other series the association has been commoner in women.[104] The

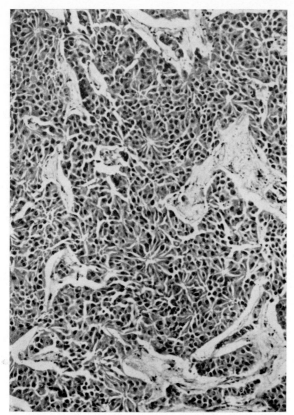

Fig. 10.41.§ This thymic tumour of 'organoid' appearance, with formation of rosettes, is comparable to some carcinoid tumours. The absence of lymphocytes is noteworthy. The patient was a man, aged 38. *Haematoxylin–eosin.* × 120.

tumours are mixed lymphocytic and epithelial thymomas (see page 908): none of the histological subtypes is significantly more frequent than the others. The usual epithelial component is the cell with a vesicular nucleus and 'watery'-looking, ill-defined cytoplasm (Fig. 10.29); a common finding is the presence of quite numerous microcysts, which often contain lymphocytes. Spindle cell thymomas are rarely associated with myasthenia gravis; however, there may be extensive areas of spindle cell change as a consequence of preoperative radiotherapy (see page 909). Lymphoid follicles with germinal centres are occasionally found within the thymomas but are much commoner in the adjoining thymic tissue.[104] Circumvascular cuffing with lymphocytes (Fig. 10.38), similar to that in experimentally induced autoimmune disease, is often seen in the tumours and their vicinity. The proportion of lymphocytes in the thymomas varies and appears not to be related to the severity of the myasthenia. It is probable that similar immuno-logical mechanisms operate in thymomatous myasthenia gravis as in the non-thymomatous disease (see page 905): in both types of case there is histological and serological evidence of a chronic auto-immune process. As mentioned above (page 906), it is uncertain whether the myasthenic state results from production of a neuromuscular blocking agent by the abnormal thymus[70] or from a fault in immune function.[105] Another unexplained accompaniment of myasthenia gravis associated with thymoma is the unusually high incidence of autoantibodies and of inflammatory changes in skeletal and cardiac muscle.[106]

The prognosis in relation to the thymoma, as distinct from the myasthenic condition, is good. This is because the tumour is usually still confined to one lobe when its presence is recognized: it is therefore amenable to surgical excision, which is more successful than radiotherapy in the treatment of thymomas. There is no evidence that an adequately resected thymoma recurs.

Hypoplastic Anaemia

Hypoplastic anaemia (see page 460) develops in about 5 per cent of patients with thymoma.[107] In some 70 per cent of these cases the tumour is a mixed lymphocytic and epithelial thymoma of the spindle cell type; in most of the rest it is of the type that characteristically is associated with myasthenia gravis (see above). The relation between hypoplastic anaemia and thymoma is far from clear. As with myasthenia gravis there are two possibilities: the anaemia may be due to the secretion by the tumour of a substance that has a depressant effect on erythropoiesis; alternatively, it may be a manifestation of autoimmunity. In some cases the anaemia has become less severe or has disappeared following resection of the thymoma.

Myasthenia gravis and hypogammaglobulinaemia may be present with hypoplastic anaemia in association with a thymoma. Such findings emphasize the overlap between these various systemic diseases and thymomas.

Cushing's Syndrome

The association of thymic tumours with Cushing's syndrome is well known, although infrequent.[108] The tumours in these cases are formed almost exclusively of small epithelial cells that are quite unlike those of any of the varieties of the mixed lymphocytic and epithelial thymoma (see page 909): the histological picture is comparable to that of the so-called thymic carcinoid (see page

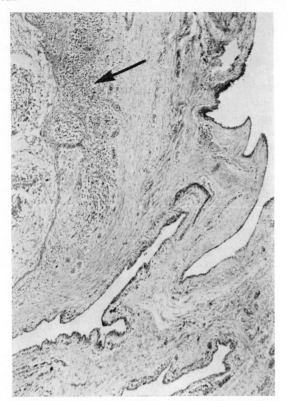

Fig. 10.42.§ Part of the wall of a large multilocular thymic cyst lined by squamous epithelium. The arrow indicates an area of chronic inflammation related to the presence in the tissues of altered cyst contents. *Haematoxylin–eosin.* × 70.

915). Studies on extracts of the tumours show that they produce a corticotrophin-like substance.[109]

Multiple Endocrine Adenomas (Pluriglandular Syndrome)

A thymoma of the type associated with Cushing's syndrome (see above) is present in some cases of pluriglandular endocrine adenomatosis (see page 1367 and Chapter 29).[110]

Hypogammaglobulinaemia

About 10 per cent of patients with acquired hypogammaglobulinaemia have a thymoma.[111, 112] The tumour is usually a spindle cell thymoma (see page 909). The explanation of its association with the immune defect is not known: the currently favoured hypothesis is that the tumour cells secrete a substance that causes faulty synthesis of immunoglobulin.

Myositis, Dermatomyositis and Myocarditis

The association of a thymoma with myositis, dermatomyositis or myocarditis is a rare but well-recognized condition.[113] Since myasthenia gravis is present in a proportion of these cases, and since patients with myasthenia gravis—particularly those with a thymoma—are significantly more liable than others to develop inflammatory lesions of skeletal and cardiac muscle,[106] it is probably inappropriate to consider the association of thymoma with myositis to be pathogenetically distinct from the association of thymoma with myasthenia gravis. Indeed, in those cases in which myositis and myocarditis have been associated with thymoma in the absence of clinical manifestations of myasthenia gravis it has been suggested that the condition is a subclinical variant of the latter.[114] The tumours in these cases have been mixed lymphocytic and epithelial thymomas.

Systemic Lupus Erythematosus

Systemic lupus erythematosus is one of the rarer systemic accompaniments of thymoma.[115] The tumour in these cases is of the mixed lymphocytic and epithelial type, with spindle metamorphosis of the latter component.

It has been known for systemic lupus erythematosus to develop following resection of a thymoma in a case of myasthenia gravis.[116]

Pemphigus

There have been several reports of the occurrence of bullous skin lesions in patients with thymoma. The finding in these cases of an epithelial antigen, such as has been recognized in association with pemphigus vulgaris, and the occasional presence of myasthenia gravis[117] indicate that the relation between the tumour and the disease of the skin is more than coincidental. This view is supported by the occasional association of pemphigus and non-thymomatous myasthenia gravis.

Other Systemic Diseases

Other diseases that have been reported in association with thymoma include Sjögren's syndrome,[118] rheumatoid arthritis, acute leukaemia and thyrotoxicosis.[104, 119, 120] The thymomas associated with leukaemia have been of the mixed lymphocytic and epithelial type: they have shown no evidence of leukaemic infiltration.

The incidence of cancer in general is higher in patients with a history of thymoma than in other people.[121] The explanation of this observation is uncertain.

REFERENCES

INTRODUCTION

1. Norris, E. H., *Contr. Embryol. Carneg. Instn*, 1938, **27**, 191.
2. Gilmour, J. R., *J. Path. Bact.*, 1941, **52**, 213.
3. Good, R. A., Papermaster, B. W., *Advanc. Immunol.*, 1964, **4**, 1.
4. Micklem, H. S., Clarke, C. M., Evans, E. P., Ford, C. E., *Transplantation*, 1968, **6**, 299.
5. Nakamura, K., Metcalf, D., *Brit. J. Cancer*, 1961, **15**, 306.
6. Miller, A. F. J. P., Osoba, D., *Physiol. Rev.*, 1967, **47**, 437.
7. Everett, N. B., Tyler, R. W., *Int. Rev. Cytol.*, 1967, **22**, 205.
8. Weismann, I., *J. exp. Med.*, 1967, **126**, 291.
9. Young, M., Turnbull, H. M., *J. Path. Bact.*, 1931, **34**, 213.
10. Selye, H., *Brit. J. exp. Path.*, 1936, **17**, 234.
11. Symmers, D., *Amer. J. Surg.*, 1934, **26**, 7.
12. Symmers, W. St C., in *Systemic Pathology*, edited by G. Payling Wright and W. St C. Symmers, 1st edn, vol. 1, page 278. London, 1966.
13. Henry, K., *Lancet*, 1966, **1**, 183.
14. Clarke, S. L., Jr, in *The Thymus—Experimental and Clinical Studies*, edited by G. E. W. Wolstenholme and R. Porter, page 3. London, 1966.
15. Loewenthal, L. A., Smith, C., *Anat. Rec.*, 1952, **112**, 1.
16. Geld, H. van der, Feltkamp, T. E. W., Lochem, J. J. van, Oosterhuis, H. J. G., *Proc. Soc. exp. Biol. (N.Y.)*, 1964, **115**, 782.
17. Hammar, J. A., *Anat. Anz.*, 1905, **27**, 23, 41.
18. Geld, H. W. R. van der, Strauss, A. J. L., *Lancet*, 1966, **1**, 157.
19. Henry, K., *Brit. J. Dis. Chest*, 1972, **66**, 291.
20. Henry, K., *Clin. exp. Immunol.*, 1968, **3**, 509.
21. Middleton, G., *Aust. J. exp. Biol. med. Sci.*, 1967, **45**, 189.
22. Hammar, J. A., *Z. mikr.-anat. Forsch.*, 1926, **6**, 107.
23. Sloan, H. E., *Surgery*, 1943, **13**, 154.
24. Boyd, E., *Amer. J. Dis. Child.*, 1932, **43**, 1162.
25. McEndey, D. P., Boon, M. C., Furth, J., *Cancer Res.*, 1944, **4**, 377.
26. Good, R. A., Varco, R. L., *J.-Lancet*, 1955, **75**, 245.
27. Miller, J. F. A. P., *Lancet*, 1961, **2**, 748.
28. Miller, J. F. A. P., *Nature (Lond.)*, 1961, **195**, 1318.
29. Dukor, P., Miller, J. F. A. P., House, M., Allmann, V., *Transplantation*, 1965, **3**, 639.
30. Miller, J. F. A. P., Mitchell, G. F., *Nature (Lond.)*, 1967, **216**, 367.
31. Roitt, I. M., Greaves, M. F., Torrigiani, G., Brostoff, J., Playfair, J. H. L., *Lancet*, 1969, **2**, 367.
32. Gowans, J. L., Knight, E. J., *Proc. roy. Soc. B*, 1964, **159**, 257.
33. Henry, K., Goldman, J. M., in *Recent Advances in Pathology*, No. 9, edited by C. V. Harrison and K. Weinbren, page 30. Edinburgh, London and New York, 1975.
34. Oort, J., Turk, J. L., *Brit. J. exp. Path.*, 1965, **46**, 147.
35. Ford, W. L., *Brit. J. exp. Path.*, 1969, **50**, 257.

THYMIC APLASIA AND HYPOPLASIA

36. Vaal, O. M. de, Seynhaeve, V., *Lancet*, 1959, **2**, 1123.

37. Gitlin, D., Vawter, G., Craig, J. M., *Pediatrics*, 1964, **33**, 184.
38. Glanzmann, E., Riniker, P., *Ann. paediat. (Basel)*, 1950, **175**, 1.
39. Hoyer, J. R., Cooper, M. D., Gabrielsen, M. D., Good, R. A., *Medicine (Baltimore)*, 1968, **47**, 201.
40. Fireman, P., Johnson, H. A., Gitlin, D., *Pediatrics*, 1966, **37**, 485.
41. DiGeorge, A. M., in discussion of: Cooper, M. D., Peterson, R. D. A., Good, R. A., *J. Pediat.*, 1965, **67**, 907.
41a. DiGeorge, A. M., *Birth Defects orig. Article Ser.*, 1968, **4**, 116.
42. Cleveland, W. N., Fogel, B. J., Brown, W. T., Kay, H. E. M., *Lancet*, 1968, **2**, 1211.
43. Nezelof, C., Jammet, M. L., Lortholary, P., Labrune, B., Lamy, M., *Arch. franç. Pédiat.*, 1964, **21**, 897.
44. Peterson, R. D. A., Kelly, W. D., Good, R. A., *Lancet*, 1964, **1**, 1189.
45. Louis-Bar, *Confin. neurol. (Basel)*, 1941–42, **4**, 32.
46. Wiskott, A., *Mschr. Kinderheilk.*, 1937, **68**, 212.
47. Aldrich, R. A., Steinberg, A. G., Campbell, D. C., *Pediatrics*, 1954, **13**, 133.
48. Levin, A. S., Spitler, L. E., Stites, D. P., Fudenberg, H. H., *Proc. nat. Acad. Sci. (Wash.)*, 1970, **67**, 821.
49. Bruton, D. C., *Pediatrics*, 1952, **9**, 722.
50. Good, R. A., Varco, R. L., *J.-Lancet*, 1955, **75**, 245.
51. Hughes, W. S., Creda, V. A., Holtzapple, P., Brooks, F. P., *Ann. intern. Med.*, 1971, **74**, 903.

THYMIC HYPERPLASIA

52. Boyd, E., *Amer. J. Dis. Child.*, 1932, **43**, 1162.
53. Hohn, E. O., *J. Endocr.*, 1959, **19**, 282.
54. Sloan, H. E., *Surgery*, 1943, **13**, 154.
55. Bearne, J. G., *Brit. J. exp. Path.*, 1968, **49**, 136.

THE THYMUS AND MYASTHENIA GRAVIS

56. Weigert, C., *Arch. Psychiat. Nervenkr.*, 1901, **34**, 1063.
57. Keynes, G., *Brit. J. Surg.*, 1954-55, **42**, 449.
58. Sloan, H. E., *Surgery*, 1943, **13**, 154.
59. Goldstein, G., *Clin. exp. Immunol.*, 1967, **2**, 103.
60. Henry, K., *personal observation*.
61. Castleman, B., *Ann. N.Y. Acad. Sci.*, 1966, **135**, 496.
62. Henry, K., *Brit. J. Dis. Chest*, 1972, **66**, 291.
63. Anderson, J. R., Vetters, J. M., in *Myasthenia Gravis*, edited by R. Greene, chap. 7. London, 1969.
64. Goldstein, G., *Lancet*, 1966, **2**, 1164.
65. Simpson, J. A., *Scot. med. J.*, 1960, **5**, 419.
66. Sahay, B. M., Blendis, L., Greene, R., *Brit. med. J.*, 1965, **1**, 762.
67. Viets, H. R., Schwab, R. S., *Thymectomy for Myasthenia Gravis—A Record of Experiences at the Massachusetts General Hospital*. Springfield, Illinois, 1960.
68. Anderson, J. R., Vetters, J. M., in *Myasthenia Gravis*, edited by R. Greene, chap. 7. London, 1969.
69. Strauss, A. J. L., Smith, C. W., Cage, G. W., Geld, H. W. R. van der, Macfarlin, D. E., Barlow, M., *Ann. N.Y. Acad. Sci.*, 1966, **135**, 557.
70. Goldstein, G., Mackay, I. R., in *The Human Thymus*, edited by G. Goldstein and I. R. Mackay, chap. 3. London, 1969.
71. Alpert, L. I., Papatestas, A., Kark, A., Osserman, R. S., Osserman, K., *Arch. Path.*, 1971, **91**, 55.

INFECTIONS AND THE THYMUS

72. Symmers, W. St C., in *Systemic Pathology*, edited by G. Payling Wright and W. St C. Symmers, 1st edn, vol. 1, page 279. London, 1966.

TUMOURS OF THE THYMUS

73. Castleman, B., *Tumors of the Thymus Gland* (Atlas of Tumor Pathology, sect. 5, fasc. 19), page 14. Washington, D.C., 1955.
74. Leading Article, *Brit. med. J.*, 1966, **1**, 834.
75. Bernatz, P. E., Harrison, E. G., Clagett, O. T., *J. thorac. cardiovasc. Surg.*, 1961, **42**, 424.
76. Iverson, L., *Amer. J. Path.*, 1956, **32**, 695.
77. Lowenhaupt, E., *Cancer (Philad.)*, 1948, **1**, 547.
78. Thomson, A. D., Thackray, A. C., *Brit. J. Cancer*, 1957, **11**, 348.
79. Castleman, B., *Tumors of the Thymus Gland* (Atlas of Tumor Pathology, sect. 5, fasc. 19), page 23. Washington, D.C., 1955.
80. Lattes, R., *Cancer (Philad.)*, 1962, **15**, 1224.
81. Friedman, N., *J. thorac. cardiovasc. Surg.*, 1967, **53**, 163.
82. Lowenhaupt, E., Brown, R., *Cancer (Philad.)*, 1951, **4**, 1193.
83. Nickels, J., Franssila, K., Hjelt, L., *Acta path. microbiol. scand. A*, 1973, **81**, 1.
84. Knight, S., Bradley, J., Oppenheim, J. J., Ling, N. R., *Clin. exp. Immunol.*, 1968, **3**, 323.
85. Gravanis, M. B., *Amer. J. clin. Path.*, 1968, **49**, 690.
86. Schlumberger, H. G., *Arch. Path. (Chic.)*, 1946, **41**, 398.
87. Castleman, B., *Tumors of the Thymus Gland* (Atlas of Tumor Pathology, sect. 5, fasc. 19), page 69. Washington, D.C., 1955.
88. Cohen, R. B., Castleman, B., *Cancer (Philad.)*, 1960, **13**, 812.
89. Rosai, J., Higa, E., *Cancer (Philad.)*, 1972, **29**, 1061.
90. Hall, G. F. M., *Brit. J. Surg.*, 1948–49, **36**, 321.
91. Benton, C., Gerard, P., *J. thorac. cardiovasc. Surg.*, 1966, **51**, 428.
92. Barnes, R. D. S., O'Gorman, P., *J. clin. Path.*, 1962, **15**, 264.
93. Benton, C., Gerard, P., *J. thorac. cardiovasc. Surg.*, 1966, **51**, 428.
94. Henry, K., *Brit. J. Dis. Chest*, 1972, **66**, 291.
95. Middleton, G., *Brit. J. Cancer*, 1966, **20**, 41.
96. Adams, J. E., *Amer. J. clin. Path.*, 1963, **40**, 173.
97. Anagnostou, D., Harrison, C. V., *J. clin. Path.*, 1972, **25**, 306.
98. Castleman, B., Iverson, L., Pardo Menendez, V., *Cancer (Philad.)*, 1956, **9**, 822.

THYMIC CYSTS

99. Pachter, M. R., Lattes, R., *Dis. Chest*, 1963, **44**, 416.
100. Castleman, B., *Tumors of the Thymus Gland* (Atlas of Tumor Pathology, sect. 5, fasc. 19), page 76. Washington, D.C., 1955.
101. Dyer, N. H., *Thorax*, 1967, **22**, 408.
102. Dubois, P., *Gaz. méd. Paris*, 1850, **25**, 392.

THYMOMAS AND SYSTEMIC DISORDERS

103. Castleman, B., *Tumors of the Thymus Gland* (Atlas of Tumor Pathology, sect. 5, fasc. 19), page 64. Washington, D.C., 1955.
104. Lattes, R., *Cancer (Philad.)*, 1962, **15**, 1224.
105. Alpert, L. I., Papatestas, A., Kark, A., Osserman, R. S., Osserman, K., *Arch. Path.*, 1971, **91**, 55.
106. Genkins, G., Mendelow, H., Sobel, H. J., Osserman, K. E., in *Myasthenia Gravis—The Second International Symposium Proceedings*, edited by H. R. Viets, page 519. Springfield, Illinois, 1961.
107. Hirst, E., Robertson, T. I., *Medicine (Baltimore)*, 1967, **46**, 225.
108. Cohen, R. B., Castleman, B., *Cancer (Philad.)*, 1960, **13**, 812.
109. Lemon, F. C., Fine, B. M., Grasso, S. G., Kinsell, L. W., *J. clin. Endocr.*, 1966, **26**, 1.
110. Rosai, J., Higa, E., Davie, J., *Cancer (Philad.)*, 1972, **29**, 1075.
111. Good, R. A., Varco, R. L., *J.-Lancet*, 1955, **75**, 245.
112. Peterson, R. D. A., Cooper, M. D., Good, R. A., *Amer. J. Med.*, 1965, **38**, 579.
113. Klein, H. O., Lennartz, K. J., *Dtsch. med. Wschr.*, 1966, **91**, 1727.
114. Fisher, E. R., in *The Thymus in Immunobiology*, edited by R. A. Good and A. E. Gabrielson, chap. 36. New York, 1964.
115. Singh, B. N., *Aust. Ann. Med.*, 1969, **18**, 55.
116. Galbraith, R. F., Sommerskill, W. H. J., Murray, J., *New Engl. J. Med.*, 1964, **270**, 229.
117. Peck, S. M., Osserman, K., Weiner, L. B., Lefkovits, A., Osserman, R. A., *New Engl. J. Med.*, 1968, **279**, 951.
118. Birch, C. A., Cooke, K. B., Drew, C. E., London, D. R., Mackenzie, D. H., Milne, M. D., *Lancet*, 1964, **1**, 693.
119. Anderson, V., Pedersen, H., *Acta med. scand.*, 1967, **182**, 581.
120. Benton, C., Gerard, P., *J. thorac. cardiovasc. Surg.*, 1966, **51**, 428.
121. Souadjian, J. V., Silverstein, M. N., Titus, J. L., *Cancer (Philad.)*, 1968, **22**, 1221.

ACKNOWLEDGEMENTS FOR ILLUSTRATIONS

Figs 10.1, 2, 17, 29, 30, 35, 37, 38, 39A, 41, 42. Photographs by Mr W. Hinks, Royal Postgraduate Medical School, London.

Fig. 10.15. Reproduced by permission of the editors, Professor C. V. Harrison and Professor K. Weinbren, and publishers, Churchill Livingstone, from: Henry, K., Goldman, J. M., in *Recent Advances in Pathology*, No. 9, page 61, Fig. 11; Edinburgh, London and New York, 1975.

Fig. 10.16. Photomicrograph provided by Professor C. L. Berry, The London Hospital Medical College, London.

Figs 10.18, 24, 25, 26A, 38. Reproduced by permission of the editor, Dr R. Greene, and publishers, William Heinemann Medical Books Ltd, from: Henry, K., in *Myasthenia Gravis*, chap. 6, Figs 10, 12, 19, 13 (a) and 16; London, 1969.

Fig. 10.37. Specimen provided by Dr D. A. Harrison, Northern General Hospital, Sheffield.

Index to Volume 2

prepared by the editor and Jean N. Symmers

Some entries include a cross-reference to another part of the index where the subject is covered in more detail or under a preferred synonym. To lessen the possible inconvenience of this practice, if there is a major account of the topic its page is indicated in parentheses: for example—

thrombocytopenia   440, **491**, *and see* purpura (492)
torulosis, *see* cryptococcosis (621)

Multiple Page Entries. When more than one page reference is given in an entry, bold type is used to indicate a main account of the topic, if appropriate.

Illustrations and Tables. Reference to an illustration or table is indicated by noting its number in parentheses after the number of the page on which it appears. In general, illustrations and tables are not included in the index as they are referred to on the page of the text to which the relevant entries in the index relate.

Footnotes. Reference to a footnote is indicated by the appropriate symbol (asterisk, dagger, *etc.*) after the page number. When necessary, [L] or [R] is added after the symbol to indicate whether the footnote is in the left-hand column or the right-hand column.

Cases. In some instances of reference to a particular case of a disease the word *case* is added in parentheses after the text of the entry.

Alternative Spellings. Terms that in American-English usage are generally spelt more simply than is traditional in Britain, such as edema (oedema), etiology (aetiology) and hemoglobin (haemoglobin), should be looked for in the spelling that accords with the latter practice.

The spellings catabolism, leucocyte, leucopenia, leucoplakia and the like are used in this book rather than katabolism, leukocyte, leukopenia and leukoplakia. It is equally in accordance with current practice in Britain that the spelling leukaemia is preferred.

Index to Volume 2

A

E

lymphomas—*continued*
Hodgkin's disease, *see* Hodgkin's disease (*main entry*) (784–818)
hydantoin therapy, relation to 699
hypogammaglobulinaemia complicated by 770, 902
immunoblastic 849
immunoblastic lymphadenopathy complicated by 703
immunodeficiency predisposing to 770
immunoglobulin-producing 823
immunosuppression, therapeutic, predisposing to 770, 820
infection, predisposition to 774
intestines, origin in 820
Kaposi's sarcoma complicated by 713
Lennert's 807
lesions, distribution at necropsy 831 (Table 9.15)
liver, origin in 820
Louis-Bar's syndrome complicated by 770
lungs, origin in 820
lymphadenitis, acute mesenteric, simulated by 575
persistent, following vaccination, mistaken for 645
'lymphoblastic' 778 (Table 9.5, footnote [†])
lymphocytic, *see* lymphocytic lymphoma (*main entry*) (821–844)
macrofollicular 835
macroglobulinaemia, primary, complicated by 498, 707, 770
mistaken for 706
secondary, accompanying 707
malabsorption syndromes predisposing to intestinal lymphomas 845
'Mediterranean' 845
mesenteric lymphadenitis, acute, simulated by 575
mycosis fungoides 853
necropsy, distribution of lesions 831 (Table 9.15)
necrosis 552
'non-Hodgkin's lymphomas' 819*
other than Hodgkin's disease 819–858
plasmacytoid 779 (Table 9.6, footnote [**])
in 'Mediterranean lymphoma' 846
pleomorphic, anaplastic 851
complicating Hodgkin's disease 811
pregnancy 768
prognosis 771, 819
treatment as factor 773
protein deposition in 823
sclerosing lymphocytic, diffuse 822
sclerotic, nodular 822
sex incidence 768
Sézary's syndrome 856
sinus histiocytosis with massive lymphadenopathy, simulating 566
skin 853
solitary 545*
spleen, benign (hamartoma) 739
malignant, origin in 820
splenomegaly, tropical idiopathic, complicated by 744
staging, clinical 772
pathological 773
steatorrhoea, idiopathic, predisposing to intestinal lymphomas 844
stomach, origin in 820
syncytial 852 (Fig. 9.267)
syndrome, bilateral hilar lymphoma [sarcoidosis] 746
synonyms 778–781
T-cell, cutaneous 856

lymphomas—*continued*
T zone 822
terminology 819
thymus 917
treatment, infection complicating 776
prognostic factor 773
undifferentiated 778, 850
vaccination, persistent lymphadenitis following, mistaken for 645
Wiskott–Aldrich syndrome complicated by 770, 902
lymphomas other than Hodgkin's disease 819–858
lymphomyeloid complex 506
lymphopathia venerea 635
lymphopenia, cortisol causing 520
lymphoma accompanied by 771
'stress' causing 520
in Wiskott–Aldrich syndrome 902
lymphopoiesis, in bone marrow 509
control of 520
in germinal centres 512
in lymphoid follicles 512
in spleen 721
in thymus 508, 899
lymphoreticular system 504–891
definition 506
diseases, nomenclature 536
lymphoreticulosis, benign infectious 638
benign inoculation 638
'lymphosarcoma' (obsolescent term) 819, **821**
first accounts 537
lysosomal diseases 758
lysozyme, in serum, in monocytic leukaemia 482

M

macrocytosis, in blood 450 (Fig. 8.9D)
macroglobulinaemia 446, **498, 706**
cryoglobulinaemia associated with 499
platelet dysfunction in 495
primary 706
lymphoma complicating 770
splenomegaly accompanying 738
secondary 707
complicating lymphoma 771
macronormoblasts, in haemolytic anaemia 473
macrophages, alveolar 526
in blood 439
dendritic 514
endothelial 526
endothelioid metamorphosis 526
epithelioid metamorphosis 521, **526**
giant cell metamorphosis 530
immunity and 521
'killer' cells 521
leishmanial parasitization of 661
microglial cells 527
monocytes 527
osteoclasts as macrophages 526
peritoneal 526
pigmented, in fatal granulomatous disease of childhood 709, **710**
in 'round cell infiltrates' 517
viral infection and 522
Madurella grisea 629

splenomegaly—*continued*

brucella infection 590
causes, multiple coexistent 743
ceroid storage disease 767
classification 742
congestive 724*, **730**
cryptogenic 744
Egyptian 737
endocarditis, infective 734
Felty syndrome 690
follicular lymphoma 836
gangliosidosis, generalized 763
Gaucher's disease 760
glycogenosis, type IV, cirrhosis causing splenomegaly 758
haemangioma 739
haemodilution accompanying 725
haemolytic anaemia, chronic, causing 473
'hairy cell leukaemia' 862
hamartoma 739
Hand–Schüller–Christian disease 764
hereditary spherocytosis causing 466
histiocytic medullary reticulosis 860
histoplasmosis 735
Hodgkin's disease 793
hydantoin lymphadenopathy accompanied by 698, 738
hyperlipaemia, idiopathic, in children, causing 765
hyperlipidaemia, mixed, causing 766
hypersplenism accompanying 724, 744
idiopathic, non-tropical 725
tropical 743
leishmanial 736
immunoblastic lymphadenopathy accompanied by 703, 738
infectious lymphocytosis 651
infectious mononucleosis 476, 650, **736**
kala azar 736
leishmaniasis 736
leucopenia accompanying 477
leukaemia 740
chronic lymphocytic 488
chronic myeloid 485
lipidoses 759
lymphomas 784
follicular lymphoma 836
Hodgkin's disease 793
other than Hodgkin's disease 820
macroglobulinaemia, primary, accompanied by 738
malaria 736
mononucleosis, infectious 476, 650, **736**
Niemann–Pick disease 761
Oroya fever 668
paratyphoid 734
plasma volume 430
polycythaemia vera 474, 740
primary 725
pyruvate kinase deficiency associated with 468
Q fever 634
reticulosis, histiocytic medullary 860
rheumatoid arthritis 690
salmonella infection 734
sarcoidosis 747
schistosomiasis 737
secondary 725
septicaemia 734
sickle cell disease 469

splenomegaly—*continued*

spherocytosis, hereditary 466
splenectomy in diagnosis of 744
splenoma, intrasplenic 739
Stengel–Wolbach sclerosis 686
Still–Felty syndrome 477
thalassaemia 454
thrombocythaemia, primary 728
thrombocytopenia accompanying 494
thyrotoxicosis 725
toxoplasmosis 737
tropical idiopathic 743
trypanosomiasis 737
American 666
tuberculosis 735
typhoid 734
volume, blood 430
plasma 430
splenunculi 726
Sporothrix schenckii 622
asteroids 750
Splendore–Hoeppli phenomenon 679*, **750**
sporotrichosis 622
glanders mistaken for 595
infarction of lymph nodes simulated by 552
lymphadenitis 622
lymphangitic form 622
Mycobacterium fortuitum lymphangitis simulating 608
solitary form 622
Splendore–Hoeppli phenomenon in 679*, **750**
Sporozoa 668
spot, Mongolian, in Niemann–Pick disease 762
staging, of Hodgkin's disease 772 (Table 9.4)
of lymphomas 772
clinical 772
pathological 773
of mycosis fungoides, internal involvement 855
staining, vital 524
staphylococcal infection, lymphadenitis in 573, 593
Staphylococcus aureus, infection by, in fatal granulomatous disease of childhood 708
fulminating, splenectomy predisposing to 723
lymphoma predisposing to 775, 776
lymphadenitis caused by 573
chronic suppurative 593
non-suppurative 593
'starry sky', of Burkitt's lymphoma 830
of follicular hyperplasia in lymph nodes 554, 555 (Fig. 9.32)
in lymphocytic lymphomas, simulating Burkitt's lymphoma 830
status thymicolymphaticus 894
steatorrhoea, idiopathic, complicated by intestinal lymphoma 844
accompanying 'Mediterranean lymphoma' 846
stem cells 519
in leukaemia 482
Stengel–Wolbach sclerosis **685**, 750
Sternberg cells 794
Sternberg–Reed cells, of Hodgkin's disease **794**, 799, 800, 802
resemblance to, in brucella infection 592
in granulomatous thymoma, so-called 911
in hydantoin lymphadenopathy 699 (Fig. 9.150)
in infectious mononucleosis 650
in mycosis fungoides 854, 855